Revision Surgery of the Foot and Ankle

Mark J. Berkowitz
Michael P. Clare • Paul T. Fortin
Lew C. Schon • Roy W. Sanders
Editors

Revision Surgery of the Foot and Ankle

Surgical Strategies and Techniques

Springer

Editors
Mark J. Berkowitz
Department of Orthopedic Surgery
Cleveland Clinic
Cleveland, OH
USA

Paul T. Fortin
Department of Orthopedic Surgery
Oakland University William Beaumont
Royal Oak, MI
USA

Roy W. Sanders
Florida Orthopedic Institute
Temple Terrace, FL
USA

Michael P. Clare
Florida Orthopaedic Institute
Temple Terrace, FL
USA

Lew C. Schon
Medstar Union Memorial Hospital
Baltimore, MD
USA

ISBN 978-3-030-29968-2 ISBN 978-3-030-29969-9 (eBook)
https://doi.org/10.1007/978-3-030-29969-9

This Springer imprint is published by the registered company Springer Nature Switzerland AG
The registered company address is: Gewerbestrasse 11, 6330 Cham, Switzerland

Preface

Numerous excellent and comprehensive textbooks covering the field of foot and ankle surgery are available today. The best of these provide clear and concise, step-by-step instruction on how to perform the extensive array of surgical procedures that make up a typical practice. However, none to my knowledge exclusively addresses the countless unique challenges involved in *revision* surgery of the foot and ankle.

As anyone who has practiced foot and ankle surgery can attest, revision procedures are anything but routine and often do not proceed in "cookbook" fashion. In fact, the techniques described for primary foot and ankle procedures often are not applicable in the revision setting. Poorly placed incisions, compromised soft tissue, bone loss, failed internal fixation, and deformity not uncommonly render primary techniques ineffective and require alternative strategies and approaches.

This project was undertaken with the young foot and ankle surgeon in mind. In fact, its origins go back 15 years to my time as a novice foot and ankle surgeon in the US Army, freshly graduated from residency and without the benefit of fellowship training. During this exciting but stressful time, the traditional textbooks of foot and ankle surgery served as excellent resources for primary procedures. However, I found few resources available to provide guidance when tackling a complicated revision case. In order to fill this void and bring greater attention and granularity to the topic of revision foot and ankle surgery, an Instructional Course Lecture was developed and first presented at the 2015 AAOS Annual Meeting in Las Vegas. The success of this ICL directly lead to the development of the current textbook.

The current text aims to serve as a "go-to" resource for the early-career foot and ankle surgeon treating patients whose initial surgical treatment has failed. You will notice that it is presented in bullet format and is case-based. This format is intentional as it is not intended to be an exhaustive resource on all aspects of foot and ankle surgery. Rather, this book is intended to serve as a source of ideas for creative problem-solving, a necessary skill for the revision surgeon. It is hoped that the cases, techniques, and strategies presented in each chapter will stimulate the reader's own critical thinking and provide a template for successfully addressing even the most challenging revision situation.

Although we are excited to finally make the first edition of *Revision Surgery of the Foot and Ankle* available, we are already looking to make improvements to subsequent editions. Specifically, in subsequent editions, we will incorporate video clips demonstrating the revision techniques presented in the text. The goal will be to make this text increasingly useful and practical for the foot and ankle surgeon who is planning a revision procedure. Finally, we deeply appreciate and welcome feedback from our readers and will use their comments and suggestions to make future editions even better.

Cleveland, OH, USA Mark J. Berkowitz, MD, MBA

Acknowledgments

I would like to thank all of my coeditors who so graciously agreed to participate in this humble project, without whom, it never would have materialized. Each one of them has served as a mentor to me, either directly or from afar. Collectively, these individuals are true masters at revision foot and ankle surgery, and many of the creative strategies and techniques presented in this book were developed by these individuals. I have never stopped learning from these gentlemen, and I am confident that you will find their insight equally helpful in your practice.

All of the editors as a group are grateful to the numerous authors and contributors who have made this book come to fruition. Their time, energy, expertise, and commitment to this project brought needed valuable attention to the topic revision surgery of the foot and ankle. We sincerely appreciate all their hard work and dedication. Needless to say, without them, this book would not have been possible.

Contents

Part III Sports

Part IV Arthritis and Reconstruction

Contributors

John G. Anderson, MD Orthopaedic Associates of Michigan, Grand Rapids, MI, USA

Gonzalo F. Bastías, MD Department of Orthopedic Surgery, Foot and Ankle Unit, Clínica Las Condes, Las Condes, Chile

Department of Orthopedic Surgery, Universidad de Chile Complejo Hospitalario San José, Santiago, Chile

Douglas N. Beaman, MD Mid Columbia Medical Center, Department of Orthopaedic Surgery, The Dalles, OR, USA

Mark J. Berkowitz, MD, MBA Director, Foot and Ankle Center, Cleveland Clinic, Department of Orthopaedic Surgery, Orthopaedic and Rheumatologic Institute, Cleveland, OH, USA

Donald R. Bohay, MD Orthopaedic Associates of Michigan, Grand Rapids, MI, USA

Karim Boukhemis, MD University of California at Davis, Department of Orthopaedics, Sacramento, CA, USA

Taylor N. Cabe, BA Hospital for Special Surgery, Foot and Ankle Service, New York, NY, USA

Michael P. Clare, MD Florida Orthopaedic Institute, Tampa, FL, USA

Camille L. Connelly, MD Skagit Northwest Orthopedics, Mount Vernon, WA, USA

Sophia Davis, DO Orlando Orthopaedic Center, Orlando, FL, USA

Mark C. Drakos, MD Hospital for Special Surgery, Foot and Ankle Service, New York, NY, USA

Paul T. Fortin, MD Oakland University William Beaumont, School of Medicine, Royal Oak, MI, USA

Eric Giza, MD University of California at Davis, Department of Orthopaedics, Sacramento, CA, USA

Steven L. Haddad, MD Orthopaedic Foot and Ankle Sugery, Illinois Bone and Joint Institute, LLC, Glenview, IL, USA

Todd A. Irwin, MD OrthoCarolina Foot and Ankle Institute, Carolinas Medical Center, Charlotte, NC, USA

Qin Jianzhong, MD Second Affiliated Hospital of Soochow University, Department of Orthopaedics, Su Zhou, China

Sydney C. Karnovsky, BA Hospital for Special Surgery, Foot and Ankle Service, New York, NY, USA

John Ketz, MD Strong Memorial Hospital, University of Rochester, Department of Orthopaedics, Rochester, NY, USA

Christopher D. Kreulen, MD, MS University of California at Davis, Department of Orthopaedics, Sacramento, CA, USA

Brandon Levy, MD Kingsbrook Jewish Medical Center, Division of Orthopedic Surgery, Brooklyn, NY, USA

Elisabeth Manke, MD University Hospital Carl Gustav Carus at TU Dresden, University Center of Orthopaedics and Traumatology, Dresden, Germany

Arthur Manoli II, MD Wayne State University, Detroit, MI, USA

Department of Orthopaedic Surgery, Michigan State University, East Lansing, MI, USA

Department of Orthopaedic Surgery, Michigan International Foot and Ankle Center, St. Joseph Mercy Hospital—Oakland, Pontiac, MI, USA

John D. Maskill, MD Orthopaedic Associates of Michigan, Grand Rapids, MI, USA

Roshan T. Melvani, MD MedStar Union Memorial Hospital, Department of Orthopaedic Surgery, Baltimore, MD, USA

Stuart D. Miller, MD MedStar Union Memorial Hospital, Department of Orthopaedic Surgery, Baltimore, MD, USA

Alireza Mousavian, MD Ghaem Hospital, Mashhad University of Medical Sciences, Department of Orthopedic Surgery, Mashhad, Iran

Jakrapong Orapin, MD Faculty of Medicine, Ramathibodi Hospital, Mahidol University, Department of Orthopaedic Surgery, Bangkok, Thailand

Stefan Rammelt, MD, PhD University Hospital Carl Gustav Carus at TU Dresden, University Center of Orthopaedics and Traumatology, Dresden, Germany

David R. Richardson, MD University of Tennessee-Campbell Clinic, Department of Orthopaedic Surgery & Biomedical Engineering, Memphis, TN, USA

Justin Roberts, MD The Orthopaedic Clinic Association, Phoenix, AZ, USA

Andrew K. Sands, MD Weill Cornell Medical College, New York Presbyterian – Lower Manhattan Hospital, Department of Orthopedic Surgery, New York, NY, USA

Roy W. Sanders, MD Department of Orthopaedic Surgery, Orthopaedics Johns Hopkins School of Medicine, Baltimore, MD, USA

Florida Orthopaedic Institute, Tampa, FL, USA

Department of Orthopaedics, Tampa General Hospital, Tampa, FL, USA

Lew C. Schon, MD, FACS Department of Orthopaedic Surgery, MedStar Union Memorial Hospital, Baltimore, MD, USA

Georgetown School of Medicine, Washington, DC, USA

Johns Hopkins University, Baltimore, MD, USA

Fischell Literati Faculty, University of Maryland, Fischell Department of Bioengineering, College Park, MD, USA

Thomas I. Sherman, MD Orthopedic Associates of Lancaster, Lancaster, PA, USA

Brian Steginsky, DO Orthopaedic Foot and Ankle Sugery, Illinois Bone and Joint Institute, LLC, Glenview, IL, USA

Brandon A. Taylor, MD Orthopaedic Specialists of Palm Harbor, Palm Harbor, FL, USA

Part I

Forefoot

Revision of Failed 1st MTPJ Fusion

1

Mark J. Berkowitz and Camille L. Connelly

Key Takeaway Points

- The goal of reconstruction is to establish a stable 1st ray with a balanced metatarsal cascade to reestablish an even forefoot weight-bearing pattern.
- Lesser metatarsal osteotomies may be necessary to establish a balanced metatarsal cascade after revision 1st MTPJ fusion.
- For an accurate assessment of fusion positioning intraoperatively, align the arthrodesis along a flat plate to stimulate weight-bearing.
- Bone loss should be estimated preoperatively to plan for structural autograft or allograft needs.
- The general indication for an interposition bone-block arthrodesis is bone loss greater than 10 mm.

Introduction

1st MTPJ arthrodesis is the "gold standard" operative treatment for end-stage hallux rigidus, severe hallux valgus, and salvage procedures of the 1st MTPJ [1, 2]. Historically, rates of fusion and patient satisfaction both exceed 90 percent [3–6]. Revision or salvage fusions, however, are less predictable, especially in cases of severe bone loss, with rates of fusion in the literature from 79 to 99 percent [7–9].

Failures of a primary arthrodesis can occur due to nonunion, malunion, or infection. Additionally, a salvage 1st MTPJ fusion may be indicated to address failed hallux valgus, 1st MTPJ arthroplasty, or failed resection arthroplasty surgery. Revision arthrodesis often must address substantial bone loss from previous 1st MT osteotomies, implant removal, or avascular necrosis. Shortening of the 1st ray causes weight-bearing loads to be transferred laterally to the lesser metatarsals resulting in painful metatarsalgia and increasing deformity [1, 3, 7–10]. Restoration of 1st MT length and plantigrade positioning are crucial to address transfer metatarsalgia [1, 8, 9]. In the setting of revision arthrodesis, and especially with the use of interposition bone-block arthrodesis, average time to union can exceed 12 weeks, and prolonged immobilization should be considered until radiographic union is achieved [7].

M. J. Berkowitz
Director, Foot and Ankle Center, Cleveland Clinic, Department of Orthopaedic Surgery, Orthopaedic and Rheumatologic Institute, Cleveland, OH, USA

C. L. Connelly (✉)
Skagit Northwest Orthopedics, Mount Vernon, WA, USA

M. J. Berkowitz et al. (eds.), *Revision Surgery of the Foot and Ankle*,
https://doi.org/10.1007/978-3-030-29969-9_1

Evaluation and Assessment

For the symptomatic 1st MTPJ and/or resulting transfer metatarsalgia, conservative measures including carbon fiber inserts, orthotics, accommodative shoes, and NSAIDs should be attempted before considering revision surgery.

A thorough history and physical examination should be performed. Previous surgeries on the extremity should be noted as well as any history of wound healing issues or infection and documentation of any current implants. Patient factors should also be considered including general health, current tobacco use, and ability to comply with postoperative limitations. Regarding cases of atrophic nonunion consider bone homeostasis and vitamin D levels. Additionally, counsel patients that revision fusions may require a longer time to union, with additional postoperative immobilization and patient compliance.

A physical examination should be completed with attention to the forefoot alignment, pain, evidence of transfer metatarsalgia, and abnormal callous formation. Carefully consider the complaints the patient presented with, and discuss with the patient if additional osteotomies of the lesser MTs or hindfoot realignments may be needed to restore a plantigrade foot.

Skin quality and vascular status should be noted. Scar locations should be noted regarding incision planning, and the overall alignment of the foot should be carefully evaluated for any significant hindfoot deformity that may require either concurrent or staged procedures to address. Preoperative weight-bearing radiographs of the foot (AP, lateral, and oblique) should be obtained to evaluate foot alignment, cascade, 1st ray bone loss, nonunion, AVN, osteolysis, presence of current implants, and broken hardware. If current infection is suspected, then ESR, CRP, and WBC levels should be obtained.

Surgical Planning

First metatarsal positioning is crucial to reestablish even forefoot weight-bearing [10, 11]. A 1st MTPJ fusion with excessive dorsiflexion resulting in a cock-up deformity will cause shoe impingement and pain at the dorsal IPJ and transfer metatarsalgia, while a plantarflexion malunion will result in a painful plantar IPJ callus, sesamoiditis, and a need to vault over the toe with gait. The 1st MTPJ angle necessary to achieve a plantigrade foot will vary with the overall geometry of the foot [11]. Therefore, it has been advocated to position the hallux such that the distal phalanx pulp rests just off (1–3 mm) a flat plate (surgical set box top) with the ankle at 90 degrees [8, 10, 11]. The authors have found this provides a simple and reproducible intraoperative approximation of final weight-bearing position.

The metatarsal cascade is used to gauge hallux length. Typically, when there is less than 5 mm shortening, an in situ fusion can be performed [10]. A deficit of 5–10 mm can be managed with an in situ fusion in conjunction with lesser metatarsal shortening osteotomies to rebalance the foot. Severe 1st ray bone loss, defined as greater than 10 mm shortening, should be addressed with a bone-block structural interposition arthrodesis with or without additional lesser metatarsal osteotomies as needed to restore a balanced cascade [1, 3, 4, 8–10].

Intraoperative considerations include the challenges of navigating a revision surgical field in addition to considerations for utilizing additional biology in the form of bone graft, restoration of 1st MT length, choice of fusion site preparation, and fixation technique. Additionally, the decision to use autograft versus allograft and the potential for donor site morbidity or infection transmission risks must be weighed.

The authors prefer to utilize a lag screw and dorsal compression/neutralization plate construct when able. This fixation is supported in the biomechanical literature demonstrating superior strength to competing screw and/or wire constructs [12].

In cases requiring structural bone graft, autograft or allograft may be used. Traditionally tricortical iliac crest autograft has been the most utilized source of structural graft; however the recent literature supports high fusion rates and safety using allograft [1, 8, 9]. For interposition grafts, the authors prefer to utilize allograft with the addition of bone marrow aspirate to provide osteoconductive, osteoinductive, and osteogenic properties while limiting donor site morbidity. Additionally, the authors prefer to utilize a cannulated conical reaming system, when able, to prepare both the joint surfaces and the interposition bone graft to maximize surface area and facilitate positioning of the fusion [6].

Case Examples

Case 1.1 Failed 1st MTPJ Fusion After Implant Arthroplasty

History

- Failed 1st MTPJ fusion after metal hemiarthroplasty
- Continued and worsening pain and limited range of motion 2 years after metal hemiarthroplasty for hallux rigidus (Fig. 1.1a, b)

Reasons for Failure

- Implant loosening
- Restricted and painful 1st MTPJ ROM

Surgical Plan

- The surgeon should be prepared to use structural bone graft if a large gap exists after implant removal.

Approach

- The patient is positioned supine on the operative table with a thigh tourniquet, with an ipsilateral hip bump, and with the ipsilateral iliac crest prepped in sterilely to obtain bone marrow aspirate or structural graft.
- A dorsal incision is made over the 1st MTPJ, incorporating previous scars when possible. The extensor hallucis longus is retracted laterally and a capsulotomy performed.
- When necessary, a Z-lengthening of the EHL is performed.

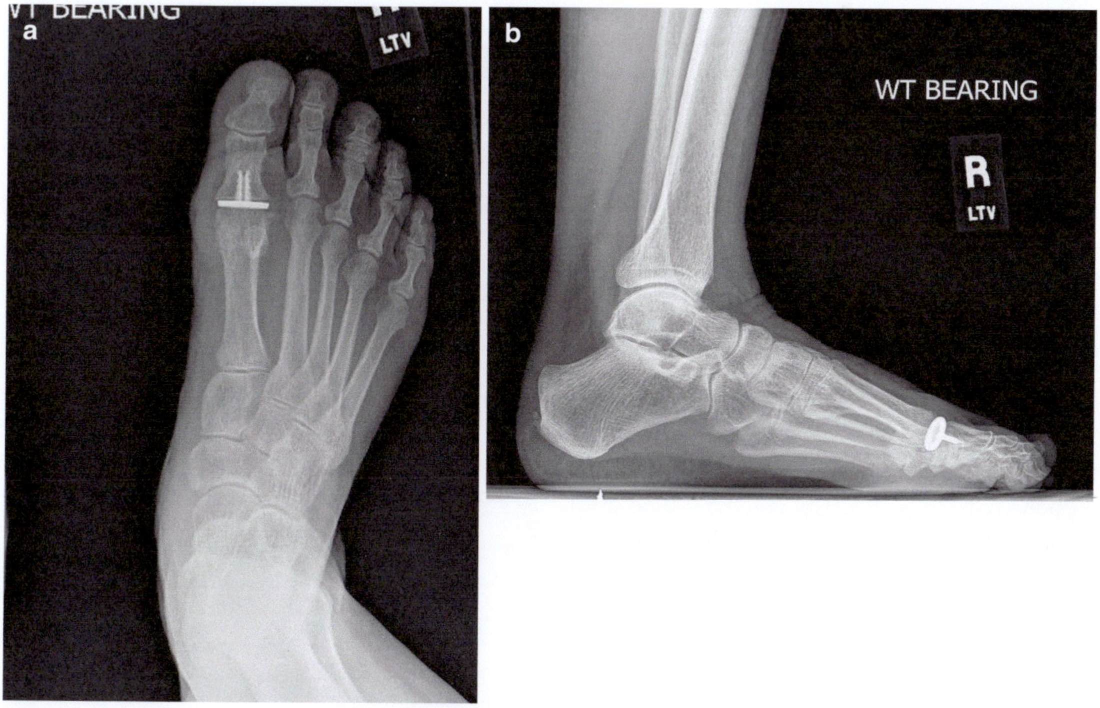

Fig. 1.1 Preoperative anterior-posterior (**a**) lateral (**b**) radiographs demonstrate a metal 1st MTPJ hemiarthroplasty implant

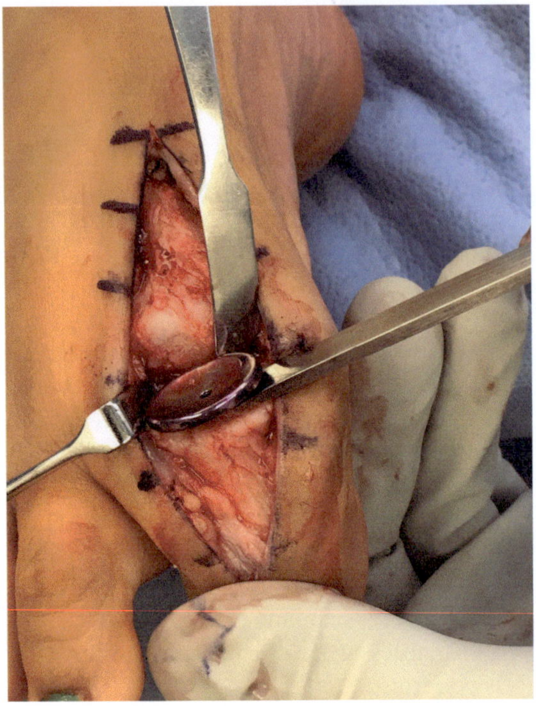

Fig. 1.2 An osteotome is used here to demonstrate and remove a grossly loose metallic hemiarthroplasty implant

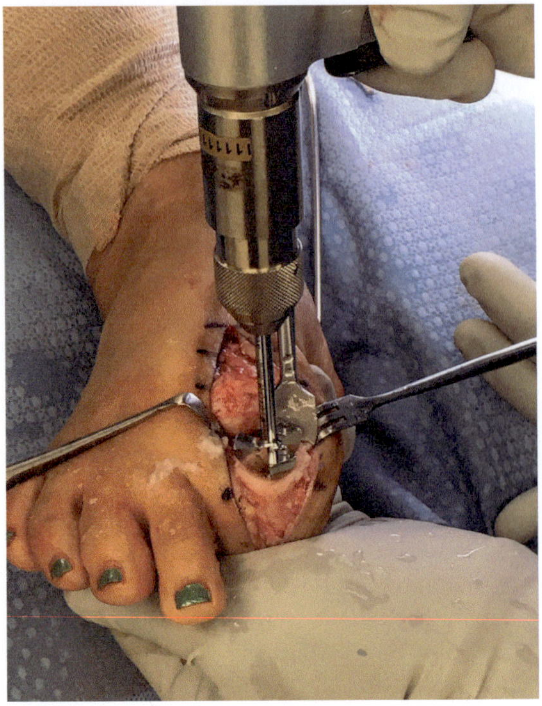

Fig. 1.3 A cannulated reamer set is used to prepare the joint surfaces

- The 1st MTPJ is mobilized allowing exposure of the hemiarthroplasty implant. The implant (Fig. 1.2) is noted to be loose and is removed using an osteotome.
- The joint surfaces are prepared using conical reamers (Fig. 1.3) and a 1.5 mm wire pass drill to increase bony ingrowth. Drilling is completed under cooling to prevent thermal necrosis.
- After joint preparation, the toe is positioned, and the gap measured (Fig. 1.4). With the gap measuring 1 cm, a decision for structural bone grafting is made.
- A femoral head allograft is prepared with conical reamers until fitting the contours of the bone gap (Figs. 1.5, 1.6, and 1.7). Iliac crest aspirate is harvested and mixed with the structural bone graft. Demineralized cortical fibers are also packed on each surface of the joint and the structural bone graft implanted.
- The toe is provisionally pinned and alignment checked against a flat plate. The guide pin is exchanged for a cannulated lag screw. A dorsal neutralization plate is applied under compression with a combination of cortical and locking screws.

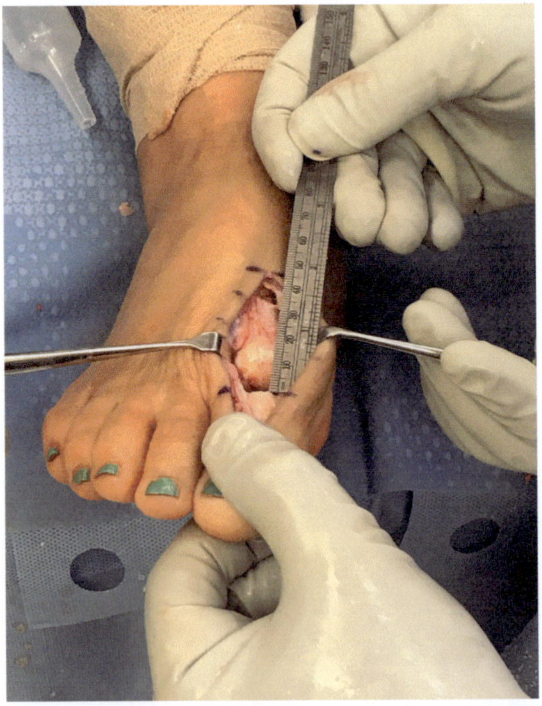

Fig. 1.4 After joint preparation, the toe is pulled to the desired position and the gap measured to determine need or size of an interposition bone graft

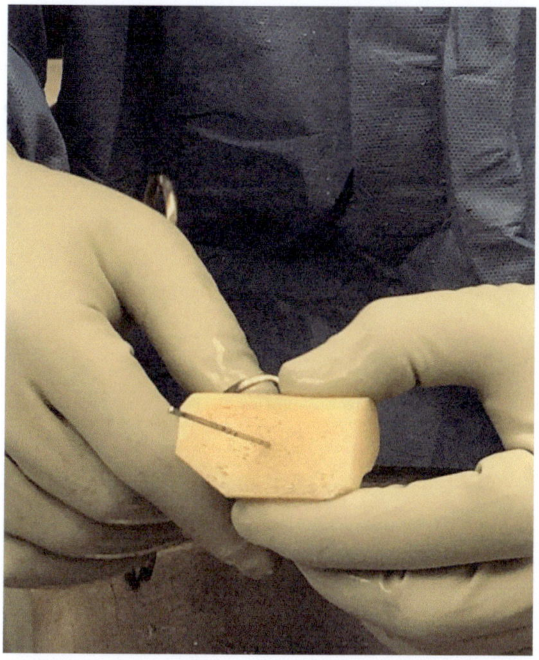

Fig. 1.5 A femoral head allograft is thawed and sectioned. A K-wire is placed centrally in the graft for shaping with the conical reamers

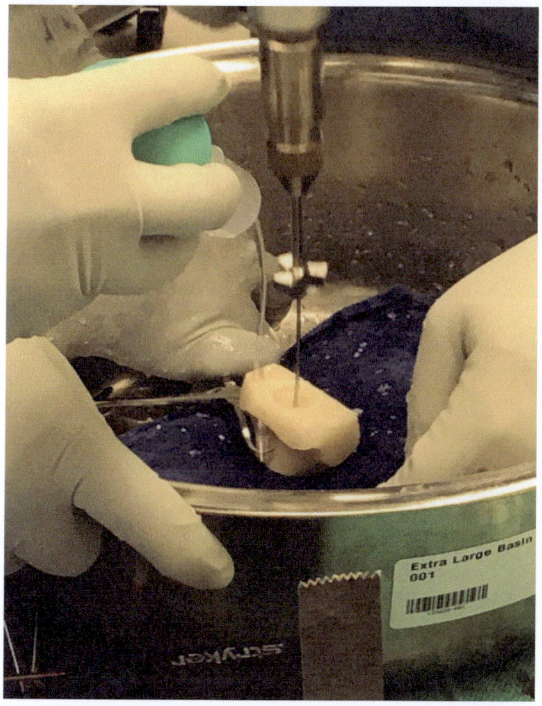

Fig. 1.6 Conical reamers are used to create an interposition bone-block corresponding to the gap measured and sizes used in preparation of the 1st MT head and base of the proximal phalanx

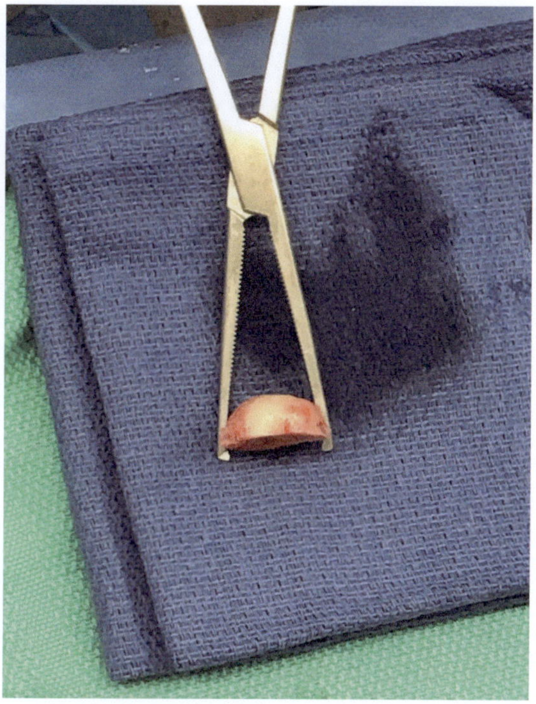

Fig. 1.7 The final interposition allograft fashioned with concave and convex ends

- The tourniquet is released prior to closure and hemostasis achieved. The wound is closed in layers.
- A bulky dressing and splint are applied. The post-op splint is changed to a non-weight-bearing short leg cast at the first post-op appointment. Sutures are removed 2–3 weeks post-op, and another non-weight-bearing short leg cast is placed. The patient is kept non-weight-bearing in a short leg cast until radiographic evidence of healing (Fig. 1.8a, b), generally 6–10 weeks, with transition to a boot and progressive weight-bearing at that point.

Implants

- Lag screw and neutralization plate construct of choice. This case featured:
  - OrthoHelix 1st MTPJ fusion plate
  - OrthoHelix 4 mm lag screw

Pearls and Pitfalls

- Carefully debride the joint of synovitis, fibrous tissue, and avascular bone to expose healthy bleeding surfaces.

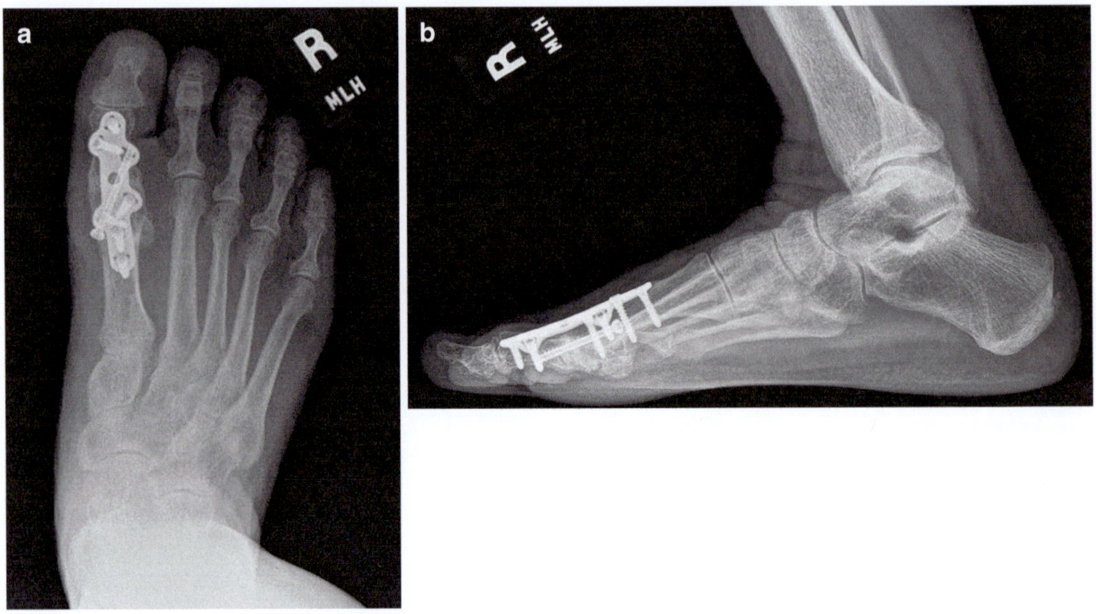

Fig. 1.8 Postoperative AP (**a**) and lateral (**b**) radiographs demonstrate a healed interposition allograft arthrodesis with lag screw and dorsal plate construct

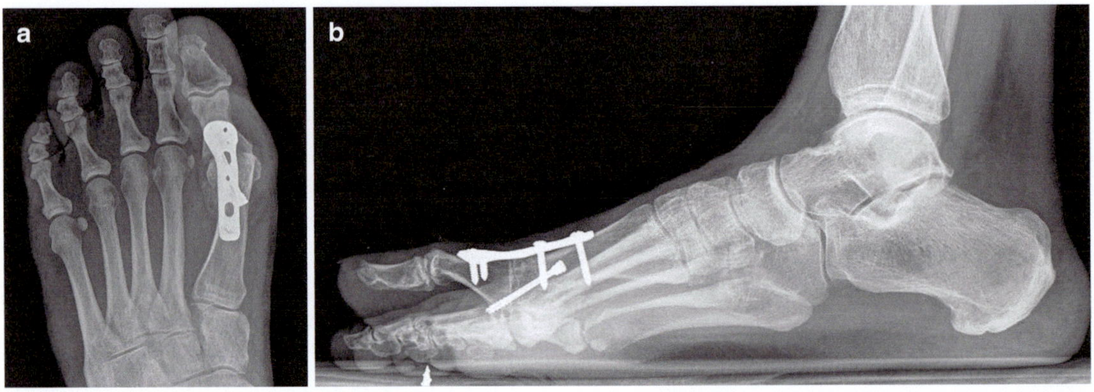

Fig. 1.9 Preoperative AP (**a**) and lateral (**b**) radiographs demonstrate a dorsiflexion malunion of a 1st MTPJ arthrodesis

- Avoid malposition of the hallux by utilizing fluoroscopy and a flat plate intraoperatively.
- A combination of lag screws, pins, and non-locking and locking implants may be required to achieve stable fixation in poor bone quality.
- Restore 1st MT length without comprising vascularity. Performing surgery without tourniquet or releasing the tourniquet prior to interposition bone-block placement may help avoid vascular compromise from over lengthening.
- A bone-block interposition graft is at higher risk for nonunion with two potential failure interfaces and may require prolonged immobilization.

Case 1.2 Malunion of a 1st MTPJ Fusion

History

- Dorsiflexion malunion of a 1st MTPJ fusion resulting in painful transfer metatarsalgia (Fig. 1.9a, b)

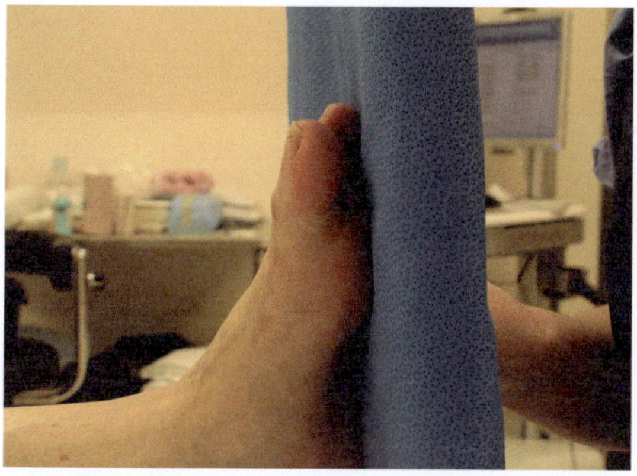

Fig. 1.10 A dorsiflexion malunion is demonstrated by stimulated weight-bearing against a flat plate. Excessive dorsiflexion leads to dorsal IPJ pain and callus, shoe impingement, and transfer metatarsalgia

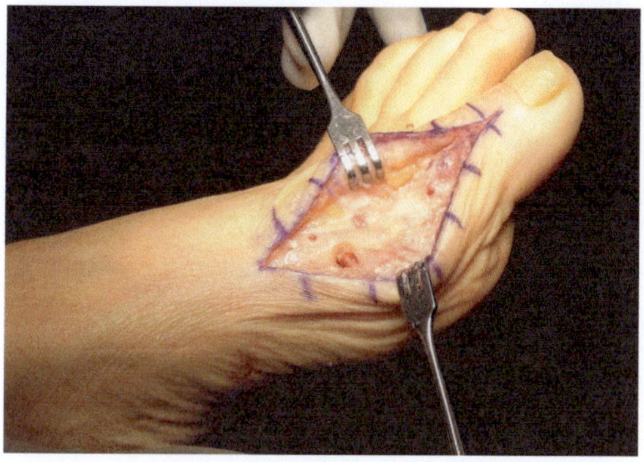

Fig. 1.11 Dorsiflexion malunion 1st MTPJ after implant removal

Reason for Failure

- Malunion with excessive dorsiflexion and valgus alignment resulting in transfer metatarsalgia (Fig. 1.10)

Surgical Plan

- Revision of malunion site with a dorsal opening wedge osteotomy with nonstructural bone graft

Approach

- The patient is positioned supine on the operative table with a thigh tourniquet, with an ipsilateral hip bump, and with the ipsilateral iliac crest prepped in sterilely to obtain bone marrow aspirate or graft.

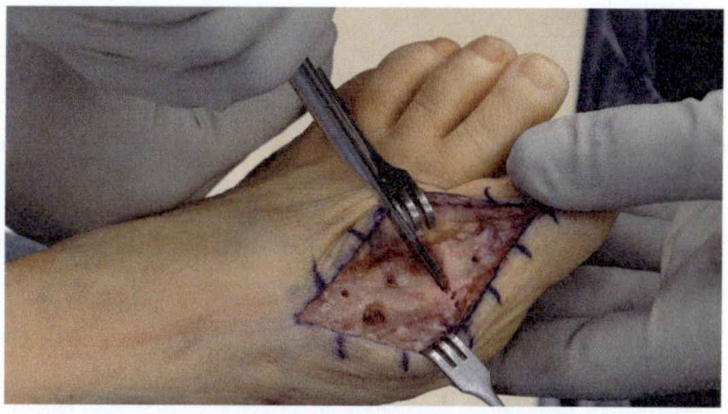

Fig. 1.12 An osteotome is used to open the malunion site

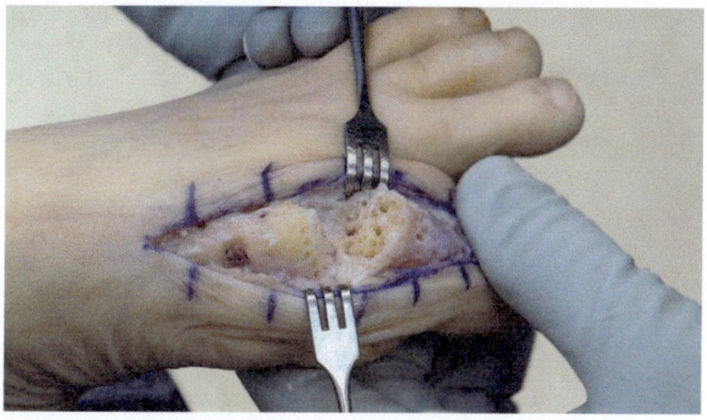

Fig. 1.13 After joint surface preparation

- The patient's previous dorsal incision is reopened. Full-thickness flaps are raised, and the EHL is mobilized and protected.
- The hardware is removed (Fig. 1.11). In this case, a bur is used to assist in locating and removing a buried headless lag screw.
- The fusion is inspected and an osteotome used to perform an osteotomy through the original fusion site (Fig. 1.12). The fusion is mobilized and the bone surfaces prepared with a combination of osteotomes, curettes, rongeurs, motorized bur, and a 1.5 mm wire (Fig. 1.13).
- After preparation, the joint is flexed into the corrected position, creating a gap dorsally.
- The position is then pinned with two K-wires and checked on a flat plate intraoperatively for appropriate weight-bearing characteristics and alignment (Fig. 1.14).
- Iliac crest bone aspirate is harvested and mixed with allograft bone and packed densely into the dorsal gap (Fig. 1.15).
- The position is secured with a 1st MTPJ fusion plate and lag screw (Fig. 1.16). Appropriate positioning and placement of hardware is con-

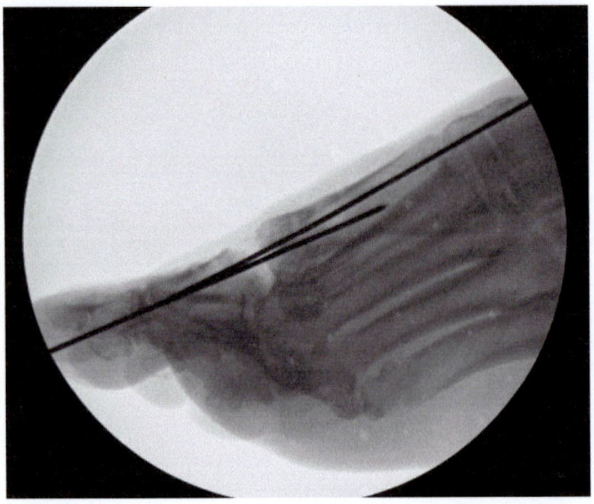

Fig. 1.14 Intraoperative fluoroscopic imaging demonstrating K-wire placement and alignment of the dorsal opening wedge osteotomy

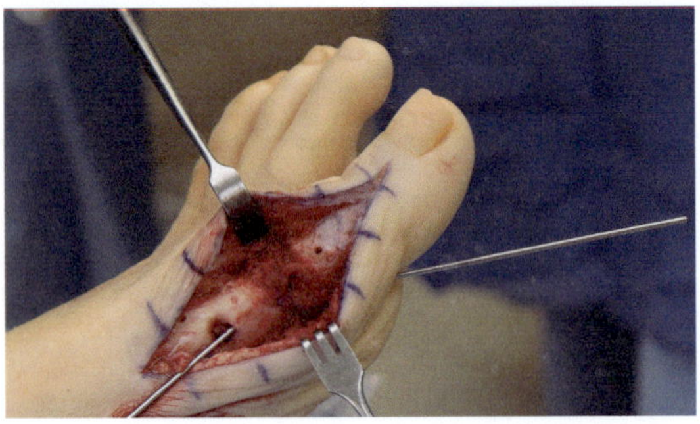

Fig. 1.15 A dorsal opening wedge is created through the joint, pinned with K-wires, and filled with allograft soaked in bone marrow aspirate

firmed on fluoroscopy (Fig. 1.17) and again with the flat plate (Fig. 1.18).
- The tourniquet is released and hemostasis obtained. The wound is closed in layers and bulky dressing and splint applied.
- The patient is kept non-weight-bearing in a short leg cast until radiographic evidence of healing (6–10 weeks) with transition to a boot and progressive weight-bearing at that time (Fig. 1.19a, b).

Implants
- Lag screw and neutralization plate construct of choice. This case featured:
  - OrthoHelix MaxLock 1st MTPJ fusion plate
  - OrthoHelix 4 mm cannulated lag screw

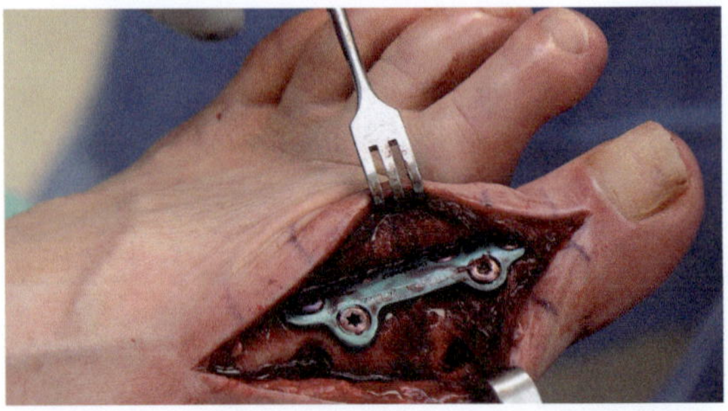

Fig. 1.16 Final fixation is placed

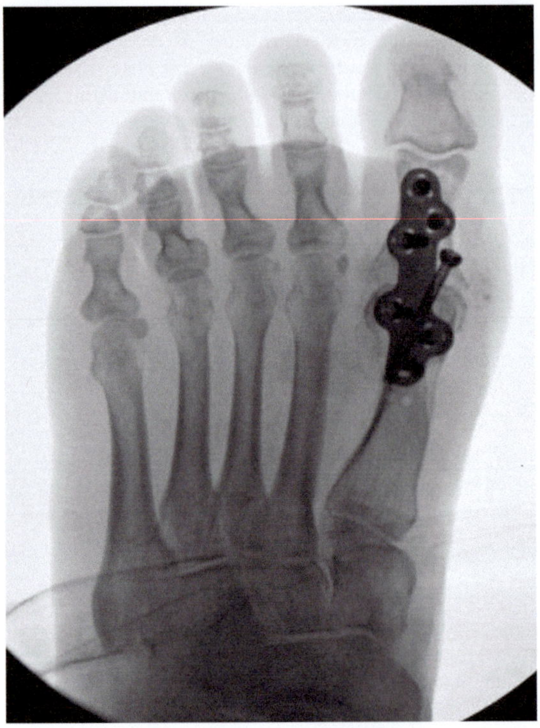

Fig. 1.17 Intraoperative imaging showing final plate and lag screw construct

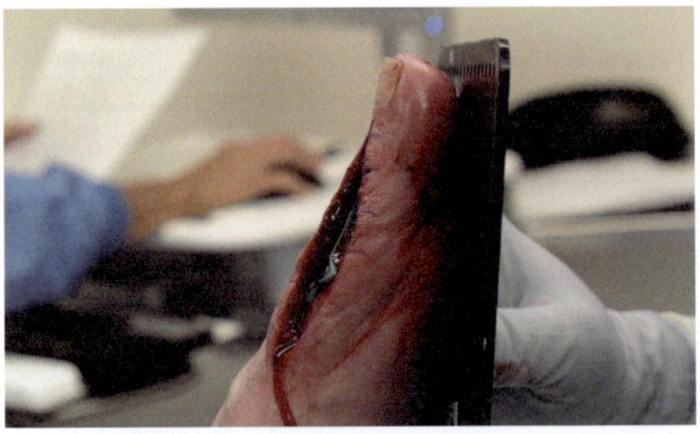

Fig. 1.18 Simulated weight-bearing position of the revision 1st MTPJ fusion against a flat plate

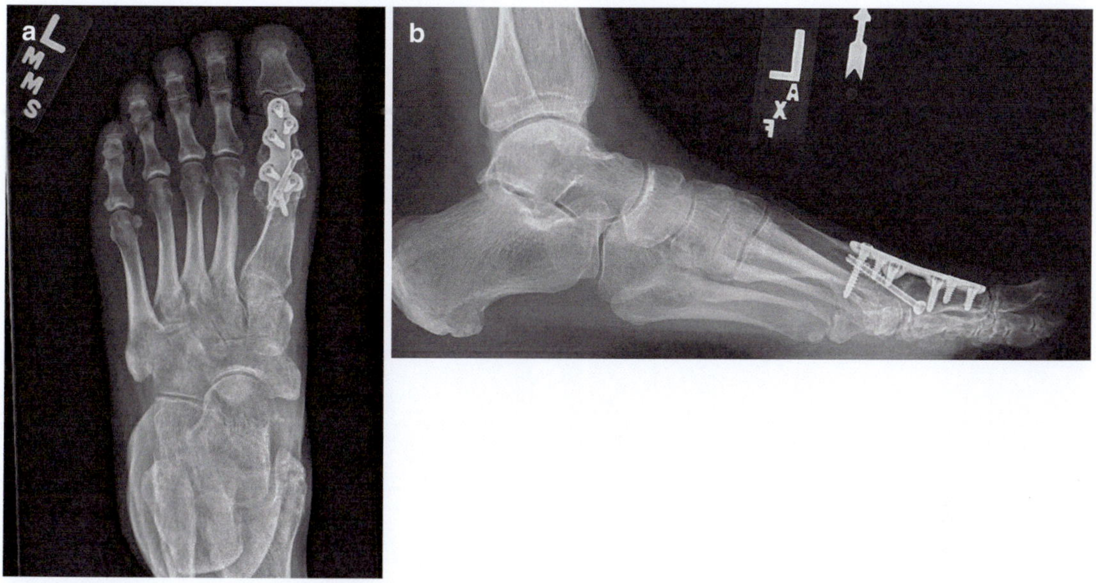

Fig. 1.19 Postoperative radiographs AP (**a**) and lateral (**b**) demonstrate a healed 1st MTPJ fusion in improved alignment after revision with a dorsal opening wedge and nonstructural allograft

Pearls and Pitfalls

- Avoid malposition of the hallux by utilizing fluoroscopy and a flat plate intraoperatively. To approximate weight-bearing, the flat plate should be used with the ankle at 90 degrees. The tip of the hallux should be 2–3 mm off the flat plate and lying adjacent to but not touching the second toe [1, 9].
- Simple flat cut opening or closing wedge osteotomies can be created at the apex of the original fusion to correct plantarflexion and dorsiflexion malunions.
- Opening wedge defects are packed with allograft or autograft at the surgeon's discretion.

Case 1.3 Nonunion of 1st MTPJ Fusion

History

- 1st MTPJ fusion for hallux rigidus with early implant failure and plate breakage noted on follow-up (Fig. 1.20a, b, c).
- Patient had been on an immediate WBAT protocol.
- Patient is now 3 years out from index surgery with continued pain, nonunion, and broken hardware.

Reasons for Failure

- Early weight-bearing and implant failure?
- Poor biology?
- Inadequate fixation?

Surgical Plan

- Revision fusion with nonstructural graft and rigid fixation

Approach

- The patient is positioned supine on the operating room table with a thigh tourniquet and ipsilateral iliac crest prepped into the sterile field.
- The prior dorsal incision is reopened over the 1st MTPJ. The extensor hallucis longus is retracted laterally and capsulotomy performed, exposing the hardware.
- The plate is noted to be broken (Fig. 1.21) and screws loose. All hardware is removed allowing visualization of the nonunion site, which is grossly mobile (Fig. 1.22). The nonunion site is debrided aggressively with a curette, creating two concave bone defects on both the proximal phalanx and the first metatarsal head.
- No significant longitudinal bone loss was encountered.

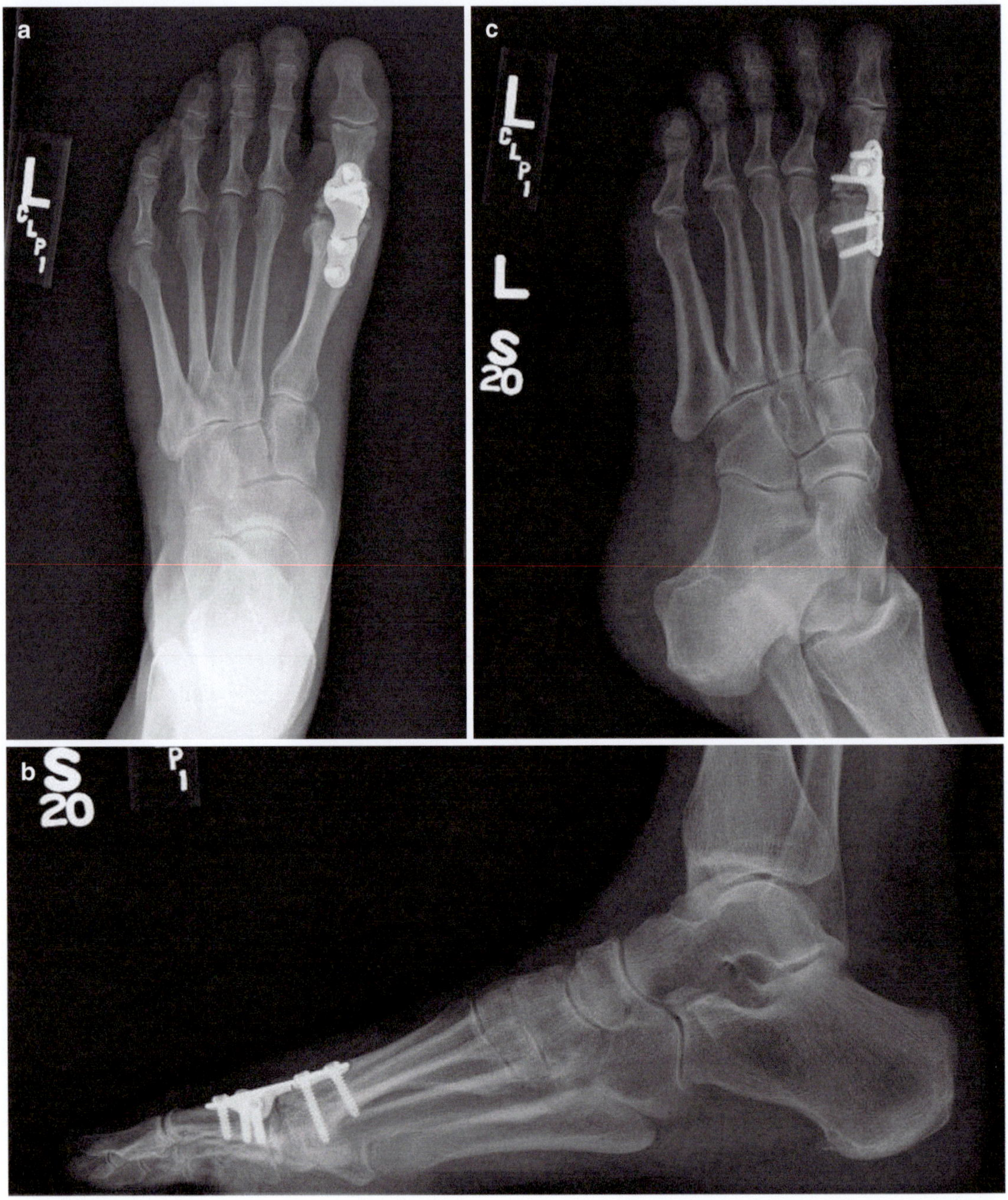

Fig. 1.20 AP (**a**), lateral (**b**), and oblique (**c**) radiographs demonstrate a broken plate and nonunion of a 1st MTPJ arthrodesis

- The joint surfaces are prepared with a 1.5 mm wire pass drill and a 4 mm bur back to punctate bleeding bone.
- Iliac crest bone marrow aspirate is harvested and mixed with cancellous or demineralized cortical fiber allograft. This is packed densely into each concave bone defect (Fig. 1.23).
- The joint is then realigned and held with guide pins (Fig. 1.24a, b, c) and inspected against a flat plate (Fig. 1.24d). Two crossed cannulated

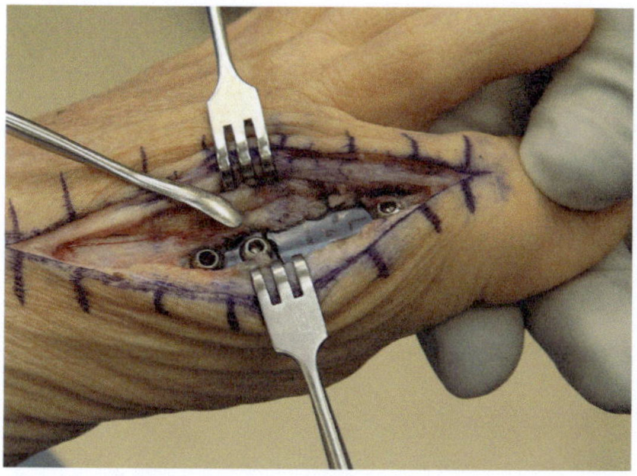

Fig. 1.21 Broken plate in a nonunion of a 1st MTPJ fusion

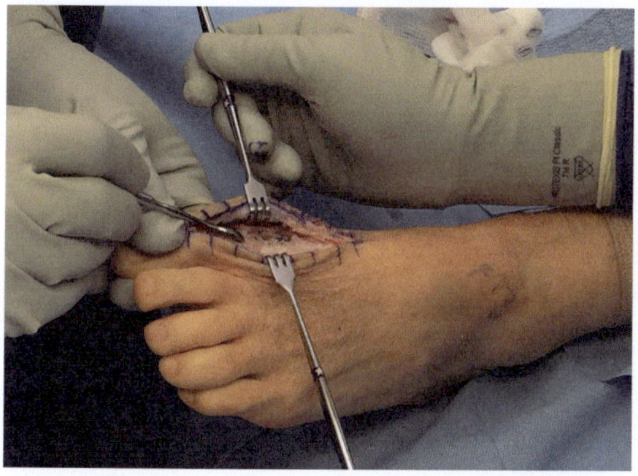

Fig. 1.22 Removal of hardware and exposure of nonunion

lag screws are placed over the wires (Fig. 1.25), and a dorsal neutralization plate is placed (Fig. 1.26).

- Final intraoperative imaging is inspected demonstrating appropriate alignment and stable fixation (Fig. 1.27a, b).
- The tourniquet is released and hemostasis obtained. The wound is closed in layers and a bulky dressing and splint applied.

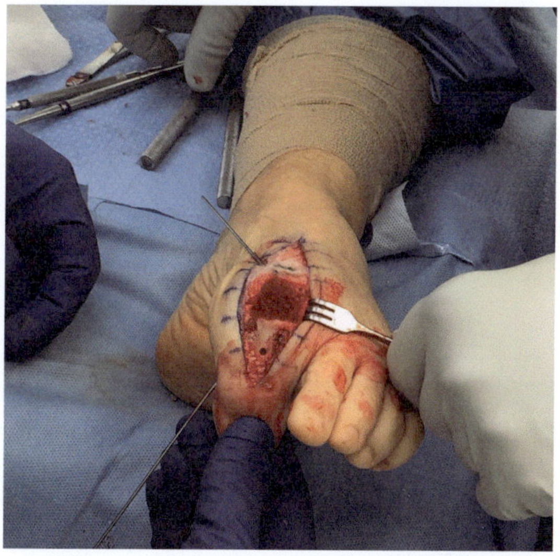

Fig. 1.23 Bone defects are packed with nonstructural bone graft

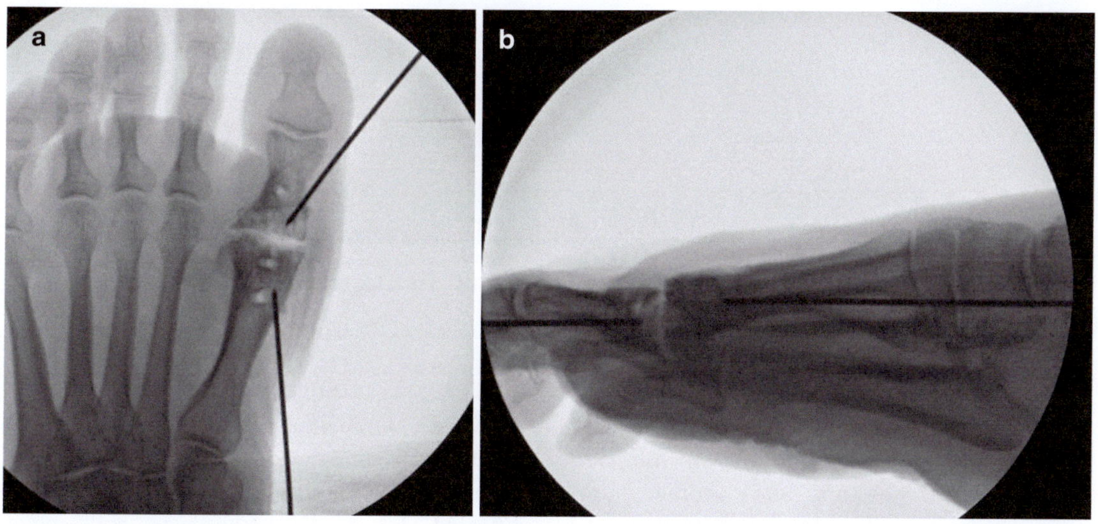

Fig. 1.24 Intraoperative fluoroscopic images demonstrate guide pin alignment for a planned crossed screw construct (**a**). Wires are positioned medial to lateral with one wire dorsal based and the other plantar based to avoid screw interference (**b**). The final crossed wire construct (**c**) and screw placement (**d**)

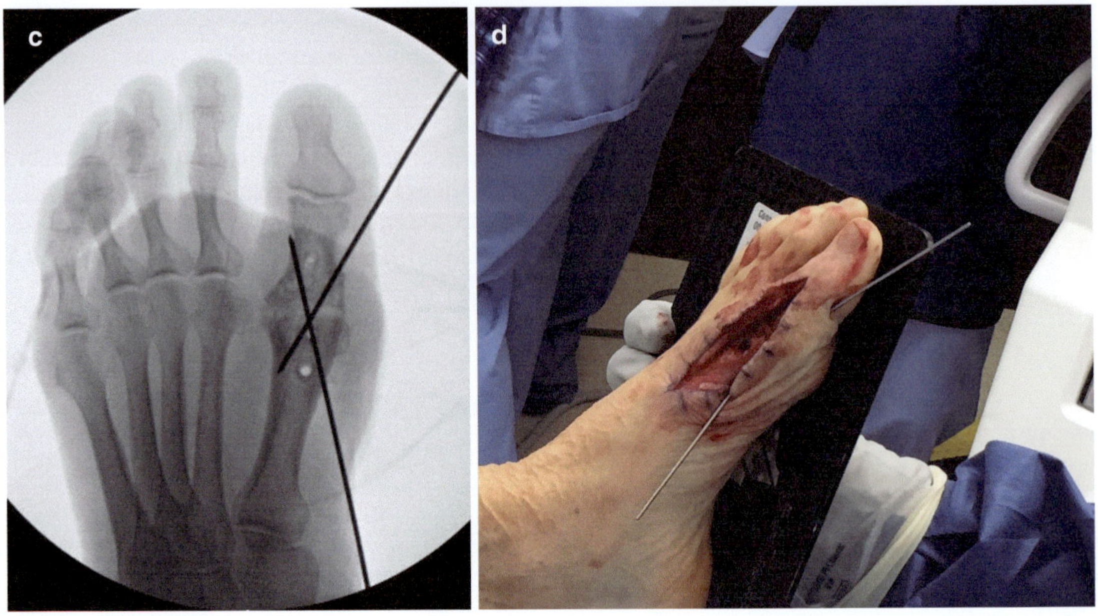

Fig. 1.24 (continued)

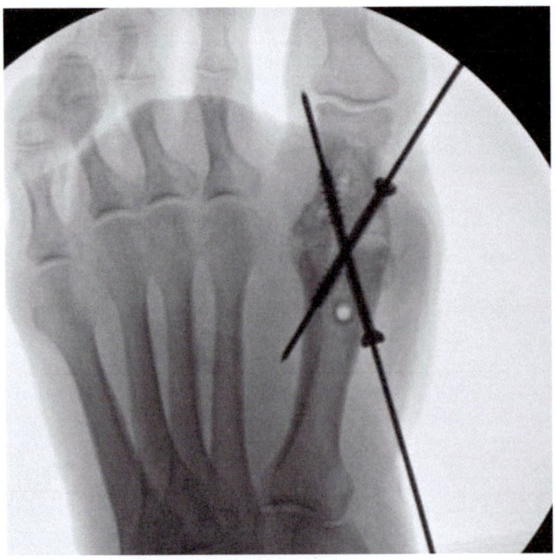

Fig. 1.25 Cannulated screw fixation

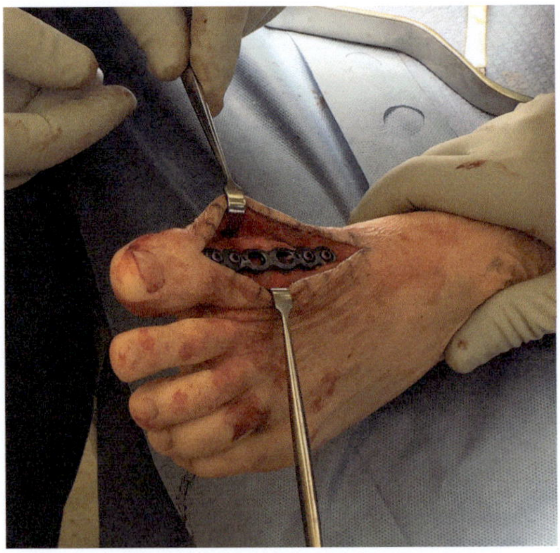

Fig. 1.26 Final lag screw and dorsal plate fixation

- The post-op splint is changed to a non-weight-bearing short leg cast at the first post-op appointment. Sutures are removed 2–3 weeks post-op, and another non-weight-bearing short leg cast is placed until 6 weeks post-op. At 6 weeks, an XR is taken out of the cast, and the patient is placed into a boot with progressive weight-bearing.
- Final follow-up radiographs demonstrating a healed 1st MTPJ arthrodesis and intact implants (Fig. 1.28a, b).

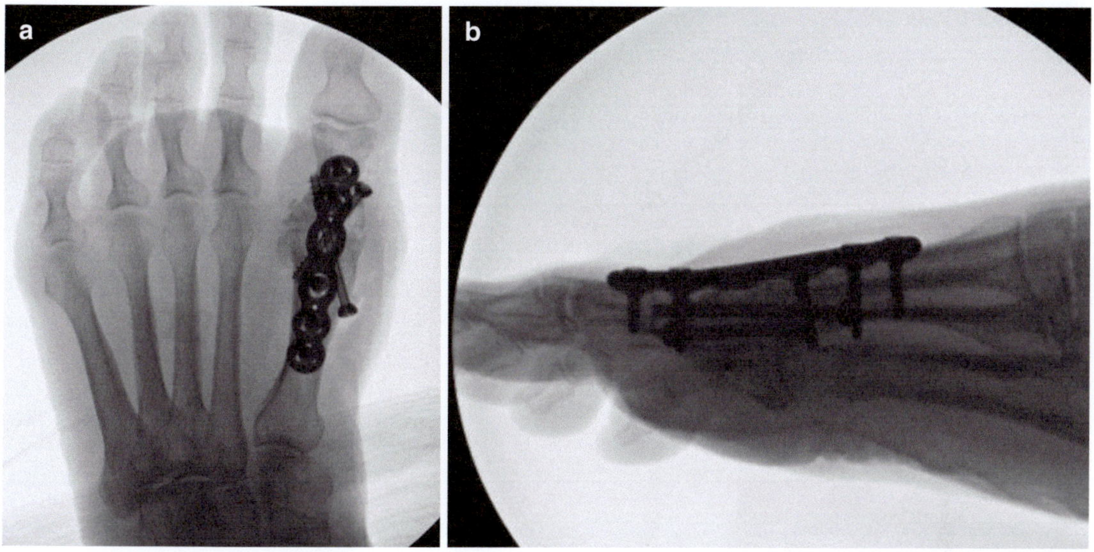

Fig. 1.27 Intraoperative imaging AP (**a**) and lateral (**b**) demonstrating the final fixation construct with crossed lag screw and a dorsal neutralization plate

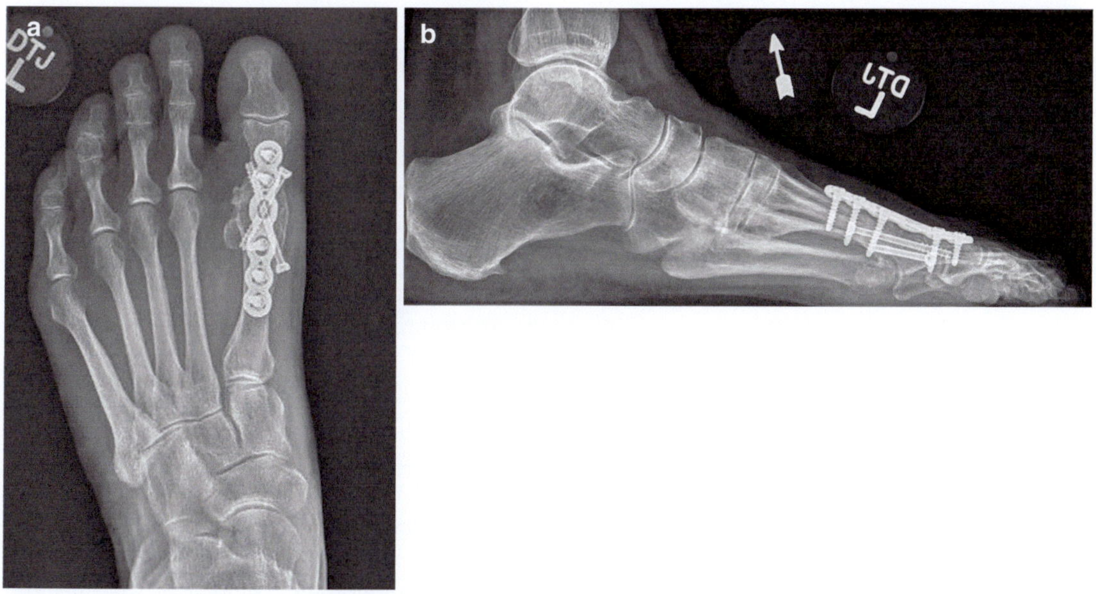

Fig. 1.28 Final follow-up AP (**a**) and lateral (**b**) radiographs demonstrating a healed 1st MTPJ arthrodesis with intact implants

Implants

- Lag screw and neutralization plate construct of choice. This case featured:
  - OrthoHelix 1st MTPJ fusion plate
  - OrthoHelix 4 mm cannulated lag screw

Case 1.4 Nonunion of 1st MTPJ Fusion

History

- 1st MTPJ fusion for hallux rigidus with nonunion (Fig. 1.29a, b)
- Patient with continued pain, nonunion

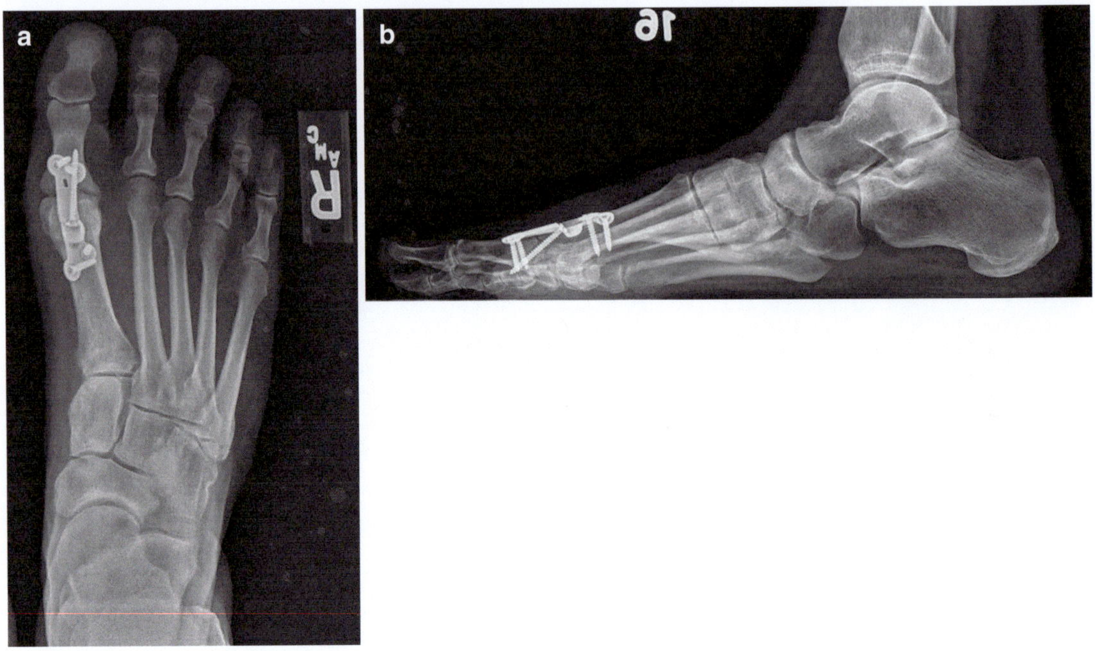

Fig. 1.29 AP (**a**) and lateral (**b**) radiographs of a 1st MTPJ fusion with a slotted plate lag screw technique that has gone on to nonunion

Reasons for Failure

- Poor biology?
- Inadequate fixation?

Surgical Plan

- Revision fusion with nonstructural graft and rigid fixation

Approach

- The patient is positioned supine on the operating room table with a thigh tourniquet and ipsilateral iliac crest prepped into the sterile field.
- The prior incision is reopened over the 1st MTPJ. The extensor hallucis longus is retracted laterally and capsulotomy performed, exposing the hardware (Fig. 1.30a).
- The plate is noted to be broken at the lag screw slot (Fig. 1.30b). All hardware is removed allowing visualization of the nonunion site, which is grossly mobile (Fig. 1.30c). The nonunion site is debrided.
- No significant longitudinal bone loss was encountered.
- The joint surfaces are prepared with a 1.5 mm wire pass drill and a 4 mm bur back to punctate bleeding bone.
- Iliac crest bone marrow aspirate is harvested and mixed with cancellous or demineralized cortical fiber allograft. This is packed densely into the bone defect.
- The joint is then realigned and held with guide pins that are exchanged for a cannulated lag screws and dorsal neutralization plate construct.
- The tourniquet is released and hemostasis obtained. The wound is closed in layers and a bulky dressing and splint applied.
- The patient is maintained non-weight-bearing until radiographic evidence of healing (Fig. 1.31a, b) and then placed into a boot with progressive weight-bearing.

Implants

- Lag screw and neutralization plate construct of choice. This case featured:
  - OrthoHelix 1st MTPJ fusion plate
  - OrthoHelix 4 mm cannulated lag screw

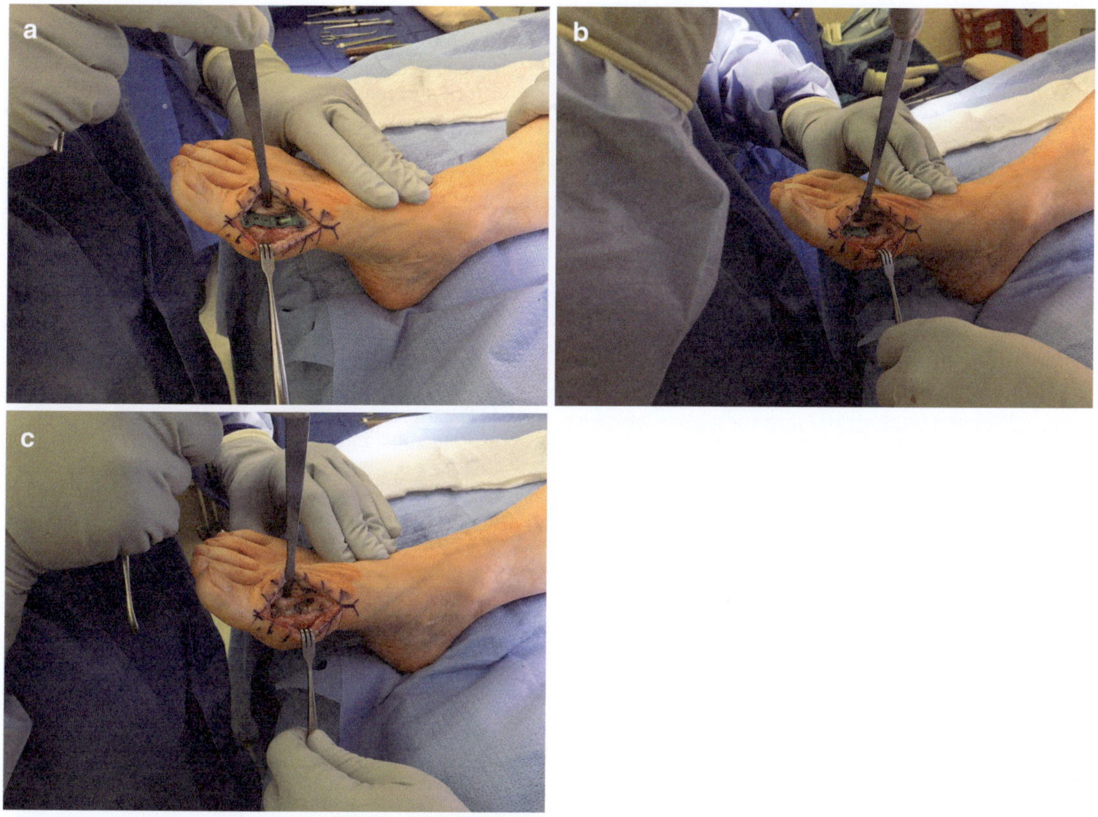

Fig. 1.30 Intraoperative photographs demonstrating the plate and screws (**a**) and location of the broken plate at the lag screw slot (**b**) and the appearance of the nonunion with all hardware removed (**c**)

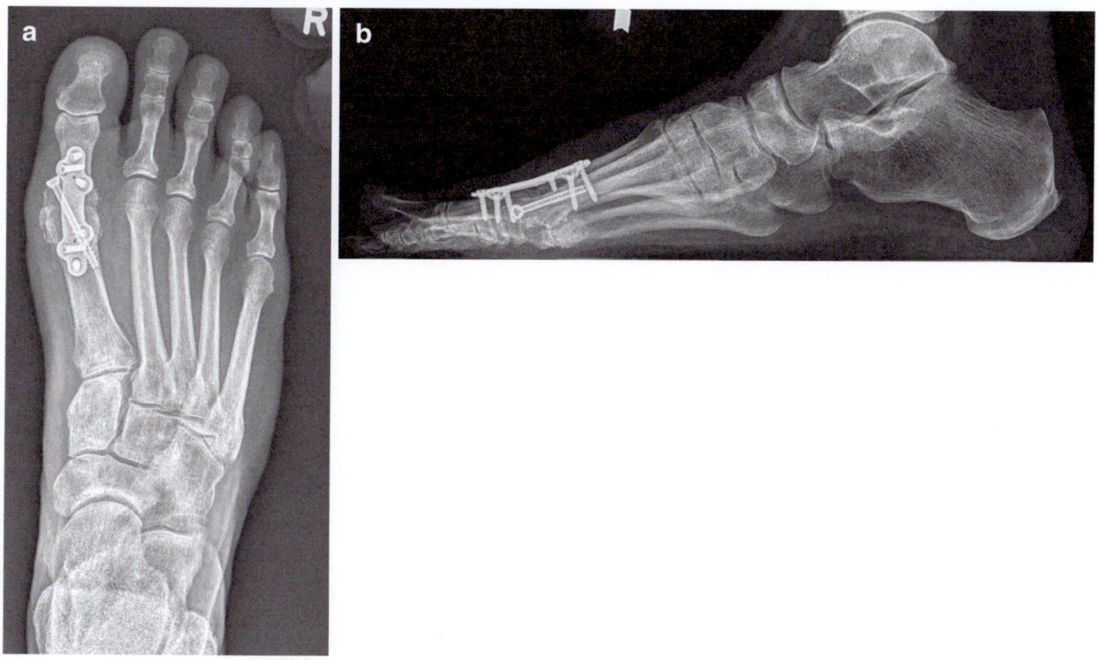

Fig. 1.31 Follow-up AP (**a**) and lateral (**b**) radiographs of a healed 1st MTPJ arthrodesis with an independent lag screw and dorsal plate construct

Summary

Salvage arthrodesis continues to be a technically challenging but successful long-term option for 1st MTPJ fusion failures. Constructing a stable 1st ray with a balanced metatarsal cascade is vital to reestablish an even forefoot weight-bearing pattern. Attention should be paid to positioning a plantigrade 1st ray, to maintaining or restoring 1st MT length, and to addressing lesser metatarsal or claw toe deformities as needed. Consideration should be given to the use of biologic adjuncts (bone graft) and the establishment of rigid fixation. In the setting of revision arthrodesis, and especially with the use of interposition bone-block arthrodesis, prolonged immobilization should be considered until radiographic union is achieved.

References

1. Bei C, Gross C, Adams S, et al. Dual plating with bone block arthrodesis of the first metatarsophalangeal joint: a clinical retrospective review. Foot Ankle Surg. 2015;21:235–9.
2. Brodsky JW, Passmore RN, Pollo FE, et al. Functional outcome of arthrodesis of the first metatarsophalangeal joint using parallel screw fixation. Foot Ankle Int. 2005;26:140–6.
3. Bhosale A, Munoruth A, Blundell C, et al. Complex primary arthrodesis of the first metatarsophalangeal joint after bone loss. Foot Ankle Int. 2011;32(10):968–72.
4. Brodsky JW, Baum BS, Pollo FE, et al. Prospective gait analysis in patients with first metatarsophalangeal joint arthrodesis for hallux rigidus. Foot Ankle Int. 2007;28(2):162–5.
5. Coughlin MJ, Shunas PS. Hallux rigidus: grading and long-term results of operative treatment. J Bone Joint Surg Am. 2003.;85-A;85:2072–88.
6. Rammelt S, Panzner I, Mittlmeier T. Metatarsophalangeal joint fusion: why and how? Foot Ankle Clin N Am. 2015;20:465–77.
7. Brodsky JW, Ptaszek AJ, Morris SG. Salvage first MTP arthrodesis utilizing IBCG: clinical evaluation and outcome. Foot Ankle Int. 2000;21:290–6.
8. Luk P, Johnson J, McCormick J, et al. First metatarsophalangeal joint arthrodesis technique with interposition allograft bone block. Foot Ankle Int. 2015;36:936–43.
9. Myerson MS, Schon LC, McGuigan FX, et al. Result of arthrodesis of the hallux metatarsophalangeal joint using bone graft for restoration of length. Foot Ankle Int. 2000;21:297–306.
10. Winters BS, Czachor B, Raikin SM. Metatarsophalangeal fusion techniques with first metatarsal bone loss/defects. Foot Ankle Clin N Am. 2015;20:479–91.
11. Leaseburg JT, DeOrio JK, Shapiro SA. Radiographic correlation of hallux MP fusion position and plate angle. Foot Ankle Int. 2009;30:873–6.
12. Politi J, John H, Njus G, et al. First metatarsal-phalangeal joint arthrodesis: a biomechanical assessment of stability. Foot Ankle Int. 2003;24:332–7.

2 Management of Failed Hallux Valgus

Thomas I. Sherman, Qin Jianzhong, Alireza Mousavian, Jakrapong Orapin, and Lew C. Schon

Key Takeaway Points

- The initial surgery preceding a recurrent hallux valgus deformity is often retrospectively found to have been inadequately powered for the initial deformity.
- Excessive dorsiflexion and shortening of the first metatarsal are the most frequently encountered hallux valgus malunion deformities, often leading to transfer metatarsalgia symptoms.
- Nonunion is a relatively uncommon complication; however, an infectious etiology must always be ruled out.
- Avascular necrosis in the pre-collapse phase is difficult to differentiate from expected clinical and radiographic findings following hallux valgus surgery.
- Hallux varus may be effectively treated with tendon transfer procedures if the deformity is flexible; however, arthrodesis is most reliable when there is underlying arthrosis or stiffness.

T. I. Sherman (✉)
Orthopedic Associates of Lancaster, Lancaster, PA, USA

Q. Jianzhong
Second Affiliated Hospital of Soochow University, Department of Orthopaedics, Su Zhou, China

A. Mousavian
Ghaem Hospital, Mashhad University of Medical Sciences, Department of Orthopedic Surgery, Mashhad, Iran

J. Orapin
Faculty of Medicine, Ramathibodi Hospital, Mahidol University, Department of Orthopaedic Surgery, Bangkok, Thailand

L. C. Schon
Department of Orthopaedic Surgery, MedStar Union Memorial Hospital, Baltimore, MD, USA

Georgetown School of Medicine, Washington, DC, USA

Johns Hopkins University, Baltimore, MD, USA

Fischell Literati Faculty, University of Maryland, Fischell Department of Bioengineering, College Park, MD, USA

Introduction

Regardless of the etiology, a failed hallux valgus correction presents a frustrating and often challenging scenario for both the patient and surgeon. Although hallux valgus correction surgery is a commonly performed procedure, complications are not infrequent. Rates are estimated to range from 10% to 55% [1]. There are several reasons that a hallux valgus surgery may result in failure. General surgical complications such as infection, neuroma, symptomatic hardware, stiffness, and painful scarring may occur. Complications more unique to hallux valgus corrective surgery include recurrence, malunion, nonunion, avas-

M. J. Berkowitz et al. (eds.), *Revision Surgery of the Foot and Ankle*,
https://doi.org/10.1007/978-3-030-29969-9_2

cular necrosis, and hallux varus. The management of these complications is the focus of this chapter.

Evaluation

The approach to a patient with a failed hallux valgus surgery begins with a detailed history. It is imperative that patients' primary, current complaint is elucidated. It is quite possible that patients' concerns may be disparate from the objective assessment of the problematic toe. Furthermore, the surgeon must also clarify the chief complaint that predated the patient's initial surgery and discern as to what degree previous surgeries addressed or failed to address that complaint. This is imperative to understanding patients' concerns and developing appropriate expectations.

A thorough physical examination is absolutely necessary. The area of patients' pain and discomfort must be localized. Findings most relevant to the various causes of failure are hallux position, lesser toe deformities, plantar metatarsal calluses, stiffness, and instability. Complete assessment of hallux position will reveal not only deformities in the coronal plane, such as recurrence or hallux varus, but also malrotation and deformities in the sagittal plane. Lesser toe deformities may occur with abnormal stress transference from the pathomechanics of a mal-aligned hallux. Keratoses may form on the plantar aspects of the distal lesser metatarsals due to stress transfer and overloading of the lesser metatarsals if the first metatarsal has been excessively shortened or dorsiflexed. Careful attention must also be given to assessing the neurovascular status, particularly in patients with diabetes and tobacco users.

Complete review of weight-bearing radiographs is required. The presence of hardware, arthritis, avascular necrosis, and alignment of both the hallux and the lesser metatarsals in coronal and sagittal planes should be noted. Analysis of the intermetatarsal angle (IMA) may be challenging following previous surgery, as the translation of the distal fragment distorts the diaphyseal long axis of the metatarsal. Thus, it is preferable to establish the axis of the first metatarsal using a distal reference point via the center-of-head technique rather than the center of the distal meta-diaphyseal junction mode of measurement (Fig. 2.1). The former technique provides a distal reference point for establishing the axis of the first metatarsal while mitigating the potential distortive effects that a previous osteotomy has on the distal meta-diaphyseal junction reference point [2]. Additionally, careful analysis of sesamoid position will also aid in determining the position of the first metatarsal, as the sesamoids will be well localized and centered under a properly aligned first metatarsal. Conversely, they will be relatively laterally translated with recurrence and relatively medially translated in hallux varus cases. The presence of arthrosis must also be noted. Additionally, the tarsometatarsal (TMT) joint should be carefully analyzed, particularly on the lateral radiograph. Instability is evident by plantar gapping and/or relative dorsal translation of the first metatarsal (Fig. 2.2).

Recurrence

Introduction

Recurrence following hallux valgus corrective surgery is a well-recognized complication. The reported rates of recurrence vary by series and surgical technique. In one large review, the rate of surgical revision for recurrence was 1.85% following a distal chevron osteotomy, 2.92% following a Lapidus-type procedure, and 2.94% after a closing base wedge osteotomy [3]. Determining accurate recurrence rates is limited by the multifactorial etiologies that contribute to failures due to recurrence, as well as the vastly different procedure types that are used to correct hallux valgus. Nevertheless, recognizing contributing factors to recurrence and understanding their effects are paramount to treating this difficult problem.

Causes of Failure

Recurrence may occur due to patient characteristics, factors related to the previous surgery, and features of the deformity itself. Relevant patient

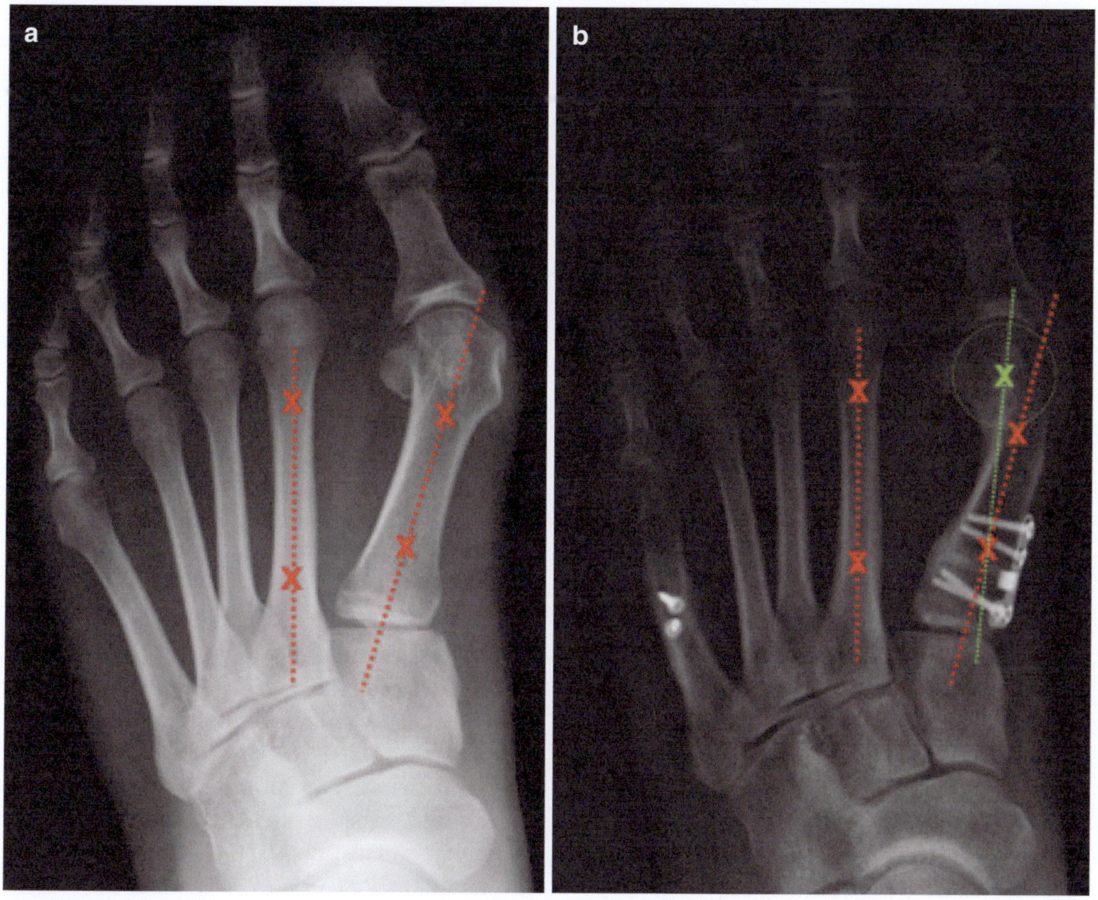

Fig. 2.1 The distal meta-diaphyseal junction reference point (red line) is accurate for measuring the IMA in patients that have not undergone previous osteotomies, (**a**) but the center-of-head distal reference point (green line) more accurately characterizes the IMA in patients that have had previous osteotomies (**b**)

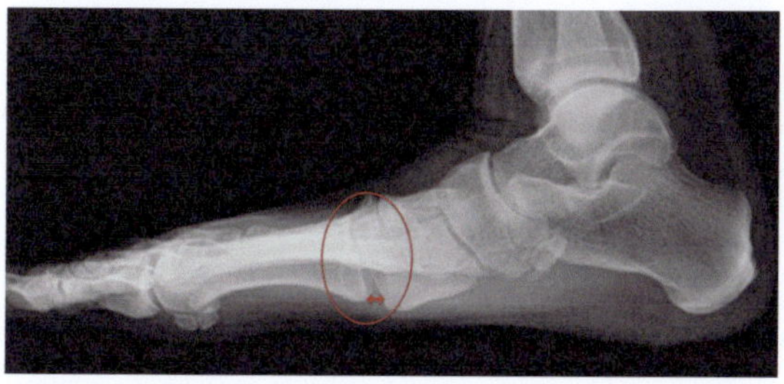

Fig. 2.2 Lateral radiograph demonstrating severe plantar gapping (arrows) of the first TMT joint (oval) and dorsal translation of the first metatarsal

factors that contribute to recurrence include ligamentous laxity, systemic disorders such as rheumatoid arthritis, spasticity, and underlying MTP arthrosis. Equally relevant is patients' understanding of recurrence risk and their perception and expectations, as many instances of recurrence are iatrogenic.

In general, the initial corrective surgery must be considered in the context of the deformity. That is, each surgery has its maximal capacity for correction, and recurrence may occur if complete correction is not obtained by way of addressing a deformity too severe for the selected procedure. It is also possible that the correction may be compromised in the immediate postoperative period by loss of fixation or noncompliance with postoperative strapping, which may result in attenuation of the reconstructed medial structures.

Recurrence often results from insufficient correction of the IMA. To this end, the surgeon must recognize that concomitant metatarsus adductus often conceals the full extent of the radiographic deformity, and thus, the measured IMA underestimates the true angle. The mechanism by which metatarsus adductus contributes to hallux valgus is not fully understood but is likely at least in part owed to the loss of the normal dynamic medial buttress afforded by the abductor hallucis as it translates plantar with congenital adduction of the first metatarsal [4]. Furthermore, concomitant metatarsus adductus results in a minimal first intermetatarsal space and thus limits the amount of lateral translation of any metatarsal osteotomy [5]. Because the goal of any primary or revision hallux valgus surgery is to restore the normal weight-bearing tripod of the foot, any additional pathology that disrupts the normal plantigrade position of the foot must also be addressed. Examples of such deformities include ankle equinus, hindfoot valgus, and the uncommon scenario of first tarsometatarsal joint instability. The surgeon was also evaluating the distal metatarsal articular angle (DMAA), as patients with an increased lateral slope of the first metatarsal articular surface will experience an increase in the severity of their deformity with isolated correction of the IMA. Here, concomitant correction of the increased DMAA is also required.

Evaluation and Surgical Planning

When evaluating patients with a recurrent deformity, it is helpful to review the previous operative report if possible. This may reveal a potential technical problem that was incurred or details regarding potentially incompetent soft tissue. It is also important to determine whether the recurrence occurred insidiously or if there was never satisfactory correction of the deformity. The latter suggests that an insufficient procedure was performed. Additionally, it is important to determine whether there were any complications or unusual circumstances encountered during the postoperative course.

Physical examination is important to the determination of the appropriate treatment. A comprehensive evaluation is necessary. It is important to identify any associated deformities, such as significant hindfoot valgus, which may require intervention especially if there is associated medial column collapse. Additionally, the presence of a plantar flexion contracture should be examined, as restoration of a plantigrade foot is required in addition to correcting the recurrence. Pain and/or instability of the medial column, including the first TMT joint, should prompt the surgeon to consider an arthrodesis at this level with simultaneous correction of the IMA. The lesser metatarsophalangeal joints must also be carefully evaluated for signs of pathology due to stress transference from the dysfunctional first ray. In such situations, consideration should be given to performing metatarsal shortening osteotomies. The first MTP joint must be carefully assessed. If there is a painful arc of motion, severe stiffness, or tenderness at the sesamoids, arthrodesis is advisable. Additionally, patients with destructive osteoarthritis or inflammatory arthritis may benefit from a fusion or an interpositional arthroplasty. Patients with advanced neurologic conditions such as Parkinson's disease or those with spasticity are likewise often best served with a fusion.

The IMA must be assessed, as insufficient correction is the most common cause for recurrence in the author's experience. The first MTP joint should be inspected for evidence of arthrosis. Additionally, the concentricity of the joint should also be evaluated. This is particularly important in cases where the IMA is relatively neutral but a deformity persists, which may be due to a laterally deviated articular surface defined by an elevated DMAA. Normal is considered 6 degrees or less [6]. If this encountered, a biplanar distal chevron osteotomy with a medial closing wedge component is recommended [7]. Consideration may be given to modifying the osteotomy with the plantar limb oriented more horizontal so that a medial wedge only need be removed from the dorsal aspect, which is more technically facile [7]. Evidence for prior metatarsal stress fractures should be noted and may indicate the need for load redistribution. Finally lesser MTP deviations and dislocations are important to note as they may contribute to symptom that requires surgical correction.

Radiographic assessment should include evaluation for metatarsus adductus. Multiple techniques are available for this purpose, and the author's preferred method is illustrated in Fig. 2.3. In general, a metatarsus adductus angle greater than 20 degrees is considered abnormal [5]. An elevated metatarsus adductus angle artificially diminishes the IMA. To account for this, it may be advisable to calculate a "corrected IMA" by adding the magnitude of the metatarsus adductus angle greater than 15 degrees to the IMA. For example, the "corrected IMA" in the setting of a metatarsus adductus angle of 21 degrees and an IMA of 12 degrees is 18 degrees.

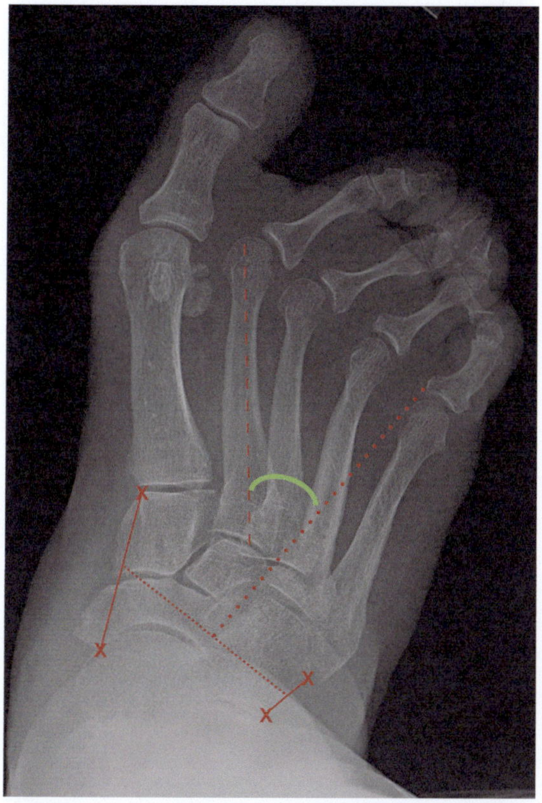

Fig. 2.3 Anteroposterior radiograph demonstrating measurement of the metatarsus adductus angle. A line (solid line) is drawn connecting the distal and most proximal aspects of the cuboid and another (solid line) from the distal medial cuneiform to the most proximal point of the navicular. A line (small dashed line) is then drawn that connects the midpoints and another line (dotted line) perpendicular to this one. The angle between the lattermost line (dotted line) and another (large dashed line) defining the axis of the second metatarsal characterizes the metatarsus adductus angle (green arc)

Cases

Case 2.1

History

- A 69-year-old female with well-controlled rheumatoid arthritis reports first MTP joint pain, as well as second and third metatarsalgia following a modified Lapidus procedure (first TMT arthrodesis) and second metatarsal shortening osteotomy 9 years prior. She reports recurrence began 6 months after surgery.
- Physical examination reveals crossover of the hallux plantar to the second digit, and a restricted and painful arc of motion with the hallux passively corrected.
- Radiographs demonstrate osseous fusion of the first TMT joint (Fig. 2.4). The IMA is 11 degrees, HVA is 38 degrees, DMAA is 4 degrees, and there is relative lateral translation of the sesamoids. The metatarsus adductus angle is 22 degrees.

Reason Case Failed

- Recurrence is likely multifactorial secondary to underlying metatarsus adductus, insufficient IMA correction, and soft tissue insufficiency due to rheumatoid arthritis.

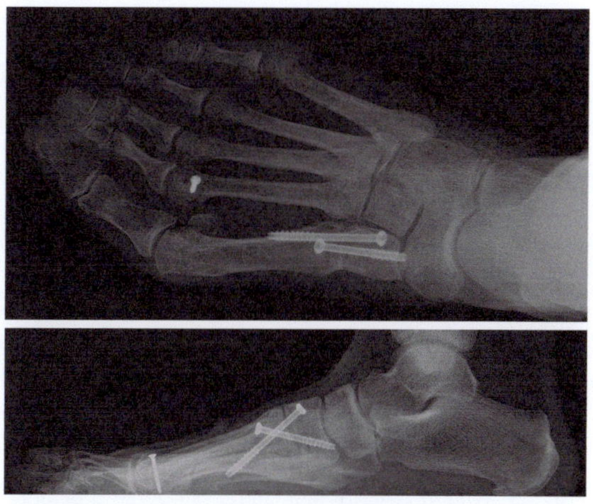

Fig. 2.4 Anteroposterior and lateral radiographs demonstrating a recurrent hallux valgus following a previous modified Lapidus procedure

Surgical Plan

- Given symptomatic arthritis at the first MTP and underlying rheumatoid arthritis, the surgical plan is a first MTP arthrodesis.

Approach

- A dorsal approach centered over first MTP joint is used, and the extensor hallucis longus (EHL) is retracted laterally. The joint surfaces are prepared through meticulous debridement of the remaining cartilage and subchondral bone with the use of a rongeur, curettes, and pneumatic 4 mm burr. Each side is peppered with a 0.045 inch Kirschner wire.

Implants

- A 3.0 mm partially threaded cannulated screw (Arthrex, Naples, FL) is initially used to obtain compression, followed by a dorsal first MTP fusion locking plate (Arthrex, Naples, FL) (Fig. 2.5).

- Appropriate positioning of the first MTP is imperative in the setting of previous ipsilateral first TMT fusion. Intraoperative assessment using a metal tray or container lid to simulate weight-bearing is required to determine the appropriate position in the sagittal plane.

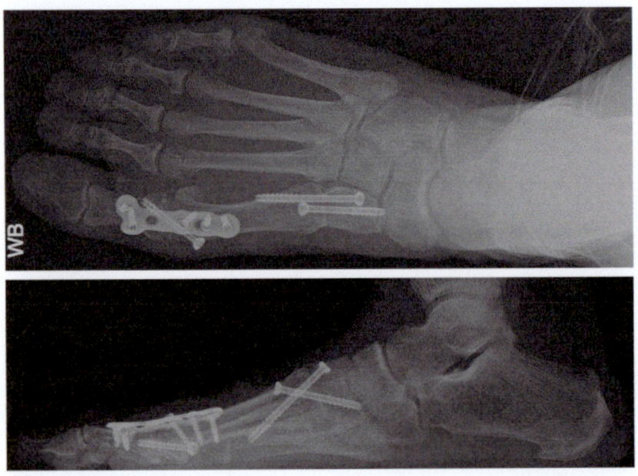

Fig. 2.5 Anteroposterior and lateral radiographs demonstrating correction of the recurrence following a first MTP arthrodesis 6 months postoperative

Case 2.2

History

A 55-year-old healthy male reports first metatarsal dorsomedial eminence pain, pain at the plantar second metatarsal, and a bunionette deformity following a modified Lapidus procedure performed 4 years prior. The patient reports the foot was never straight after the surgery and the deformity gradually recurred to be more severe than it was prior to surgery over the subsequent several years.

Physical examination reveals crossover of the hallux plantar to the second digit, and a painless arc of motion with the hallux passively corrected. There is tenderness underlying the second metatarsal head.

Radiographs demonstrate osseous fusion of the first TMT joint (Fig. 2.6). The IMA is 14 degrees, HVA is 34 degrees, DMAA is 8 degrees, and there is relative lateral translation of the sesamoids. The metatarsus adductus angle is 16 degrees. There is arthritis of the second MTP joint.

Reason Case Failed

Recurrence is secondary to insufficient IMA correction. Transfer second metatarsalgia and arthritis secondary to the pathomechanics of the first ray.

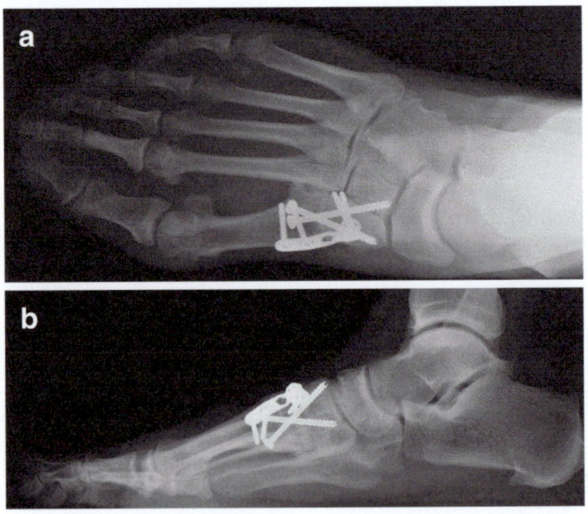

Fig. 2.6 Anteroposterior (**a**) and lateral (**b**) radiographs of a patient with recurrent hallux valgus following a previous modified Lapidus procedure

Surgical Plan

Plan for correction of the IMA with a medial opening wedge osteotomy, with partial removal of hardware and a biplanar distal chevron osteotomy with a medial closing wedge component to correct the elevated DMAA, which is further elevated by correcting the IMA. Second metataralgia corrected with debridement and dorsal rotation of plantar cartilage.

Approach

The previous medial incision extending from the first MTP joint to the first TMT joint is utilized (Fig. 2.7). The first MTP capsule is incised longitudinally. The joint is inspected and is without arthrosis. The dorsomedial plate at the TMT joint is removed. The proximal osteotomy is templated on biplanar fluoroscopy with Kirschner wires placed perpendicular to the first metatarsal coro-

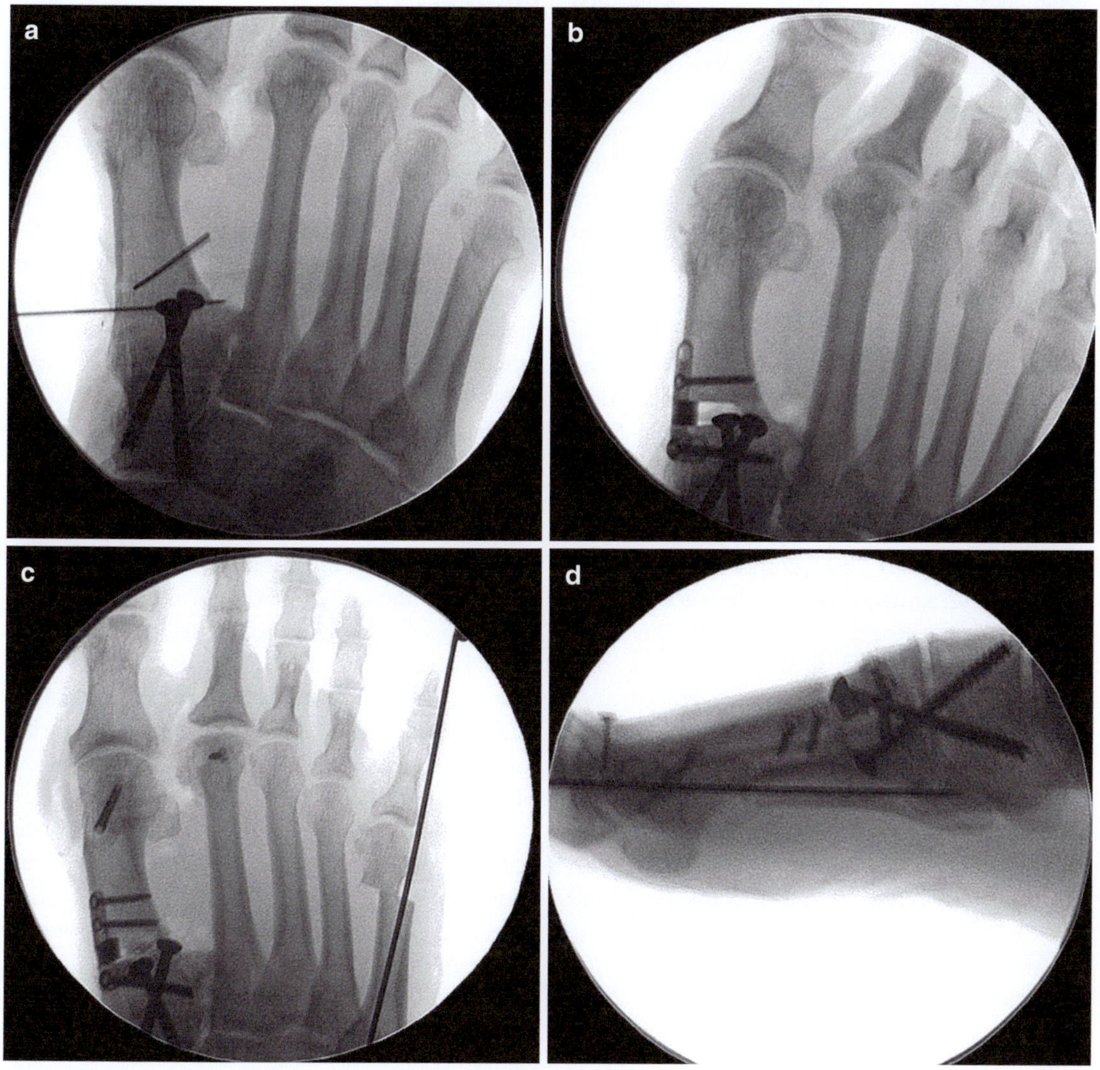

Fig. 2.7 Intraoperative fluoroscopy demonstrating correction of an elevated IMA and DMAA following a modified Lapidus procedure. The proximal osteotomy is templated following removal of hardware (**a**). Correction of the IMA is achieved with the appropriate wedge plate (**b**). Final correction of the deformity and the DMAA with fixation followed by a distal osteotomy with a medial closing wedge component (**c**). Lateral view demonstrating appropriate hardware position and no iatrogenic sagittal plane deformity (**d**)

nal and sagittal axes. The osteotomy is carried out with a 10 mm sagittal saw with care to leave the lateral cortex intact. It is carefully hinged open with osteotomes, and an appropriately sized 4.5 mm medial opening wedge plate (Arthrex, Naples, FL) is used to achieve correction of the IMA. It is packed with bone from the resected medial eminence.

- A distal chevron osteotomy is performed with the apex 2 mm distal to the center of the first metatarsal. The dorsal limb is made more vertical and the plantar more horizontal. A 2 mm medial wedge is removed from the dorsal limb to correct the DMAA. The capital fragment is translated lateral 3 mm with the use of a towel clamp. Fixation is provided by a dorsal to plantar screw perpendicular to the plantar limb of osteotomy. The capsule is imbricated after excising an apex-plantar V from the plantar limb.
- A second metatarsal shortening derotational osteotomy (see section on lesser metatarsal revision surgery) is performing through a dorsal approach centered over the second MTP joint. The extensor digitorum brevis is transected just proximal to its insertion. The EDL is retracted lateral. The capsule is incised longitudinally, and the collateral ligaments released proximal and distal. The second toe is hyper-plantarflexed, and an oblique osteotomy is performed parallel to the axis of the foot. Screw fixation is used.
- A percutaneous distal osteotomy of the bunionette deformity is performed.

Implants

- A 4.5 mm medial opening wedge plate with non-locking screws (Arthrex, Naples, FL) and a 2.5 mm headless compression screw (Arthrex, Naples, FL) are used on the first metatarsal. A 2.0 mm "snap-off" screw (Arthrex, Naples, FL) is used for fixation of the second metatarsal.

Pearls and Pitfalls

- The medial opening wedge osteotomy must be performed perpendicular to the first metatarsal axis to avoid inadvertent plantar flexion or dorsiflexion.
- The lateral cortex must be preserved to maintain stability.
- An already elevated DMAA will be exaggerated by a medial opening wedge osteotomy and must be compensated by a distal medial closing wedge osteotomy.

Hallux Varus

Introduction

The hallux varus deformity is one in which the hallux assumes a medially deviated position. Although these deformities may be congenital, the cause is most commonly iatrogenic. Hallux varus may occur after a multitude of different hallux valgus corrective surgeries but was classically associated with the McBride procedure. Considering hallux varus following this procedure provides a framework for understanding the dynamic forces that contribute to the development of hallux varus deformities in general. The McBride procedure in part consists of transfer of the adductor tendon to the first metatarsal neck as well as fibular sesamoid resection and, by default, release of the lateral head of the flexor hallucis brevis (FHB). Frequently, this surgery resulted in the hallux deviating medially due to the unopposed pull of the abductor hallucis and medial head of the FHB. The metatarsophalangeal (MTP) joint became hyperextended due to the deficient flexors, and the interphalangeal (IP) joint flexed due to the resulting imbalance of the FHL and the EHL without the pull of the EHB.

Despite a historical association with the McBride procedure, hallux varus is a recognized complication of most hallux valgus corrective surgeries, including distal metatarsal osteotomies, proximal metatarsal osteotomies, and interposition arthroplasty techniques.

Causes of Failure

Hallux varus may result due to a multitude of surgical factors, including overtightening of the medial capsule and excessive medial translation of the tibial sesamoid, overcorrection of the IMA through metatarsal osteotomies, overrelease of the lateral ligamentous complex, and extreme resection of the medial eminence [8, 9]. The reported frequency of postoperative hallux varus ranges from 2% to 13% and is likely more common after a proximal metatarsal osteotomy as opposed to a distal osteotomy [10]. Determining the factors that contributed to the development of a hallux varus deformity in each case is paramount to revision surgical decision making.

Most hallux varus deformities are well tolerated, particularly those in which the deformity is 10 degrees or less, although some contend that even deformities upward of 16 degrees or more are seldom problematic [9, 11]. When hallux varus deformities are symptomatic, it is most often due to pain from deranged joint mechanics and problematic shoewear; however, cosmesis may also be the primary complaint.

Evaluation and Surgical Planning

The first step in the evaluation of patients with a symptomatic hallux varus deformity is determining whether it is a flexible deformity. Additionally, Hawkins classified hallux varus deformities into two groups consisting of static and dynamic types [12]. Static deformities are characterized by overcorrection of the toe without muscular imbalance. Dynamic ones result from muscle imbalance that causes alteration of the normal adductor complex function. It is also helpful to determine whether the deformity is one confined to the MTP joint in the axial plane or involving both the first MTP joint and IP joint in both the axial and sagittal planes. The IP joint was commonly involved in hallux varus cases following the McBride procedure. This was due to EHB deficiency and the metatarsal head protruding through the incompetent plantar plate in place of the excised fibular sesamoid and the long flexor tendon becoming stretched around it, thus becoming an omnipresent, unbalanced flexor. Consequently, the MTP joint may be extended and the IP joint flexed, resulting in the characteristic "cock-up" or "snake in the grass deformity." Such deformities have the potential to become rigid overtime and thus may also require correction with fusion of the IP joint. Additionally, some reconstructive options require rerouting of the entire extensor hallucis longus (EHL) tendon to provide a dynamic correction, which may cause an imbalance at the IP joint. Thus, the surgeon should carefully examine the IP joint in patients with hallux varus and must also consider the effects of reconstructive options on the IP joint.

There are other physical examination findings characteristic of hallux varus deformities. In many patients, the EHL tendon may be palpated in a medially translated position and may also be quite taut. A medially deviated tibial sesamoid is often palpable plantar. A dorsal callus may develop on the medial aspect of the IP joint due to the malpositioning of the toe and may represent the primary source of pain [13]. It is imperative to examine the foot in a non-weight-bearing and weight-bearing mode to see the full impact of the deformity. One must check the reducibility of the deformity while standing to appreciate the forces required to achieve a surgical correction.

Radiographs should carefully be reviewed. The hallux valgus angle should be measured and is by definition negative in varus deformities. The IMA should also be assessed, which will typically be 5 degrees or less, particularly in cases where excessive translation of the osteotomy occurred. It is crucial to use the "center-of-head" technique to account for distortion of the long axis of the first metatarsal by previous osteotomies. The location of the sesamoids must be determined, which will often be medially translated. Additionally, the presence of arthrosis should be evaluated. The lesser metatarsals and toes must also be appraised for pathology that may result from stress transference from the deranged first ray.

In most cases, a trial of taping, splinting, and modified shoewear should be attempted. In one study, the success rate of this treatment was 22% [13]. When nonsurgical treatment fails, operative interventions should be considered. Surgical interventions are dictated by the nature of the deformity with corrective options consisting of medial soft tissue release, tendon transfers, metatarsal osteotomies, arthrodesis, and resection arthroplasty. In general, for cases in which there is underlying symptomatic degenerative changes at the MTP joint, arthrodesis is the most predictable surgical option, though resection arthroplasty such as the Keller or interpositional arthroplasty procedures may be considered, particularly in lower demand individuals. Deformities without degenerative changes may be amenable to reconstructive options as directed by the characteristics of each deformity.

Soft tissue procedures in isolation are best indicated in the setting of a flexible hallux varus without a negative intermetatarsal angle. A transfer of the EHL tendon was described by Johnson for iatrogenic hallux varus [14]. Here, a longitudinal dorsal incision is made between the first and second metatarsals on the dorsolateral aspect of the EHL, extending to its insertion on the distal phalanx. The entire tendon is released as distal as feasible and then rerouted to provide a dynamic corrective force. Concomitant IP fusion was performed in this initial description, as this procedure was described for hallux varus following the McBride procedure, in which there was typically clawing of the IP joint. In cases without IP joint deformity, a split EHL transfer may be preferable as it mitigates the resulting imbalance at the IP joint from a complete EHL release. Using this technique, the lateral portion of the EHL is used for dynamic correction of the adduction [15, 16]. The lateral half or two-thirds of the tendon is passed plantar to the intermetatarsal ligament from proximal to distal. In this way, the ligament provides a mechanical advantage to the tendon by serving as a pulley to the tendon. The tendon is then secured to the proximal phalanx after being passed plantar to dorsal or lateral to medial through a vertical or transverse osseous tunnel, respectively, created in the proximal aspect of the proximal phalanx. Fixation of the tendon may be achieved by suturing the tendon to itself or the adjacent periosteum, oversewing it to a button, or, alternatively, use of a suture anchor or interference screws. Additional medial soft tissue releases may also be performed as needed, and fixation reinforcement may be provided by temporary, trans-articular Kirschner wire with the toe held in a reduced position.

A modification of this technique was described by Lau and Myerson [17]. Here, the authors recommended use of the lateral half of the EHL to provide a corrective moment, by detaching the lateral portion proximally and leaving the insertion intact. The rationale for this modification was that tensioning of the transferred portion of the tendon also tensions the non-transferred portion of the tendon in the original description and disrupts its normal function at the IP joint. Thus, the authors recommended detaching the lateral half of the tendon proximal at the level of the TMT joint and then passing the tendon plantar to the intermetatarsal ligament directed distal to proximal. The tendon can then be attached to the first metatarsal 1.5 cm proximal to the first MTP joint. In this way, the transferred tendon serves a static tenodesis mechanism.

Additional tendon transfer options include a reverse transfer of the abductor hallucis tendon and an extensor hallucis brevis (EHB) tendon transfer [18, 19]. For the transfer of the abductor hallucis, a medial incision is made, and the abductor is resected widely off the proximal phalanx and medial sesamoid. Proximal dissection of the tendon to the level of the muscle is performed. A distal turndown of the tendon is completed to extend the length of the tendon. The tendon is passed plantar to the EHB muscle and then under the intermetatarsal ligament into an anchor on the base of the lateral aspect of the proximal phalanx. This is a technically challenging procedure.

For transfer of the EHB, a dorsal incision is used, and the EHB tendon is transected proximal at the musculotendinous junction so as to provide a tendon length of approximately 1.5 cm. It is then passed distal to proximal, plantar to the intermetatarsal ligament, and then fixated to the first metatarsal 1.5 cm proximal to the MTP joint. Fixation is provided by suturing of the tendon to itself after passage through a bone tunnel or with use of a suture anchor. Prior to fixation, the tendon is maximally tensioned to provide correction without interfering with normal motion. Additionally, medial joint releases may be performed including the medial capsule and/or the abductor tendon complex.

In situations with a negative IMA, a corrective "reverse osteotomy" of the first metatarsal should be planned. A reverse chevron osteotomy has demonstrated favorable results for this purpose [10, 20]. Here, when possible, the first metatarsal is approached through the previous incision. If this is not possible, an incision made in the mid-axis of the distal metatarsal should be used. A longitudinal medial capsulotomy is performed. Care should be taken to avoid excessive soft tissue stripping so as to mitigate comprise of the vascular supply to the metatarsal head. A 60-degree distal chevron osteotomy is performed with the proximal aspects of the osteotomy exiting proximal to the synovial capsular fold so as to avoid postoperative arthrofibrosis. Once the osteotomy is completed, the distal capital fragment is held with a towel clip and is translated medially. The degree of translation is dependent on the needed correction, and intraoperative fluoroscopy is used to assess this. Fixation options include Kirschner wires, small screws, and absorbable pins. The medial capsule may be loosely approximated, and a lateral plication through a separate dorsal first webspace incision may be included if necessary.

A reverse SCARF osteotomy, performed in combination with a proximal phalanx medial opening wedge, has also been described with limited reports but satisfactory results [21]. Others have reported success augmenting the lateral restraints of the MTP joint with implanted suture and button devices [22, 23]. Others have reported use of medial bone grafting in cases with excessive medial bone resection [24].

In cases of hallux varus with concomitant MTP arthritis and stiffness, an arthrodesis procedure is indicated. Arthrodesis following failed hallux valgus corrective surgeries has demonstrated clinical success and long-standing durability [25]. Previous studies have demonstrated reliable clinical results with this intervention, as well as restoration of normal IMA and HVA [26].

Cases

Case 2.3

History

- The patient is a 14-year-old female who previously underwent a hallux valgus correction with a distal chevron osteotomy and lateral distal soft tissue release 2 years prior. Initial preoperative radiographs demonstrate a mild hallux valgus deformity (A), and immediate postoperative radiograph (B) demonstrates correction of the deformity with an IMA of 4 degrees, a HVA of 8 degrees, and a DMAA of 4 degrees (Fig. 2.8).
- She developed an iatrogenic hallux varus deformity 6 months later.
- Physical examination reveals a hallux varus deformity with a flexible MTP joint. The IP joint is supple. There are no signs of generalized ligamentous laxity.
- Radiographs demonstrate a negative HVA of 8 degrees and an IMA of 2 degrees (Fig. 2.9).

Reason for Failure

- Recurrence is likely multifactorial secondary to slight overcorrection of the IMA and overzealous lateral soft tissue release.

Surgical Plan

- Reverse distal chevron osteotomy to correct IMA and medial capsule release

Approach

- A medial approach through previous medial incision is used. A longitudinal capsulotomy is made in line with the incision. A 60-degree distal chevron osteotomy with the apex 2 mm distal to the center of the metatarsal head is completed. The capital fragment is translated medial under fluoroscopic guidance approxi-

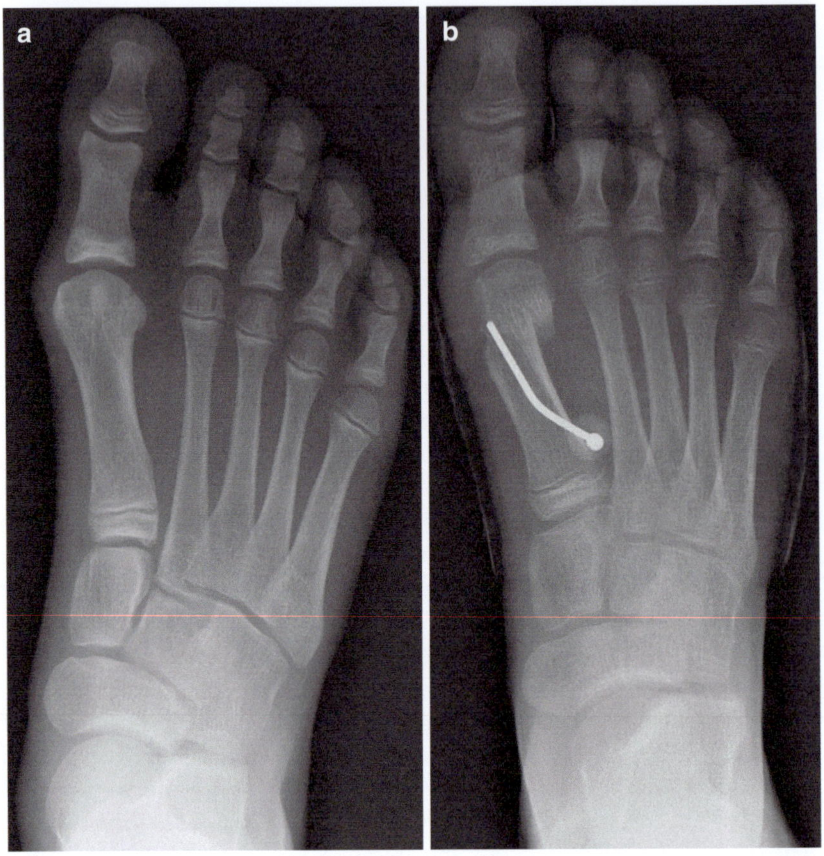

Fig. 2.8 Anteroposterior radiographs of a skeletally immature individual with hallux valgus prior to correction (**a**) and immediately postoperative with correction and percutaneous Kirschner wire fixation (**b**)

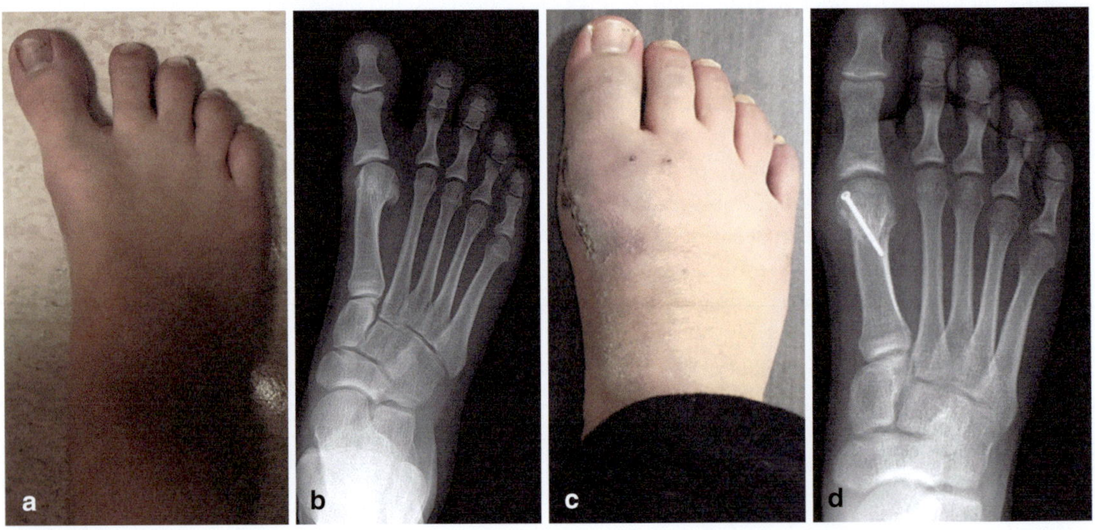

Fig. 2.9 Preoperative clinical photograph (**a**) and anteroposterior radiograph (**b**) and 8-week postoperative clinical photograph (**c**) and anteroposterior radiograph (**d**) following reverse distal chevron osteotomy

mately 2 mm and appropriate clinical position assessed in a simulated weight-bearing position. Screw fixation is utilized. The medial capsule is sutured in a loosely re-approximated fashion (Fig. 2.9).

Implants

- A 2.4 mm fully threaded non-cannulated interfragment screw (Arthrex, Naples, FL) is advanced perpendicular to the osteotomy.

Pearls and Pitfalls

- Fluoroscopic guidance is required to determine appropriate translation of the osteotomy.
- The medial capsule should not be repaired with tension.

Malunion

Introduction

Malunion is a recognized complication of any metatarsal osteotomy performed for hallux valgus correction. The two most commonly encountered malunion types are dorsiflexion deformities and excessive shortening of the first metatarsal. Although many malunions may be asymptomatic, they also have the potential to be problematic. Symptomatic malunions may manifest with pain and/or dysfunction at the first ray or the lesser metatarsals due to the pathomechanics resulting from the deranged first ray.

Surgical intervention is indicated when symptoms persist despite nonoperative management. The goal of any revision surgery for malunion is correcting the digit to a neutral, plantigrade position so as to relieve pain and restore normal function.

Dorsiflexion malunion deformities are traditionally associated with proximal metatarsal osteotomies commonly employed for correction of moderate and severe hallux valgus. To this end, in a review of 75 patients (109 feet) who underwent a proximal crescentic osteotomy with distal soft tissue release, Mann et al. reported a dorsiflexion deformity in 28% of feet [27]. Similarly, up to 17% of patients undergoing proximal chevron osteotomies are reported to develop dorsiflexion malunion deformities [28, 29]. Although less frequently encountered than with proximal metatarsal osteotomies, dorsiflexion malunion deformities may also occur following distal osteotomies, such as with chevron, Mitchell, and Wilson osteotomies [30]. They are also not infrequently encountered following TMT arthrodeses [31].

Dorsiflexion malunion deformities most typically result from either improper orientation of the osteotomy or loss of fixation in the early postoperative period due to premature weight-bearing prior to stable osseous union [32]. Typical symptoms related to a dorsiflexion malunion are pain at the first metatarsophalangeal joint due to dorsal impingement, transfer metatarsalgia from altered mechanics, and arch pain secondary to medial column instability [33].

Causes of Failure

Shortening of the first metatarsal following a corrective osteotomy for hallux valgus may result from bone loss inherent to the kerf of the saw blade, impaction of cancellous bone at the osteotomy, or improper coronal orientation of the osteotomy [34, 35]. With few exceptions, almost all osteotomies have the potential to result in shortening of the first metatarsal. The degree of shortening associated with different osteotomy types varies, however. In one series of 25 patients undergoing a proximal chevron osteotomy for correction of moderate and severe hallux valgus, the average magnitude of first metatarsal shortening was 2.6 mm [36]. Glazebrook et al. reported the first metatarsal was shortened on average by 5.6% after a proximal chevron osteotomy in their cohort [37]. Similarly, shortening has also been associated with distal chevron osteotomies and is typically reported to range from 2 to 6 mm on average [38–41].

Excessive shortening of the first metatarsal may manifest as transfer metatarsalgia due to the pathomechanics of the disrupted weight transfer mechanism. As the patient progresses from heel strike to toe off during the gait cycle, the windlass mechanism is less effective at plantar flexing a shortened first ray. Consequently, more weight is transferred to the central metatarsals, resulting in complaints of lesser metatarsalgia. Accordingly, Jung and Schon demonstrated plantar forefoot pressures are significantly increased under the second metatarsal after shortening and dorsiflexion malunions of the first metatarsal in a simulated cadaver model [42].

Evaluation

Patients with suspected malunions mandate a careful and thorough history and physical evaluation. Malunions should be evaluated for in patients who had previously undergone hallux valgus corrective surgery with complaints related to metatarsalgia. Findings associated with lesser metatarsal overload include intractable plantar keratosis, plantar plate ruptures, stress fracture, synovitis, and pain at the plantar metatarsal heads due to stress overload. Patients with dorsiflexion malunions may also demonstrate restricted dorsiflexion and pain elicited at the extremes of this motion at the first MTP joint.

Radiographs should be carefully assessed. Dorsal malunions may be subtle, and detection may be facilitated by assessing for deviation in parallelism of the dorsal cortices of the first and second metatarsals. Detection of first metatarsal shortening is also challenging, as characterizing the relative length relationship of the first metatarsal to the lesser metatarsals is notoriously difficult and unreliable. Various techniques have been described including use of lines tangent to the distal metatarsal head surfaces as well as with use of concentric arches [43]. Use of comparative radiographs to the asymptotic contralateral side may be aid in detection of suspected shortening.

Surgical Planning

Dorsiflexion Malunion

Nonoperative management is the preferred first-line treatment for patients with symptomatic dorsiflexion malunions. Most commonly, use of comfortable, modified shoewear and use of orthotic devices are recommended. Shoes with a wide toe box, a soft upper, and low heel are advisable. Additionally, a metatarsal pad may be effective for alleviating associated complaints related to transfer metatarsalgia. When patients continue to have pain despite these interventions, surgery should be considered.

As stated, the goal of any revision surgery for malunion is correcting the first ray to a neutral, plantigrade position so as to restore the normal weight-bearing tripod of the foot. First MTP arthrodesis may be considered in patients with concomitant symptomatic hallux rigidus. When painless motion is maintained at the first MTP, the dorsiflexion malunion deformity can be corrected by use of a dorsal opening wedge osteotomy or plantar closing wedge osteotomy. Although either technique is a viable option, a plantarflexion closing wedge osteotomy has the disadvantage of introducing the potential to shorten the first ray [33]. Moreover, the osteotomy site is under primarily tensile forces, which increases the risk of a cock-up deformity. Thus, in our experience, a dorsal opening wedge osteotomy with bone graft mitigates these risks and is the preferred option for correction of a dorsal malunion deformities.

Shortening Malunion

Surgical correction of a shortened first metatarsal is often a relatively more challenging problem. These procedures are technically demanding and less reliable in our experience. For instance, structural bone block often undergoes some resorption at its interface, which is often asymmetric. This may lead to angular deformities, particular dorsiflexion deformities, as the dorsal aspect of the graft is under the most compressive forces. Additionally, lengthening of the first metatarsal may result in increased contact pressure of the first MTP and symptomatic stiffness, propagation of hallux rigidus, or exacerbation of underlying arthritis. Additionally, soft tissue complications, such as wound healing, are also not infrequently encountered, as they are inherently stretched with corrective surgery. Thus careful assessment of the neurovascular status of patients with this problem is imperative before proceeding with surgical revision.

The most commonly employed revision techniques are either one-stage lengthening with intercalary bone graft [44, 45] or gradual lengthening by callotasis [46, 47]. The major theoretical advantages of gradual distraction over acute lengthening is mitigating risk of soft tissue compromise and neurovascular complications as well as the potential for more aggressive lengthening [48, 49]. Its potential disadvantages are the increased time required, pin-tract infection, and patient compliance. In our experience, single-stage revision is preferable for most patients and also affords the surgeon the opportunity to more easily correct concomitant angular deformities and address pathology of the lesser toes. To this end, in a comparison of single-stage metatarsal lengthening with intercalary bone graft to a gradual distraction technique, the authors found that there was little difference between the groups in terms of the magnitude of length gained or complication rates, and they concluded single-stage techniques are preferable especially when 15 mm or less of lengthening is needed [50, 51].

Cases

Case 2.4

History

- The patient is a 44-year-old female with complaints of callus and pain under the second and third metatarsal heads, as well as an inability to place her hallux on the ground. She previously underwent a hallux valgus corrective procedure 5 years ago with a distal metatarsal shortening osteotomy.
- Physical examination reveals a dorsomedial surgical scar overlying the first metatarsal, callus under the second and third metatarsal heads, and the hallux in a dorsally translated position (Fig. 2.10).

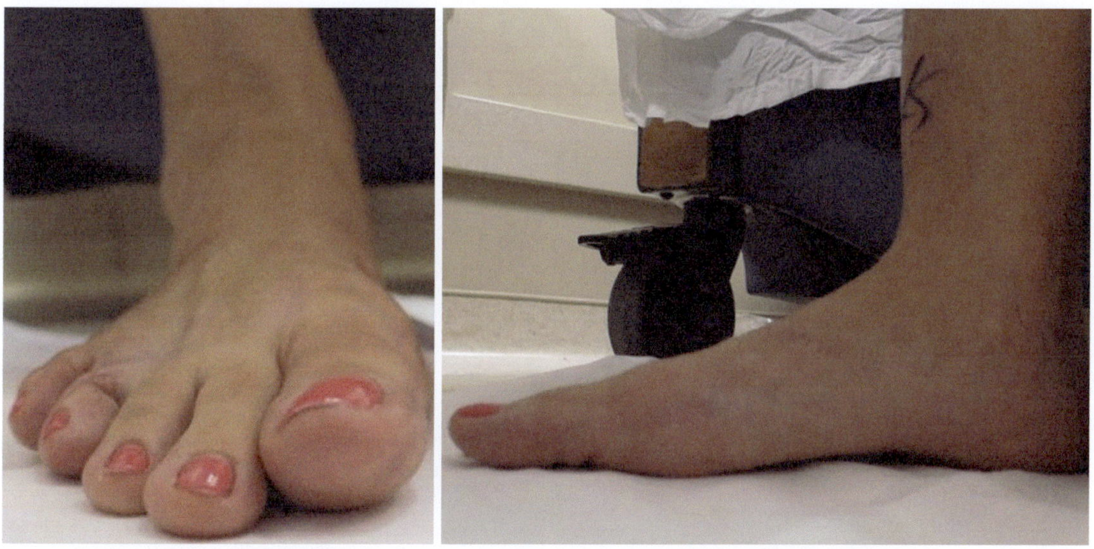

Fig. 2.10 Preoperative clinical photographs demonstrating relative dorsal translation of the hallux

Reason for Failure

- Iatrogenic dorsiflexion of the distal fragment of the metatarsal osteotomy

Surgical Plan

- Dorsal opening wedge osteotomy of the first metatarsal with iliac crest bone grafting

Approach

- The malunion and intended osteotomy site is identified with a Kirschner wire (Fig. 2.11a).
- An oscillating saw is used to perform the transverse osteotomy from medial to lateral leaving the plantar cortex intact (Fig. 2.11b).
- An articulating distractor is used, and the osteotomy is "greensticked" through intact plantar cortex (Fig. 2.11c). An opening wedge plate (Arthrex, Naples, FL) is positioned on the dorsal aspect of the first metatarsal, and the appropriate size needed to correct the deformity is selected (Fig. 2.11d). Cancellous bone graft from the iliac crest is harvested using a large bore needle (Fig. 2.11e) and is used to fill the osteotomy site (Fig. 2.11f). Fluoroscopy is used to confirm appropriate plate position, adequate plantarflexion of the first ray (Fig. 2.11g), as well as appropriate orientation in the coronal plane (Fig. 2.11h). The "thumb test" is used to palpate the plantar aspect of the metatarsal heads to ensure the foot is in a plantigrade position.

Implants

- A low profile 3.5 mm wedge plate (Arthrex, Naples, FL) positioned on the dorsal cortex

Pearls and Pitfall

- Extreme care must be taken to ensure the plantar cortex is left intact.

Case 2.5

History

- The patient is a 17-year-old female with a severely shortened first ray and recurrent hallux valgus with mild arthritic changes at the first MTP joint following a first metatarsal osteotomy and distal soft tissue release for hallux valgus correction performed 3 years prior. No fixation was provided per the operative report. The patient complains of pain at

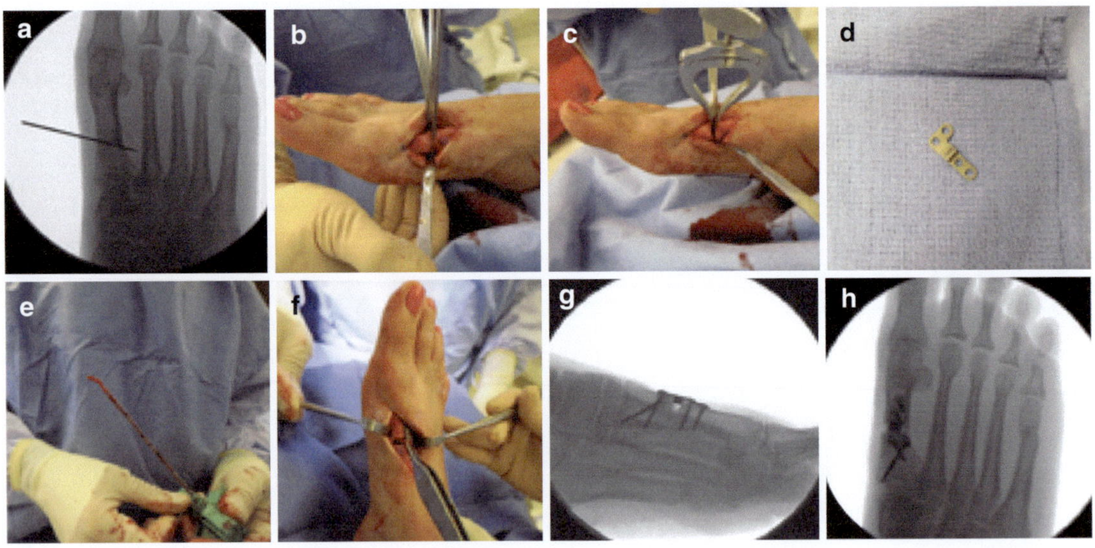

Fig. 2.11 Surgical technique for correction of dorsiflexion malunion following previous distal first metatarsal osteotomy for hallux valgus

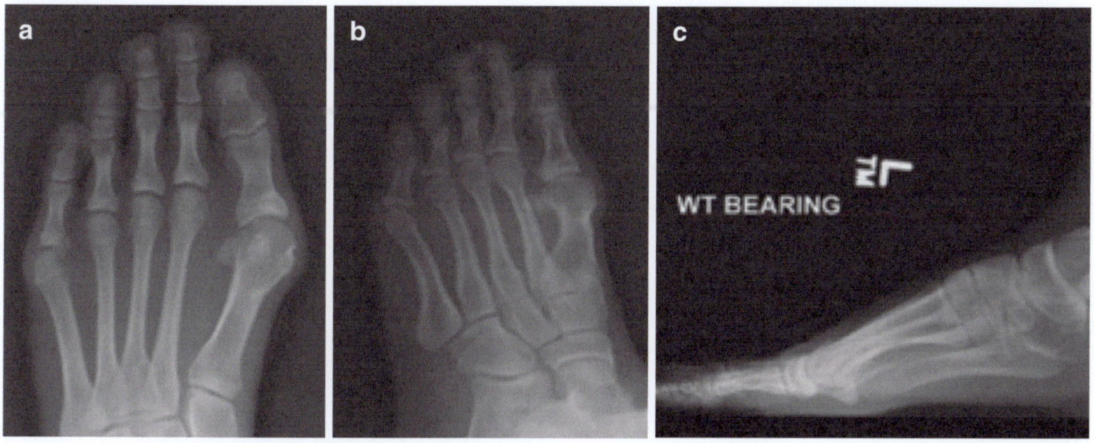

Fig. 2.12 Anteroposterior (**a**), oblique (**b**), and lateral (**c**) radiographs demonstrating excessive shortening following a distal metatarsal osteotomy for hallux valgus correction, in which no fixation was used

the dorsomedial eminence of the first MTP joint and underlying the second metatarsal.

- Physical examination reveals the hallux crossing dorsal to the second digit and pain at the limits of first MTP dorsiflexion to 25 degrees.
- Radiographs demonstrate significant shortening of the first metatarsal with a HVA of 30° and an IMA of 13° (Fig. 2.12).

Reason for Failure

- Excessive shortening of the metatarsal and insufficient correction of the IMA

Surgical Plan

- Medial proximal opening wedge osteotomy with local bone grafting of the resected eminence to the osteotomy site and distal soft tissue procedure

Approach

- The surgery is performed in the supine position with the toes oriented vertical. The previous incision on the medial border of the first ray is used. A Kirschner wire templates the osteotomy with the trajectory such that the lateral tip is oriented as close to the metatarsocuneiform joint as possible (Fig. 2.13a). An oscillating saw is used to create the osteotomy with care to preserve the lateral cortex (Fig. 2.13b). A distractor is used to "greenstick" the osteotomy (Fig. 2.13c). Biplanar fluoroscopy is used to assess correction, and an appropriately sized 6 mm wedge plate (Arthrex, Naples, FL) is selected (Fig. 2.13d). Care is taken to ensure the screws through the proximal aspect of the plate are not intra-articular. Additional lateral fixation is provided with a Kirschner wire due to inadequate periosteal hinging of the osteotomy. The medial eminence and dorsal prominence are removed using a saw through distal extension of the medial approach. This bone is packed into the osteotomy site.

Implants

- A low profile 6.5 mm wedge plate (Arthrex, Naples, FL) positioned on the medial cortex

Pearls and Pitfalls

- Extreme care must be taken to ensure the lateral cortex is left intact. In the event of an inadvertent lateral cortex penetration or poor periosteal tissue, the osteotomy is closed (undistracted) and a small oblique K-wire inserted to support the hinge. Then the osteotomy is re-distracted and the plate inserted. The screws should be oriented so as to avoid intra-articular penetration (Fig. 2.13).

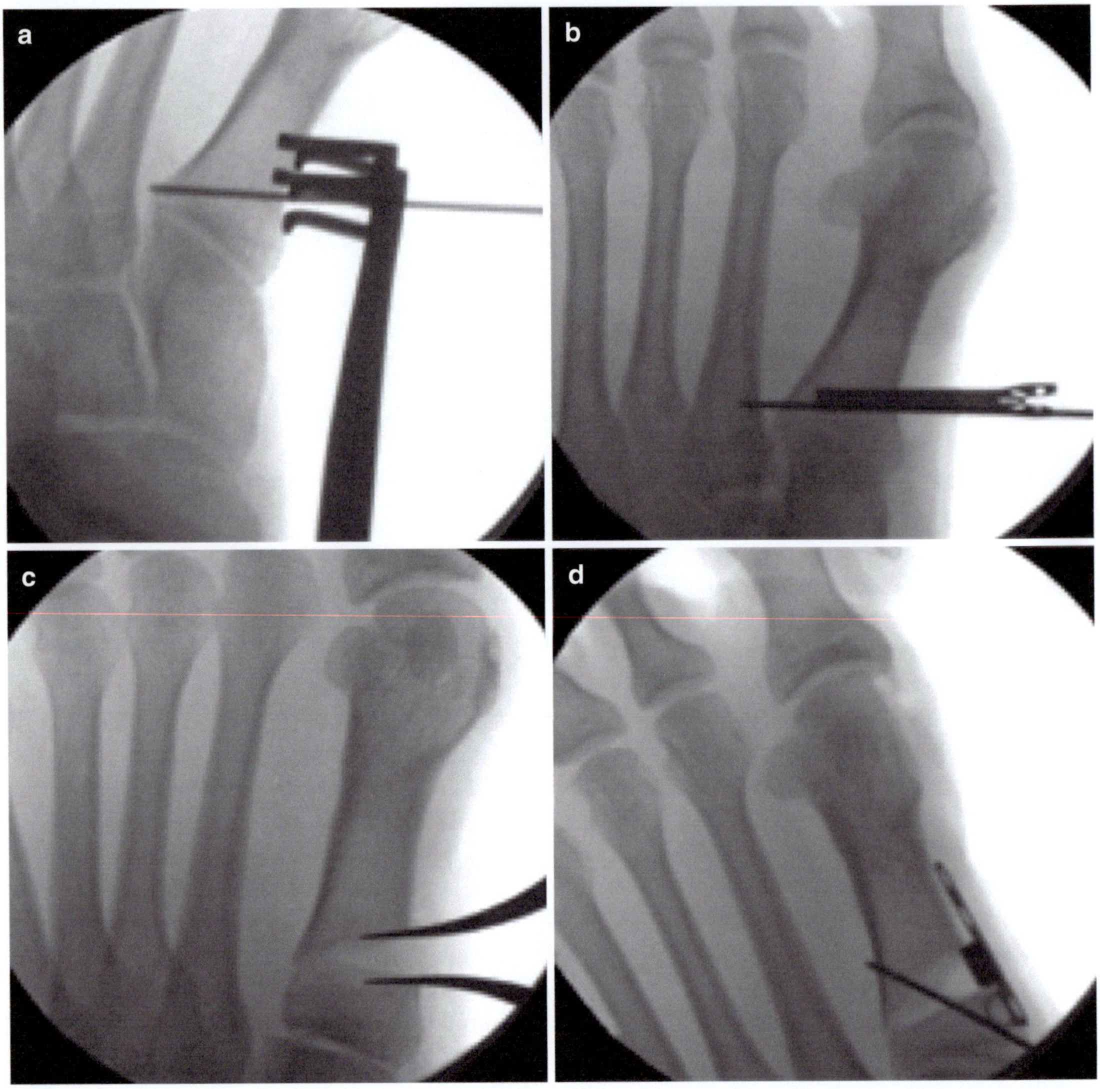

Fig. 2.13 A Kirschner wire (**a**) was introduced across the metatarsal as close to the metatarsocuneiform joint as possible to plan for the osteotomy. An oscillating saw (**b**) was used to create the osteotomy site without violating the lateral cortex to allow for a greenstick fracture. The osteotomy was distracted hinging off the lateral cortex which unfortunately becomes unstable and gaps (**c**). An oblique K-wire is placed with the distraction released to preserve the hinge, and then with the osteotomy re-distracted, the arthrex block plate was placed to produce an angular correction of the first metatarsal (**d**). The site is subsequently grafted

Postoperative Care

The foot is wrapped with a well-padded sterile dressing with an applied varus force to the hallux. The foot is placed in a postsurgical shoe and is instructed to remain primarily non-weight-bearing with the exception of heel weight-bearing for transfers. Sutures are removed at 10 days at the first follow-up visit. In most cases, heel and "outside of the foot" weight-bearing is permitted after the first visit in the rigid, postoperative shoe. Radiographs are repeated at 6 weeks postoperatively. If there is evidence of bony consolidation, the patient may bear full weight in the postoperative shoe. Transition to a regular shoe is initiated at 12 weeks with gradual return to activity as tolerated.

Avascular Necrosis

Introduction and Causes of Failure

Reports of avascular necrosis (AVN) of the first metatarsal head following hallux valgus corrective surgery vary, but in general, its incidence is relatively uncommon. AVN has been linked historically and anecdotally with distal metatarsal osteotomies performed in conjunction with lateral soft tissue releases, which have been espoused by some to unavoidably compromise the blood supply. However, it has been established both clinically and anatomically that concomitant distal metatarsal osteotomies and soft tissue releases may be safely performed [52–55].

Furthermore, it should be noted that even with blood flow disruption, clinical AVN is not inevitable [56–58]. It stands to reason, however, that minimizing soft tissue stripping is important for mitigating this complication, particularly when performing a lateral soft tissue release. More specifically, avoiding injury to the plantar lateral corner of the distal metatarsal when performing both a lateral release and metatarsal osteotomy cuts is most important to mitigating the occurrence of AVN [54]. It should be noted, however, that thermal necrosis from the saw blade can contribute to jeopardizing the blood supply. Also, stretching of the nutrient artery and disruption of the intraosseous supply can occur with performance of the osteotomy. Nevertheless, AVN is a rare occurrence, and symptomatic AVN is even more infrequent.

Evaluation

The most typical complaints of patients with AVN are nonspecific and vary with the timing and stage of the disease. There is often disparity between radiographic findings and patients' clinical picture in that many patients with AVN remain subclinical. In general, the radiographic stages of AVN are pre-collapse, collapse, and osteoarthritis [59]. Radiographic signs during the pre-collapse stage are often difficult to differentiate from normal postoperative radiographic findings following a distal osteotomy. That is, subchondral lucencies and cysts are characteristic during the pre-collapse stage, but most patients' radiographs will reveal such changes, especially in the first 2 months postoperative [58]. These changes likely represent an expected response to the vascular insult of the osteotomy. Additionally, mottling of the head may persist, but generally resolves by the first year. If these changes continue after the first year, they tend to correlate to decreased motion, but not necessarily progression to advanced AVN collapse nor clinical symptoms [58]. Thus, typical signs of bone remodeling are unidentifiable from early, pre-collapse AVN on radiographs and not predictive of more advanced collapse.

AVN may not be definitively identifiable until the early collapse phase, where loss of sphericity becomes apparent. Thus, MRI or bone scan may be considered for further investigation if there is suspicion for symptomatic AVN in the pre-collapse stage, but it should be noted that evidence of vascular insult on MRI and bone scan is not atypical in patients even without symptoms [57, 60]. Thus, serial radiographs are most useful for patient's presenting with continued MTP joint pain following a hallux valgus corrective surgery, with advanced collapse and osteoarthritis that are readily identified on radiographs. In patients with end-stage findings, consideration should be given to the possibility of infectious etiologies which can be assessed with serum erythrocyte sedimentation rate (ESR), complete blood count (CBC) with differential, and C-reactive protein (CRP) levels and ultimately aspiration or biopsy.

Symptomatic patients in the early stages of AVN will typically present with nonspecific complaints of pain and swelling. Often the pain is disproportionate to the radiographic findings. As the process progresses, patients will complain of arthrosis-related symptoms, and if shortening occurs, they may also complain of transfer metatarsalgia.

Surgical Planning

Surgical intervention is dictated by the patient's complaints more so than the radiographic findings, especially in the earliest stages. As stated, early, pre-collapse AVN does not correlate to progression, and thus, there is no imperative for early surgical intervention for the purposes of mitigating progression. For patients with persistent pain despite modified activity and shoewear, joint debridement may be considered. Experience with core decompression in other joints for this problem may be extrapolated to the first metatarsal in the pre-collapse and early collapse phases [61].

The more reliable option in our experience is either a first MTP resection arthroplasty or arthrodesis. A resection arthroplasty may be considered in patients who wish to maintain motion at the first MTP joint [62]. Here, a 2–3 mm wedge of subchondral bone and cartilage is resected from the proximal phalanx with care to preserve the plantar plate attachment. The first metatarsal head is debrided of nonviable bone. An autograft "anchovy" comprised of the dorsal MTP capsule and extensor hallucis brevis tendon is harvested. The tendon is transected approximately 3 cm proximal to the joint, and dissection is carried out distally incorporating the capsule. A pedicle of this tissue at the lateral MTP joint is left intact, and the tissue is draped over the metatarsal head and secured to the plantar plate with absorbable braided suture. Such a procedure has the added benefit of not relying on osseous healing in a region with already compromised healing capacity from previous vascular insult. However, it should only be performed when there is not significant shortening of the first metatarsal.

Additional options include arthrodesis [25, 63]. If shortening has not occurred, an in situ arthrodesis procedure with cancellous autograft from the iliac crest (preferably), distal tibia, or calcaneus may be considered. Other allograft bone can be used as supplement as well. Care should be taken to meticulously prepare the arthrodesis surfaces, typically with a 4 mm burr used with irrigation. Alternatively, commercially available conical cup and cone reamers are good options. The bone should be perforated with a small Kirschner wire or drill so as to incite bleeding and may help revitalize the bone. Next compression is applied with the surgeon's preference for fixation, which may include a screw construct if there is good bone fixation or plate/screw construct when there is a more tenuous bony purchase. Autograft or allograft material is packed in any small voids and around the fusion site.

In situations where extensive bone loss has occurred, the use of structural autograft or allograft should be considered to restore length [64]. Here, the surfaces are similarly debrided to a viable surface. Use of a saw is often advisable to provide for flat surfaces so as to facilitate apposition of the allograft. Bulk femoral head allograft can be cut to the appropriate length and contoured as needed. Alternatively, structural iliac crest autograft can be used [64, 65]. If the former is utilized, consideration should be given to infusing the graft with concentrated bone marrow aspirate to optimize the local biology at the fusion site [66]. The use of a Hintermann articulating distractor or smooth tipped lamina spreader is useful for applying distraction across the debrided joint while positioning of the graft. Fixation may be supplied with an all screw construct, plate and screw construct, or plate construct.

Ajis and colleagues also reported success using an osteochondral distal metatarsal allograft for salvage of advanced avascular necrosis with shortening [67]. We do not have experience with this technique, but it may be considered as an alternative, particularly in patients with significant shortening.

Cases

Case 2.6

History

- The patient is a healthy 31-year-old female with continued pain at the first metatarsal. She previously underwent a distal chevron osteotomy 1 year prior. She developed pain and stiffness postoperatively. Hardware was removed; however, her symptoms persisted.

- Physical examination reveals a medial surgical scar overlying the first metatarsal, no callus or tenderness under the lesser metatarsal heads, and the hallux relatively shortened.
- Radiographs at 6 months demonstrate expected mottling of the metatarsal head and slight recurrence (Fig. 2.14a). At 18 months, following hardware removal, there is complete collapse of the metatarsal head and shortening (Fig. 2.14b).

Reason for Failure

- Iatrogenic avascular necrosis. A potential contributing factor is excessive soft tissue stripping and an aggressive lateral release.

Surgical Plan

- In situ arthrodesis with iliac crest bone grafting and bone marrow aspirate concentrate injection. A distraction arthrodesis is considered; however, the patient does not have symptoms of transfer metatarsalgia and is not bothered by the shortening.

Approach

- The previous medial incision is used. The joint bone surfaces are meticulously derided and contoured with the use of a rongeur, curette, and 4 mm burr. The bone edges are drilled to ensure bleeding, signifying bone viability. Core bone plugs from the iliac crest are placed in-between the bone edges. Cross screw fixation is used, and bone marrow aspirate concentrate from the iliac crest is injected percutaneously following well-sealed closure. Radiographs at 6 months postoperative arthrodesis procedure reveal osseous union (Fig. 2.14c).

Implants

- Two partially threaded 4.0 cannulated partially threaded screws (Zimmer, Warsaw, IN)

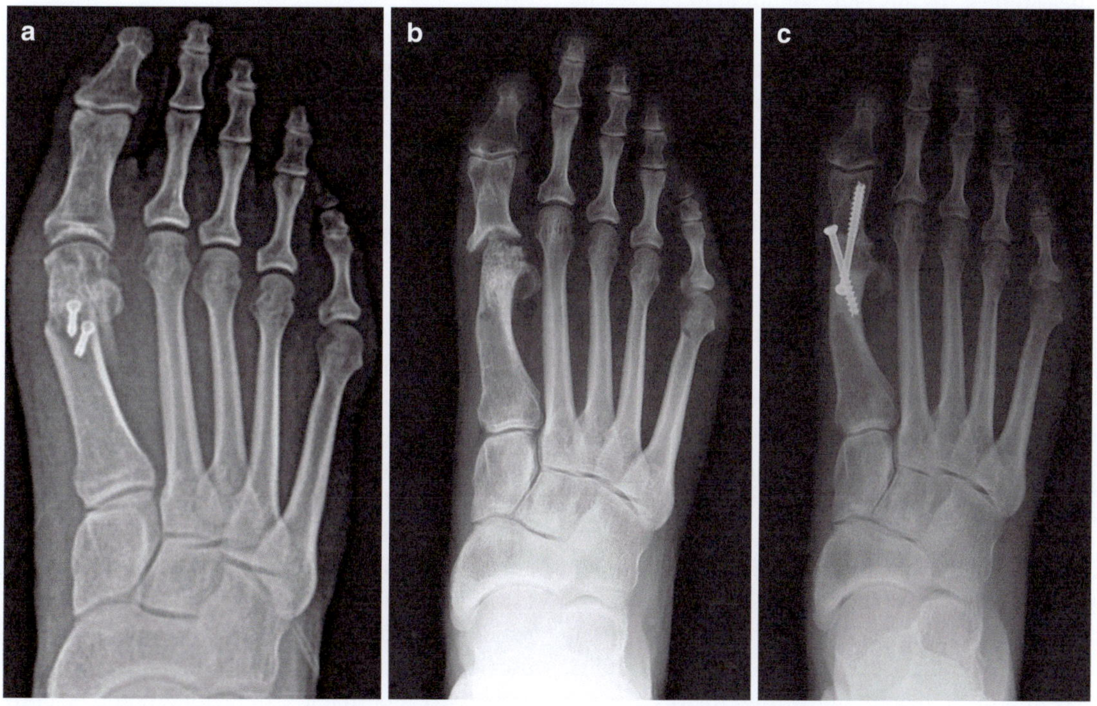

Fig. 2.14 Six-month post-surgical radiographs demonstrate typical mottling (**a**). There is shortening and advanced AVN 18 months after the initial surgery (**b**). This was effectively managed with a fusion of the MTP joint (**c**)

Pearls and Pitfalls

- Bone must be debrided to viable bleeding surfaces.
- Position of the fusion must be assessed to avoid malposition.
- Shortening may result in transfer metatarsalgia.
- Lengthening may result in nonunion.

Nonunion

Introduction and Causes of Failure

Inherent to any osteotomy is the risk of nonunion. Fortunately, this complication is infrequently encountered following hallux valgus corrective surgery. Nonunions of the first metatarsal should be considered in the context of the biomechanics of the first metatarsal. That is, the first metatarsal is a long bone that withstands significant loads perpendicular to its long axis. Thus, osteotomies are exposed to substantial bending and shear forces. To this end, nonunion rates vary by the type of osteotomy, but in general nonunions following proximal first metatarsal osteotomies are more frequent than those after distal metatarsal osteotomies. This is in part owed to the fact that there is less stress and shear imparted to the distal metatarsal with weight-bearing, as there is a nominal moment arm at the distal location compared to the proximal aspect of the first metatarsal [68]. That is, the greater the moment arm, the more proximal the osteotomy. The orientation of the osteotomy is also critical to its inherent stability. Those that are perpendicular to the first metatarsal axis are subject to greater deforming forces as they do not directly transfer forces from the distal fragment to the proximal one. Such osteotomies require rigid fixation, as they are unable to independently resist deforming forces [69]. As implant design and manufacturing have advanced and greater options for fixation have become available, osteotomy stability has improved, thereby mitigating the occurrence of nonunion even with use of inherently unstable osteotomy types. Another advantage of the distal osteotomies is the intrinsic stability of the dense cancellous bone surfaces versus the cortical diaphyseal surfaces more proximally which are more prone to invaginate when opposed. There is also the influence of osteotomy location on vascular supply. In general, distal metatarsal osteotomies, performed at the metaphysis, benefit from a robust blood supply to encourage routine healing, whereas the vasculature of bone diaphyses is generally more tenuous.

Nevertheless, nonunion is a risk of any hallux valgus corrective surgery utilizing an osteotomy. The etiology of nonunions varies, and determining the underlying cause and risk factors is imperative to effective management. Nonunions can often be successfully managed without surgery if identified early and there is no associated deformity. However, if shortening or angular displacement has occurred, surgical intervention is often indicated.

Evaluation

In general, nonunions are classified according to the underlying etiology. These include hypertrophic, atrophic, and infectious types. Hypertrophic nonunions typically result from insufficient fixation or early loss of fixation. This leads to excessive motion at the osteotomy and loss of compression. As a result there is abundant vascular infiltration and radiographically evident abundant callus formation. If this scenario is identified in the early postoperative period, and patient compliance is of concern, improved external immobilization with a cast may be considered.

Atrophic nonunions are attributable to "poor biology." Risk factors include diabetes, tobacco use, hypothyroidism, hypoparathyroidism, vitamin D deficiency, vascular insufficiency, and those with immunocompromised states. Consideration should be given to evaluating patients with atrophic nonunions for these conditions and even referral to an endocrinologist. All potentially modifiable risk factors should be optimized prior to surgical intervention. Nonunions may be precipitated by the presence of an infection. A careful history regarding postoperative complications, including the use of antibiotics or delayed wound healing, should be performed. If there is suspicion of an infectious etiology, aspiration or biopsy and obtaining a serum erythrocyte sedimentation rate (ESR), complete blood count (CBC) with differential, and C-reactive protein (CRP) levels should be considered prior to proceeding with definitive management.

Nonunions of distal metatarsal osteotomies, particularly distal chevron osteotomies, are exceedingly rare as most are intrinsically stable, in an area of robust blood supply, and subject to less deforming forces by virtue of their location. If a nonunion following a distal metatarsal osteotomy is encountered, it is typically associated with proximal translation of the apex of the osteotomy [70]. In the setting of a distal metatarsal nonunion, there is often associated dorsal displacement and valgus angulation. Such malpositioned nonunions or even delayed unions require surgical revision. Careful attention to an associated malpositioning is required for surgical planning purposes. Broken hardware is a signal of nonunion.

Proximal metatarsal nonunions are more frequently encountered than those at the distal aspect. A nonunion at a previous proximal crescentic osteotomy is often associated with dorsal translation and angulation, as well as varus orientation [27, 71]. Oblique osteotomies, such as the Mau and Ludloff types, are more intrinsically stable than the proximal crescentic type but are not immune to malunions and nonunions [69]. However, given their broad surface area and potential for excellent compression with internal fixation, nonunion is quite rare. Similarly, the SCARF osteotomy is generally considered very reliable, but has a delayed union rate reported up to 5% in some reports [72, 73].

Surgical Planning

The general tenants of nonunion management are the same for nonunions following osteotomies for correction of hallux valgus. These include debridement of nonviable bone and interposed material, grafting, revision of any associated deformity, and rigid fixation. All bone edges should be meticulously debrided and viability determined through induction of bleeding at the bone edges. Drilling or penetrating the bone edges is advisable for this purpose. Next, a means of fixation should be determined. In general, it is advisable to have several options of plate fixation available. In the case of a distal chevron osteotomy nonunion, consideration may be given to use of an intraosseous sliding plate to maximize mechanical stability. Locking screw constructs are advisable in patients with compromised bone quality, of which many patients may have secondary to disuse osteopenia. Definitive fixation should not be attempted until any associated malpositioning is corrected.

Bone grafting options are vast. It is the senior's author preference to use autograft as well as supplement areas with concentrated bone marrow aspirate concentrate [66]. Viable sources of bone graft include the iliac crest, proximal tibia, distal tibia, and calcaneus, which can be harvested with little associated morbidity [74–77]. A multitude of options for allograft bone, as well as cellular and acellular bone stimulating graft material (rhPDGF, rhBMP), are also available and have demonstrated efficacy for foot and ankle applications [78–81]. Review of the various graft options is beyond the scope of this manuscript and should be familiar to the surgeon. Regardless of the surgeon's choice for grafting material, sufficient volume is required to pack the area to optimize union rates [82].

Following surgery, consideration may be given to the use of bone stimulators. Types of external stimulation include inductive coupling, combined magnetic field, capacitive coupling, and ultrasound. There is a paucity of literature for their use in the setting of hallux values nonunion revision, but success has been reported with their use for other conditions of the foot and ankle [83].

Cases

Case 2.7

History

- The patient is a healthy 48-year-old female with pain and deformity at the first MTP joint following a distal chevron osteotomy 1 year prior.
- Radiographs after the initial surgery are unremarkable (Fig. 2.15a). At 6 months postoperative (Fig. 2.15b), there is lack of healing medial, and at 12 months, there is obvious deformity and nonunion (Fig. 2.15c).
- Physical examination reveals a dorsomedial surgical scar overlying the first metatarsal, no callus or tenderness under the lesser metatarsal heads, and the hallux relatively shortened (Fig. 2.16). The first MTP joint is supple with 60 degrees active and passive dorsiflexion without increased pain and tenderness.
- Serum laboratory infection markers are unremarkable.

Reason for Failure

- Idiopathic distal chevron atrophic nonunion

Surgical Plan

- Nonunion revision with iliac crest bone grafting and bone marrow aspirate concentrate injection with plate fixation

Approach

- The previous dorsomedial incision is used. The nonunion bone surfaces are debrided and contoured with the use of a rongeur and curette. The bone edges are drilled to ensure bleeding, signifying bone viability. Core bone plugs from the calcaneus are placed in the osteotomy site. Radiographs at 12 months revealed osseous union, and the patient was asymptomatic for 13 years. Fourteen years later (Fig. 2.17a), the patient progressively developed pain under her second metatarsal, and the hardware was bothersome. She elected to undergo plate removal and a second metatarsal shortening osteotomy for complaints of transfer metatarsalgia (Fig. 2.17b).

Implants

- T-type locking plate (Synthes, Paoli, PA)

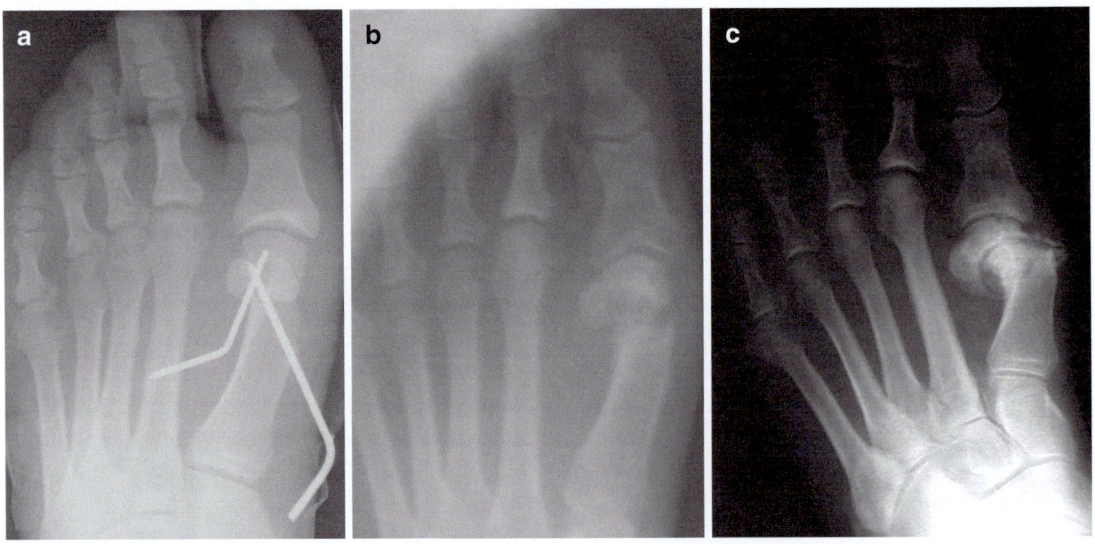

Fig. 2.15 Anteroposterior radiographs immediately following a distal chevron osteotomy with percutaneous fixation (**a**), at 6 months postoperative demonstrating mild shortening and lack of healing, particularly medial (**b**), and 1 year postoperatively, demonstrating moderate shortening with medial translation and angulation (**c**)

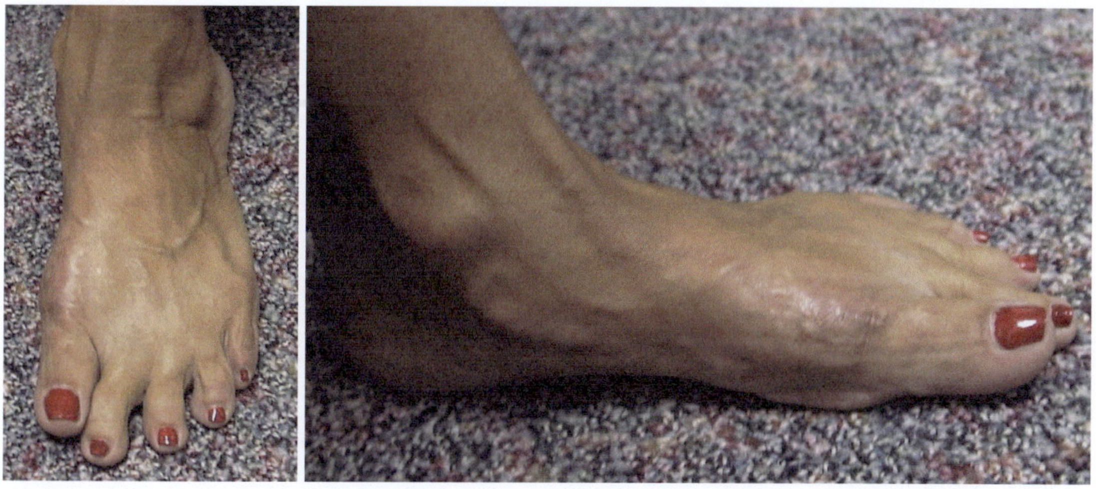

Fig. 2.16 Clinical photographs demonstrating shortening of the first metatarsal and significant swelling at the first MTP joint

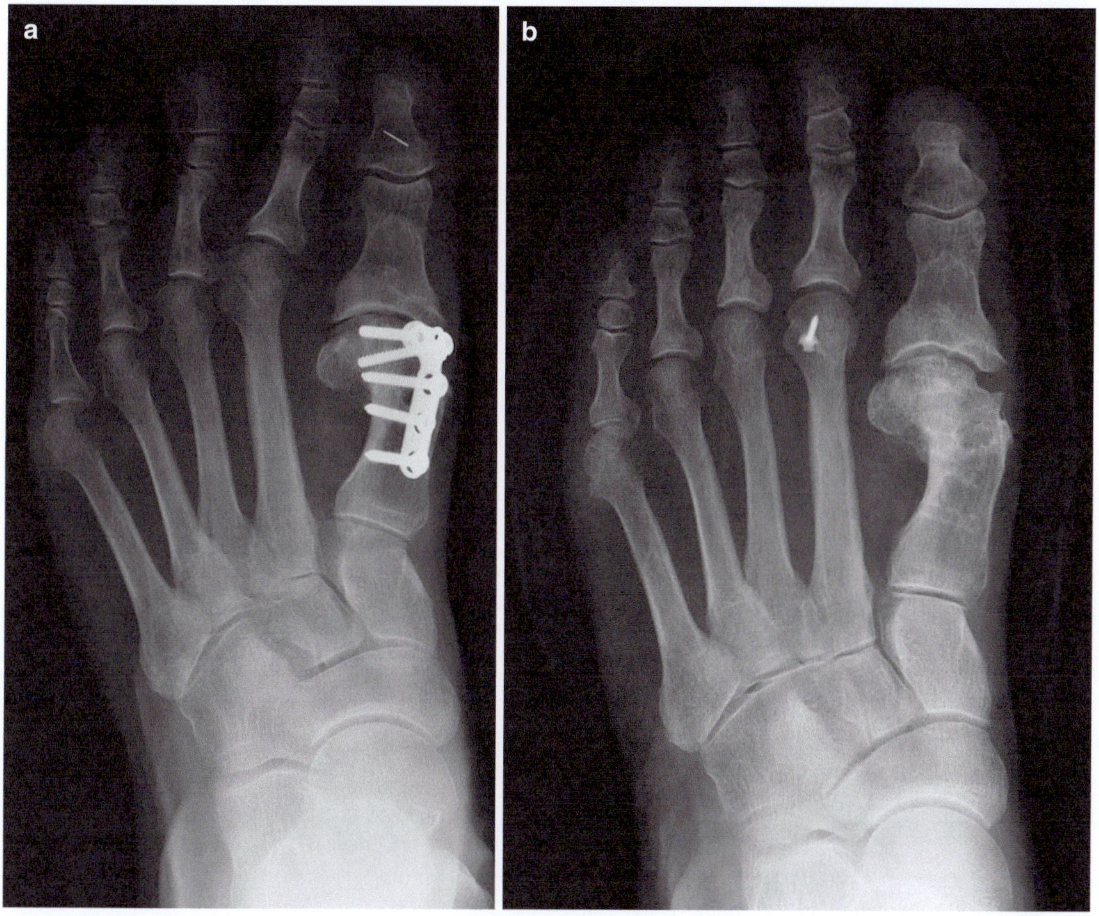

Fig. 2.17 Anteroposterior postoperative radiographs at 14 years (**a**) and 15.5 months after second metatarsal osteotomy and plate removal (**b**)

Pearls and Pitfalls

- Bone must be debrided to viable bleeding surfaces.
- The plate may be applied to the distal fragment and then reduced to the proximal fragment.
- A multitude of small Kirschner wires should be available to assist in achieving provisional fixation.

References

1. Scioli MW. Complications of hallux valgus surgery and subsequent treatment options. Foot Ankle Clin. 1997;2:719–39.
2. Coughlin MJ, Saltzman CL, Nunley JA. Angular measurements in the evaluation of hallux valgus deformities: a report of the ad hoc committee of the American Orthopaedic Foot & Ankle Society on angular measurements. Foot Ankle Int. 2002;23(1):68–74.
3. Lagaay PM, Hamilton GA, Ford LA, Williams ME, Rush SM, Schuberth JM. Rates of revision surgery using Chevron-Austin osteotomy, Lapidus arthrodesis, and closing base wedge osteotomy for correction of hallux valgus deformity. J Foot Ankle Surg. 2008;47(4):267–72.
4. Coughlin MJ. Hallux valgus. J Bone Joint Surg Am. 1996;78(6):932–66.
5. Aiyer A, Shub J, Shariff R, Ying L, Myerson M. Radiographic recurrence of deformity after hallux valgus surgery in patients with metatarsus Adductus. Foot Ankle Int. 2016;37(2):165–71.
6. Richardson EG, Graves SC, McClure JT, Boone RT. First metatarsal head-shaft angle: a method of determination. Foot Ankle. 1993;14(4):181–5.
7. Corte-Real NM, Moreira RM. Modified biplanar chevron osteotomy. Foot Ankle Int. 2009;30(12):1149–53.
8. Donley BG. Acquired hallux varus. Foot Ankle Int. 1997;18(9):586–92.
9. Trnka HJ, Zettl R, Hungerford M, Mühlbauer M, Ritschl P. Acquired hallux varus and clinical tolerability. Foot Ankle Int. 1997;18(9):593–7.
10. Lee KT, Park YU, Young KW, Kim JS, Kim KC, Kim JB. Reverse distal chevron osteotomy to treat iatrogenic hallux varus after overcorrection of the intermetatarsal 1-2 angle: technique tip. Foot Ankle Int. 2011;32(1):89–91.
11. Johnson KA, Cofield RH, Morrey BF. Chevron osteotomy for hallux valgus. Clin Orthop Relat Res. 1979;142:44–7.
12. Hawkins FB. Acquired hallux varus: cause, prevention and correction. Clin Orthop Relat Res. 1971;76:169–76.
13. Skalley TC, Myerson MS. The operative treatment of acquired hallux varus. Clin Orthop Relat Res. 1994;306:183–91.
14. Johnson KA, Spiegl PV. Extensor hallucis longus transfer for hallux varus deformity. J Bone Joint Surg Am. 1984;66(5):681–6.
15. Fuhrmann RA. Split transfer of the extensor hallucis longus tendon in flexible hallux varus deformity. Oper Orthop Traumatol. 2008;20(3):274–82.
16. Coughlin M, Anderson R. Hallux valgus. In: Coughlin M, Saltzman C, Anderson R, editors. Mann's surgery of the foot and ankle. 9: Elsevier; 2013. p. 300–6.
17. Lau JT, Myerson MS. Modified split extensor hallucis longus tendon transfer for correction of hallux varus. Foot Ankle Int. 2002;23(12):1138–40.
18. Leemrijse T, Hoang B, Maldague P, Docquier PL, Devos BB. A new surgical procedure for iatrogenic hallux varus: reverse transfer of the abductor hallucis tendon: a report of 7 cases. Acta Orthop Belg. 2008;74(2):227–34.
19. Myerson MS, Komenda GA. Results of hallux varus correction using an extensor hallucis brevis tenodesis. Foot Ankle Int. 1996;17(1):21–7.
20. Choi KJ, Lee HS, Yoon YS, Park SS, Kim JS, Jeong JJ, et al. Distal metatarsal osteotomy for hallux varus following surgery for hallux valgus. J Bone Joint Surg Br. 2011;93(8):1079–83.
21. Kannegieter E, Kilmartin TE. The combined reverse scarf and opening wedge osteotomy of the proximal phalanx for the treatment of iatrogenic hallux varus. Foot (Edinb). 2011;21(2):88–91.
22. Gerbert J, Traynor C, Blue K, Kim K. Use of the Mini TightRope® for correction of hallux varus deformity. J Foot Ankle Surg. 2011;50(2):245–51.
23. Hsu AR, Gross CE, Lin JL. Bilateral hallux varus deformity correction with a suture button construct. Am J Orthop (Belle Mead NJ). 2013;42(3):121–4.
24. Rochwerger A, Curvale G, Groulier P. Application of bone graft to the medial side of the first metatarsal head in the treatment of hallux varus. J Bone Joint Surg Am. 1999;81(12):1730–5.
25. Grimes JS, Coughlin MJ. First metatarsophalangeal joint arthrodesis as a treatment for failed hallux valgus surgery. Foot Ankle Int. 2006;27(11):887–93.
26. Geaney LE, Myerson MS. Radiographic results after hallux metatarsophalangeal joint arthrodesis for hallux varus. Foot Ankle Int. 2015;36(4):391–4.
27. Mann RA, Rudicel S, Graves SC. Repair of hallux valgus with a distal soft-tissue procedure and proximal metatarsal osteotomy. A long-term follow-up. J Bone Joint Surg Am. 1992;74(1):124–9.
28. Sammarco GJ, Conti SF. Proximal Chevron metatarsal osteotomy: single incision technique. Foot Ankle. 1993;14(1):44–7.
29. Easley ME, Trnka HJ. Current concepts review: hallux valgus part II: operative treatment. Foot Ankle Int. 2007;28(6):748–58.
30. Mitchell LA, Baxter DE. A Chevron-Akin double osteotomy for correction of hallux valgus. Foot Ankle. 1991;12(1):7–14.

31. Myerson M. Metatarsocuneiform arthrodesis for treatment of hallux valgus and metatarsus primus varus. Orthopedics. 1990;13(9):1025–31.
32. Becker A. First metatarsal malunion. Foot Ankle Clin. 2009;14(1):77–90.
33. Harper MC. Dorsal closing wedge metatarsal osteotomy: a trigonometric analysis. Foot Ankle. 1990;10(6):303–5.
34. Goldberg A, Singh D. Treatment of shortening following hallux valgus surgery. Foot Ankle Clin. 2014;19(2):309–16.
35. Shahid MS, Lee P, Evans S, Thomas R. A comparative study of bone shortening and bone loss with use of saw blades versus burr in hallux valgus surgery. Foot Ankle Surg. 2012;18(3):195–7.
36. Markbreiter LA, Thompson FM. Proximal metatarsal osteotomy in hallux valgus correction: a comparison of crescentic and chevron procedures. Foot Ankle Int. 1997;18(2):71–6.
37. Glazebrook M, Copithorne P, Boyd G, Daniels T, Lalonde KA, Francis P, et al. Proximal opening wedge osteotomy with wedge-plate fixation compared with proximal chevron osteotomy for the treatment of hallux valgus: a prospective, randomized study. J Bone Joint Surg Am. 2014;96(19):1585–92.
38. Holden D, Siff S, Butler J, Cain T. Shortening of the first metatarsal as a complication of metatarsal osteotomies. J Bone Joint Surg Am. 1984;66(4):582–7.
39. Laughlin TJ. Complications of distal first metatarsal osteotomies. J Foot Ankle Surg. 1995;34(6):524–31. discussion 93-4
40. Mann RA, Donatto KC. The chevron osteotomy: a clinical and radiographic analysis. Foot Ankle Int. 1997;18(5):255–61.
41. Kinnard P, Gordon D. A comparison between Chevron and Mitchell osteotomies for hallux valgus. Foot Ankle. 1984;4(5):241–3.
42. Jung HG, Zaret DI, Parks BG, Schon LC. Effect of first metatarsal shortening and dorsiflexion osteotomies on forefoot plantar pressure in a cadaver model. Foot Ankle Int. 2005;26(9):748–53.
43. Hardy RH, Clapham JC. Observations on hallux valgus; based on a controlled series. J Bone Joint Surg Br. 1951;33-B(3):376–91.
44. Kim JS, Baek GH, Chung MS, Yoon PW. Multiple congenital brachymetatarsia. A one-stage combined shortening and lengthening procedure without iliac bone graft. J Bone Joint Surg Br. 2004;86(7):1013–5.
45. Marcinko DE, Rappaport MJ, Gordon S. Post-traumatic brachymetatarsia. J Foot Surg. 1984;23(6):451–3.
46. Kawashima T, Yamada A, Ueda K, Harii K. Treatment of brachymetatarsia by callus distraction (callotasis). Ann Plast Surg. 1994;32(2):191–9.
47. Masuda T, Matoh N, Nakajima T, Tomi M, Ohba K. Treatment of brachymetatarsia using a semicircular lengthener. 1-3 years results in 6 patients. Acta Orthop Scand. 1995;66(1):43–6.
48. Robinson JF, Ouzounian TJ. Brachymetatarsia: congenitally short third and fourth metatarsals treated by distraction lengthening--a case report and literature summary. Foot Ankle Int. 1998;19(10):713–8.
49. Wada A, Bensahel H, Takamura K, Fujii T, Yanagida H, Nakamura T. Metatarsal lengthening by callus distraction for brachymetatarsia. J Pediatr Orthop B. 2004;13(3):206–10.
50. Choi IH, Chung MS, Baek GH, Cho TJ, Chung CY. Metatarsal lengthening in congenital brachymetatarsia: one-stage lengthening versus lengthening by callotasis. J Pediatr Orthop. 1999;19(5):660–4.
51. Kim HT, Lee SH, Yoo CI, Kang JH, Suh JT. The management of brachymetatarsia. J Bone Joint Surg Br. 2003;85(5):683–90.
52. Jones KJ, Feiwell LA, Freedman EL, Cracchiolo A. The effect of chevron osteotomy with lateral capsular release on the blood supply to the first metatarsal head. J Bone Joint Surg Am. 1995;77(2):197–204.
53. Kuhn MA, Lippert FG, Phipps MJ, Williams C. Blood flow to the metatarsal head after chevron bunionectomy. Foot Ankle Int. 2005;26(7):526–9.
54. Malal JJ, Shaw-Dunn J, Kumar CS. Blood supply to the first metatarsal head and vessels at risk with a chevron osteotomy. J Bone Joint Surg Am. 2007;89(9):2018–22.
55. Peterson DA, Zilberfarb JL, Greene MA, Colgrove RC. Avascular necrosis of the first metatarsal head: incidence in distal osteotomy combined with lateral soft tissue release. Foot Ankle Int. 1994;15(2):59–63.
56. Mann RA. Complications associated with the Chevron osteotomy. Foot Ankle. 1982;3(3):125–9.
57. Resch S, Stenström A, Gustafson T. Circulatory disturbance of the first metatarsal head after Chevron osteotomy as shown by bone scintigraphy. Foot Ankle. 1992;13(3):137–42.
58. Thomas RL, Espinosa FJ, Richardson EG. Radiographic changes in the first metatarsal head after distal chevron osteotomy combined with lateral release through a plantar approach. Foot Ankle Int. 1994;15(6):285–92.
59. Meier PJ, Kenzora JE. The risks and benefits of distal first metatarsal osteotomies. Foot Ankle. 1985;6(1):7–17.
60. Wilkinson SV, Jones RO, Sisk LE, Sunshein KF, Van Manen JW. Austin bunionectomy: postoperative MRI evaluation for avascular necrosis. J Foot Surg. 1992;31(5):469–77.
61. Fu FH, Gomez W. Bilateral avascular necrosis of the first metatarsal head in adolescence. A case report. Clin Orthop Relat Res. 1989;246:282–4.
62. Aynardi MC, Atwater L, Dein EJ, Zahoor T, Schon LC, Miller SD. Outcomes after interpositional arthroplasty of the first metatarsophalangeal joint. Foot Ankle Int. 2017;38(5):514–8.
63. Trnka HJ. Arthrodesis procedures for salvage of the hallux metatarsophalangeal joint. Foot Ankle Clin. 2000;5(3):673–86. ix
64. Myerson MS, Schon LC, McGuigan FX, Oznur A. Result of arthrodesis of the hallux metatarsophalangeal joint using bone graft for restoration of length. Foot Ankle Int. 2000;21(4):297–306.

65. Brodsky JW, Ptaszek AJ, Morris SG. Salvage first MTP arthrodesis utilizing ICBG: clinical evaluation and outcome. Foot Ankle Int. 2000;21(4):290–6.
66. Hernigou P, Poignard A, Beaujean F, Rouard H. Percutaneous autologous bone-marrow grafting for nonunions. Influence of the number and concentration of progenitor cells. J Bone Joint Surg Am. 2005;87(7):1430–7.
67. Ajis A, Seybold JD, Myerson MS. Osteochondral distal metatarsal allograft reconstruction: a case series and surgical technique. Foot Ankle Int. 2013;34(8):1158–67.
68. Stokes IA, Hutton WC, Stott JR. Forces acting on the metatarsals during normal walking. J Anat. 1979;129(Pt 3):579–90.
69. Acevedo JI, Sammarco VJ, Boucher HR, Parks BG, Schon LC, Myerson MS. Mechanical comparison of cyclic loading in five different first metatarsal shaft osteotomies. Foot Ankle Int. 2002;23(8):711–6.
70. Vora AM, Myerson MS. First metatarsal osteotomy nonunion and malunion. Foot Ankle Clin. 2005;10(1):35–54.
71. Veri JP, Pirani SP, Claridge R. Crescentic proximal metatarsal osteotomy for moderate to severe hallux valgus: a mean 12.2 year follow-up study. Foot Ankle Int. 2001;22(10):817–22.
72. Bock P, Kluger R, Kristen KH, Mittlböck M, Schuh R, Trnka HJ. The scarf osteotomy with minimally invasive lateral release for treatment of hallux Valgus deformity: intermediate and long-term results. J Bone Joint Surg Am. 2015;97(15):1238–45.
73. Coetzee JC. Scarf osteotomy for hallux valgus repair: the dark side. Foot Ankle Int. 2003;24(1):29–33.
74. Raikin SM, Brislin K. Local bone graft harvested from the distal tibia or calcaneus for surgery of the foot and ankle. Foot Ankle Int. 2005;26(6):449–53.
75. O'Malley MJ, Sayres SC, Saleem O, Levine D, Roberts M, Deland JT, et al. Morbidity and complications following percutaneous calcaneal autograft bone harvest. Foot Ankle Int. 2014;35(1):30–7.
76. Geideman W, Early JS, Brodsky J. Clinical results of harvesting autogenous cancellous graft from the ipsilateral proximal tibia for use in foot and ankle surgery. Foot Ankle Int. 2004;25(7):451–5.
77. Biddinger KR, Komenda GA, Schon LC, Myerson MS. A new modified technique for harvest of calcaneal bone grafts in surgery on the foot and ankle. Foot Ankle Int. 1998;19(5):322–6.
78. Daniels TR, Younger AS, Penner MJ, Wing KJ, Le IL, Russell IS, et al. Prospective randomized controlled trial of hindfoot and ankle fusions treated with rhPDGF-BB in combination with a β-TCP-collagen matrix. Foot Ankle Int. 2015;36(7):739–48.
79. Dekker TJ, White P, Adams SB. Efficacy of a cellular bone allograft for foot and ankle arthrodesis and revision nonunion procedures. Foot Ankle Int. 2017;38(3):277–82.
80. DiGiovanni CW, Lin SS, Baumhauer JF, Daniels T, Younger A, Glazebrook M, et al. Recombinant human platelet-derived growth factor-BB and beta-tricalcium phosphate (rhPDGF-BB/β-TCP): an alternative to autogenous bone graft. J Bone Joint Surg Am. 2013;95(13):1184–92.
81. Jones CP, Loveland J, Atkinson BL, Ryaby JT, Linovitz RJ, Nunley JA. Prospective, multicenter evaluation of allogeneic bone matrix containing viable osteogenic cells in foot and/or ankle arthrodesis. Foot Ankle Int. 2015;36(10):1129–37.
82. DiGiovanni CW, Lin SS, Daniels TR, Glazebrook M, Evangelista P, Donahue R, et al. The importance of sufficient graft material in achieving foot or ankle fusion. J Bone Joint Surg Am. 2016;98(15):1260–7.
83. Streit A, Watson BC, Granata JD, Philbin TM, Lin HN, O'Connor JP, et al. Effect on clinical outcome and growth factor synthesis with adjunctive use of pulsed electromagnetic fields for fifth metatarsal nonunion fracture: a double-blind randomized study. Foot Ankle Int. 2016;37(9):919–23.

Revision Intermetatarsal Neurectomy

3

David R. Richardson and Brandon A. Taylor

Key Takeaway Points

- Failure of the initial excision may result from incorrect diagnosis, inadequate excision, or formation of a stump neuroma.
- Symptoms usually recur within the first 12 months.
- History and physical examination are the mainstays of diagnosis.
- Conservative treatment usually is warranted, but it has a high failure rate. Corticosteroid injection may be beneficial but should be limited.
- Results of revision intermetatarsal neurectomy are satisfactory but less gratifying than those of primary excision.

D. R. Richardson (✉)
University of Tennessee-Campbell Clinic, Department of Orthopaedic Surgery & Biomedical Engineering, Memphis, TN, USA
e-mail: drrichardson@campbellclinic.com

B. A. Taylor
Orthopaedic Specialists of Palm Harbor, Palm Harbor, FL, USA

The Problem: Recurrent Intermetatarsal Neuroma

Causes for Failure

Presumed recurrence may be due to a previous wrong diagnosis, inadequate resection, or inadequate preparation and placement of the nerve trunk following resection [1–4].

Differential Diagnosis Includes

- Distal resection of a previous neuroma
- Failure to excise the correct structure (e.g., lumbrical)
- Adjacent web space neuroma
- Metatarsophalangeal joint synovitis
- Freiberg osteochondrosis
- Stress fracture of the metatarsal neck
- Tarsal tunnel syndrome
- Peripheral neuropathy
- Lumbar radiculopathy
- Unrelated soft-tissue tumor (e.g., ganglion, synovial cyst, lipoma)
- Histologic changes in a primary interdigital neuroma occur distal to the transverse intermetatarsal ligament and represent an entrapment neuropathy resulting in perineural fibrosis [5, 6].
- Recurrence following interdigital neuroma resection represents a true histopathologic

M. J. Berkowitz et al. (eds.), *Revision Surgery of the Foot and Ankle*,
https://doi.org/10.1007/978-3-030-29969-9_3

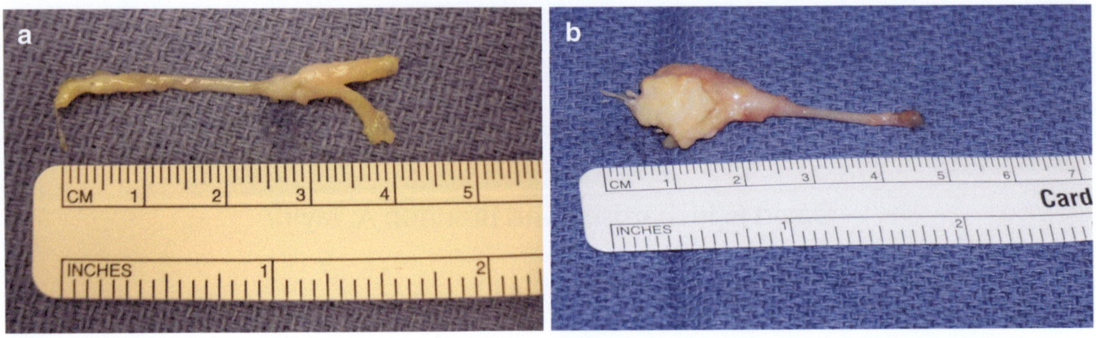

Fig. 3.1 Recurrence following previous resection of an interdigital neuroma represents a true histopathologic stump neuroma (haphazard proliferation of axions). (**a**) Primary interdigital neuroma. (**b**) Recurrent (stump) neuroma

stump neuroma (haphazard proliferation of axions) [6] (Fig. 3.1).

- Stump (true) neuromas tend to form at the transected end of nerves, and proliferation is directed toward the skin or distal portion of the transected nerve [7, 8].

Clinical Evaluation of Pathology (History)

- Two-thirds of patients present with symptoms of "recurrent" neuroma within 12 months of their index surgery [2].
  - This probably represents an original misdiagnosis or resection of the wrong structure or original inadequate resection [9, 10].
- An incisional neuroma of a branch of the superficial peroneal nerve may occur and will result in primarily dorsal pain.
- It is important to obtain a thorough, detailed history and physical examination in patients suspected of having a recurrent interdigital neuroma [4, 5, 11–15].
- Patients with a stump neuroma often complain of plantar pain (burning, aching, electrical) radiating proximally (unlike an original Morton neuroma in which the pain radiates distally).
- Patients often describe a sensation of "walking on a rock," with pain relieved by removing tight shoes and walking on soft surfaces [2].
  - However, unlike an original Morton neuroma in which the symptoms can be quite vague, a true stump neuroma usually results in very localized, reproducible pain.
- If the patient denies digital numbness, even in the immediate postoperative period following the index procedure, a true stump neuroma is doubtful.
- If this history is given, it is necessary to rule out other causes in the differential, including an inadequate original resection.

Clinical Evaluation of Pathology (Physical)

- Plantar tenderness in the web space is the most common physical examination finding [5, 6, 12, 13, 15].
  - This tenderness usually is more localized, reproducible, and intense than with an original Morton neuroma.
- Pain is aggravated by ambulation and shoe wear and relieved with rest [2, 3, 13, 14, 16].
- Patients likely have a positive "Tinel sign," although the pain often radiates proximally.
- Plantar flexion of the corresponding metatarsophalangeal (MTP) joint can help differentiate joint synovitis from a neuroma.
  - This maneuver causes increased pain with a synovitic joint, but pain is uncommon in patients with a neuroma.
- The Mulder test often is useful [5, 6, 11–15].
  - This test is best performed with the patient positioned prone with the knees flexed 90°.

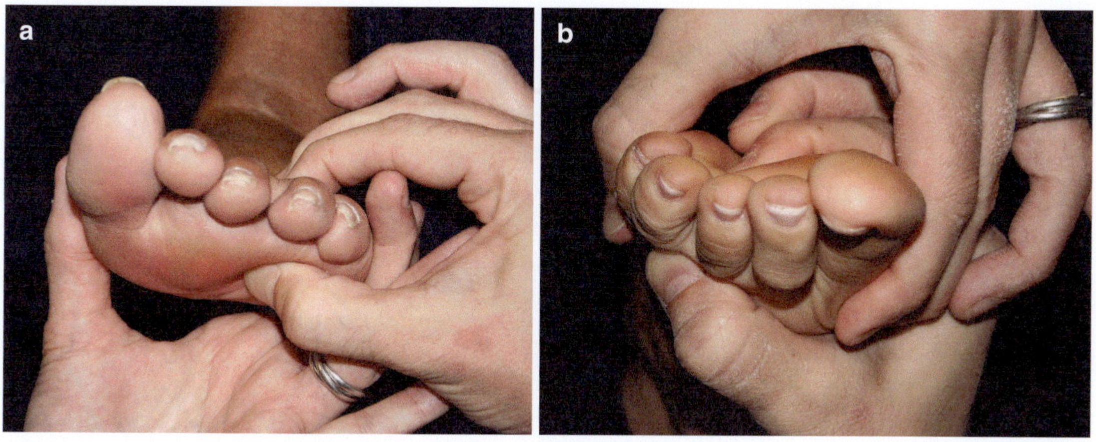

Fig. 3.2 The Mulder test (**a**) is useful, but the "click" is less pronounced in patients with previous neuroma excision. Performing the test with the patient prone may be beneficial (**b**)

  - Pain often is more pronounced and the "click" less pronounced in patients with recurrent neuromas compared to those with primary Morton neuromas (Fig. 3.2).
- Metatarsal fat pad atrophy may occur after primary neuroma excision (perhaps due to poor technique) but also may result from aging, trauma, medications, or other conditions.
- Fat pad atrophy increases the risk of continued pain after surgery and must be discussed with the patient.

Radiologic Studies

- The diagnosis of recurrent intermetatarsal neuroma is primarily a clinical exercise, relying on history and physical examination [2, 5, 11, 13–15].
- Standing anteroposterior (AP), lateral, and oblique radiographs are necessary to assess the MTP joint and osseous structures.
- Electromyographic nerve conduction studies rarely are useful in diagnosing a recurrent intermetatarsal neuroma, but they may be beneficial in patients with suspected concomitant tarsal tunnel syndrome or lumbar radiculopathy [3, 10].
- If the clinical examination is ambiguous, an MRI or ultrasound (US) may help with conditions such as a stress fracture or a space-occupying lesion causing neuritic pain. Ultrasound appears more helpful than MRI in the diagnosis of a recurrent neuroma.
  - However, both of these imaging modalities have a high false-negative rate (approximately 20%), especially for small neuromas [17, 18].

Nonoperative Options

- Nonoperative treatment results in varying degrees of relief, but only 20%–30% of patients get complete, lasting resolution of symptoms [13].
- Approximately 40% of those treated conservatively experience enough symptomatic relief to avoid surgery; therefore, nonoperative treatment is recommended before surgical intervention.
- Wide, soft inner-soled, stiff, laced shoes with a low heel are recommended [13–15].
- An accommodative orthotic with a metatarsal support can be placed proximal to the point of maximal tenderness [12–14, 19] (Fig. 3.3).
- A corticosteroid injection may provide symptomatic relief for up to 2 years in approximately 30% of patients [2, 4, 12, 20] (Fig. 3.4).
  - This injection can be both diagnostic and therapeutic; however, caution is required to ensure that the medication is placed around

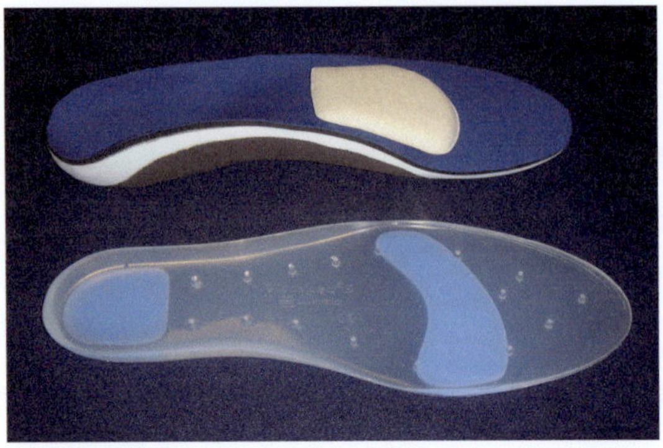

Fig. 3.3 Conservative treatment should include accommodative orthotics and a metatarsal pad placed proximal to the point of maximal tenderness

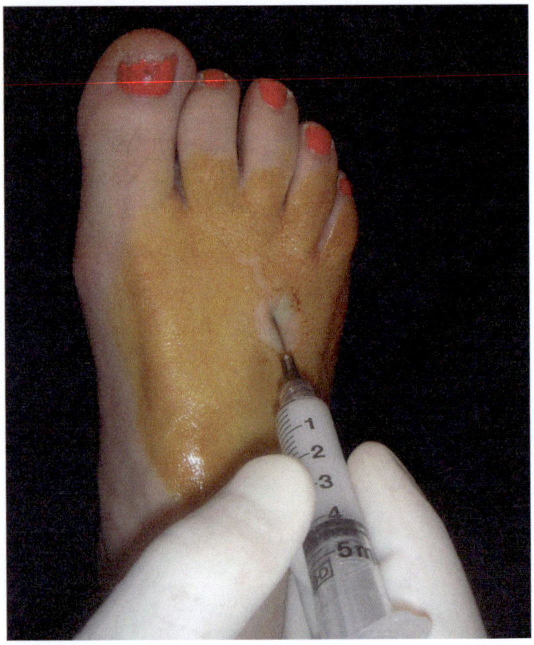

Fig. 3.4 A corticosteroid injection can provide temporary, or even long-lasting, relief

the neuroma (not intraneural) and the MTP joint is avoided.
  - Ultrasound guidance may help direct the injection and document appropriate placement.
  - Injections should be attempted with caution because fat pad atrophy, skin discoloration, or MTP joint instability may occur.
  - No more than two injections should be attempted

- We use a mixture of 40 mg Depo-Medrol:1 cc 0.25% Marcaine and a dorsal approach for the injection.

Operative Options

Surgical Planning

Contraindications and Precautions

- Pain control after surgical intervention is less predictable in patients being treated for chronic pain, diagnosed with a mood disorder, taking preoperative narcotics, or using tobacco products. Obesity has not been associated with worse outcomes [21–23].
- A lengthening procedure should be considered in those with a tight gastroc-soleus complex (Silfverskiöld test).
- Absolute and relative surgical contraindications are the same as for any forefoot surgery, e.g., peripheral vascular disease, poorly controlled diabetes mellitus (A1C >8), and local infection [23].

Goals of Procedure

- The goal of revision intermetatarsal neurectomy is relief of pain and dysfunction. It must be made clear to the patient that intermetatarsal neurectomy is more unpredictable in terms of permanent, complete symptomatic relief than many other surgeries about the foot and ankle. Revision surgery adds to the unpredictability, and results appear to be worse than after primary excision; however, the literature suggests reasonable results in patients in whom conservative treatment has failed [11].

Advantages

- The advantages of revision neuroma excision include improved outcomes compared to conservative treatment.

Key Principles

- As far as is possible, the primary diagnosis must be ensured to be correct, and secondary conditions (e.g., neuropathy, radiculopathy, gastroc-soleus contracture) must be treated as effectively as possible.

- Patient education is critical to prevent unrealistic expectations and prepare for possible complications.
  - The patient should be aware that numbness is expected and "mild aching" pain often exists, especially after increased activity [5, 11–15, 19].
  - The sharp, stabbing pain should be significantly improved.
  - If a plantar incision is planned, the patient should be aware that the scar often is sensitive for several months postoperatively [2, 19, 24].

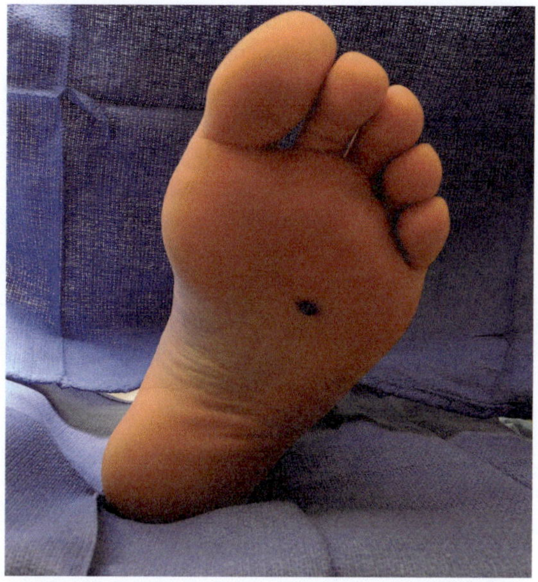

Fig. 3.5 For a plantar approach, the surgeon should be seated at the end of the operative table. A 4-cm incision is made centered over the point of maximal tenderness

Preoperative Preparation and Patient Positioning

- An ankle or forefoot black is administered using a 50/50 mixture of a long- and short-acting anesthetic (e.g., lidocaine and Marcaine).
  - Approximately 20–30 cc is used for an ankle block, while 10–20 cc is adequate for a forefoot block.
- An examination under anesthesia should be performed because a Mulder click may be present, especially in those with an inadequate resection at index procedure, or an interspace mass may be more easily appreciated [14].
- Instruments needed include a Freer elevator, Weitlaner or neuroma retractor, hemostats, small retractor.
- A sterile ankle tourniquet is used with cast padding and an Esmarch wrap.
- With a plantar incision, care must be used to position the incision proximal to the metatarsal heads and centered on the neuroma [2, 19, 24].

Positioning

- After standard preparation and draping, a 3-inch bump is placed under the distal leg, proximal to the ankle, such that the heel is floating. This will allow the ankle to be flexed as needed for visualization.
- If the surgery is to be performed with the patient supine using a dorsal approach, the surgeon should sit or stand proximal to the foot with an assistant at the end of the bed to help with retraction. If the surgery is to be performed with the patient supine through a plantar approach (easier if only local anesthesia administered), in addition to the bump under the heel, patient is placed in a mild Trendelenburg position (Fig. 3.5).
- If a plantar approach is used (preferable for visualization but patients often need general anesthesia), the patient is placed prone with a 3-inch bump under the distal leg just proximal to the ankle. The patient's feet must be at the distal end of the operative table to allow the surgeon to stand (or sit) at the foot of the bed.
- Surgical loupes are recommended.

Operative Technique

Dorsal Approach

- This approach is reserved for revision cases in which inadequate or incomplete resection is suspected. Because of the convergence of the metatarsals at their base, it is very difficult to identify a true stump neuroma and dissect the common digital nerve adequately proximal.

- A dorsal incision is made 4 cm proximal to the web, extending distally to the web space.
- The incision is slightly oblique from proximal-lateral to distal-medial but does not follow the extensor tendons (as this would be too laterally oriented in the proximal direction).
- The dorsal sensory nerves are retracted to the side of least resistance.
- The lumbrical tendon is to the lateral side of the dissection.
- The dorsal interosseous fascia and muscle belly are identified proximally and followed distally to the bursa overlying the transverse metatarsal ligament.
- A neuroma or Weitlander retractor is placed to distract the metatarsals and improve visualization.
- The bursa is incised to expose the transverse metatarsal ligament.
- The interspace is manually palpated to insure that the transverse metatarsal ligament has been released (it can reconstitute or scar after the index procedure).
- A Freer elevator is placed under the transverse ligament (or scar tissue) to protect the underlying structures, and then the ligament is released with a no. 15 blade knife.
- The lumbrical tendon is in the lateral aspect of the dissection just plantar the intermetatarsal ligament.
- The neurovascular bundle is identified medial and plantar to the lumbrical.
- Despite the size of the nerve or obvious presence of a neuroma, the nerve should be resected as planned.
- Structures that may be mistaken for the nerve (and therefore may be resected from the previous index procedure) include the lumbrical tendon, which passes to the medial portion of the adjacent proximal phalanx (extension expansion) and therefore is lateral to the nerve or the common digital artery which usually crosses proximal-medial to distal-lateral lying dorsally over the nerve [2, 13, 14].
- The nerve is identified proximally and followed distally to the stump (or Morton) neuroma.
- The transverse head of the adductor hallucis may need to be retracted to gain access to the plantar-directed common digital nerve.
- Any branches of the common digital nerve are divided to allow it to retract 1–2 cm.
- The common digital nerve itself is divided while both sides are gently held with an Adson forceps, and the damaged portion of the nerve is removed.
- If the recurrence was due to incomplete resection at the index procedure, the distal remaining nerve is circumferentially dissected to the bifurcation and divided just distal to the bifurcation.
- The proximal portion of the nerve is transposed into the intrinsic musculature of the foot (usually the interosseous muscle) [25].
- If desired, a 6-0 nylon epineural stitch can be used to secure the distal aspect of the remaining nerve into muscle belly.
- The specimen is sent for pathologic examination if desired.
- The tourniquet is released, and hemostasis is obtained.
- The wound is irrigated with sterile saline and closed with an interrupted 4-0 nylon suture in an everted, non-tensioned manner.
- A Xeroform gauze is placed on the wound, followed by a mildly compressive forefoot dressing.

Plantar Approach (Preferred for Recurrence due to True Stump Neuroma)

- If a longitudinal incision is preferred, a 4-cm longitudinal incision is made centered over the previously determined point of maximal tenderness. The incision usually begins 1 cm proximal to the first web space and extends 4 cm proximally. The incision is made between the metatarsal heads, which must be carefully located and marked before the incision is made (Fig. 3.5).
- If a transverse incision is preferred, a 4-cm transverse plantar incision is made over the point of maximal tenderness. This usually is 1 cm proximal to the weight-bearing pad and parallel to the natural crease.
- The metatarsal heads are repeatedly palpated to provide a reference point for dissection.
- A small Weitlaner retractor is placed to retract the fat overlying the plantar aponeurosis.

- Careful dissection using tenotomy scissors is needed to expose the septa of the plantar fascia.
- The interval between the longitudinal limbs of the plantar fascia septa is exposed.
- Using a no. 15 blade knife, the aponeurosis is incised longitudinally.
- The bands of the plantar fascia are retracted medially and laterally with a Senn retractor, and the interspace is carefully explored to identify the common digital nerve and vessel.
- The common digital nerve will lie just dorsal (deep) to the plantar fascia and just plantar (superficial) to the flexor digitorum brevis muscle or tendon.
- Tenotomy scissors are used to bluntly spread until the common digital nerve is identified proximally.
- The dissection then proceeds distally to identify the stump neuroma and proximally to expose 2 cm of the common digital nerve.
- The intermetatarsal ligament often is scarred or reconstituted, but does not need to be resected because the stump neuroma is well proximal and plantar.
- The transverse head of the adductor hallucis may need to be retracted to gain access to the plantar directed common digital nerve.
- Any branches of the common digital nerve are divided to allow retraction of 1–2 cm.
- The stump neuroma itself is removed, while both sections are gently held with an Adson forceps, and the damaged portion of the nerve is removed (Fig. 3.6).
- The proximal portion of the nerve is transposed into the intrinsic musculature of the foot (usually the interosseous muscle) [25].
- If desired, a 6-0 nylon epineural stitch can be used to secure the distal aspect of the remaining nerve into muscle belly.
- The tourniquet is released, and hemostasis is obtained.
- The wound is irrigated with sterile saline and closed with an interrupted 4-0 nylon suture in an everted, non-tensioned manner (Fig. 3.7).
- A Xeroform gauze is placed on the wound, followed by a mildly compressive forefoot dressing (Fig. 3.8).
- A short leg posterior splint is worn for 10–14 days.

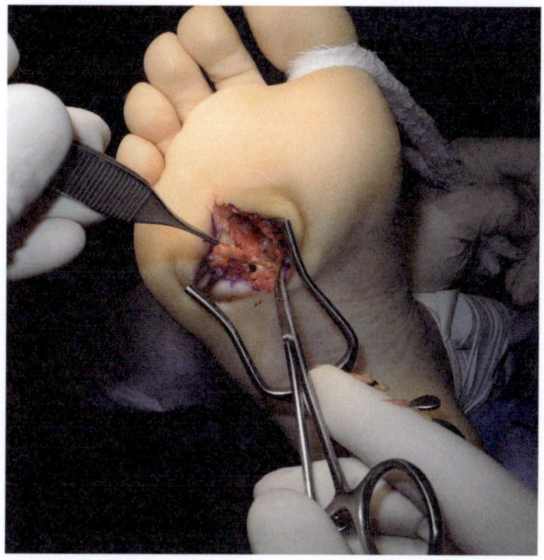

Fig. 3.6 The stump neuroma is removed, while the proximal segment is gently held with an Adson forceps. The proximal segment is transposed into intrinsic musculature

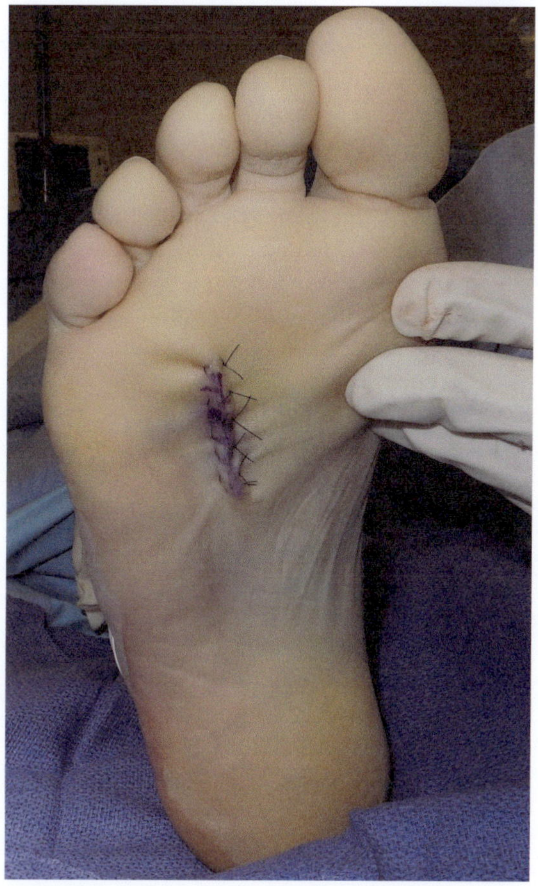

Fig. 3.7 Strict hemostasis is obtained, and a non-tensioned everted closure is created with 4-0 nylon suture

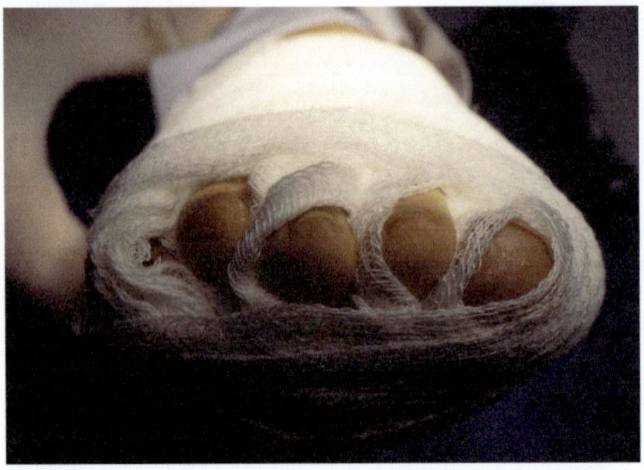

Fig. 3.8 A mildly compressive dressing is applied

Tips and Pearls

- History and physical are the primary basis for diagnosis and treatment.
- Attempt conservative treatment before surgery; 6 months is reasonable, but this depends on patient personality and symptom severity, as well as whether the index procedure resulted in symptom relief.
- Discuss possible complications, especially the relatively high risk of incomplete symptom relief and recurrence [5, 11–13, 19].
- For a plantar incision, avoid placing the incision directly under the metatarsal heads.
- Transect the common digital nerve 2 cm proximal to the stump neuroma, and transpose the nerve into the intrinsic musculature of the foot [25].
- Obtain hemostasis prior to closure.
- Keep patients non-weight-bearing until the wound is healed.

Hazards and Pitfalls

- Good to excellent results may be less frequent than previous literature suggests.
- Avoid a plantar incision in those known to form keloid or with thick callosities. Hypersensitivity may occur.
- Avoid hematoma formation to lessen risk of wound problems and infection.

Complications/Bailout/Salvage

- Complications include those associated with most surgeries, such as infection, wound complications, and continued pain, and those particular to surgery of the nerves and foot in particular, such as numbness, "shocking" pain, limited shoe wear, and activity limitations.
- Resect the nerve (whether intact due to prior incomplete resection or transected) proximally despite gross appearance. A "normal" appearing nerve may still have cellular pathology.
- The salvage procedure is revision surgery as described above. Caution is advised if the patient has failed two previous resections.
- Conservative treatment should be attempted before any revision, and a full workup for other etiologies should again be undertaken.

Postoperative Care

- After a mildly compressive dressing and short leg splint are placed, the operative limb should be elevated the majority of time for 3 days.
- Sutures should remain until the wound is completely healed (2–3 weeks).
- A stiff-soled shoe is worn for 2 weeks after suture removal, and then the patient is transitioned into a wide toe box shoe until asymptomatic.

Outcomes

- Long-term numbness should be expected.
- Shoe wear restrictions are a common complaint after revision neuroma excision [2, 4, 6, 14].
- Recovery from revision surgery often takes longer than patients expect (often 4 months).
- Reported good-to-excellent outcomes of surgical treatment of interdigital neuromas are variable but range from 50% to 85% [1, 5, 12, 13, 15, 20, 26, 27].

  - Our experience is on the less encouraging side, with 50% good and excellent results at average 67-month follow-up [14, 15].
- Good-to excellent results after revision surgery may be less than those of primary excision [4, 6, 11].
- In patients with significant preoperative symptoms, revision surgery offers a reasonable expectation of benefit.

Case Examples

Case 3.1

History

A 34-year-old male with no significant medical conditions complained of right foot pain that had been present for several years. He was initially seen 2 years earlier by a foot specialist who diagnosed bilateral third web space neuromas. The patient is a nonsmoker and has no previous history of trauma. Initially, he wore metatarsal pads to off-load the painful area, but this was of minimal benefit and, in fact, at times made symptoms worse. Because the patient and his surgeon believed that conservative treatment was not going to be successful and because the left side was more symptomatic, a left-sided neuroma excision was performed. At the same time, he had an injection to the third web space on the right (contralateral) side. Following this, pain on the right side worsened somewhat, and shoe modification and padding did not provide any significant relief. Approximately 1 year later, he proceeded to undergo a right third-web neuroma resection. He states that he continued to have pain even immediately after surgery. HK felt it was the same type and intensity of pain as prior to surgery. With weight-bearing, he localized his pain to the third space and under the third and fourth metatarsal head area. He states that he never walks barefoot as this "makes it much worse." He feels as though he is always walking on a "soft pebble," but the longer he stands, the more it feels like a "large, sharp, very uncomfortable pebble." He complains of numbness and tingling in the third and fourth digits. He has tried multiple different types of shoes, and none of them really make him pain free. He has a few pairs of tennis shoes that are more comfortable but really continues to have pain with any shoe wear. He has no night pain. The pain is only with weight-bearing.

Physical Examination

The patient is a 6′1″, 240-pound male, well-developed, well-nourished, and very pleasant. He is cooperative with the examination. Examination of bilateral lower extremities demonstrates 2+ pedal pulses, with no evidence of radiculopathy or peripheral neuropathy. Both feet demonstrate normal sensation in all distributions except for decreased sensation on the medial side of the fourth toe and the lateral side of the third toe on the left foot. He has normal, pain-free ankle, hindfoot, and midfoot motion and neutral hindfoot alignment. Plantar fat pads are normal, and there are no plantar callouses. There is no tenderness under the first, second, and fifth metatarsal heads but mild tenderness under the third and fourth metatarsal heads. He is most exquisitely tender to plantar palpation in the interspace between the third and fourth metatarsal heads. He does have some irritation and some discomfort with range of motion of the third and fourth MTP joints, particularly with extension, but has no deformity of the MTP joints. He has a negative nerve percussion response; however, deep plantar palpation in the interspace between the third and fourth metatarsals just proximal to the metatarsal heads reproduces his pain (see Fig. 3.2). He has a positive Mulder click with axial compression of the web space (see Fig. 3.2).

Reasons for Failure

Failure to resect primary neuroma (perineural fibrosis): Following the right-sided third-web neuroma excision, there was no significant change in symptoms. Furthermore, no improvement was noticed in the months following the index procedure, as he had experienced on the left after surgery. His physical examination was consistent with a primary third-web neuroma rather than a synovitis or bursitis or stump neuroma.

Surgical Plan

Primary interdigital neuroma excision: Treating the ongoing symptoms with revision neuroma excision was believed most appropriate, because further nonoperative treatment had limited chance of adequate symptom relief. After a lengthy discussion with the patient regarding risks and potential for incomplete pain relief, he wished to proceed with surgery.

Approach

Dorsal third-web space approach: See Operative Technique: Dorsal approach for primary neuroma excision

Implants

None

Pearls and Pitfalls

Pearls

- Carefully review the history and previous treatment.
- Consider and eliminate other diagnoses in the differential diagnosis.
- Exhaust nonoperative treatment options.

Pitfalls

- Resection of the wrong structure (e.g., lumbrical)
  - In this case, the common digital nerve was intact and a primary neuroma encountered (Fig. 3.9).

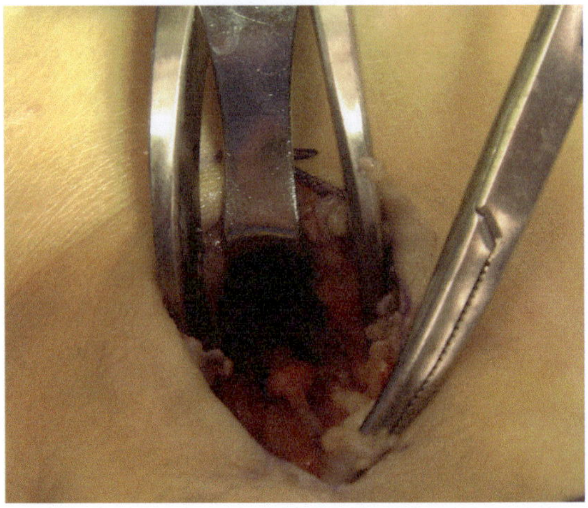

Fig. 3.9 Primary neuroma found during revision surgery; the wrong structure (lumbrical) was resected at the initial surgery

Case 3.2

History

A 43-year-old male with no medical conditions complains of right foot pain ongoing for several years. He was initially seen by the senior author 2 years earlier. He is a nonsmoker and has no previous history of trauma. After failure of conservative treatment consisting of shoe modification, metatarsal pads, anti-inflammatories, and an ultrasound-guided (note: we no longer routinely use US-guided corticosteroid injection), he elected to proceed with surgical resection of the intermetatarsal neuroma. He had an uneventful postoperative course and returned to full activity with minimal pain approximately 3 months after surgery. He continued to be minimally symptomatic until 4 months before presentation with complaints of increasing pain with weight-bearing, especially when not wearing shoes. He states that he has tried NSAIDs, shoe modifications, and orthotics. He was offered another steroid injection, which was refused. We, therefore, modified his metatarsal pad, believing it was too distal, and he was prescribed a tapered dose of methylprednisolone. Laboratory analysis was negative for an inflammatory arthropathy. He returned after 6 weeks stating that there was no change in symptoms. He complained of a sharp pain between his third and fourth metatarsals that radiated proximally. He continued to have numbness in the third and fourth digits and wished to proceed with revision surgery though a plantar approach.

Physical Examination

This 5′7″, 140-pound male is well-developed, well-nourished, and very pleasant. He is cooperative with the examination. Examination of the lower extremities demonstrates 2+ pedal pulses, with no evidence of radiculopathy or peripheral neuropathy or multiple joint pain. He has normal sensation in all distributions of his right foot except for decreased sensation on the medial side of the fourth toe and the lateral side of the third toe, which is quite dense. He has normal, pain-free ankle, hindfoot, and midfoot motion and neutral hindfoot alignment with no plantar callouses and adequate plantar fat pads. He is non-tender under his metatarsal heads. He is most exquisitely tender to plantar palpation in the interspace between the third and fourth metatarsals, proximal metatarsal heads. This is reproducible and recreates his symptoms. He does not have irritation with range of motion of the third and fourth MTP joints and no deformity of these joints. He has a positive nerve percussion response in the third web space.

Reasons for Failure

Formation of stump neuroma: Following his right-sided third-web neuroma excision, he experienced significant relief of symptoms which continued for 18 months. He now experiences sharp, proximally radiating neuritic pain. His physical examination is consistent with a third-web stump neuroma.

Surgical Plan

Revision surgery with stump-neuroma excision: Treating the ongoing symptoms with stump-neuroma excision through a plantar approach was believed to be most appropriate, because further nonoperative treatment had limited chance of adequate symptom relief. After a lengthy discussion with the patient regarding risks, potential for incomplete pain relief, and painful plantar scar, he wished to proceed with surgery.

Approach

Plantar third web space approach: See Operative Technique: Plantar Approach

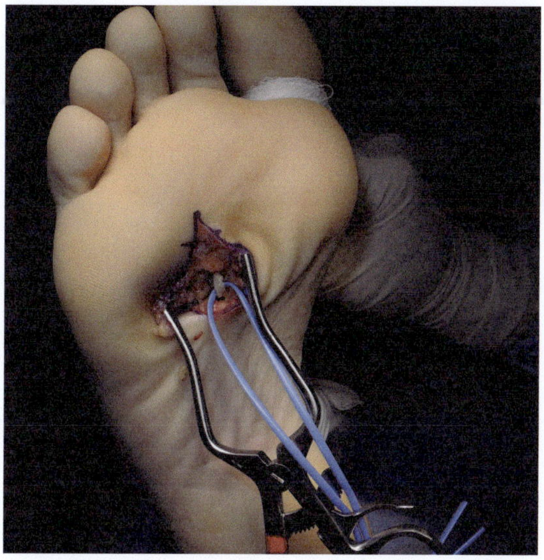

Fig. 3.10 Common digital nerve scarred to the third metatarsal

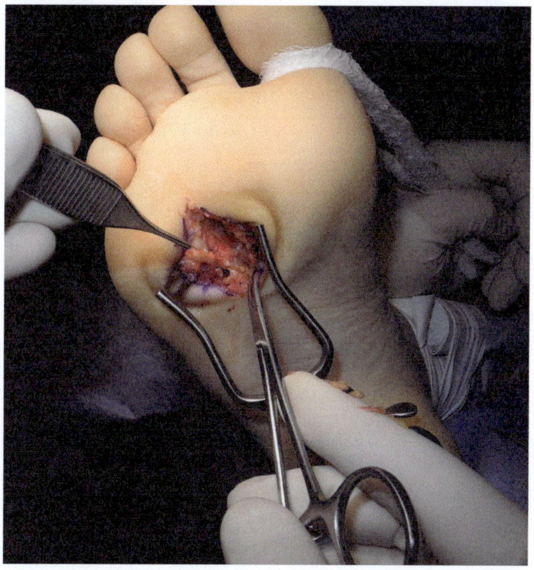

Fig. 3.11 Release is done distally and dissection proximally

- Identify common digital nerve (Fig. 3.10), which was found to be scarred to the third metatarsal.
- Release distally and dissect proximally (Fig. 3.11).
- Resect at least 2 cm proximally (see Fig. 3.1b).
- Cauterize the terminal aspect of the nerve and bury it in intrinsic musculature.
- Close with interrupted 4–0 nylon suture in an everted, non-tensioned manner (see Fig. 3.7).

Implants

None

Pearls and Pitfalls

Pearls

- Carefully review the history and previous treatment.
- Consider and eliminate other diagnoses in the differential diagnosis.
- Exhaust nonoperative treatment options.
- The stump neuroma is almost always found scarred to the lateral aspect of the third metatarsal, lumbrical, or flexor digitorum longus (look medial during dissection) (see Fig. 3.10).
- Obtain strict hemostasis before closure leading to avoid wound problems.
- Maintain non- or heel-weight-bearing status to prevent wound issues or painful plantar scar.

Pitfalls

- Inadequate resection of the primary neuroma at the index procedure or of the stump neuroma at revision.
- Failure to transpose the common digital nerve stump into intrinsic musculature.

Case 3.3

History

A 47-year-old female presents with left foot pain that has been present for several years. She has a medical history of depression, anxiety, tobacco abuse (1 ppd. cigarettes), atrial fibrillation, asthma, and rheumatoid arthritis. She is prescribed lisinopril, digoxin, aspirin, and Tylenol with codeine (prescribed for left foot pain) and methotrexate. She had a left third-web resection 2 years before presentation with significant but incomplete pain relief for approximately 1 year. She has had increasing pain without significant relief after shoe modification, metatarsal pads, and physical therapy. She agreed to an ultrasound-guided corticosteroid injection which proved moderately effective for 2 months. She is unable to walk barefoot and still has pain with shoe wear as well. She complains of occasional burning pain at night. She has numbness in her left third and fourth digits. She agreed to a smoking cessation program, weaning off narcotic pain medicine, and an ultrasound-guided corticosteroid injection which proved moderately effective for 2 months. After 3 months, she states that she has decreased her tobacco use to 1/4 ppd. and is off narcotic pain medication. Her rheumatologist modified her drug regimen, adding hydroxychloroquine. She remains "miserable" with her left foot pain that is localized and reproducible in the plantar aspect of the third web space. She denies significant right foot pain.

Physical Examination

This 5′3″, 155-pound female is well-developed, well-nourished, pleasant, and cooperative with the examination. Examination of the lower extremities demonstrates 2+ pedal pulses, with no evidence of radiculopathy; however, her examination is consistent with peripheral neuropathy. She maintains protective sensation to 10 g monofilament testing and has vague multiple joint pain with range of motion and palpation. She has dense loss of sensation on the medial side of the fourth toe and the lateral side of the third toe. She has normal ankle dorsiflexion that is minimally painful and symmetric hindfoot and midfoot motion. She has neutral hindfoot alignment, no plantar callouses, and adequate plantar fat pads. She is mildly tender under the metatarsal heads and most exquisitely tender to plantar palpation in the interspace between the third and fourth metatarsals, proximal metatarsal heads (see Fig. 3.2). This is reproducible and reproduces her symptoms. She has mild irritation with range of motion of the third and fourth MTP joints but no deformity. She has a positive nerve percussion response in the third web space, but this is negative over the tarsal tunnel.

Reasons for Failure

Formation of stump neuroma, inadequate control of inflammatory arthropathy, and tobacco abuse: Following her left-sided third-web neuroma excision, she experienced significant but incomplete pain relief. Her initial improvement lasted approximately 1 year. Pain increased after this time and was not adequately controlled with nonoperative treatment. Her physical examination was consistent with formation of a third-web stump (traumatic) neuroma as well as mild synovitis of the third and fourth metatarsophalangeal joints. Her risk of continued pain increased with continued tobacco use [22], history of depression/anxiety, and chronic narcotic use [23].

Surgical Plan

Third-web interdigital stump-neuroma excision and synovectomy of third and fourth MTP joints: Treating the ongoing symptoms with revision neuroma excision was believed to be most appropriate, because further nonoperative treatment had a limited chance of adequate symptom relief. Because of her history of RA, there was concern about fat pad atrophy or distal migration of the plantar fat pad causing pain with a plantar incision. After a lengthy discussion with the patient regarding risks (increased with continued tobacco use [22]) and potential for incomplete pain relief, she wished to proceed with surgery. She understood postoperative pain control could be difficult because of her history of depression/anxiety and chronic narcotic use [23].

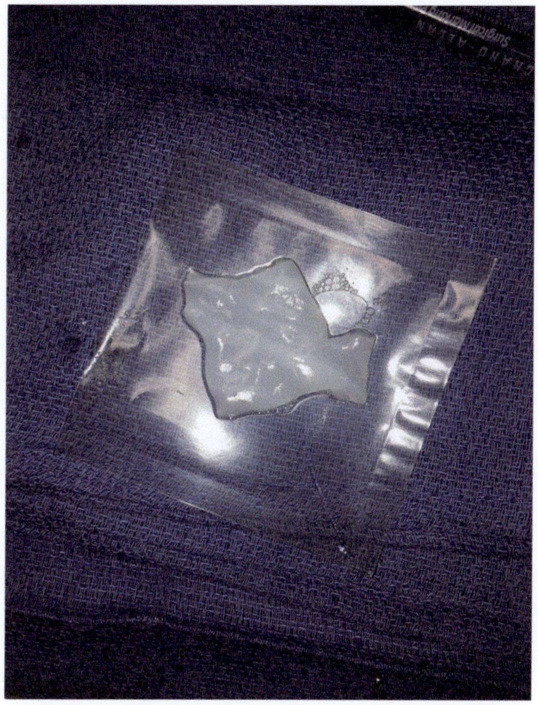

Fig. 3.12 Cryopreserved human amniotic membrane

Approach

Dorsal third-web space approach through previous incision with proximal extension: See Operative Technique: Dorsal Approach

- Stump neuroma encountered (Fig. 3.1b) scarred to the third metatarsal and flexor tendon.
- Cauterize the terminal aspect of the nerve.
- Because of the patient's history of RA, chronic pain, recurrence of neuroma (above average in size), and tobacco use, an allograft nerve wrap was believed to be appropriate (Fig. 3.12).

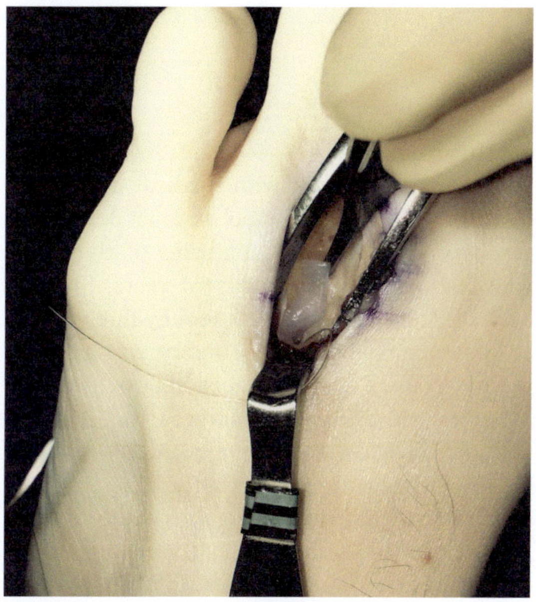

Fig. 3.13 Cryopreserved human amniotic membrane overwrap of terminal aspect of common digital nerve and suture to epineurium with 6-0 absorbable monofilament surgical suture (Monocryl)

Implants

- Cryopreserved human amniotic membrane (Fig. 3.13) overwrapped the terminal aspect of common digital nerve and was sutured to epineurium with 6-0 absorbable monofilament surgical suture (Monocryl).

Pearls and Pitfalls

Pearls

- Carefully review the history and previous treatment.
- Consider and eliminate other diagnoses in the differential diagnosis.
- Exhaust nonoperative treatment options.
- Optimize management of medical conditions (e.g., inflammatory arthropathy, tobacco abuse, depression/anxiety).
- Consider nerve wrapping in difficult cases [28, 29].
- Obtain strict hemostasis and a tight closure.
- Consider a multimodal postoperative pain control regimen consisting of a low-dose oral steroid, gabapentin, NSAID, Tylenol, and narcotic medication.

Pitfalls

- Primary or revision surgery on patients who continue to use tobacco and/or long-term narcotics may be problematic.
- Neurectomy in patients with inflammatory arthropathy may result in incomplete pain relief.

Case 3.4

History

A 72-year-old female with medical conditions consisting of a stroke without residual deficit and coronary artery disease complains of right foot pain that has been present for 4 years. She has had six surgeries on her right foot by three different physicians. The index surgery was primary third-web space neuroma excision through a dorsal approach. The second surgery was revision neuroma excision through a plantar approach. Neither of these procedures afforded significant pain relief. Subsequent surgeries were a right Keller resection arthroplasty; fourth metatarsal condylectomy; fourth metatarsal (Weil) shortening osteotomy, which proceeded to a nonunion; and fourth MT head resection. Before her Weil osteotomy, the treating surgeon stated in the clinic notes that "it seems, no matter how hard I talk, the more persistent she is...." She has been given oxycodone and hydrocodone intermittently over the last several years, although she is not currently prescribed narcotic pain medication. She is a nonsmoker. She has tried shoe modification and orthotics with MT relief with minimal reduction of her pain. Most of her complaints concern the plantar aspect of her right foot. She states she has numbness in her right lateral foot (somewhat diffusely) and occasional "shooting pain" in her right leg with ambulation. She denies significant left foot or leg pain. She has moderate low back pain with activity. She is being treated by a spine specialist and has had several steroid injections for facet arthritis. An MRI and nerve conduction study did not reveal evidence of radiculopathy. She has no inciting traumatic event to her right foot. She takes aspirin and piroxicam daily.

Physical Examination

This 5′6″, 178-pound female is well-developed, well-nourished and pleasant but anxious and persistent. She is cooperative with the examination. Examination of the lower extremities demonstrates 2+ pedal pulses, with no evidence of radiculopathy or peripheral neuropathy. She does have low back pain with palpation in the midline and with rotatory motion. She has dense loss of sensation on the medial side of the fourth toe and the lateral side of the third toe. She has ankle dorsiflexion to neutral only with her right knee extended; however, with knee flexion, her contracture improves (positive Silfverskiöld test). She has symmetric hindfoot and midfoot motion. She has mildly varus hindfoot alignment with a moderately painful plantar keratosis at the incision site. She is moderately tender under the metatarsal heads and has diffuse lateral, plantar right foot pain. She has irritation with range of motion of the third and fourth MTP joints, significant cock-up fourth-toe deformity with instability, and second, third, and fifth hammertoe deformities but maintains good correction of her hallux valgus deformity following surgery (Fig. 3.14). She has a positive nerve percussion response in the third web space as well as over the tarsal tunnel.

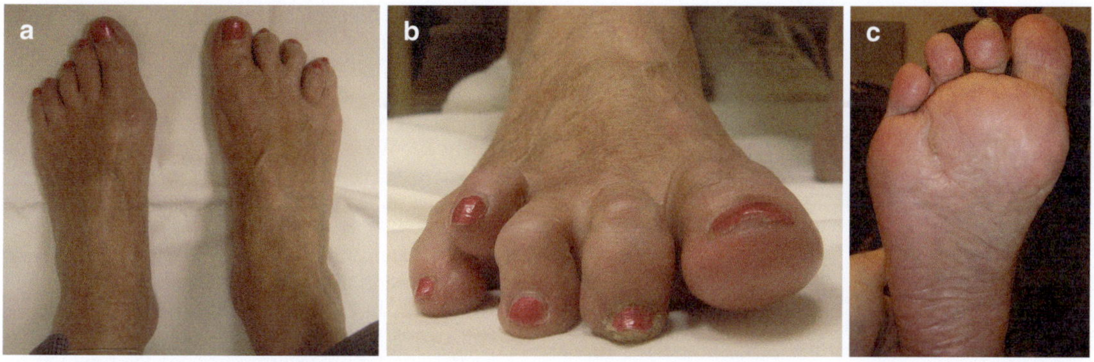

Fig. 3.14 This patient with multiple forefoot surgeries had a significant cock-up fourth-toe deformity with instability and second, third, and fifth hammertoe deformities but maintained good correction of her hallux valgus deformity after surgery (**a**–**c**)

Reasons for Failure

Patient selection, questionable initial diagnosis, and a tight gastrocnemius muscle: Since she had minimal relief of symptoms following neuroma resection and subsequent revision resection, it is likely a neuroma was not the appropriate diagnosis. Given the patients insistence on subsequent surgery, caution is needed before proceeding.

Surgical Plan

Gastrocnemius recession (Strayer procedure): It was believed that additional forefoot surgery would not be significantly beneficial; however, because she has a significant right gastrocnemius contracture, we proceeded with a Strayer procedure. She was fully weight-bearing after surgery in a walking boot with a small heel lift to relieve tension on her calf incision.

Approach

A 2-cm midline incision was used at the junction of the proximal 2/3 and distal 1/3 junction of the calf:

- Sural nerve was retracted.
- Superficial posterior fascia was released.
- Gastrocnemius fascia was recessed.
- This allowed 10 degrees of right ankle dorsiflexion.

Implants

None

Pearls and Pitfalls

Pearls

- Know when to stop. This patient had multiple procedures without significant relief.
- Carefully review the history and previous treatment.
- Consider and eliminate other diagnoses in the differential diagnosis.
- Always check for a tight heel cord before forefoot surgery.

Pitfalls

- Being pushed into surgery about which you have significant reservations.

Summary

Failure of the initial excision of an intermetatarsal neuroma may result from incorrect diagnosis, inadequate excision, or formation of a stump neuroma and symptoms usually recur within the first 12 months. History and physical examination are the mainstays of diagnosis. Conservative treatment usually is warranted, but it has a high failure rate. Corticosteroid injection may be beneficial but should be limited. Results of revision intermetatarsal neurectomy are satisfactory but less gratifying than those of primary excision. Managing expectations is important and "better," even if not symptom free, should be considered a positive outcome.

References

1. Bradley N, Miller WA, Devans JP. Plantar neuroma: an analysis and results following surgical excision of 145 patients. South Med J. 1976;69:853–4.
2. Beskin JL, Baxter DE. Recurrent pain following interdigital neurectomy—a plantar approach. Foot Ankle. 1988;9:34–9.
3. Benedetti RS, Baxter DE, Davis PF. Clinical results of simultaneous adjacent interdigital neurectomy in the foot. Foot Ankle Int. 1996;17:264–8.
4. Stamatis ED, Myerson MS. Treatment of recurrence of symptoms after excision of an interdigital neuroma. A retrospective review. J Bone Joint Surg Br. 2004;86:48–53.
5. Giannini S, Bacchini P, Ceccarelli F, Vannini F. Interdigital neuroma: clinical examination and histopathologic results in 63 cases treated with excision. Foot Ankle Int. 2004;25:79–84.
6. Johnson JE, Johnson KA, Unni KK. Persistent pain after excision of an interdigital neuroma. Results of reoperation. J Bone Joint Surg Am. 1988;70:651–7.
7. Colgrove RC, Huang EY, Barth AH, Greene MA. Interdigital neuroma: intermuscular neuroma transposition compared with resection. Foot Ankle Int. 2000;21:206–11.
8. Dellon AL. Treatment of recurrent metatarsalgia by neuroma resection and muscle implantation: case report and proposed algorithm of management for Morton's "neuroma". Microsurgery. 1989;10:256–9.
9. Amis JA, Siverhus SW, Liwnicz BH. An anatomic basis for recurrence after Morton's neuroma excision. Foot Ankle. 1992;13:153–6.
10. Wolfort SF, Dellon AL. Treatment of recurrent neuroma of the interdigital nerve by implantation of the proximal nerve into muscle in the arch of the foot. J Foot Ankle Surg. 2001;40:404–10.
11. Bucknall V, Rutherford D, MacDonald D, Shalaby H, McKinley J, Breusch SJ. Outcomes following excision of Morton's interdigital neuroma: a prospective study. Bone Joint J. 2016;98-B:1376–81.
12. Coughlin MJ, Pinsonneault T. Operative treatment of interdigital neuroma. A long-term follow-up study. J Bone Joint Surg Am. 2001;83:1321–8.
13. Mann RA, Reynolds JC. Interdigital neuroma—a critical analysis. Foot Ankle. 1983;3:328–43.
14. Richardson DR, Dean EM. The recurrent Morton neuroma: what now? Foot Ankle Clin. 2014;19:437–49.
15. Womack JW, Richardson DR, Murphy GA, Richardson EG, Ishikawa SN. Long-term evaluation of interdigital neuroma treated by surgical excision. Foot Ankle Int. 2008;29:574–7.
16. Bennett GL, Graham CE, Mauldin DM. Morton's interdigital neuroma: a comprehensive treatment protocol. Foot Ankle Int. 1995;16:760–3.
17. Sharp RJ, Wade CM, Hennessy MS, Saxby TS. The role of MRI and ultrasound in Morton's neuroma and the effect of size of lesion on symptoms. J Bone Joint Surg Br. 2003;85:999–1005.
18. Torres-Claramunt R, Ginés A, Pidemunt G, Puig L, de Zabala S. Morton's neuroma: diagnostic accuracy and correlation. Indian J Orthop. 2012;46:321–5.
19. Richardson EG, Brotzman SB, Graves SC. The plantar incision for procedures involving the forefoot. An evaluation of one hundred and fifty incisions in one hundred and fifteen patients. J Bone Joint Surg Am. 1993;75:726–31.
20. Pace A, Scammell B, Dhar S. The outcomes of Morton's neurectomy in the treatment of metatarsalgia. Int Orthop. 2010;34:511–5.
21. Bettin C, Gower K, McCormick K, et al. Cigarette smoking increases complication rate in forefoot surgery. Foot Ankle Int. 2015;36:488–93.
22. Mulligan RP, McCarthy KJ, Grear BJ, Richardson DR, Ishikawa SN, Murpjy GA. Psychological risk factors for postoperative pain in ankle and hindfoot reconstruction. Foot Ankle Int. 2016;37:1065–70.
23. Stewart MS, Bettin CC, Ramsey MT, et al. Effect of obesity on outcomes of forefoot surgery. Foot Ankle Int. 2016;37:483–7.
24. Nery C, Raduan F, Del Buono A, Asaumi ID, Maffullii N. Plantar approach for excision of a Morton neuroma: a long-term follow-up study. J Bone Joint Surg Am. 2012;94:654–8.
25. Rungprai C, Cychosz CC, Phruetthiphat O, Femino JE, Amendola A, Phisitkul P. Simple neurectomy versus neurectomy with intramuscular implantation for interdigital neuroma: a comparative study. Foot Ankle Int. 2015;36:1412–24.
26. Friscia DA, Strom DE, Parr JW, Saltzman CL, Johnson KA. Surgical treatment for primary interdigital neuroma. Orthopedics. 1991;14:669–72.
27. Lee KT, Kim JB, Young KW, Park YU, Kim JS, Jegal H. Long-term results of neurectomy in the treatment of Morton's neuroma: more than 10 years' follow-up. Foot Ankle Spec. 2011;4:349–53.
28. Campbell JT, Schon LC, Burkhardt LD. Pathologic findings in autogenous saphenous vein graft wrapping for recurrent tarsal tunnel syndrome: case report. Foot Ankle Int. 1998;19:766–9.
29. Masear VR. Nerve wrapping. Foot Ankle Clin. 2011;16:327–37.

Revision Surgery for the Failed Hammer Toe

4

Jakrapong Orapin and Lew C. Schon

Key Takeaway Points

- The initial surgeries on PIP or DIP may result in non-union and/or malunion.
- Excision of excessive bone may further complicate the surgery resulting in an unstable toe.
- Deviations may occur in any plane.
- A floppy deformed toe may catch as a sock is applied.
- A rigid deformed toe can create shoe sear problems.
- Reconstruction with revision may be performed by re-resecting the bone preserving as much stock as possible.
- To stabilize the pip joint or the bone, 1–3 intramedullary K-wires may be needed.

J. Orapin
Faculty of Medicine, Ramathibodi Hospital, Mahidol University, Department of Orthopaedic Surgery, Bangkok, Thailand

L. C. Schon (✉)
Department of Orthopaedic Surgery, MedStar Union Memorial Hospital, Baltimore, MD, USA

Georgetown School of Medicine, Washington, DC, USA

Johns Hopkins University, Baltimore, MD, USA

Fischell Literati Faculty, University of Maryland, Fischell Department of Bioengineering, College Park, MD, USA

Introduction

Hammer toe is the most common deformity of the lesser toes with a higher incidence in females with increasing age. There are multiple contributing factors including shoes with constricting toe boxes, excessively long metatarsal, hallux valgus, intrinsic muscle imbalance, neuromuscular disease, inflammatory joint disease, and muscle contracture after compartment syndrome. The second toe and metatarsal were reported as the most common site of involvement because of its longer length compared to adjacent toes and its location next to the great toe which may be deviated [1].

Hammer toe deformity can be either flexible or rigid. It can be associated with metatarsophalangeal (MTP) joint instability or osteoarthritis. The ability to passively correct the lesser toes to neutral position at the proximal interphalangeal (PIP) and distal interphalangeal (DIP) joints, as the MTP joint is held in neutral plantar flexion, is a hallmark of a flexible deformity. On the other hand, rigid deformity precludes passive correction of the toe to a straight or neutral position.

The plantar plate and collateral ligaments play a major role in stabilizing the MTP joint [2, 3]. Varus or valgus deformity may occur in combination with hammer toe when there is damage to the collateral ligaments. Likewise, plantar plate insufficiency leads to sagittal plane instability, and the toe may dorsally subluxate or dislocate.

M. J. Berkowitz et al. (eds.), *Revision Surgery of the Foot and Ankle*,
https://doi.org/10.1007/978-3-030-29969-9_4

Patients will complain about pain with constricting shoe wear from shoe rubbing or external pressure on a corn or callus at the dorsal aspect of contracted toes. Common deformity of hammer toe is plantar flexion of PIP joint that is frequently combined with hyperextension of the MTP joint. In this deformity, the DIP joint may stay in neutral, be extended, or assume a plantar flexed position.

Associated callosity under pulp of the toe and a nail deformity can also occur after prolonged friction with shoe insole. An important factor that influences this kind of deformity is the balance between intrinsic and extrinsic muscles. With a normal center of rotation, the intrinsic muscles that have insertions at the base of proximal phalanx, the extensor sling, and hood help with flexion of MTP joint and extension of IP joints. An attenuated plantar plate and capsule allow proximal phalanx to subluxate dorsally on the metatarsal head and shifts the center of rotation to the dorsal aspect [4, 5]. This effect turns intrinsic muscles into deforming forces that create the flexion deformity of the PIP joint and extension deformity on MTP joint [4, 6]. The duration of the deformity and the presence of arthritis determine the flexibility of the joint. As toe deformities become more rigid, the more difficult it is to correct the malposition by non-operative means.

Metatarsalgia is another complaint which can occur with a hammer toe deformity. After proximal phalanx shifts upward, the plantar fat pad also moves distally, and the metatarsal head encounters more pressure from ground reaction force during the third rocker gait progression. Also, a plantar callosity can develop underneath the metatarsal head due to excessive contact pressures.

Nonsurgical treatment of the hammer and the claw toes is focused on relieving pain from the pressure point and rubbing by the undersurface of shoe's upper toe box. A roomy toe box in an extra-depth shoe with soft uppers helps alleviate symptom. Gel or foam toe sleeves prevent rubbing and help redistribute pressure on dorsum of PIP joint. Taping of the proximal phalanx in figure of eight, canopy, or straight fashion helps stabilize the toe, by reducing MTP joint subluxation and stabilizing a lax plantar plate and capsule, thereby reducing synovitis and pain. A metatarsal dome or pad placed proximal to metatarsal head decreases the load and pressure. A Budin splint has a strap to hold toe in a straighter position with metatarsal pad for plantar cushioning [2, 4, 7]. Operative management is considered if symptoms continue to compromise comfort and function despite conservative management.

Surgical treatment depends on flexibility of the deformity and associated deformity of the adjacent toes. A hammer toe with flexible or semi-rigid deformity can be corrected with just capsular or collateral ligament release and may be combined with flexor tendon transfer in cases where residual MTP joint extension still occurs. A rigid hammer toe requires correction with PIP joint resection arthroplasty or arthrodesis [1, 2, 4, 7, 8]. The results can be unpredictable and leave the patient with complaints from consequence of the surgery. Complications after hammer toe repair are uncommon, but not all patients with radiographic non-union of the PIP are symptomatic. Coughlin and associates [1] reported 92% pain relief rate and 84% satisfaction rate in 118 toes of 63 patients. Although they achieved 81% fusion rate, they found equal satisfaction between fusion and fibrous union; however, 23% of patients had no toe pulp contact on weight bearing after surgery. In O'Kane and Kilmartin study [9], which focused on the outcome after excisional arthroplasty in the second toe only, out of 75 patients (100 toes), they found complications in 31 toes. These included 18 floating toes, 4 recurrent hammer toes, 3 soft tissue infections, 3 malalignments, 1 swollen toe, and the need for 2 revision surgeries. Sung et al. [10] retrospectively reviewed the outcomes after hammer toe correction with three different techniques (resection arthroplasty, arthrodesis, and interpositional implant arthroplasty) in 136 second toes and found satisfactory outcomes in pain relief, sagittal plane correction with 35–56% complication rate and 10–38% revision rate. They also concluded that implant interposition arthroplasty had the best result of transverse plane deformity correction between three procedures. Although Higgs [11] reported that non-union could result in recurrent pain and deformity, patients still have satisfactory results after surgery if the toe correction results in joint stiffness whether the fusion is achieved or not, as stated by Kelikian [12] and Coughlin [1].

Physical Assessment and Preoperative Evaluation

Examination should be done thoroughly both in standing and sitting position to see overall alignment of the toes and how they contact the ground. Resultant positions of attempted hammer toe corrections should be documented and may include frontal, coronal, sagittal, and rotational toe deformities. Also, excessive shortening may occur. Flexion of PIP joint is typical and often combines with a neutral or flexed DIP joint. Occasionally the PIP or rarely the DIP joint is hyperextended. Frequently, the MTP joint is hyperextended. Flexible deformity can be identified, with hyperextended MTP joint, by bringing down proximal phalanx to neutral position, and toe becomes straight. The role of the flexor digitorum longus (FDL) can be assessed by performing passive movement of the ankle and seeing its effect on the PIP flexion deformity. Performing the "drawer test" helps assess MTP joint instability and guide the treatment. Loss of digital strength or toe purchase, as well as instability, can be documented with the "paper pull-out test" [13]. The test can be performed, with patient standing, by placing a strip of paper underneath the affected toe, and the examiner tries to pull the paper strip out from beneath the toe while the patient is flexing the toe against paper pulling. Positive result is considered if the patient is unable to hold the paper. The stiffness of deformity should be determined both in a sitting and standing mode as a more rigid deformity will typically trigger the need for a bone and soft tissue procedure. Conversely, a previously operated toe may be floppy due to excessive bone removal or tendon lengthening.

The presence of arthritis is important to note as a failed reconstruction may have resulted in an arthritic joint. This may manifest with a stiff painful joint but also may result in a tender protruding osteophyte with or without overlying skin changes. Other sources of pain should be sorted out such as avascular necrosis, scar pain, nerve damage, vascular damage, or synovitis. Malunion or non-union of a metatarsal osteotomy may result in metatarsal over or underload. These conditions may require correction during a revision procedure.

Adjacent toe deformity should be evaluated and realigned simultaneously. Correction of adjacent toes must provide enough space after bringing down the hammer toe; otherwise recurrence of deformity can occur. Limited ankle dorsiflexion from gastrocnemius tightness and tendo Achilles contracture should be addressed and corrected at the time of revision hammer toe surgery as well.

Surgical Planning

A comprehensive examination of the affected foot and ankle combined with a weight-bearing dorsoplantar and lateral view and non-weight-bearing oblique view radiographs is needed for preoperative planning. A detailed prior operative note which includes prior implants and their brand should be reviewed if possible. Deformities in all dimensions (varus, valgus, flexion, extension, axial rotation, shortening) are addressed carefully, and an assessment of the parabolic cascade of all metatarsals has to be made. Fixed and flexible deformities have to be distinguished and approached as mentioned in preoperative evaluation above. Associated hallux valgus and adjacent toe deformities need to be corrected at the same time to decrease deforming forces that lead to recurrent deformity. Adjacent toes correction should create enough space to bring the hammer toe down to its original position.

A variety of surgical procedures for primary and secondary hammer toe procedures had been mentioned in the literatures, but proper selection for each patient can be challenging. Flexible hammer toe deformity can be corrected by soft tissue release at the MTP, PIP, and/or DIP joints. If there is subluxation or dislocation of the MTP, a flexor tendon transfer can be performed with or without a proximal phalangeal shortening or proximal phalangeal fusion. The surgeon should pay attention to avoid excessive bone cuts because a floppy or unstable toe can result. Tightening of the transferred flexor tendon around the base of the phalanx should be meticulously tailored in each patient because excessive tension can decrease MTP dorsiflexion and toe stiffness [14, 15]. Fixed deformity requires resection arthroplasty or arthrodesis and usually will not achieve sufficient correction without additional Z-extensor tendon lengthening [15], flexor tendon transfer, and metatarsal osteotomy. With fusions or osteotomies, care should be taken on amount of bone removed to achieve toe alignment. At times, recession of the gastrocnemius may be added if the patient has positive Silfverskiold test on preoperative examination.

Routinely with any surgery, the patient should be counseled about post-operative stiffness from fusion and/or scar tissue, swelling, numbness, vascular compromise, non-union, K-wire breakage or migration, infection, and floppy toe as well. Complication rates after lesser toe deformity correction can range from 21% to 56% as reported in literatures [2, 9, 10, 16, 17], and pain from friction or rubbing over bony prominence of the misaligned toe with surrounding surfaces is the most common source of dissatisfaction [18]. These complications are higher with revision cases. From this perspective, it is critical to set patient expectations as to what residual issues they may be left with following revision.

Implants for primary or revision PIP joint fusion include K-wire, interfragmentary compression screw, and numerous other special intramedullary devices. Our senior surgeon (LCS) prefers using K-wire to temporarily stabilize the PIP joint fusion for 6 weeks with satisfactory results. It is inexpensive and provides easy, stable fixation. Prolonged time to K-wire removal is associated with up to 18% complication rate including bending, breakage, loosening, migration, and pin tract infection [19–22]. Klammer and associates [19] found 47.8% versus 8.7% failure rate in alignment control in the group in which the K-wire was removed at 3 weeks and 6 weeks, respectively. In the large study of Zingas et al. [21], they found 33 broken wires in 1002 toes (565 patients) with overall failure rate of 3.2% after 6 weeks of fixation, and all failures occurred in toes where transfixion beyond the MTP joint was performed while using a 1.14 mm (0.045″) wire diameter. When using the K-wire for a revision procedure, the surgeon should be prepared to use several wires per toe depending on bone quality.

With the special PIP joint implants, one can encounter malunion, non-union, and infections. When revising these toes, more damage can occur excavating out the implant. This leads to even more difficulty with quality and quantity of remaining bone. Furthermore, they create additional fixation challenges. It is useful to identify the prior implants that were utilized and explore removal strategies with the company representatives or specialists. Occasionally, special tools are needed that may need to be delivered to the OR in advance. When revision in this scenario is performed, a bone graft may be required. This can be effectively harvested in a less invasive fashion by a JAmshiti needle or bone trephine system like the Michelle trephines. Many companies that have bone marrow harvest systems can also make available their harvesting trephine/trochar devices which nicely harvest 10–15-mm-long 2-mm-wide firm cancellous bone cylinders.

PIP Joint Non-union

PIP non-union is a frequent radiographic phenomenon after fusion, but it is not often symptomatic. Fernandez and colleagues [23] found that their patients preferred a stiff but straight lesser toes. Preserving some motion of the PIP joint sometimes causes instability or loss of correction overtime. PIP joint fusion is their choice of treatment because of better more reliable results. According to a study of Schrier and colleagues [16], 39 toes were included in resection group and 50 toes in fusion group. They often had radiologic non-union after PIP joint fusion, but the non-union rarely resulted in pain. Otherwise, they found that PIP joint fusion resulted in better improvement of sagittal alignment with statistically significant difference compared with the resection group. As stated by Nery and colleague [24], MTP joint extension and recurrent flexion deformity of the PIP joint are the most common deformities after hammer toe surgery. They also mentioned that despite 50% non-union rate, fusion is the best procedure to deal with recurrent isolated hammer toe deformity. The overall plan for these non-unions is to re-cut the bone surfaces, curette the zone of bone deficiency, realign all the elements of the associated deformity at the DIP and MTP, pack bone graft, and insert one to several K-wires.

When addressing a painful non-union after PIP joint fusion, donor sites for bone graft including iliac crest, tibial metaphysis, and/or calcaneus should be sterilely prepped. Autogenous graft is a fabulous source of structural and biologically active graft, rich in growth factors and progenitor cells. Sometimes an additional biologic adjuvant is helpful. Unfortunately, the volume that can be used in these small spaces is such that it can be difficult to justify their use. If other surgeries will be performed, bone marrow aspirate concentrate (BMAC) can be used.

PIP Joint Malalignment or Malunion

Callosity from shoe rubbing over bony prominence at the flexed or deviated PIP can cause significant pain to the patients. In addition, patients may have pain from a prominence due to a translational deformity. Sometimes the non-united swollen toe will be positioned next to adjacent toes in an acceptable deviated position. This can be called toe packing or "molding" [2, 25]. Location and cause of the deformity should be determined clinically and radiographically. Unintentionally oblique cuts of the distal aspect of proximal phalanx and the proximal aspect of middle phalanx can occur and may create problems.

When there is a malunion of the PIP, re-cutting the surfaces and performing a fusion are advised. Ideally, the first bone cutting should be at the supracondylar region of the distal aspect of the proximal phalanx and perpendicular to the proximal phalanx axis [2]. The second cut is just beyond the articular surface of the proximal aspect of the middle phalanx, and this should be parallel to the first cut. Myerson [26] recommended resection with bone cutter or sagittal saw with no more than the distal one quarter or 4 mm of the proximal phalanx. LCS recommends 2 mm for best preservation of cancellous bone stock to help avoid complications.

When there is deformity at the MTP, revision should address the issues. For toe deviation 15 degrees or less at the MTP joint, an MTP capsular and collateral release with extensor tenotomy or lengthening is warranted. With this degree of deformity, a proximal phalanx basal osteotomy (Akinette) may be a useful adjuvant. If there is more than a 15-degree deformity, an extensor digitorum brevis (EDB) transfer with or without a metatarsal osteotomy is recommended by the senior author, LCS.

Flail Toe

Recurrent hammer toe or residual deformity can occur if not enough bone resection is achieved. On the other hand, excessive resection can cause another problem that may be worse than recurrence. Patient with flail toe may experience pain, deformity, instability, and displeasing appearance of the toe. The floppy toe also has a tendency to catch while the patient puts on socks or stockings. At times barefoot walking is also difficult as the toe shifts around. The painful floppy toe can occur with other symptoms including weakness, stiffness, and metatarsalgia [8, 27, 28]. Patients who have undergone a proximal phalangectomy and syndactylization are at risk for a floppy toe with a cosmetically unacceptable outcome. Cahill and Connor [29] reported that 17 of 34 patients had a poor result, even though pain relief could be good, and cosmesis was poor.

As stated by Solan and Davies [18], it is better not to shorten the toe at the first place by avoiding excessive bone resection because flail toe is extremely difficult to manage.

PIP joint arthrodesis, as a salvage procedure, is preferable to amputation, but partial amputation occasionally is an acceptable procedure in some selected patients [18, 24, 26]. Myerson and Filippi [26, 30] proposed structural bone block graft lengthening technique for correction of short floppy toe deformity. The bicortical bone graft may be harvested from the ipsilateral calcaneus or from the iliac crest. The length of the graft is ascertained by inserting a hemostat or small laminar spreader. The graft may be mixed with BMAC. They also pointed out that toe perfusion may be compromised by lengthening. They concluded that this procedure helps restore length, stability, and better cosmesis of the toe for active patients.

DIP Joint Non-union or Malalignment

Patients undergoing PIP joint arthrodesis may develop a DIP joint flexion contracture or a mallet toe as a result of FDL tightness. Symptoms occur when the tip of the toe strikes the ground. With prolonged striking and rubbing, a painful callosity at the plantar or dorsal aspect develops. Distinguishing between a fixed or flexible deformity of the DIP joint will help guide treatment. Flexible deformity can be treated with FDL tenotomy alone. In a rigid deformity, the options include DIP fusion or condylectomy of the middle phalanx in combination with FDL tenotomy, which will help shorten and decompress the bone. Solan and Davies [18] preferred DIP joint excisional arthroplasty because DIP joint fusion often results in non-union. Coughlin [31] reported results after excisional arthroplasty in 72 toes. Major complaints of pain and callus were relieved in 97% of patients. Fusion was achieved in 70% of cases, and 99% had good-to-excellent post-operative radiographic alignment. On subjective evaluation, 62 toes (86%) were rated as satisfactory by patients. Results of the distal phalangectomy in 39 toes (26 patients) with mean age of 63 years old were mentioned by Raja and associates [32]. All patients had satisfactory pain relief, and 97% of patients were satisfied with surgery. Complications (7.5%) can include nail growth from a nail matrix remnant and a minor wound infection. Another option is to perform a terminal Symes amputation of the toe. This is a good option when the stiff DIP deformity is associated with a callused distal toe tuft and thickened deformed painful nails. Another good indication for a terminal amputation is the presence of a distal toe ulcer with or without infection.

Cases

Case 4.1 PIP Joint–Non-union

History

A 61-year-old female sustained crush injury to second toe from a falling lawnmower battery. She had open fracture that was initially treated at an outside institution with a washout and sutures. She came to our clinic at 3 months after the injury with complaint of a painful swollen toe. X-ray revealed a fracture non-union (Fig. 4.1).

On examination she had tenderness and swelling of the toe at the PIP and DIP joints with contracture and hyperextension of MTP joint. It was felt that she may have a low-grade infection based on the clinical appearance, and the implications of this were discussed with the patient. She elected to attempt a salvage procedure with dorsal capsulotomy and Z-extensor tendon lengthening EDL EDB at the MTP and a PIP and DIP fusion by a 2.0 mm screw from distal phalanx to proximal phalanx supplemented by autogenous bone graft (Fig. 4.2). Cultures and biopsy were negative.

Two months after PIP/DIP joint fusion, she still had tenderness to palpation along the toe with swelling and erythema. There was no drain-

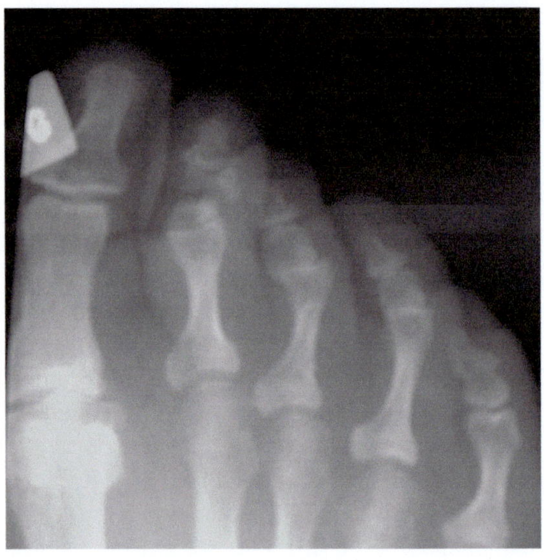

Fig. 4.1 Painful fracture non-union of the middle phalanx of the right second toe after crush injury

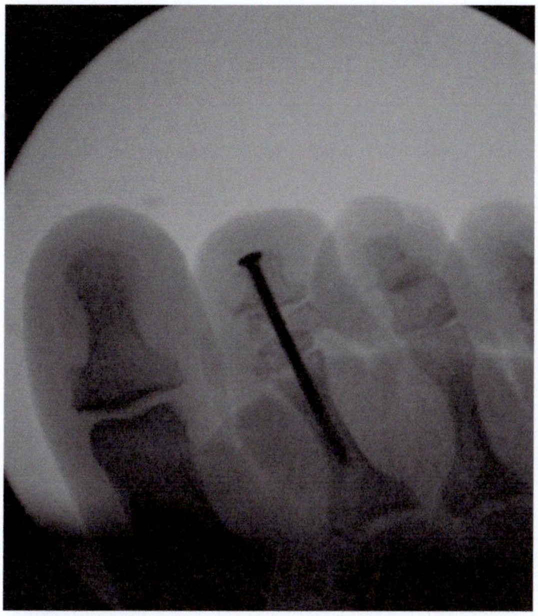

Fig. 4.2 Fusion with 2.0 mm compression screw of the PIP and DIP joints was performed with morselized bone graft augmentation

age or proximal cellulitis. The screw was showing signs of loosening, and there was no evidence of bony union. Given the condition of the chronically painful toe and the probability of infection, the patient was advised to proceed with second toe partial amputation.

Reasons for Failure

The crush toe with an open fracture resulted in local vascular damage, with bone and soft tissue compromise and a low-grade infection. As a result, there was persistent poor soft tissue and bone healing with a recurrent low-grade infection.

Surgical Plan

Amputation at the mid-proximal phalanx of the right second toe.

Approach

We used fish mouth incision at the level of distal proximal phalanx under local anesthetic block and intravenous sedation. Condyles of the proximal phalanx were cut with microsagittal saw. Skin was closed with interrupted 4–0 nylon sutures.

Implants

None

Post-operative Care

She was instructed to perform heel or lateral foot weight bearing in a post-operative shoe in the first 2 weeks, and then progressive weight bearing was allowed after 2 weeks as tolerated. Patient had been doing well after operation until her last follow-up at 8-year post-operative period (Fig. 4.3).

Pearls and Pitfalls

Severe crush injury may increase risk of chronic recalcitrant pain and non-union. Soft tissue injury and a low-grade infection can complicate a salvage attempt. Partial amputation as a last resort can provide satisfaction in selected cases.

Case 4.2 PIP Joint–Malunion/Malalignment

History

A 33-year-old female previously had hammertoe surgeries for her right second, third, fourth, and fifth toe and developed severe pain and discoloration of the toes post-operatively. After ruling out a vascular disorder with Doppler exams, she was diagnosed with a chronic regional pain syndrome and reflex sympathetic dystrophy. Eventually, the pain and discoloration improved in all the toes, but she had ongoing complaints of a painful deformity of the third toe with a tender prominence laterally at the PIP. Despite taping the toes and activity modification, she had persistent pain and dysfunction.

On examination, there was tenderness over a prominent bony edge of the PIP of the third toe. There was discomfort with stressing the PIP joint. She had a 15–20-degree varus deformity of the third toe (Figs. 4.4 and 4.5).

Reasons for Failure

Possible causes could be uneven bone cut, inadequate post-op immobilization after fusion, inadequate fixation, and subsequent PIP non-union with bony osteophyte impingement. The severe painful discolored toes may have been due to a

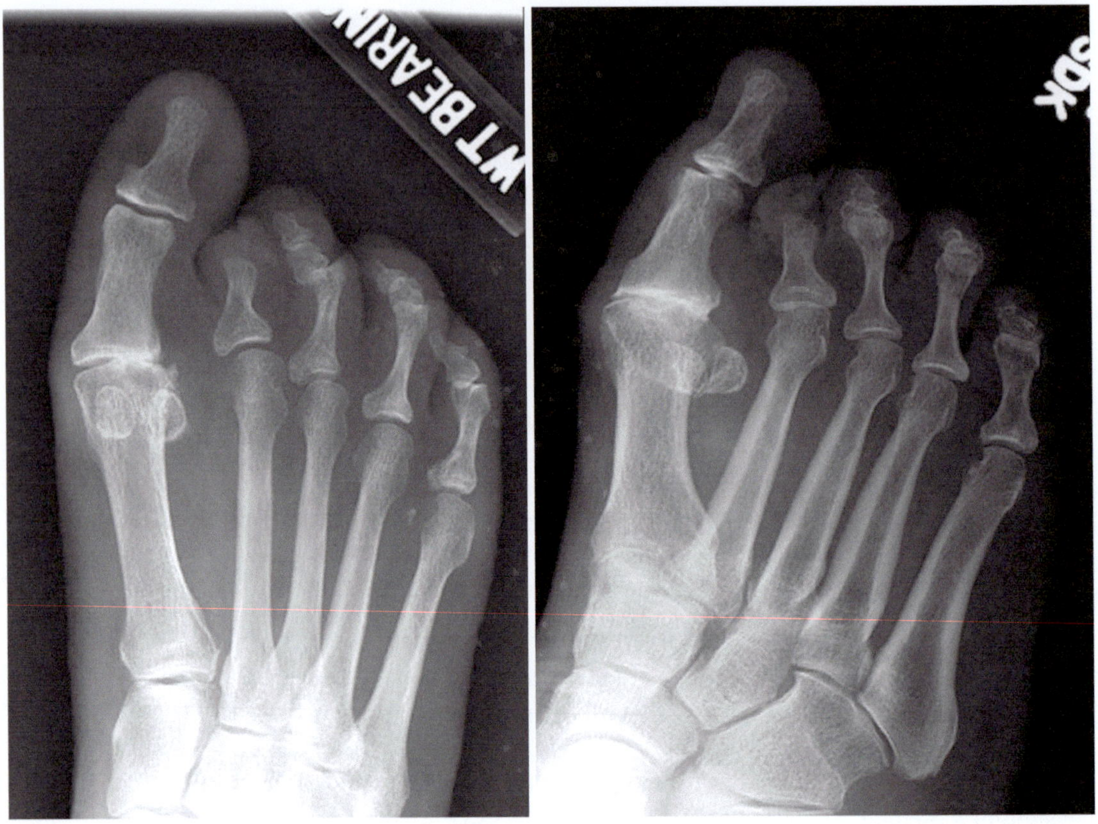

Fig. 4.3 Follow-up at 8 years after amputation through the PIP joint, minimal toe drifting was observed without ulcer

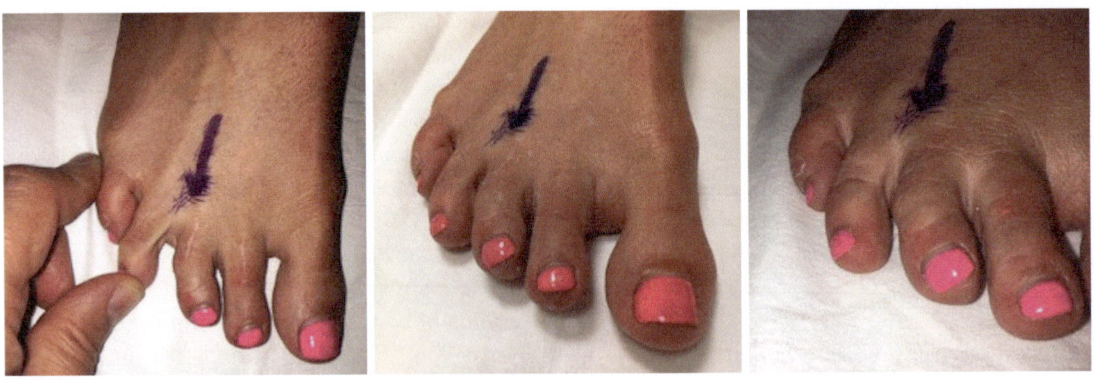

Fig. 4.4 The patient had pain and varus deformity from a non-united PIP fusion of the right third toe. She had no corn or ulcer on toe examination

neurovascular sensitivity such as Raynaud's or *erythromelalgia*, tourniquet application, or a local anesthetic administration with vascular compromise due to needle trauma or surgical trauma.

Surgical Plan

Revision fusion of the PIP joint of the right third toe without use of tourniquet and without digital nerve anesthetic blocks.

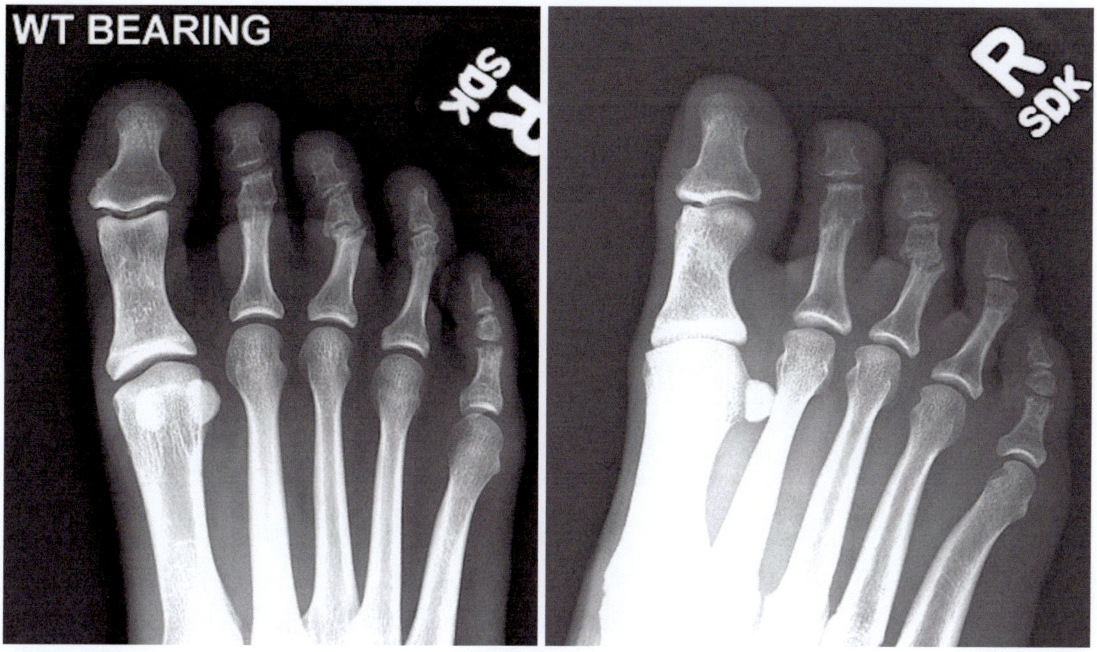

Fig. 4.5 Her dorsal-plantar and oblique foot radiographs represented non-union and varus deformity from collapsing medial cortical support of the middle phalanx of the third toe

Approach
Without a tourniquet and digital nerve anesthetic blocks, a PIP joint fusion of the right third toe was performed through the prior dorsal longitudinal approach. Careful retraction and dissection was utilized to minimize neurovascular trauma. The bone was cut 1 mm from the edge with an irrigated microsagittal saw. Autogenous 2 mm diameter 12-mm-long bone graft dowels were harvested from the iliac crest with a trephine. Three K-wires were placed for better stability (Fig. 4.6) Bone marrow aspirate was concentrated and injected into the surgical site after closure.

Implants
0.045″ K-Wire

Post-operative Care
Weight bearing was allowed after operation as tolerated in hard-soled shoe on the heel and outside of the foot avoiding pressure on the third toe for 2 months. A non-restrictive dressing was applied. To further minimize the potential for sympathetic dystrophy or the neurovascular reaction, the patient was encouraged to move and massage the foot and ankle except the third toe. By 2-month post-operative period, the patient was doing well; good bone bridging was achieved at fusion site without evidence of implant loosening or infection. Patient continued to do well several years post-op.

Pearls and Pitfalls
Articular surface bone cut should be perpendicular to the long axis of the phalanx. Additional fixation with three K-wires was determined to be necessary based on stability perceived at the time of surgery. Additional cylindrical autogenous bone graft dowels may increase rate of healing.

Case 4.3 Flail Toe #1

History
The patient is a 22-year-old woman who had a left second hammer toe surgery at an outside hospital. She had a non-union and malalignment of the second toe after the attempted PIP fusion. She had pain and problems from toe rubbing on the

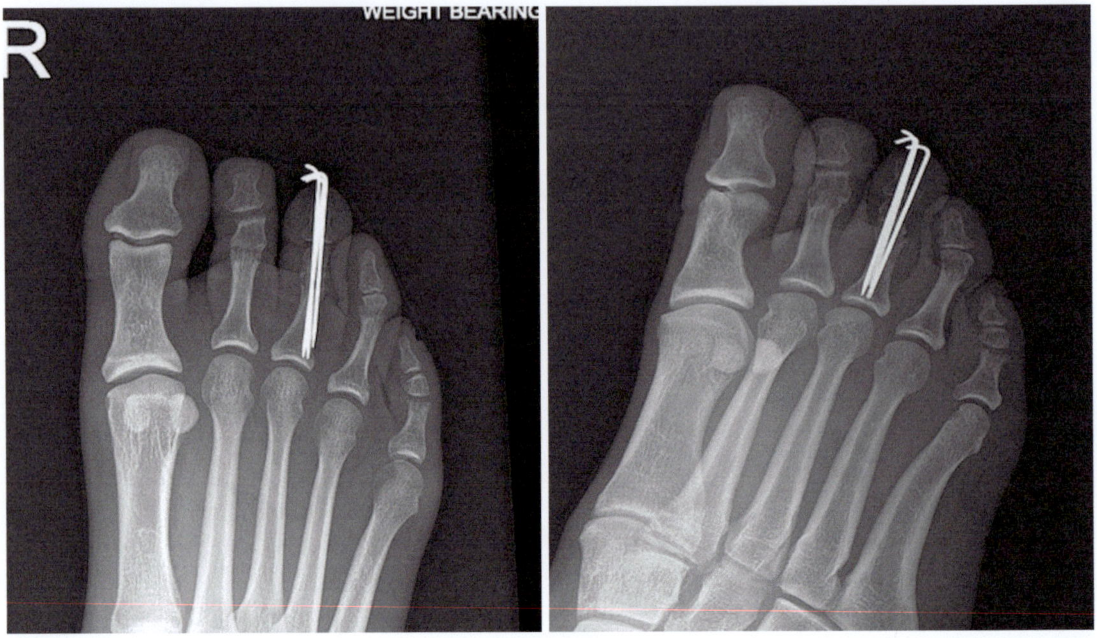

Fig. 4.6 Revision of the PIP joint fusion of right third toe was performed, three K-wires were fixed for better stability, and bone graft from iliac crest and bone marrow aspirate concentrate were added to improve healing

toe box of the shoe despite modifications to accommodate the deformity. Her left foot examination showed shortening and lateral deviation of the second toe compared to contralateral side (Fig. 4.7a). The second toe was floppy and unable to touch the ground (Fig. 4.7b). Her radiographs showed non-union of the PIP fusion and lateral deviation of the middle phalanx (Fig. 4.8).

Reasons for Failure

Non-union, due to excessive bony resection from the proximal and middle phalanx. Inadequate stability of the fixation may lead to malalignment.

Surgical Plan

Revision PIP joint fusion of the left second toe with calcaneal bone graft and screw fixation.

Approach

We approached the non-union site through previous dorsal skin incision with proximal and distal extensions. Fibrous tissue around the fusion area was removed and bone ends were freshened. Calcaneal bone graft was harvested through a 3 mm second incision at the lateral aspect of the calcaneus posterior to the sural nerve. A 4 mm narrow head cannulated screw was then used to secure the toe in position and confirmed with an AP and lateral fluoroscopy. The remaining defect was then packed with cancellous bone graft. Since the second toe still rested in an extended position, we extended the incision proximally and released MTP joint capsule. The extensor digitorum longus (EDL) was identified and lengthened in Z-fashion to allow to be in a more neutral position.

Implants

I.CO.S. Cannulated screw (Integra Life Science Corporation, Plainsboro, NJ, USA) diameter 4 mm, 36 mm in length. The screw has a threaded head that allows for extra compression which increases its width. For this indication, the threaded head is removed providing a very narrow head long cannulated screw.

Post-operative Care

Three months after operative correction, she was doing well, and radiographs showed progressive union without sign of screw breakage or loosening (Fig. 4.9).

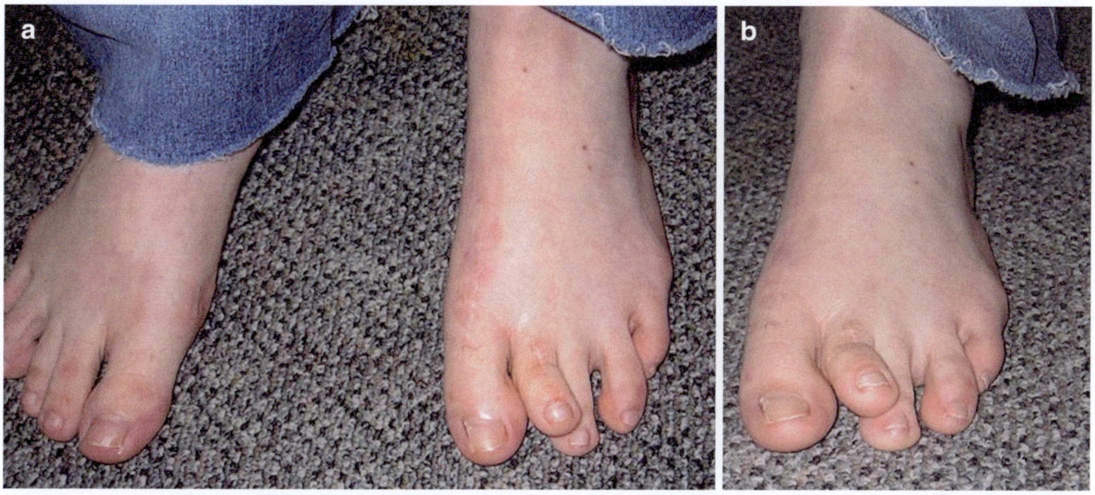

Fig. 4.7 Left second toe deformity after hammer toe surgery in 22-year-old female. (**a**) Shortening and lateral deviation of the left second toe compared with the contralateral foot. (**b**) Combined extension deformity of the PIP joint led to floating of the tip of the second toe

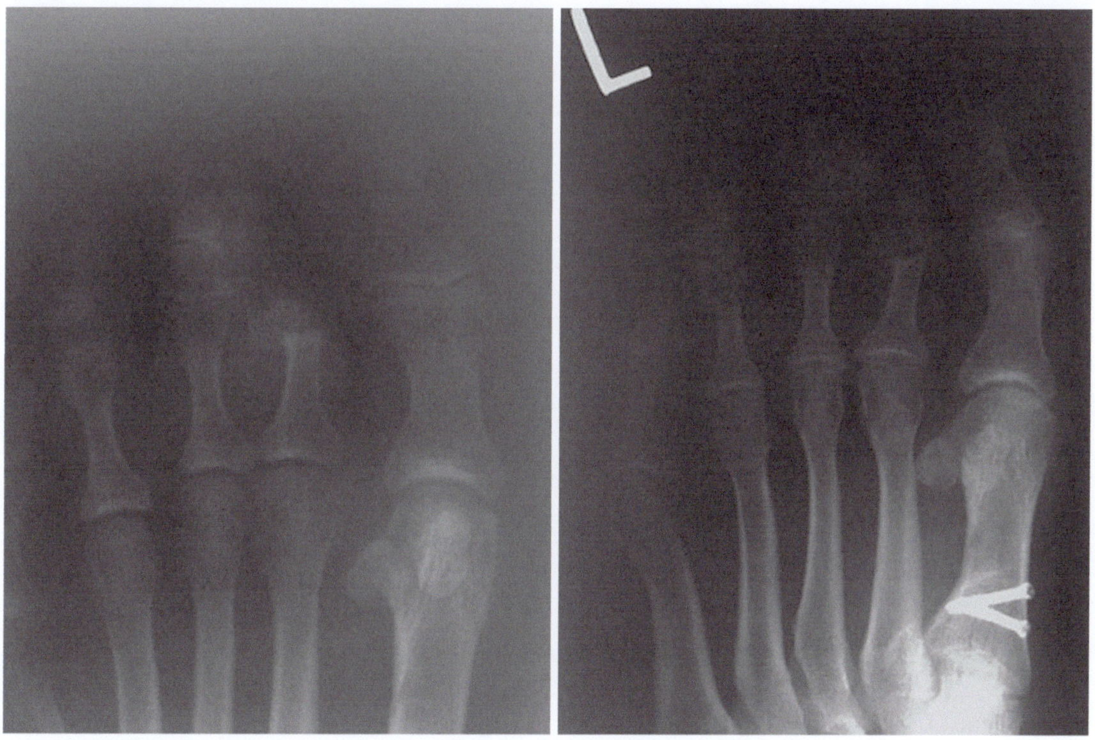

Fig. 4.8 Lateral deviation of the middle phalanx on the shortened proximal phalanx of the left second toe was shown in dorsal-plantar and oblique view radiographs

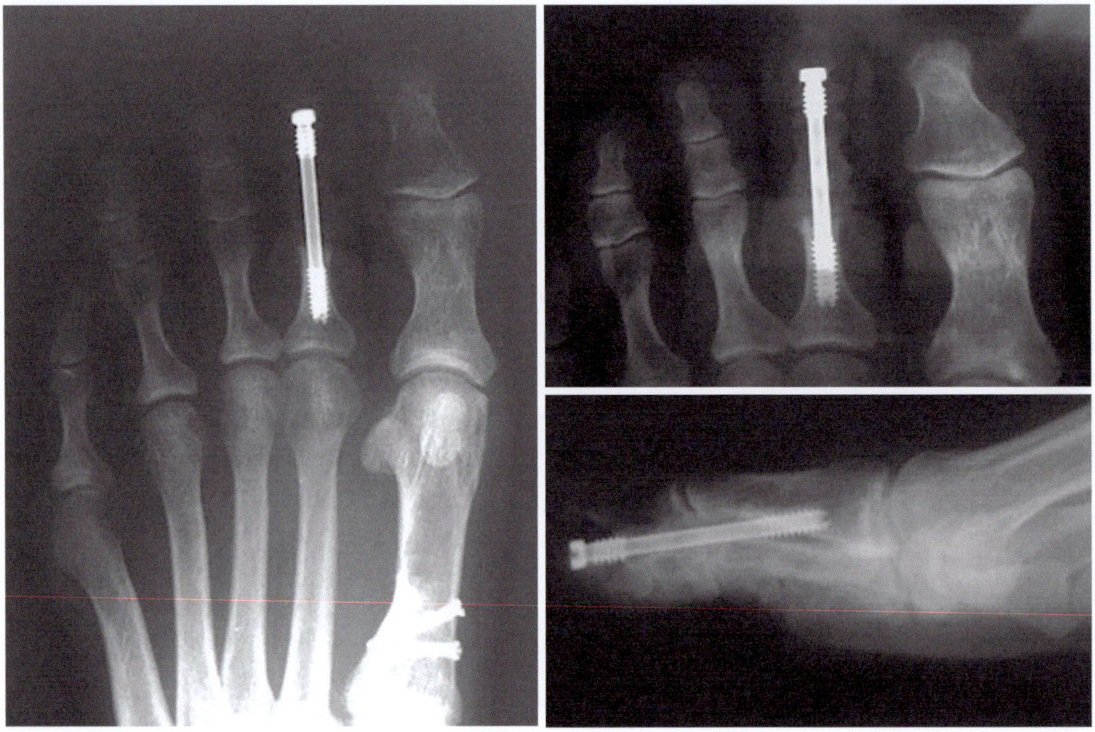

Fig. 4.9 Three months after revision fusion, radiographs showed progressive union without sign of screw loosening or breakage

Pearls and Pitfalls

Avoid excessive bone resection; using bone cutter might increase chance of more bone loss and resulting oblique uneven bone cut. Distal proximal phalanx and proximal middle phalanx should be thoroughly freshened when treating a non-union. Headless screw fixation was helpful to maintain stability. Bone graft provides biologic substrate for healing.

Case 4.4 Flail Toe #2

History

A sixty-seven-year-old female with a history of prior resection arthroplasty of her left fourth hammer toe. Post-operatively she had developed an increasingly worse deformity and painful arthritis of the PIP. This unstable, excessively mobile toe would catch while putting on socks and shoes. She decided to proceed with surgery after failing conservative modalities. Examination of her left foot showed an unstable PIP joint with floppiness of the fourth toe. There was no apparent connectivity between the middle and the proximal phalanges on palpation. She had tenderness at the distal proximal phalanx without callus or ulceration. Her preoperative radiographs showed excessive shortening of the proximal phalanx and dorsolateral deviation of the fourth toe (Fig. 4.10).

Reasons for Failure

Excessive bone removal of the proximal and middle phalanges and failure to achieve stable fibrous non-union.

Surgical Plan

Fusion of the PIP joint with cortical screw fixation combined with additional bone graft to create proper toe length, bone bridging between proximal and middle phalanges, and correct floppiness of the left fourth toe.

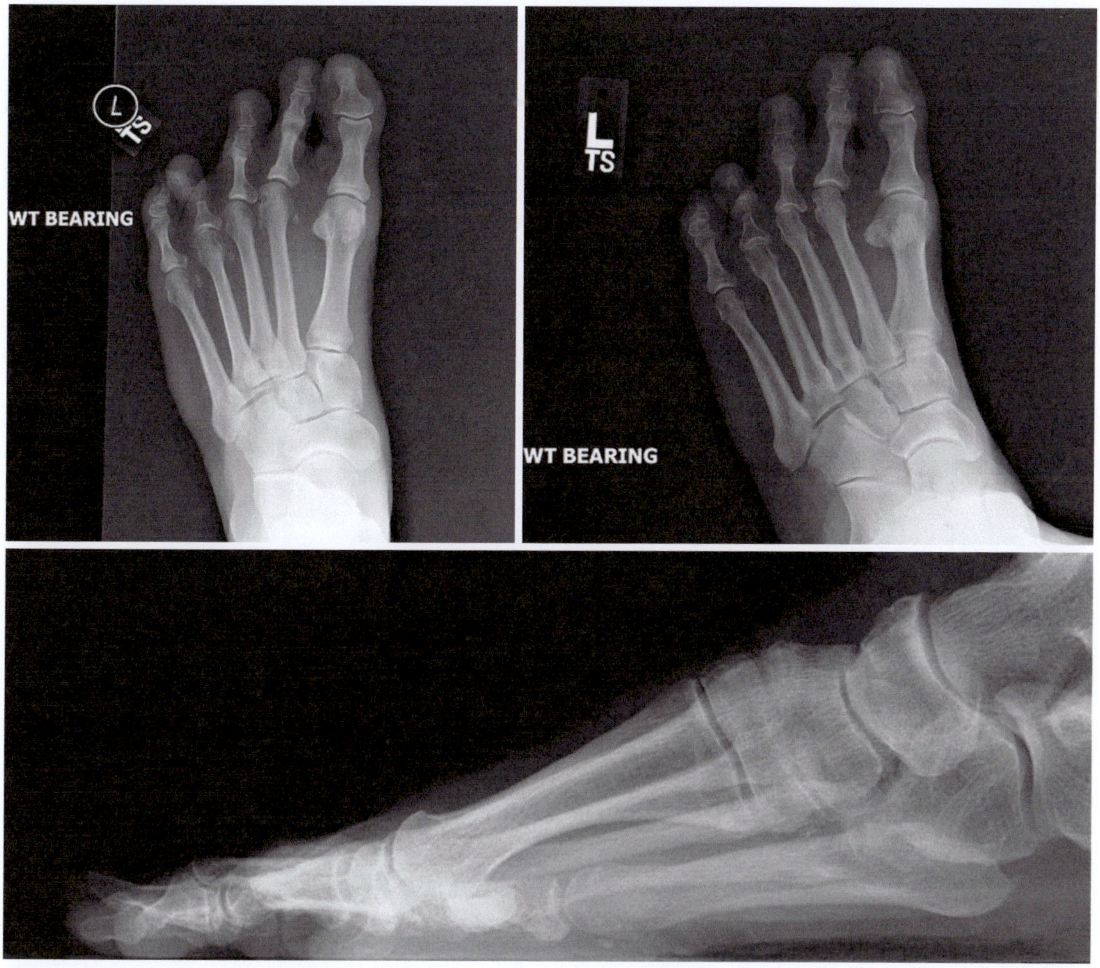

Fig. 4.10 Excessive bone resection resulted in large gap between proximal and middle phalanges with an unstable left fourth toe

Approach

A 3.5 cm dorsal incision extending from just proximal to the toe nail up to the MTP joint was made. Sharp dissection was carried down to the PIP joint. There was scar tissue encasing the degenerative joint. The joint fibrosis was excised; the proximal and distal ends for PIP joint fusion were freshened. The DIP joint had minimal or no motion to it. We used 1.5 mm drill in antegrade fashion through the middle phalanx and penetrated out the tip of the toe. Then the drill was passed from the tip of the toe retrograde up to the proximal phalanx. A 2 mm fully threaded screw, 24 mm long, was advanced under fluoroscopic guidance to secure and provide compression to the PIP fusion. We took the bone graft from the calcaneus with a 2 mm diameter trephine trocar device. The bone graft was morselized and delivered to the fusion site. The final alignment and fusion site were rechecked under fluoroscope, and then the skin was closed.

Implants

A 2 mm fully threaded non-cannulated interfragment screw, 24 mm in length.

Post-operative Care

At about 2 weeks after operation, the patient was allowed flat foot weight bearing in the post-operative shoe with no rolling through the forefoot. The toe alignment and screw fixation was well maintained (Fig. 4.11). She came back to us for her concern of infection at 3 weeks. The area of dorsal incision had dehiscence with some serosanguinous oozing. We placed silver impregnated dressing into her wound which she had changed at home for about 2 more months until complete healing. At 3 months, she was allowed weight bearing with rolling through in a hard sole shoe. She was instructed to increase her daily activities as tolerated. At 4 months, her toe was stable, well aligned, and non-tender. Radiographs showed intact arthrodesis screw and maintained toe alignment with improvement of PIP joint fusion (Fig. 4.12). Four years after operation, she returned to our clinic with a new complaint on the second hammer toe with good clinical result on the operated fourth toe (Fig. 4.13).

Pearls and Pitfalls

Excessive bone resection led to floppiness and poorly cosmetic result following a PIP resection. PIP joint fusion might yield a more reliable outcome in rigid hammer toe. Wound care with silver impregnated mesh dressings permitted final healing. In an unsalvageable toe, partial toe amputation may give satisfactory results.

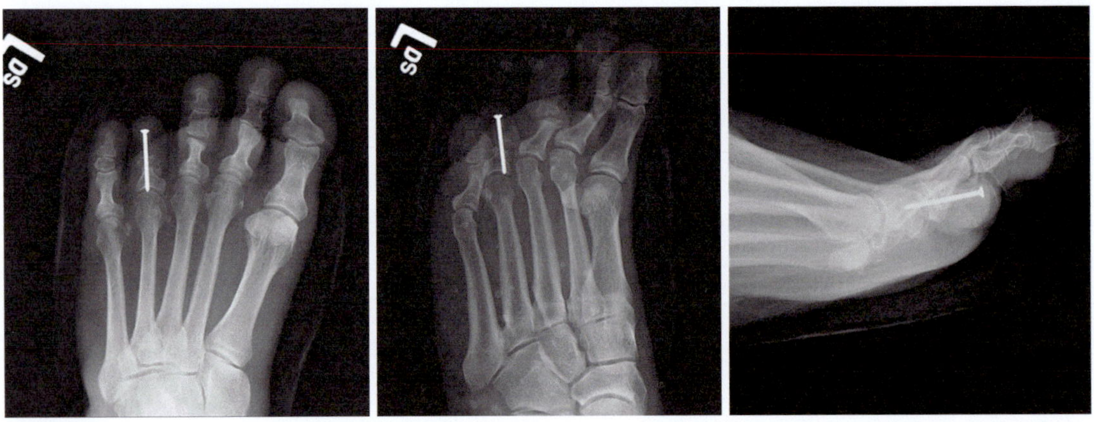

Fig. 4.11 Radiographs of the left foot at 2 weeks showed well-maintained alignment of the fourth toe and stable screw fixation

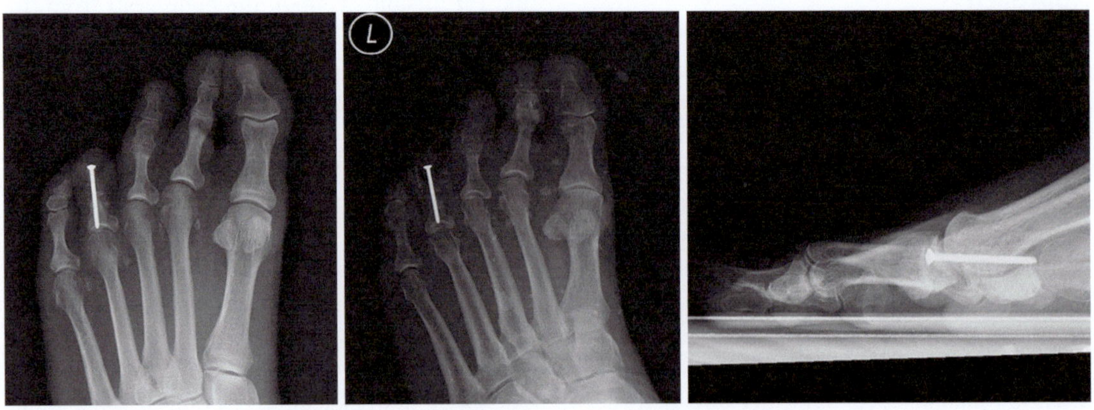

Fig. 4.12 After 4 months, radiographs showed intact arthrodesis screw and maintained toe alignment with improvement of PIP joint fusion

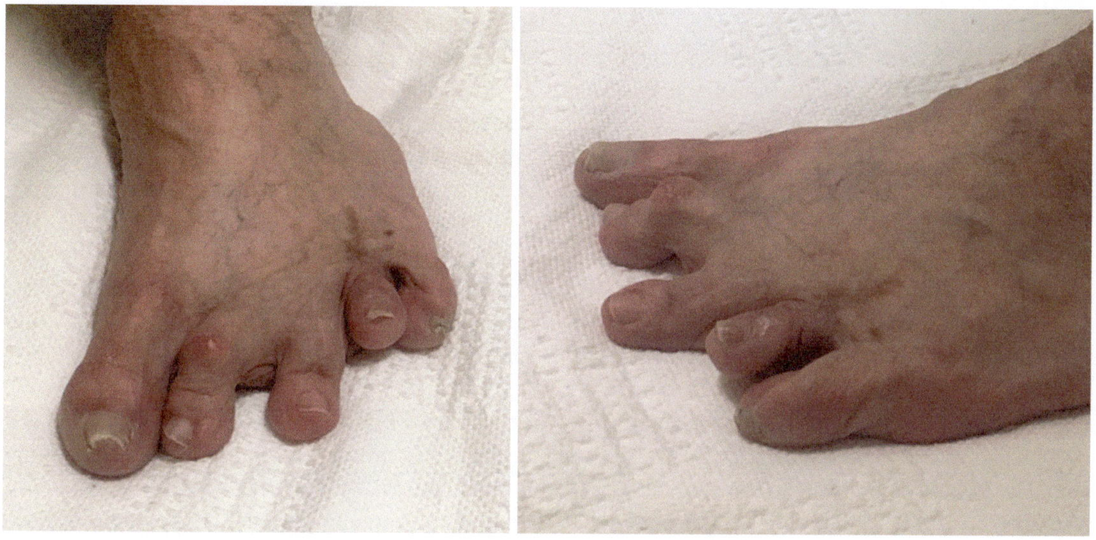

Fig. 4.13 She returned to our clinic 4 years later with a new complaint on the second hammer toe with good clinical outcome on the operated fourth toe

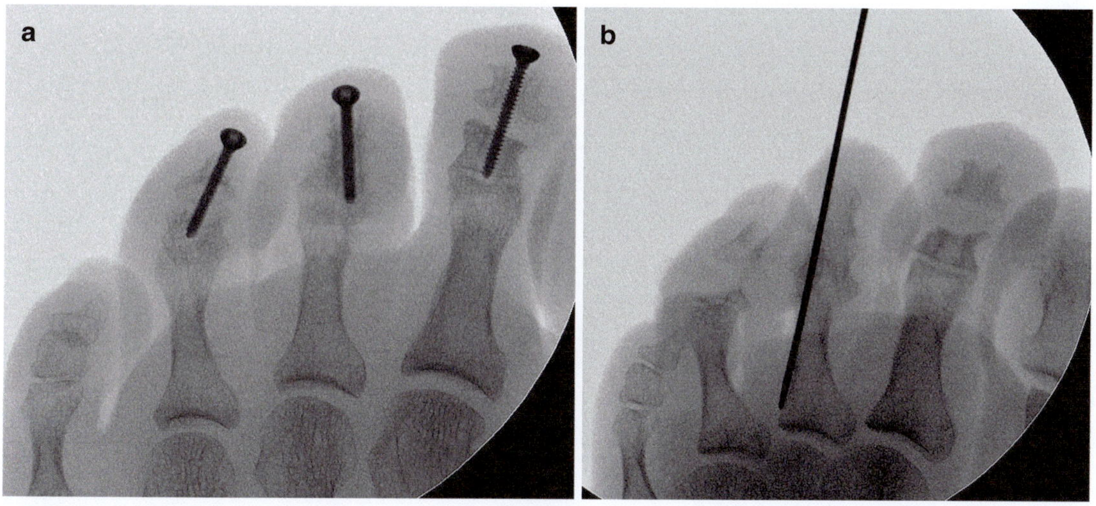

Fig. 4.14 (**a**) Screw loosening and non-union after DIP fusion of the second and fourth toe. (**b**) After the articular surfaces of the PIP joint were removed, fusion site was stabilized with K-wire

Case 4.5 DIP Joint–Non-union

History

A 44-year-old female presented at our clinic with severely painful, inflamed, and deformed DIP joints of the left second, third, fourth toe. The pain was aggravated with palpation and DIP joint range of motion. At the prior surgery, she was diagnosed with mallet toe deformities of her left second, third, and fourth toe. These had been treated with DIP joint fusions. On radiographic examination, the second, fourth toes had DIP joints and developed non-union and hardware loosening with arthritic PIP joint of the third toe (Fig. 4.14a).

Reasons for Failure

Non-union from unknown cause with screw loosening of the DIP joint of the left second and fourth toes.

Surgical Plan

Revision DIP joint fusion of the second and fourth toes and PIP joint fusion of the third toe with K-wire fixation.

Approach

We revised the fusion of the DIP joints on the second and fourth toe through previous transverse incisions and fused the PIP joint of the third toe through new transverse incision. Fusion sites were prepped by scar tissue removal (Fig. 4.14b) followed by burring until decent bleeding bone was encountered. All the toes were fixed with K-wires after packing bone graft in the fusion site. The bone was harvested from the calcaneus by using a trocar/trephine device and packing it into the fusion sites (Fig. 4.15). At the end, we injected BMAC into all fusion sites.

Implants

0.045″ K-Wire

Post-operative Period

Patient was allowed to walk with heel weight bearing in the post-operative shoe (hard sole) until 6 weeks post-operatively. At 6 weeks, she could walk with full weight bearing as tolerated without rolling through. At 3-month post-operative period, she was allowed for rolling through in normal shoe with rigid sole.

Pearls and Pitfalls

Perform meticulous curettage until bleeding bone is observed. Fixation of the fusion site may require multiple K-wires in parallel, convergent or divergent configuration to help stabilize the fusion site in situations where there is more bone loss.

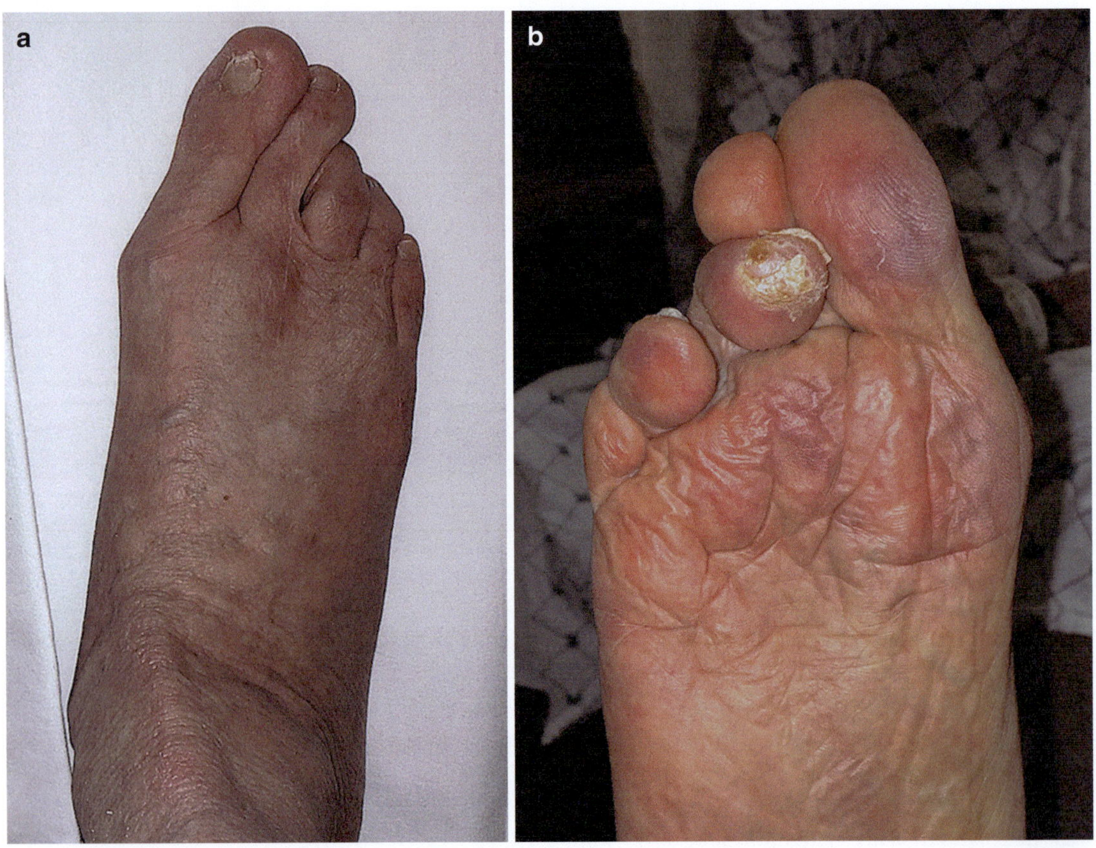

Fig. 4.15 (**a**) AP X-ray after fixing the 3rd PIP fusion with one K-wire, two K-wires were used for fixation at the second and the fourth toe to add more stability to the revision DIP fusion. (**b**) Oblique X-ray

Case 4.6 Amputation

History

The patient is 72-year-old female who presented with a major complaint of a painful callus on the lateral right foot. She also had hallux valgus and deviation of the second toe. On examination of her right foot, she had a significant hallux valgus deformity with crossover under the second toe. She also had lesser toe varus deformity (Fig. 4.16). She had a prominent bunionette deformity of the fifth toe with tenderness to palpation and a callus over the metatarsal head.

It was decided to address the hallux valgus by performing a chevron osteotomy which was fixed with a 2.0 mm screw. On the second toe, we made dorsal incision to expose metatarsal head, the shaft of proximal phalanx and the PIP joint. A PIP joint fusion and Weil osteotomy of the second toe were performed. Since the toe was still found to have a dorsal displacement and a varus deformity, we added an extensor digitorum brevis (EDB) transfer to the base of proximal phalanx. A proximal phalangeal shortening was done on the third toe with a closing wedge osteotomy. A PIP joint fusion was done on the fourth toe. Her bunionette deformity on the fifth toe was corrected with a Kramer osteotomy fixed with a K-wire. The K-wire at the fifth toe was removed at 10–14 days. All lesser toes were temporarily stabilized with K-wires which were removed at 6 weeks (Fig. 4.17). At 12 weeks, she was walking without toe off roll through in the post-operative shoe. Examination of her right foot demonstrated good healing with no point of tenderness. With standing, she had some dorsal overriding of the second toe to the third toe (Fig. 4.18a). Inspection from the plantar aspect, her fat pads looked thin with no ulcer (Fig. 4.18b). At 9-month post-operative period, she came to our clinic with a new chief complaint about right ankle pain and

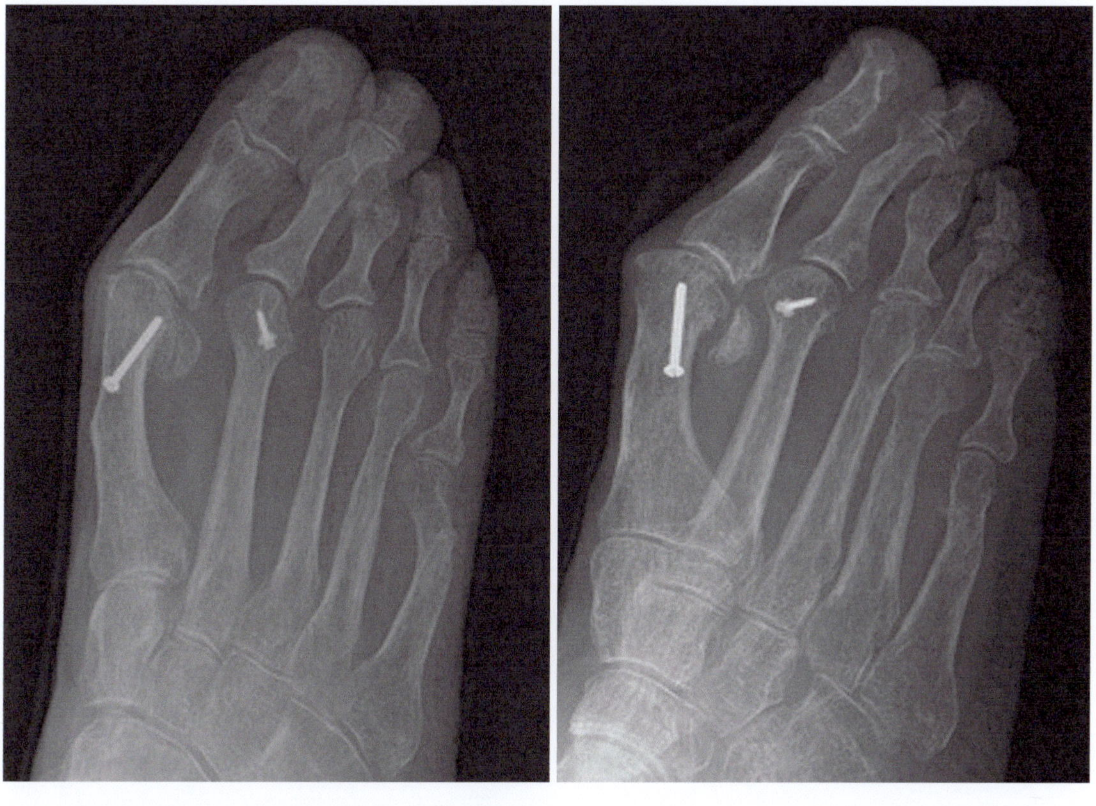

Fig. 4.16 Radiographs showed hallux valgus, crossover of the second toe with MTP joint subluxation, medial deviation of the third and fourth toes, and bunionette deformity of the fifth toe

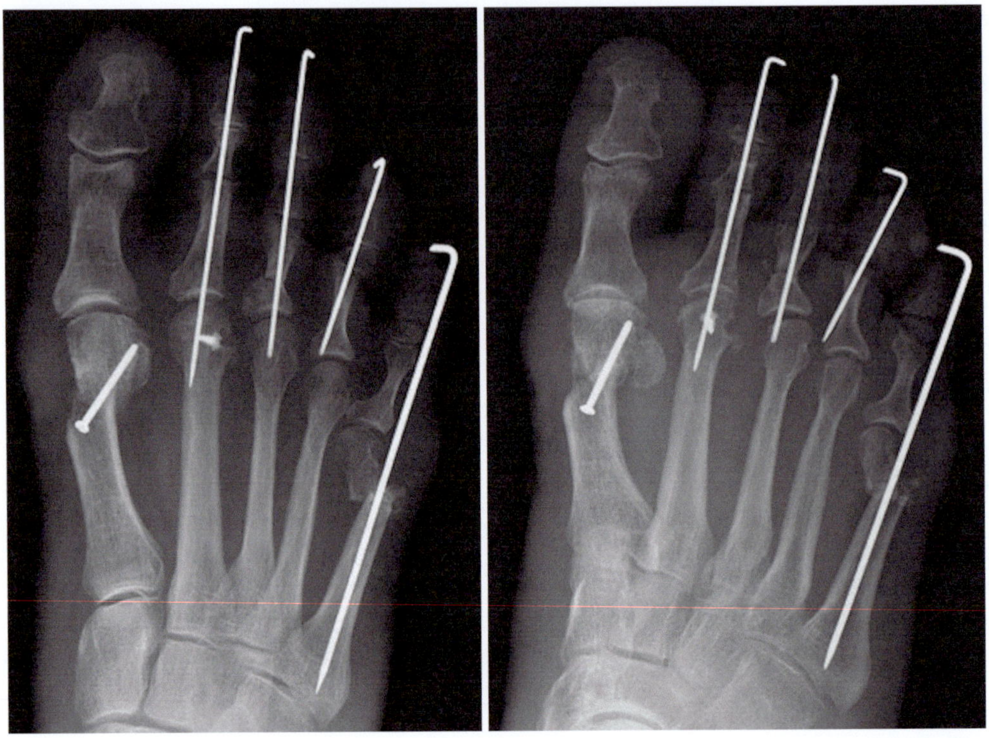

Fig. 4.17 Chevron osteotomy was performed for hallux valgus correction, and K-wire fixation was performed after correction of all lesser toes was complete

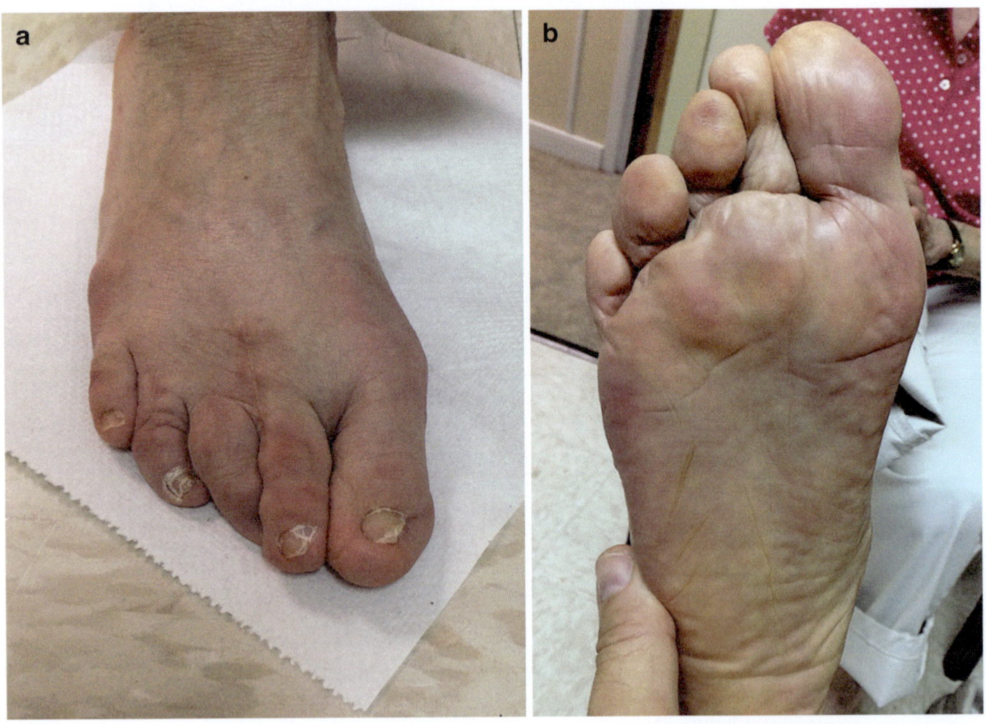

Fig. 4.18 Inspection of the right foot at 12 weeks after surgical correction of hallux valgus, lesser toe deformities, and bunionette. (**a**) DIP joint flexion deformity and medial deviation of the right third toe. (**b**) Patient had no plantar ulcer in spite of her unhealthy fat pad

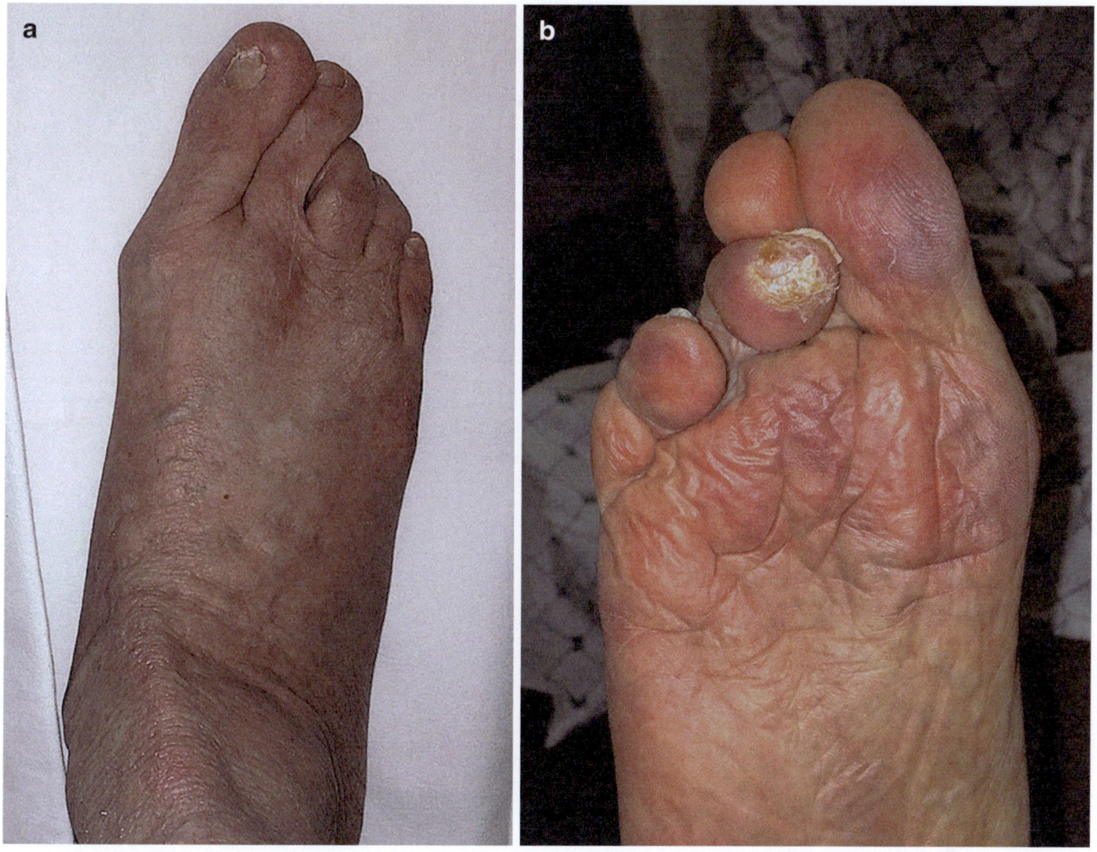

Fig. 4.19 At 9-month post-operative period. (**a**) The patient had progressive flexion deformity of DIP joint of the third toe and overriding of the second toe to the third toe. (**b**) She developed plantar ulcer and some breakdown at dorsolateral aspect of the tip of the right third toe

inversion weakness from posterior tibial tendon dysfunction. She also had progressive overriding of the second toe to the third toe (Fig. 4.19a) and plantar ulcer with some breakdown at distal dorsolateral aspect of the tip of third toe (Fig. 4.19b). Overall she was satisfied but needed treatment of her third toe. Since her hindfoot continued to collapse, we addressed both problems at once.

Reasons for Failure

Incompetent ligamentous structures with recurrent hallux valgus and medial deviation of the third DIP joint.

Surgical Plan

Amputation through the DIP joint during the surgical treatment for her posterior tibial tendon rupture.

Approach

After discussion with the patient, we proceeded with simultaneous flatfoot reconstruction and third toe amputation through the DIP joint. After we corrected flatfoot deformities with medial displacement calcaneal sliding osteotomy (MDCO), FDL transfer to navicular, posterior tibial tendon debridement, an incision was made across the tip of the toe, taking care to protect the flap plantarly. The bone was then removed at the DIP joint. This wound was then irrigated, and the skin flap was closed. The excess tissue was debrided, and this was sutured with 3-0 nylon.

Implants

None

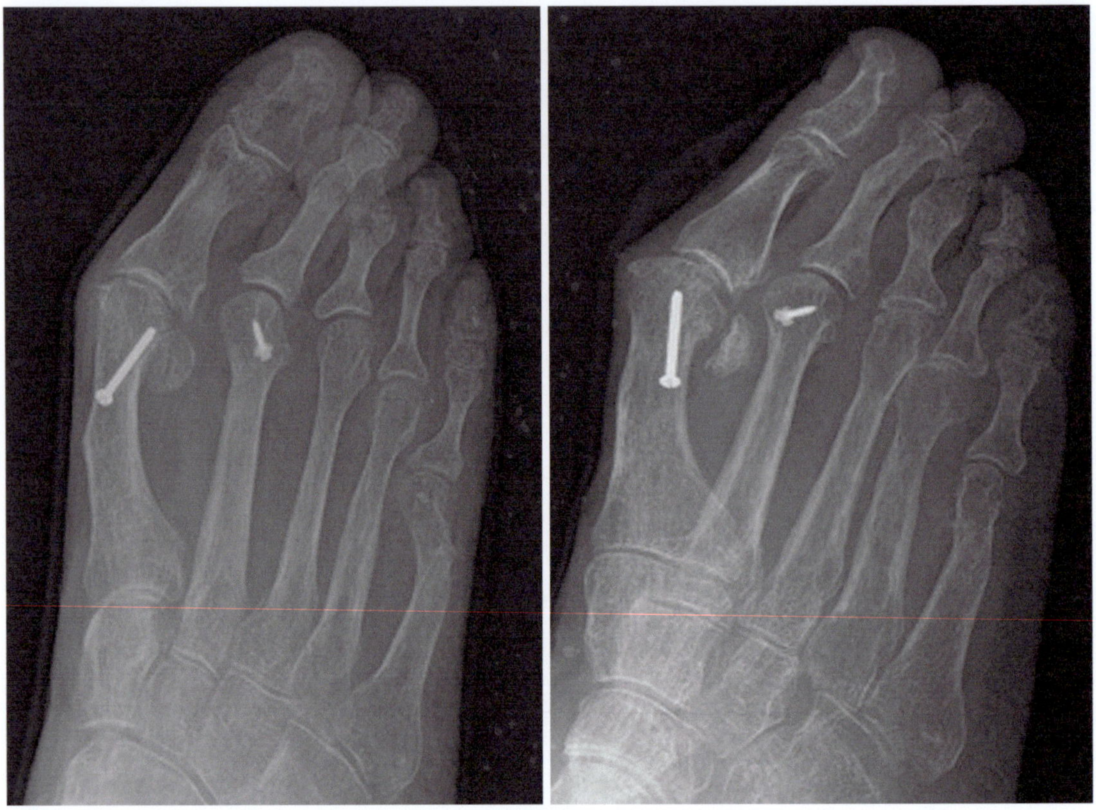

Fig. 4.20 At 12 weeks after flatfoot reconstruction and amputation through the DIP joint of the right third toe, no osteolysis found in her right foot radiographs

Post-operative Care

Patient came to visit at 2 weeks after surgery for stitch removal and dressing change. Her foot was immobilized in 20-degree plantar flexion at the ankle, and weight bearing was not allowed. At 6 weeks, her incisions were well healed, and progressive weight bearing was allowed in a boot with 20-lbs weight increment every other day as tolerated. Her ankle was then kept in a lace-up brace at 12 weeks. Surgical wound at her right third toe healed very well without recurrent ulcer and no evidence of the osteolysis in her foot radiographs (Fig. 4.20). Physical therapy prescription to work on both active and passive inversion was given.

Pearls and Pitfalls

Partial amputation may be considered as the last salvage procedure in cases with chronic pain or ulceration. Preserving plantar skin for flap coverage should always be used.

References

1. Coughlin MJ, Dorris J, Polk E. Operative repair of the fixed hammer toe deformity. Foot Ankle Int. 2000;21:94–104.
2. Coughlin MJ. Lesser toe abnormalities. J Bone Joint Surg Am. 2002;84-A(8):1445–69.
3. Myerson MS, Shereff MJ. The pathologic anatomy of claw and hammer toes. J Bone Joint Surg Am. 1989;71-A(1):45–9.
4. Shirzad K, Kiesau CD, DeOrio JK, et al. Lesser toe deformities. J Am Acad Orthop Surg. 2011;19:505–14.
5. Scheck M. Etiology of acquired hammer toe deformity. Clin Orthop Relat Res. 1977;123:63–9.
6. Ellington JK. Hammertoes and clawtoes: proximal interphalangeal joint correction. Foot Ankle Clin N Am. 2011;16:547–58.
7. Scott AT. Lesser toe deformities and sesamoid pathology. In: Parekh SG, editor. Foot and ankle surgery. New Delhi: Jaypee Brothers; 2012. p. 73–105.
8. Coughlin MJ. Lesser toe deformities. In: Coughlin MJ, Saltzman C, Anderson RB, editors. Mann's surgery of the foot and ankle. St. Louis: Mosby; 2014. p. 322–424.

9. O'Kane C, Kilmartin T. Review of proximal interphalangeal joint excisional arthroplasty for the correction of second hammer toe deformity in 100 cases. Foot Ankle Int. 2005;26(4):320–5.
10. Sung W, Weil L, Weil LS. Retrospective comparative study of operative repair of hammer toe deformity. Foot Ankle Spec. 2014;7(3):184–91.
11. Higgs SL. Hammer toe. Postgrad Med J. 1931;6:130–2.
12. Kelikian H. Deformities of the lesser toes. In: Hallux valgus, allied deformities of the forefoot and metatarsalgia. Philadelphia: W.B. Saunders; 1965. p. 292–304.
13. Bouche RT, Heit EJ. Combined plantar plate and hammertoe repair with flexor digitorum longus tendon transfer for chronic, severe sagittal plane instability of the lesser metatarsophalangeal joints: preliminary observations. J Foot Ankle Surg. 2008;47:125–37.
14. Haddad SL, Sabbagh RC, Resch S, et al. Results of flexor-to-extensor and extensor brevis tendon transfer for correction of the crossover second toe deformity. Foot Ankle Int. 1999;20(12):781–8.
15. Myers SH, Schon LC. Forefoot tendon transfers. Foot Ankle Clin N Am. 2011;16:471–88.
16. Schrier JC, Keijsers NL, Matricali GA, et al. Lesser toe PIP joint resection versus PIP joint fusion: a randomized clinical trial. Foot Ankle Int. 2016;37(6):569–75.
17. Ellington JK, Anderson RB, Davis WH, et al. Radiographic analysis of proximal interphalangeal joint arthrodesis with an intramedullary fusion device for lesser toe deformities. Foot Ankle Int. 2010;31(5):372–6.
18. Solan MC, Davies MS. Revision surgery of the lesser toes. Foot Ankle Clin N Am. 2011;16:621–45.
19. Klammer G, Baumann G, Moor BK, et al. Early complications and recurrence rates after kirschner wire transfixion in lesser toe surgery: a prospective randomized study. Foot Ankle Int. 2012;33(2):105–12.
20. Reece AT, Stone MH, Young AB. Toe fusion using Kirschner wire: a study of the postoperative infection rate and related problems. J R Coll Surg Edinb. 1987;32:158–9.
21. Zingas C, Katcherian DA, Wu KK. Kirschner wire breakage after surgery of the lesser toes. Foot Ankle Int. 1995;16:504–9.
22. Reichert K, Caneva RG. The use of Kirschner wire fixation in forefoot surgery. J Foot Surg. 1983;22:218–21.
23. Fernández CS, Wagner E, Ortiz C. Lesser toes proximal interphalangeal joint fusion in rigid claw toes. Foot Ankle Clin N Am. 2012;17:473–80.
24. Nery C, Baumfeld D. Salvage of lesser toes deformities: "revision forefoot". Tech Foot Ankle. 2017;16(1):20–7.
25. Coughlin MJ, Mann R. Lesser toe deformities. In: Coughlin MJ, Mann RA, editors. Surgery of the foot and ankle. St. Louis: Mosby; 1999. p. 320–91.
26. Myerson MS. Correction of lesser toe deformity. In: Myerson MS, editor. Reconstructive foot and ankle surgery: management of complications. Philadelphia: W.B. Saunders; 2010. p. 97–108.
27. Conklin MJ, Smith RW. Treatment of the atypical lesser toe deformity with basal hemiphalangectomy. Foot Ankle Int. 1994;15(11):585–94.
28. Daly PJ, Johnson KA. Treatment of painful subluxation or dislocation at the second and third metatarsophalangeal joints by partial proximal phalanx excision and subtotal webbing. Clin Orthop. 1992;278:164–70.
29. Cahill BR, Connor DE. A long-term follow-up on proximal phalangectomy for hammer toes. Clin Orthop. 1972;86:191–2.
30. Myerson MS, Filippi J. Bone block lengthening of the proximal interphalangeal joint for managing the floppy toe deformity. Foot Ankle Clin N Am. 2010;15:663–8.
31. Coughlin MJ. Operative repair of the mallet toe deformity. Foot Ankle Int. 1995;16(3):109–16.
32. Raja S, Barrie JL, Henderson AA. Distal phalangectomy for mallet toe. J Foot Ankle Surg. 2003;9(4):215–6.

5 Revision Surgery for the Lesser Metatarsophalangeal Joints

Gonzalo F. Bastías, Jakrapong Orapin, and Lew C. Schon

Key Takeaway Points

- Persistent metatarsalgia after Weil osteotomy is produced secondary to the relative lowering of the metatarsal head when the osteotomy is made with a single oblique cut or in an increased angle (more than 25°).
- Excessive shortening of the metatarsal head may lead to transfer metatarsalgia which can be the result of a non-harmonic parabola in the frontal or sagittal planes.
- Floating toe describes the inability of a toe to purchase the ground due to dorsiflexion of the MTP joints during static stance and is the most common complication after Weil osteotomy.
- Lesser MTP instability is well known to be associated with attenuation and tearing of the plantar plate which can lead to instability both on the sagittal and coronal planes.
- Recurrent subluxation and dislocation of the lesser MTP joints may lead to degeneration and arthritis, whose management is challenging and unpredictable.
- The main indication for revision surgery for bunionette deformity is recurrence after isolated exostectomy of the head of the fifth metatarsal or isolated soft tissue procedures.

G. F. Bastías (✉)
Department of Orthopedic Surgery, Foot and Ankle Unit, Clínica Las Condes, Las Condes, Chile

Department of Orthopedic Surgery, Universidad de Chile Complejo Hospitalario San José, Santiago, Chile
e-mail: gbastias@clinicalascondes.cl

J. Orapin
Faculty of Medicine, Ramathibodi Hospital, Mahidol University, Department of Orthopaedic Surgery, Bangkok, Thailand

L. C. Schon
Department of Orthopaedic Surgery, MedStar Union Memorial Hospital, Baltimore, MD, USA

Georgetown School of Medicine, Washington, DC, USA

Johns Hopkins University, Baltimore, MD, USA

Fischell Literati Faculty, University of Maryland, Fischell Department of Bioengineering, College Park, MD, USA

Introduction

Most surgical procedures addressing the lesser metatarsophalangeal joints (MTPJ) are used as part of the operative management of metatarsalgia, lesser toe deformity, MTPJ instability, or bunionette deformity. Even though these procedures typically lead to favorable results in many

M. J. Berkowitz et al. (eds.), *Revision Surgery of the Foot and Ankle*, https://doi.org/10.1007/978-3-030-29969-9_5

patients [1–5], there is a subset of patients that will present with recurrent pain and deformity. Requirement for revision surgery in this segment is usually the result of sub-optimal initial surgical planning, incorrect choice of primary procedure, or underestimation of the underlying progressive pathologic process.

The management of patients with recurrent pain and deformity after surgery involving the lesser MTPJ is challenging. These patients may present after one or several surgeries with worsening of the initial symptoms and a high incidence of dissatisfaction with their previous management. Many unique patient factors such as their personality, health issues, compliance, life/work demands, attitude, and general outlook play a major role. This must be coupled with nuances of the specific condition to ensure an ideal customized plan, technical execution, follow-up, and final result. Timeframe to healing and its impact on the patients function and pain must be anticipated and expressed. Outcome expectations should be addressed with understanding of risks and the possibility of incomplete recovery with residual pain, swelling, deformity, and disability.

Conservative measures such as the use of insoles with metatarsal pads and wide-box shoes should be reconsidered and implemented before proceeding with revision surgery. Chronic health conditions and recalcitrant pain should be managed by a multidisciplinary team involving the internist, physiatrists, and other subspecialists. As neurogenic pain can be difficult to improve, emphasis should be directed to neurologic pain medications and modalities.

Evaluation

A thorough and complete medical history should be obtained, including previous surgery reports and imaging studies in order to assess the previous condition of the foot and estimate any progressive condition or deformity. Special attention should be paid on previous hallux valgus or first metatarsal surgery, due to the possible influence of first ray malunion or MTPJ stiffness on lesser metatarsal pathology.

Physical examination should emphasize on locating the specific sources of pain and make them recognizable and rated by the patient. Palpation of points of tenderness, bony prominences, and intermetatarsal spaces must be performed. Joint mobilization of the entire foot but especially on the forefoot and midfoot is crucial since stiffness of the lesser MTPJ can be a common complain after previous surgery. A dorsal MTPJ drawer test should be performed for every lesser MTPJ looking for instability in the sagittal and transverse plane. Malalignment of the hallux, lesser toes, and hindfoot should be observed. Examination of the sole of the foot is of utmost importance to identify the location of plantar callosities or fat pad atrophy. Keratoses located strictly plantar to the metatarsal head reflect a functional or anatomic prominence of the corresponding metatarsal or elevation of an adjacent metatarsal during standing or the stance phase of gait. The presence of callosities more distal to the metatarsal head may be due to excessive length of the corresponding metatarsal or to shortening of an adjacent metatarsal during the propulsive phase [6]. Previous scars and approaches must be considered since they are crucial for revision surgical planning. Vascular status of the foot and digits should be noted, and peripheral pulses should be obtained especially in diabetic and smoker patients. The presence of inflammatory systemic diseases or neurologic disorders should be considered in the treatment plan.

Imaging assessment should include recent weight-bearing radiographs. Posteroanterior, oblique, and lateral views are useful to determine lesser MTPJ congruency and forefoot morphotype. Using only plain X-rays for measuring the metatarsal length may be misleading because of the high variability of radiographic measurements secondary to the observer or positioning of the foot and leg at the moment of the exam [7–9]. In addition, the use of CT scan or weight-bearing CT scan provides a valuable three-dimensional representation of the relationship between the metatarsals allowing to identify metatarsal elevation, declination, or shortening in a more detailed fashion, especially in the coronal and sagittal planes. CT scan also can give crucial information about the healing status of previous metatarsal osteotomies, bone loss, and MTPJ degenerative changes.

Magnetic resonance imaging (MRI) is useful to determine the presence of Freiberg disease or metatarsal stress fractures as well as assessing plantar plate pathology.

Surgical Planning

Recurrent Metatarsalgia/Transfer Metatarsalgia

The distal oblique metatarsal neck (Weil) osteotomy and its modifications are the most common and established procedures for the treatment of metatarsalgia [1, 10]. Nevertheless, recurrent symptoms after Weil osteotomy had been reported in between 2% and 26% of the patients [2, 8, 11, 12]. Highlander et al. reviewed 1131 Weil osteotomies reported in the literature, finding a 15% incidence of recurrent metatarsalgia [7].

The most common reason for persistent metatarsalgia after Weil osteotomy is the relative lowering of the metatarsal head that is produced when a single oblique cut is made or an increased angle (more than 25°) is used for making the osteotomy [10, 13]. According to various authors [11, 12, 14], this declination increases the pressure on the metatarsal head during the midstance, producing persistent symptoms even with a harmonized forefoot parabola according to Maestro et al. [15] on the anteroposterior plane. Plantar prominence is correlated to persistent metatarsalgia and plantar calluses [8, 11]. Modifications of the Weil osteotomy had been proposed to prevent the excessive declination of the head. Melamed et al. [16] proposed modifying the osteotomy by removing a slice or a dorsally based wedge of bone to minimize plantar displacement of the metatarsal head. The amount of the modification is variable and may be hard to control [17]. Maceira and colleagues introduced a three-step modification osteotomy aiming to recreate a more anatomic metatarsal by changing the direction of the shortening and making it coaxial to the bone instead of parallel to the plantar aspect of the foot [1]. Proximal metatarsal osteotomies had also been described for elevation of the metatarsal head in the primary setting [10, 18]. These osteotomies are usually more powerful for elevation of the metatarsal head because of their location but may be at increased risk of generating transfer metatarsalgia and should be used with caution.

In our opinion, elevation of the metatarsal head can usually be obtained by a new Weil osteotomy on the affected metatarsal, taking the precaution of removing a slice of bone to accomplish the desired elevation. Nevertheless, other distal or proximal opening or closing wedge osteotomies may be considered when considerable correction is required.

Another cause of recurrent metatarsalgia is undercorrection, mostly in the form of residual excessive metatarsal length. The appropriate amount of shortening can be underestimated intraoperatively, not accomplishing redistribution of plantar pressure in the other metatarsal heads. Stress fractures of the undercorrected metatarsal are not unusual to see and may lead to the cause of persistent symptoms [10, 19]. Revision osteotomy is recommended over the previous Weil osteotomy for additional shortening in a similar fashion as previously described.

By the other hand, excessive shortening may lead to transfer metatarsalgia which can be the result of a non-harmonic parabola in the frontal or sagittal planes. In these cases, the goal of revision surgery is to recreate a normal metatarsal parabola on both planes. On the frontal plane, adjacent metatarsals should be addressed, in order to balance the length relationship with the previously shortened metatarsal, with modified Weil osteotomies. Transfer metatarsalgia also may be caused by severe elevation of the metatarsal head in the sagittal plane. In these cases, surgical plan should include a proximal plantar translation or opening wedge osteotomy to plantarflex this metatarsal. It may also be necessary to perform multiple osteotomies to elevate the adjacent metatarsals.

Floating Toe/Metatarsophalangeal Stiffness

Floating toe describes the inability of a toe to purchase the ground due to dorsiflexion of the MTPJ (Fig. 5.1) during static stance [19] and is the most common complication after Weil osteotomy with a reported overall incidence of 36% [7]. The etiology of the floating toe is multifactorial, and it has been widely studied. As in recurrent metatarsalgia, the relative lowering of the head after conventional Weil osteotomy has a role in the dorsal subluxation of the MTPJ due to the depression of the center of rotation in relation to the intrinsic tendons, which exert an extensor pull on the MTPJ [1, 16, 20]. This malposition of the intrinsic muscles also has a role on postoperative stiffness and is the probable reason why floating toes and stiffness are related. As established previously, Weil osteotomy modifications improve this issue and minimize or prevent plantar displacement of the metatarsal head.

Concomitant hammer toe surgery with Weil osteotomy also increases the incidence of floating toe [21]. PIP joint arthrodesis or arthroplasty especially when situated without recreation of the natural flexion of the PIP exacerbates the elevation deformity. Other factors that may lead to developing a floating toe are plantar plate insufficiency and the dorsal approach to the joint that may lead to both capsular and skin contractures.

Multiple reports [2, 12, 21, 22] have shown that even in the presence of floating toes, Weil osteotomy is effective on reducing metatarsalgia symptoms, and they are usually reported as asymptomatic. Nevertheless, the symptoms of floating toe may be correlated with the severity of the deformity [7], but this has not been quantified on any report on the literature. In our experience, severe floating toes create shoe wear problems and can be annoying to the patient.

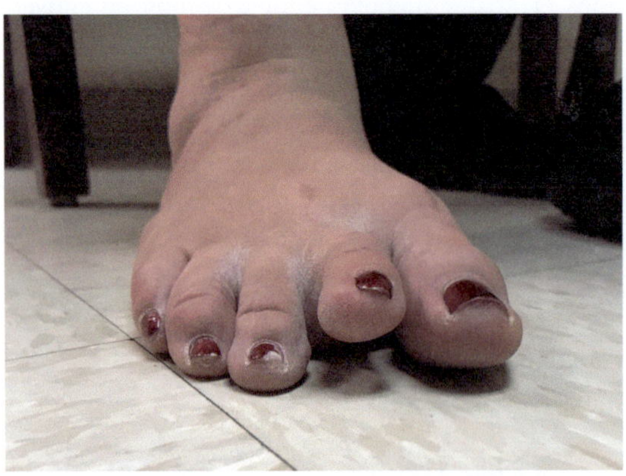

Fig. 5.1 Floating toe

A stepwise approach must be considered for the surgical correction of the floating toe considering all the factors involved in its etiology. In cases where the floating toe is not dislocated at the MTPJ, we proceed to repair of the plantar plate. If the plantar plate tissues are degenerative and not usable for a reconstruction or if there is a MTPJ dislocation, we perform a flexor-to-extensor tendon transfer.

Chronic Lesser MTP Instability: Sagittal/Coronal Malalignment

Lesser MTP instability is well-known to be associated with attenuation and tearing of the plantar plate [23, 24] which can lead to instability both on the sagittal and coronal planes. The collateral ligaments also contribute to instability of the joint in both planes [25].

Direct plantar plate repair in association with Weil osteotomy is currently a popular procedure for the primary management of lesser MTP instability [3, 26, 27]. It can be performed in conjunction with collateral capsule plication or release and tendon transfers in cases where the plantar plate is not amenable for repair or reconstruction. Unfortunately, at the moment of revision surgery, the extensor digitorum brevis (EDB) and the flexor digitorum longus (FDL) which are commonly used to stabilize the lesser MTPJ may not be available because they were used or transected during a previous surgery.

Even though recurrence after plantar plate repair is rare [3, 24], the most common cause of failure is underestimation of the tear grade or quality of the tissue. Another common cause of failure is not addressing concomitant first ray deformities and disorders as hallux valgus/rigidus in the first surgery, which leads to recurrent instability of the lesser MTPJ.

Revision surgery in these cases should include an indirect stabilization of the joint with tendon transfers and correction of the first ray deformities.

Lesser MTP instability is a progressive pathology that has several grading systems that take into account the physical examination and plantar plate pathologic features [23, 26, 28]. Most of these classifications correlate low-grade instability with mild deformity and coronal malalignment, whereas higher-grade instability is associated with dorsal subluxation/dislocation representing the sagittal instability that characterizes the natural progression of the deformity.

The most typical clinical representation of coronal instability and malalignment is the medial deviation or crossover toe [3, 28]. Although less common, a lateral deviation or valgus toe may also exist specially in association with hallux valgus deformity [24].

Our preferred technique for revision surgery for coronal instability is the use of the EDB transfer in association with Weil osteotomy.

EDB transfer was first described by Haddad and colleagues [28] to control coronal plane motion more effectively and to decrease the potential stiffness associated with the flexor-to-extensor transfer. In their description of the technique, they described superior results in cases of mild crossover toe, dorsomedial deviation, and flexible overlapping toe in comparison to FDL transfer. In cases of rigid deformities, however, flexor-to-extensor transfer provides more postoperative stability on the sagittal plane and should be the preferred procedure. Presence of an interdigital neuroma is considered a contraindication for EDB transfer since it requires surgical sectioning of the intermetatarsal ligament precluding its use as a pulley for the reconstructed EDB tendon. We prefer an alternative technique using a suture anchor to secure the tendon to the lateral (in the case of a medially deviated toe) or medial cortex (in the case of a valgus toe) of the proximal phalanx. In cases of recurrent coronal malalignment after EDB transfer and MTP soft tissue releases, a basilar proximal phalangeal osteotomy (Akinette) has been described with good results reported [29, 30].

Flexor-to-extensor transfer is a useful and effective procedure in the management of lesser MTP instability and lesser toe deformities [4, 28, 31–33]. Sagittal plane stability can be restored with flexor transfer as reported in a biomechanical cadaveric study by Bhatia and associates [34] after sectioning the plantar plate and collateral ligaments.

FDL tendon transfer has been commonly related with postoperative MTPJ stiffness [28, 31, 33]. Nevertheless, its influence on patient satisfaction is not entirely clear, and it seems that regaining stability of the MTPJ comes at the cost of increased stiffness and this is better tolerated than persistent instability or subluxation [31].

Indications for flexor-to-extensor tendon transfer in revision surgery include flexible or rigid persistent subluxation/dislocation after previous soft tissue release or isolated Weil osteotomy and deviation deformity where EDB transfer is not possible [35].

Lesser MTPJ Osteoarthritis

The management of lesser MTPJ osteoarthritis is challenging and unpredictable. One of the most common etiologies of lesser MTPJ arthritis [36] is degeneration secondary to recurrent subluxation and dislocation.

Rheumatoid arthritis usually involves the forefoot, producing progressive deformity and lateral dislocation of the MTPJ. Fortunately, with the widespread use of disease-modifying rheumatic pharmacologic treatment, the number of severe cases is decreasing, and low-grade arthritis is much more commonly seen.

Freiberg's disease is another common cause of lesser MTPJ arthropathy, consisting on an avascular necrosis of the metatarsal head leading to progressive degenerative changes and ultimately arthritis in the final stages. This pathology affects mainly the second metatarsal but also has been described on the third and fourth metatarsal [37, 38]. Other less common causes of lesser MTPJ osteoarthritis include metabolic disorders such as Charcot neuroarthropathy and gout.

Multiple surgical alternatives have been described for lesser MTPJ osteoarthritis [36, 38–43]. Joint preserving alternatives include cheilectomy and dorsiflexion or shortening metatarsal osteotomies. Preoperative assessment using MRI as well as the macroscopic intraoperative evaluation of the remaining cartilage of the metatarsal head and first phalangeal base should lead the decision-making process. In early stages, where the involvement of the joint surface is limited, debridement with resection of osteophytes and removal of loose bodies is a reasonable option with good results reported in the literature [36, 38]. Advanced degenerative changes should be approached with a dorsal wedge metatarsal osteotomy as first described by Gauthier [44]. Resection of a 1–2 mm dorsal wedge (Fig. 5.2) is useful to dorsally translate the plantar aspect of the metatarsal, reorienting healthy cartilage into the joint [10, 39, 45]. Joint sparing procedures have the most predictable results and should be considered in conjunction with flexor-to-extensor tendon transfer in patients with subluxated/dislocated MTPJ to obtain joint congruency. Concomitant deformities of the hallux as well as any first ray insufficiency should be addressed at the time of revision surgery.

Salvage options include excision/interpositional arthroplasty, MTPJ arthrodesis, and metatarsal realignment. These techniques have unpredictable results [36, 42, 46] and should be reserved only in cases of intractable chronic metatarsalgia in low-demand patients.

Recurrent Bunionette Deformity

The bunionette deformity is characterized by a painful prominence of the fifth metatarsal head secondary to a valgus deviation of the fifth metatarsal and medial displacement of the fifth toe resulting in bursal inflammation and callosity [47]. Recurrence is the main indication for revision surgery for a bunionette deformity, especially after isolated exostectomy of the head of the fifth metatarsal or isolated soft tissue procedures. In general, exostectomy is not effective for bunionettes with associated intractable plantar keratosis under the fifth metatarsal head, as the exostectomy does not correct the position of the metatarsal head or the 4–5 intermetatarsal angle [48]. In the same way, isolated resection of the bursa and callosities without bony correction does not address the underlying pathology.

Our preferred method for primary and revision correction of the bunionette deformity is the Kramer technique, which utilizes a percutaneous distal oblique fifth metatarsal osteotomy that allows bony translation to correct the angular deformity [49].

Percutaneous or minimally invasive distal metatarsal osteotomies, such as the Kramer procedure, have been described as effective method of correcting the deformity and relieving symp-

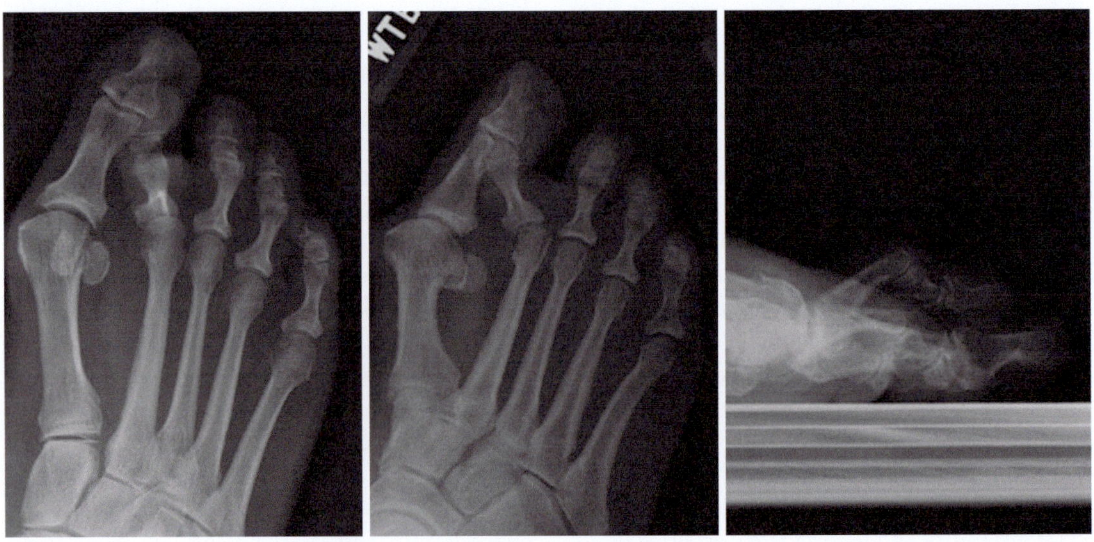

Fig. 5.2 Patient with second cock-up and crossover toe

tomatic deformities with a low incidence of recurrence and complications [47, 49–54].

Clinical Cases

Case 5.1 Flexor-to-Extensor Tendon Transfer

History

- The patient is a 75-year-old female with a severe bunion deformity and metatarsalgia of the second toe (Fig. 5.2).
- On examination, she had a painful bunion with second cock-up and crossover toe that was fairly flexible.
- She had a painful callus under the second metatarsal head.

Surgical Technique

- The skin is incised in line with the second ray centered over the MTP joint. We recommend incising the capsule adjacent to the extensor tendons with a longitudinal capsulotomy and perform the capsular release including the collateral ligaments of the metatarsal head that contribute to the deformity.
- A standard Weil osteotomy is performed, removing a 1 mm wedge of bone with two parallel cuts (total shortening should be 3 mm including the kerf), and then it is fixed in place with a solid 2.0 mm twist-off screw.
- Hammertoe deformity of the PIP joint must be corrected on its own, but in this case, MTP joint continued in a dorsiflexed position so it was decided to carry out the FDL tendon transfer.
- The FDL is harvested using a transverse plantar incision, 6–8 mm in length, located at the level of the MTP flexor crease (Fig. 5.3a). Bluntly dissected subcutaneous tissue and then the flexor sheath are identified and incised longitudinally. FDL tendon has to be isolated from FDB with recognition of its central raphe (Fig. 5.3b, c).
- We place the FDL under tension by threading it over a hemostat and percutaneously release its distal insertion on the distal phalanx with a stab incision over the distal flexor crease.
- The FDL is divided along its central raphe into two limbs and split to at the level of the MTP joint so it can be passed around the proximal phalanx. A path for each limb is established by blunt dissection along the lateral and medial aspect of the proximal phalanx in dorsal-plantar direction. Both FDL slips are grasped and delivered separately through the medial and lateral spaces alongside the proximal phalangeal base (Fig. 5.3d).

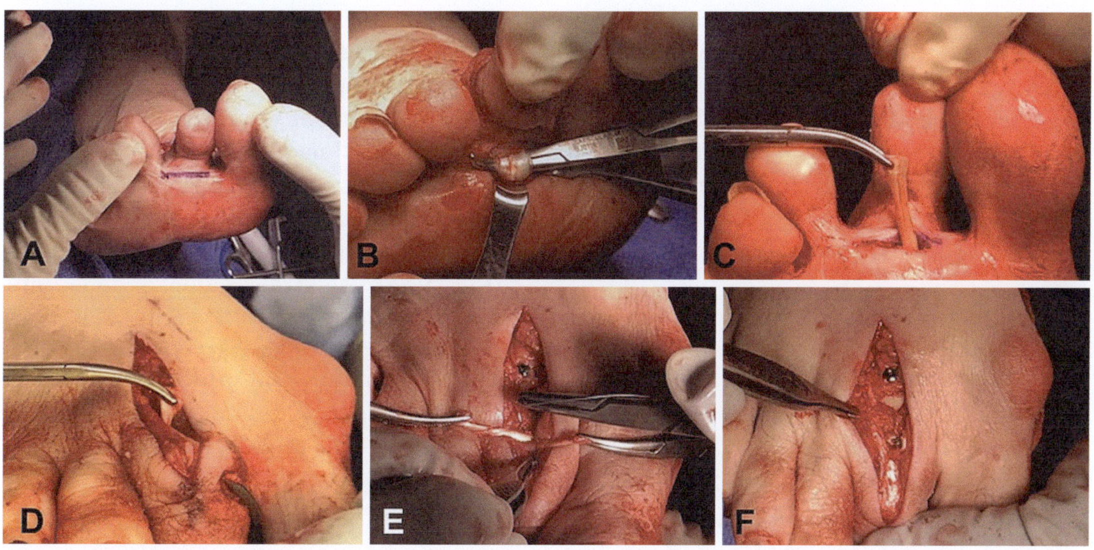

Fig. 5.3 Flexor-to-extensor transfer

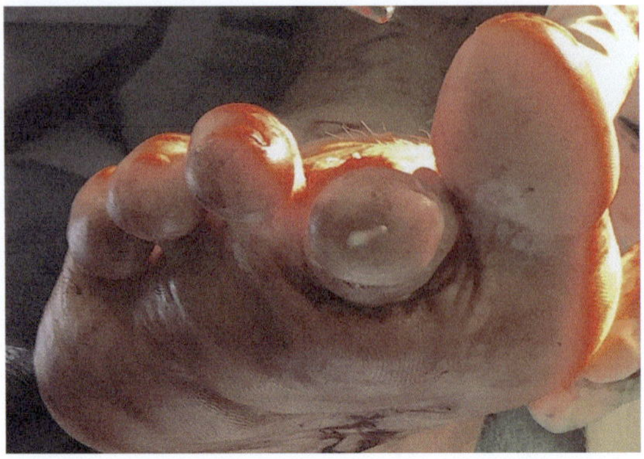

Fig. 5.4 Axial K-wire in plantar flexion position after FDL transfer

- The FDL slips are held with hemostats to prevent retraction; before fixing them together, other bony procedures including fixation, PIP resection arthroplasty, or fusion can be performed.
- The slips are crossed over the dorsum of the proximal phalanx using a nonabsorbable 4-0 Ethibond to sew to one another in a side-to-side fashion with the assistant surgeon holding down the toe to 20 degrees of plantar flexion in neutral ankle position (Fig. 5.3e, f).
- The redundant FDL can be used to reinforce the collateral ligaments if necessary. An axial K-wire is placed across the MTP joint for fixation (Fig. 5.4).
- After surgery, the patient is placed into a sterile dressing and a postoperative shoe. Heel weight-bearing of the extremity with assistive devices is indicated. The pin is removed at 6 weeks. The patient is allowed at this point to walk flat on the foot without rolling through the foot. At 12 weeks full forefoot weight-bearing is permitted.

Case 5.2 Extensor Digitorum Brevis (EDB) Transfer

History

- A 66-year-old woman with persistent metatarsalgia in addition to second and fourth hammer toes. She had a prior surgery for her deformities and developed a postoperative infection.
- On physical examination, she had a hyperextended second proximal interphalangeal joint with recent history of plantar ulcer. The patient complains of lateral deviation of the fourth toe, overload of the second metatarsal head with callus formation, and difficulties for regular shoe wear.
- X-rays are compatible with advanced osteoarthritis of first metatarsophalangeal joint but clinically without considerable symptoms (Fig. 5.5). Weil osteotomy and PIP joint fusion were performed on the second and fourth toes. EDB transfer was added for recalcitrant laterally deviation of the fourth toe.

Surgical Technique

- A longitudinal incision is firstly made above the PIP joint (Fig. 5.6a, b). The hyperextended and contracted PIP joint is addressed by doing a resection at the distal aspect of the proximal phalanx and proximal aspect of the middle phalanx (Fig. 5.6c, d).
- We proceed with soft tissue releases of the collateral ligaments at the level of the MTP joint that may be markedly contracted and stuck in a plantar flexed position after previous surgery. Weil osteotomy is then made removing a 1-mm-thick slice cut (Fig. 5.6e, f). The metatarsal head is shifted proximally and then fixed with a 2.0 mm twist-off compression screw (Fig. 5.6g, h). Finally, an axial K-wire is used for fixation of the second toe PIP joint fusion.
- In this patient, for the fourth toe, a curved incision was made above the PIP joint extending proximally and medially to be able to approach the MTP joint and intermetatarsal ligament in the third web space (Fig. 5.7a). Blunt dissection is done until we could identify the PIP joint, MTP joint, and extensor apparatus (Fig. 5.7b–d). Flexion deformity of PIP joint was corrected with fusion. We release the EDB tendon at the lateral aspect of the extensor expansion at the level of the PIP joint (Fig. 5.7e). Weil osteotomy was performed according to the same indications as the second toe (Fig. 5.7f, g).

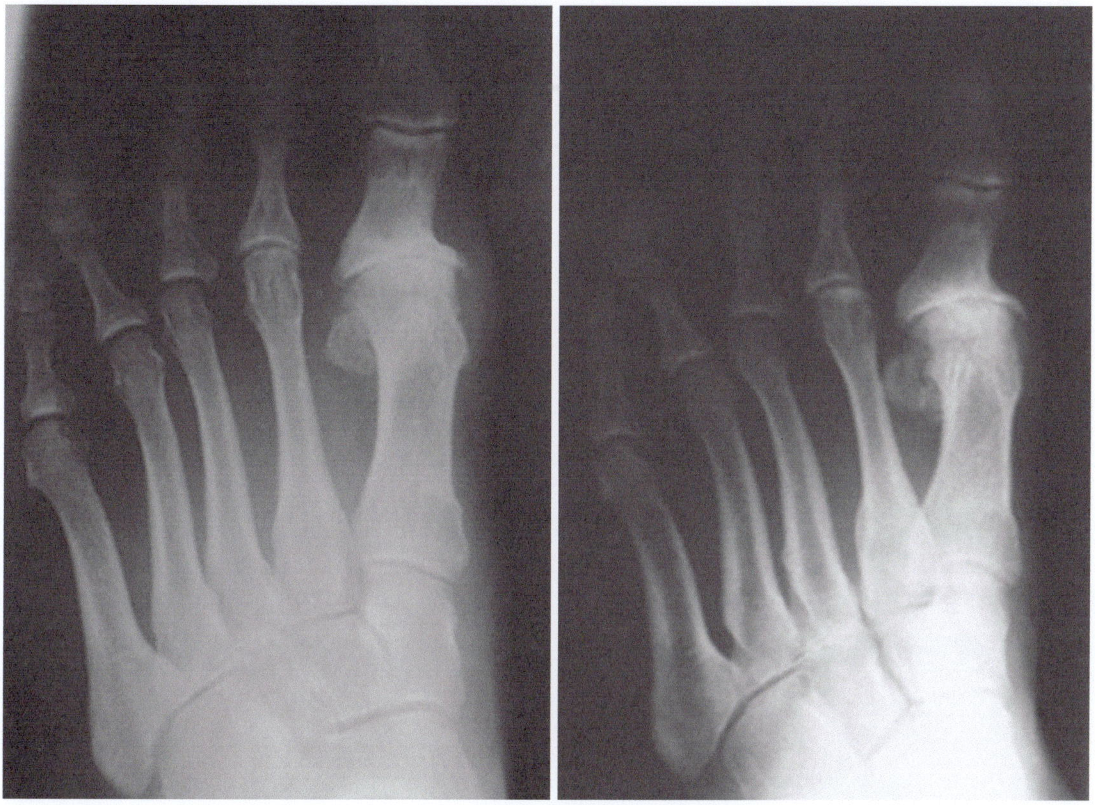

Fig. 5.5 Patient with MTP instability and lateral deviation of the second and fourth toes

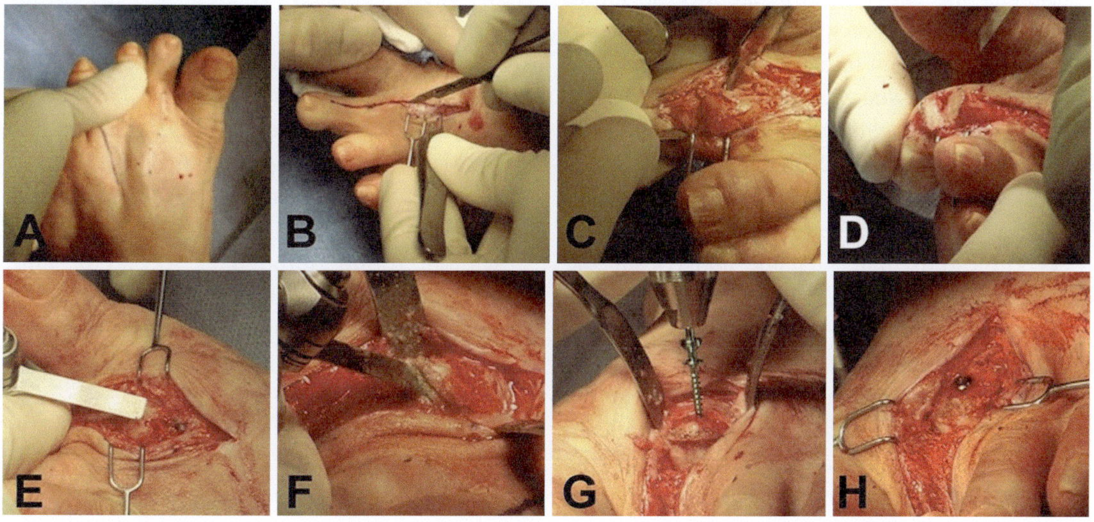

Fig. 5.6 Weil osteotomy

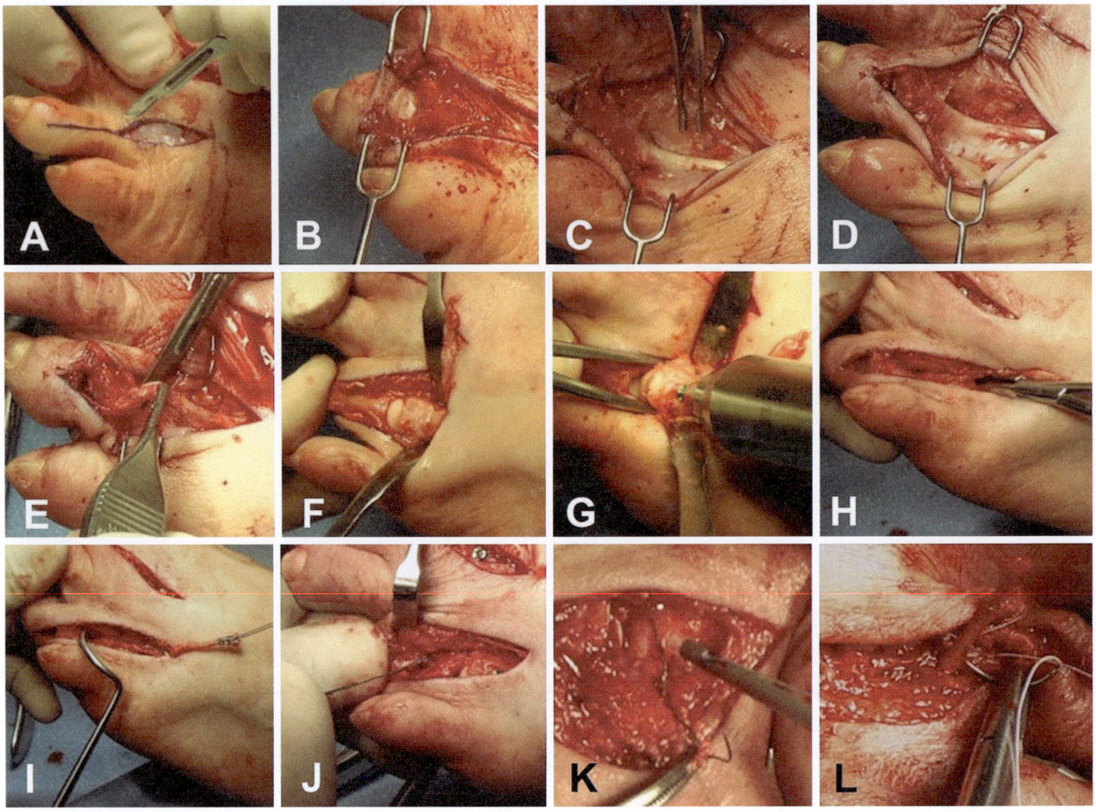

Fig. 5.7 EDB transfer

- Herein, the patient had a laterally deviating toe; the EDB tendon was brought to the medial side of the toe by threading it under the EDL tendon. Soft tissue was elevated off the side of the proximal phalanx opposite to the direction of toe deviation (Fig. 5.7h).
- An aneurysm needle was passed in a retrograde fashion from the space just created adjacent the proximal phalanx underneath the intermetatarsal ligament and delivered into the intermetatarsal space (Fig. 5.7i).
- The EDB stump was held with 2-0 Ethibond whip stitch, and then its thread was passed through the aneurysm needle. The sutures are retrieved through the needle delivering the EDB tendon into the medial space adjacent the proximal phalanx (Fig. 5.7j). A 2.4 mm micro suture anchor is used to fix the transfer (Fig. 5.7k) under maximal tension, while the toe is held in an overcorrected position. The sutures from the micro anchor are used to hold the EDB stump to lay alongside the medial cortex of the proximal phalanx (Fig. 5.7l).
- We usually use an axial K-wire fixation for the adjunct procedures (PIP fusion) but not for stabilization of an isolated EDB transfer. The foot is wrapped and placed in a postoperative shoe. K-wires are removed at 6 weeks, and the patient may begin forefoot weight-bearing without rolling through at second or third week as tolerated using the postoperative shoe. The patient was allowed to roll through the foot at 12 weeks, and regular shoes may be used at this point.

Case 5.3 Dorsiflexion Osteotomy

History

- A 47-year-old female with long history of bilateral foot pain including a mild bunion and moderate to severe second MTP synovitis

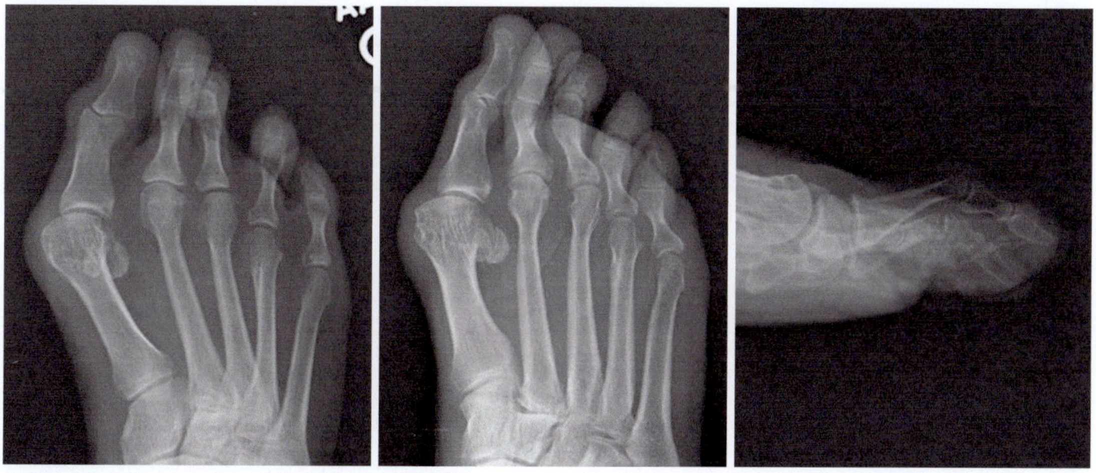

Fig. 5.8 Hallux valgus and second MTP arthritis

with toe deviation. The patient also has first and second tarsometatarsal (TMT) joint osteoarthritis.

- She originally had her left second MTP pain treated with synovectomy and pinning of the second MTP joint at an outside facility. She complained of persistent stiffness and pain in her second MTP joint.
- After failure of conservative treatment, the patient decided in favor of surgical correction of her hallux valgus deformity and second MTP arthritis (Fig. 5.8).

Surgical Technique

- A modified Lapidus procedure for the first MT and arthrodesis of the second MT were performed first in a classic fashion.
- After completing the hallux valgus correction, a longitudinal dorsal incision is made over the second metatarsal head and extended up over the proximal phalanx of the second toe. Extensive synovitis must be debrided in order to expose the metatarsal head. The second metatarsal head had a large central ulceration involving the dorsal 60% of the joint (Fig. 5.9).
- The first osteotomy cut is made at the dorsal edge of the cartilage defect, and a second converging cut is made just above the inferior edge of the ulcer (Fig. 5.10a, b). This wedge of bone which includes the arthritic section is then removed (Fig. 5.11a, b). The metatarsal head is then shifted proximally as needed, and the dorsal rim is removed perpendicular to the metatarsal anatomic axis (Fig. 5.11c–e). A twist-off screw is used to fix the metatarsal head delivering the plantar cartilage to a more dorsal orientation (Fig. 5.11f).
- This osteotomy unloads the metatarsal head but also addresses the arthritis. After skin closure, bone marrow aspirate concentrate is injected at the osteotomy sites. A sterile dressing and postoperative shoe are applied.
- The patient is indicated non-weight-bearing, and suture removal is performed at 10–14 days in conjoint with postoperative X-rays (Fig. 5.12). The patient was allowed to progressively bear weight at 6 weeks in a boot brace and wean out of the boot to a stiff-sole shoe as tolerated at 12 weeks.

Case 5.4 Proximal Phalanx Basilar Osteotomy (Akinette)

History

- A 56-year-old male patient presents with a long-standing history of progressive hallux valgus deformity with pain as well as a progressive dorsiflexion deformity of the second toe. His clinical deformity is severe with a significant medial bunion and overlapping and crossover of the second toe.

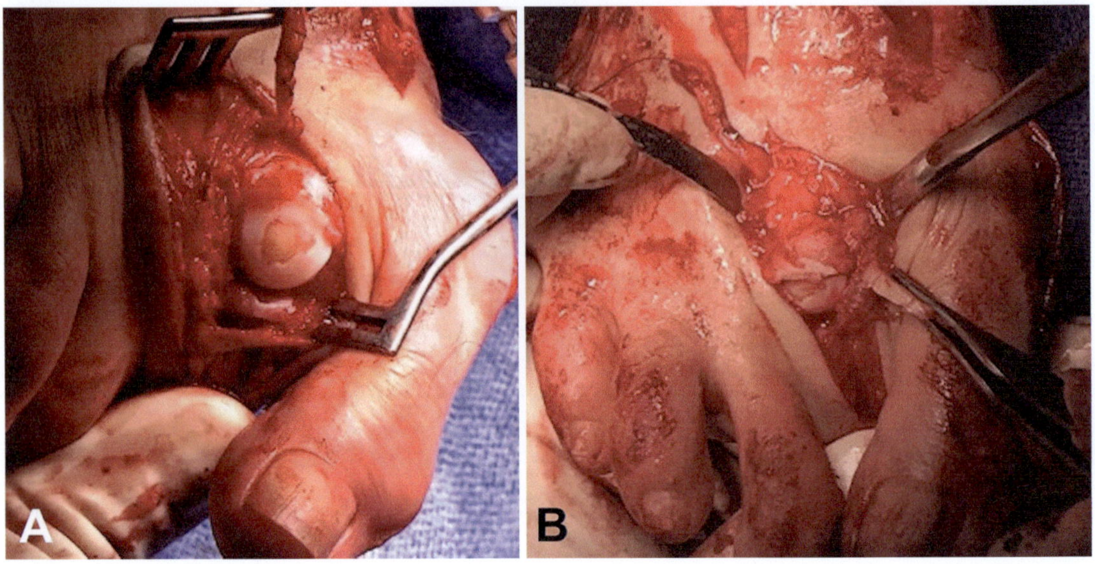

Fig. 5.9 Dorsiflexion osteotomy for second MTP arthritis

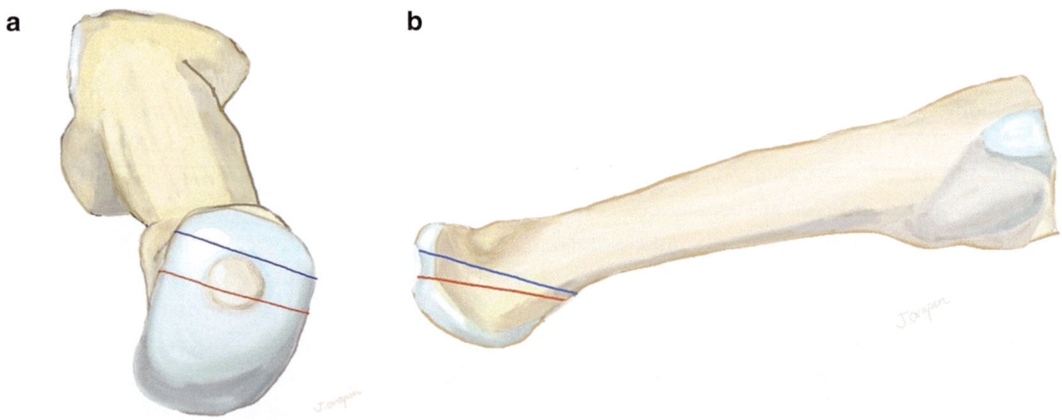

Fig. 5.10 Dorsiflexion osteotomy. Superior (blue) and inferior (red) osteotomy sites

- On physical examination, metatarsal plantar callus is noted with pain on this area and also tenderness at the second MTP joint.
- A Ludloff osteotomy was performed for correcting the hallux valgus deformity. The second toe was addressed with a Weil osteotomy combined with a capsular and soft tissue release. An axial K-wire was used to protect the MTP joint release.
- Even though the patient was doing well after hallux valgus and claw toe correction, he had a new complaint about the nail of his third toe rubbing up against the undersurface of his second toe and causing a painful callus (Fig. 5.13).
- After all conservative treatment measures failed, we proposed a closing wedge osteotomy on the lateral aspect of the third proximal phalanx to realign the third toe.

Surgical Technique

- A longitudinal incision is made over the dorsal aspect of proximal phalanx of the third toe. Blunt dissection is performed, and the slip of

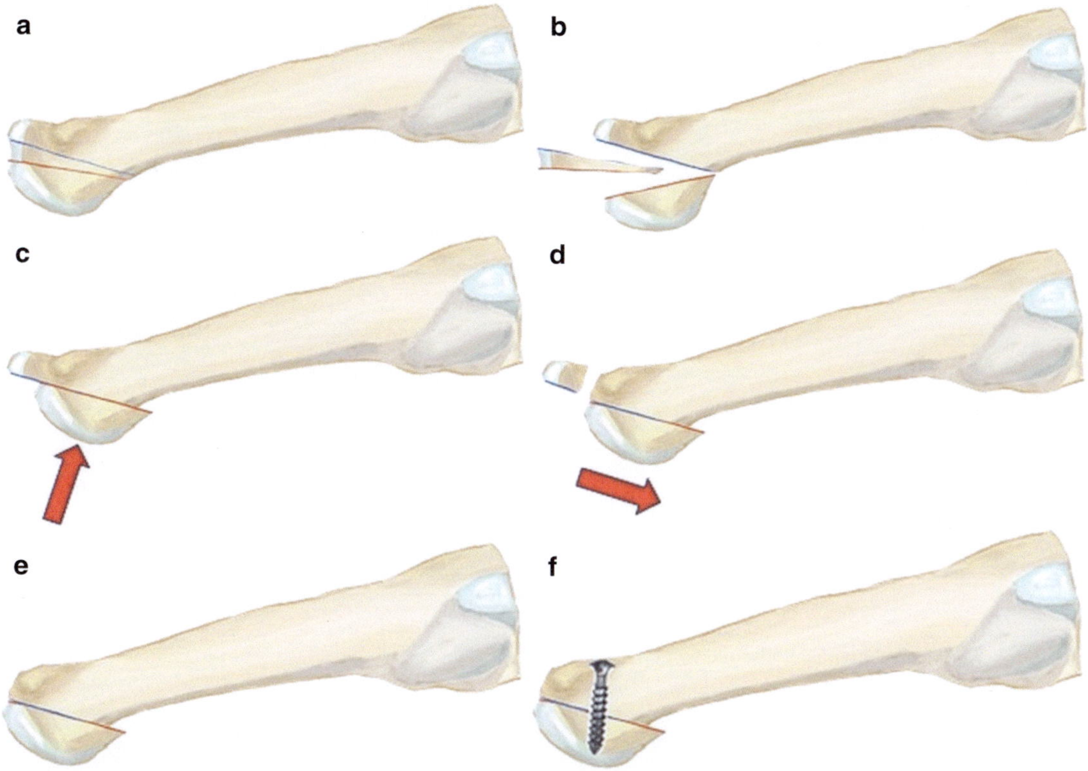

Fig. 5.11 Dorsiflexion osteotomy. Surgical technique

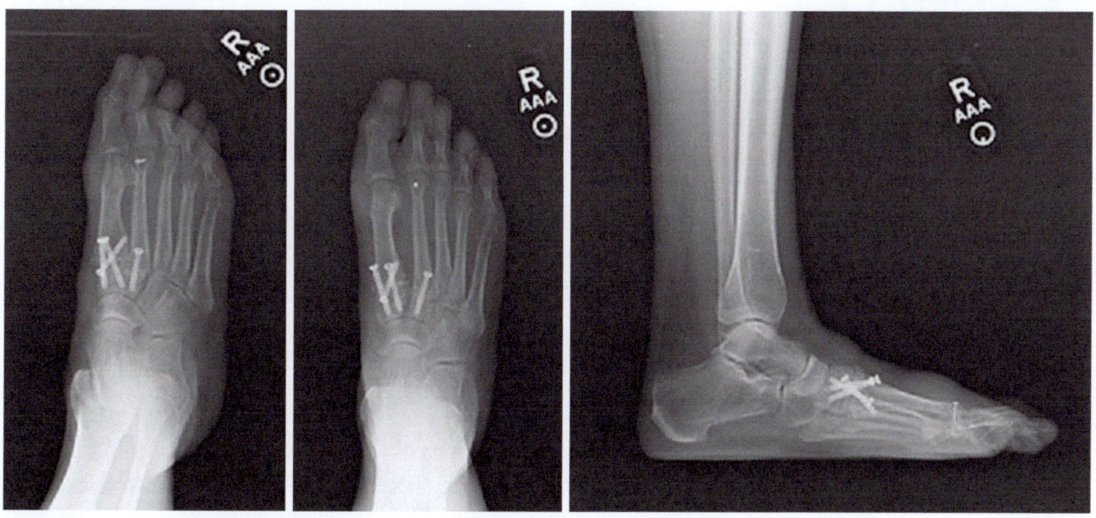

Fig. 5.12 Dorsiflexion osteotomy. Six-month follow-up postoperative X-rays

the extensor digitorum longus tendon is identified. A full-thickness incision is made at the medial aspect of the tendon, and then Hohmann retractors are applied to protect the surrounding soft tissue including plantar flexor tendon.

- Two convergent osteotomies are made on the lateral cortex of the proximal phalanx leaving

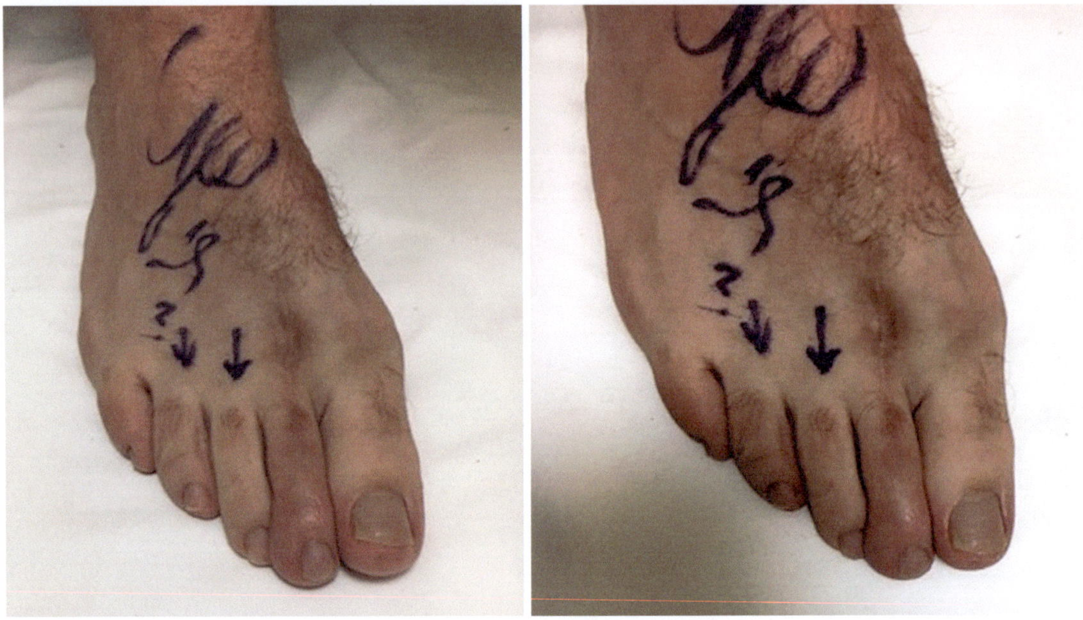

Fig. 5.13 Third toe rubbing up under the second toe

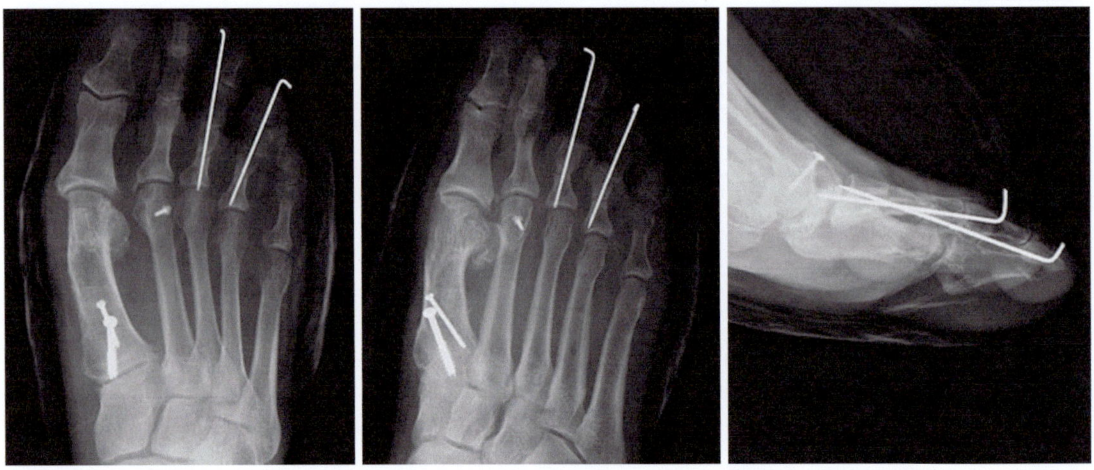

Fig. 5.14 Akinette osteotomy of the third and fourth toes. Postoperative X-rays

intact the medial cortex and periosteum. The cut is made in the diaphyseal area to maximize power of correction and avoid joint rigidity.

- The laterally based bone wedge is then removed and the osteotomy is closed. An axial K-wire is used for fixation. Intraoperative assessment was made, and a similar osteotomy was performed on the fourth toe as well (Fig. 5.14).
- Sutures are removed after 10–14 days. The patient is allowed weight-bearing at 3 weeks in a postoperative shoe. K-wires are removed at 6 weeks, and a supportive shoe with rigid sole is indicated. Full forefoot weight-bearing was permitted at 12 weeks. X-rays taken at this point showed advanced healing of the osteotomies (Fig. 5.15).
- The patient was satisfied with the procedure, and correct alignment of the lesser toes was achieved (Fig. 5.16).

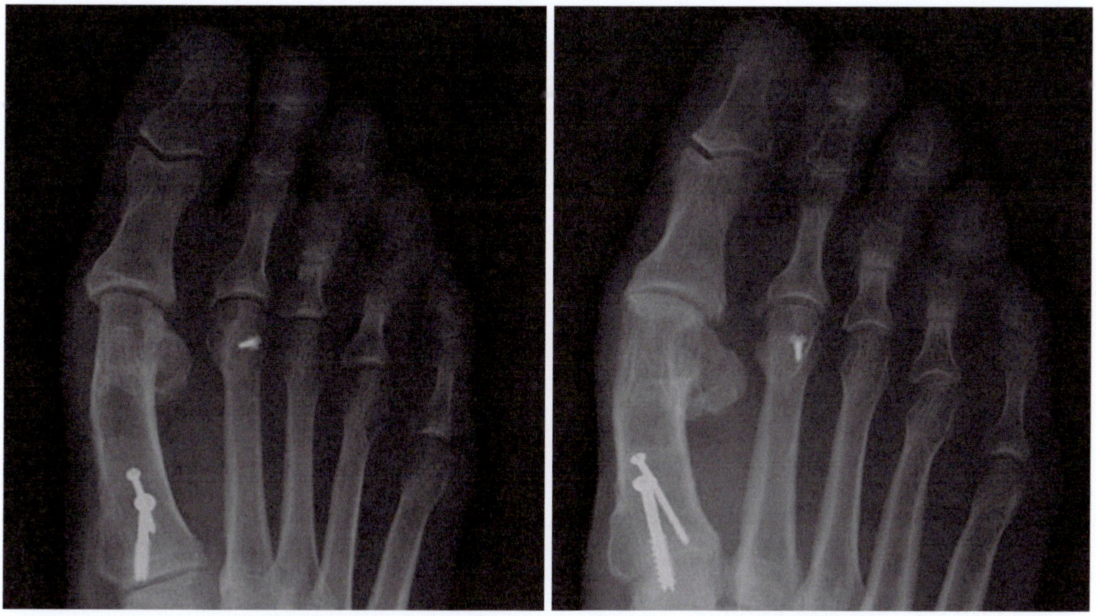

Fig. 5.15 Akinette osteotomies of the third and fourth toes. Twelve weeks postoperatively

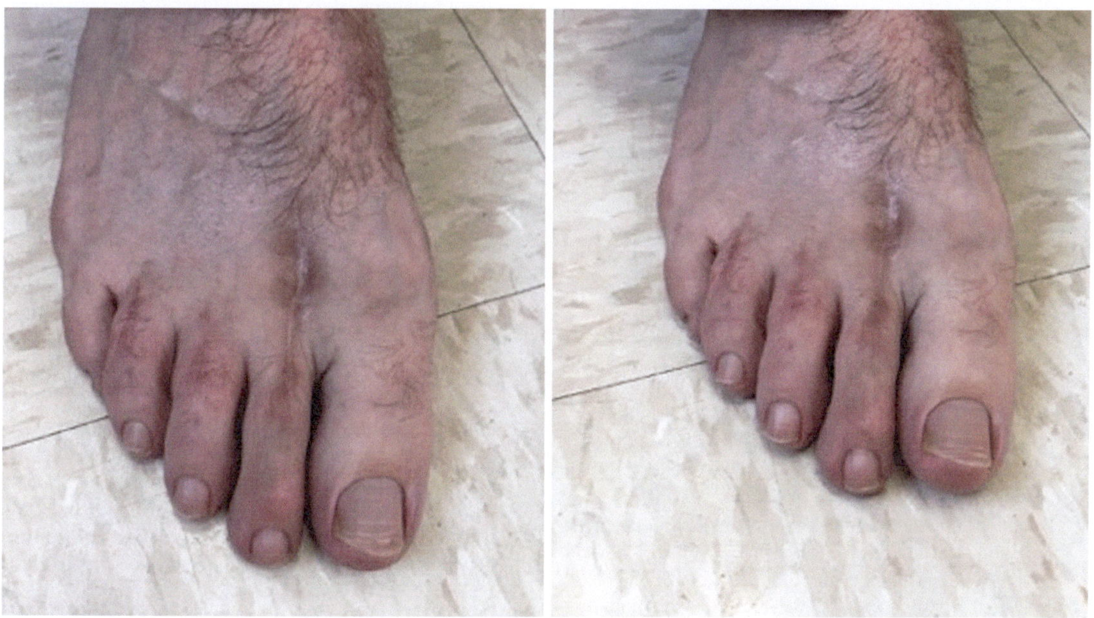

Fig. 5.16 Final clinical appearance after Akinette osteotomies

References

1. Schuh R, Trnka HJ. Metatarsalgia: distal metatarsal osteotomies. Foot Ankle Clin. 2011;16(4):583–95.
2. Hofstaetter SG, Hofstaetter JG, Petroutsas JA, Gruber F, Ritschl P, Trnka HJ. The Weil osteotomy: a seven-year follow-up. J Bone Joint Surg (Br). 2005;87-B(11):1507–11.
3. Doty JF, Coughlin MJ, Weil L Jr, Nery C. Etiology and management of lesser toe metatarsophalangeal joint instability. Foot Ankle Clin. 2014;19(3):385–405.
4. Chadwick C, Saxby TS. Hammertoes/Clawtoes: metatarsophalangeal joint correction. Foot Ankle Clin. 2011;16(4):559–71.
5. Weil L Jr, Weil LS Sr. Osteotomies for bunionette deformity. Foot Ankle Clin. 2011;16(4):689–712.
6. Maceira E, Monteagudo M. Transfer metatarsalgia post hallux valgus surgery. Foot Ankle Clin. 2014;19(2):285–307.
7. Highlander P, VonHerbulis E, Gonzalez A, Britt J, Buchman J. Complications of the Weil Osteotomy. Foot Ankle Spec. 2011;4(3):165–70.
8. Trnka HJ, Gebhard C, Muhlbauer M, Ivanic G, Ritschl P. The Weil osteotomy for treatment of dislocated lesser metatarsophalangeal joints: good outcome in 21 patients with 42 osteotomies. Acta Orthop Scand. 2002;73(2):190–4.
9. Devos Bevernage B, Leemrijse T. Predictive value of radiographic measurements compared to clinical examination in the preoperative planning for a Weil osteotomy. Foot Ankle Int. 2008;29:142–9.
10. Barouk P. Recurrent metatarsalgia. Foot Ankle Clin. 2014;19(3):407–24.
11. Khurana A, Kadamabande S, James S, Tanaka H, Hariharan K. Weil osteotomy: assessment of medium term results and predictive factors in recurrent metatarsalgia. Foot Ankle Surg. 2011;17(3):150–7.
12. Perez-Munoz I, Escobar-Anton D, Sanz-Gomez TA. The role of Weil and triple Weil osteotomies in the treatment of propulsive metatarsalgia. Foot Ankle Int. 2012;33(6):501–6.
13. Trnka HJ, Nyska M, Parks BG, Schon LC. Dorsiflexion contracture after the Weil osteotomy: results of cadaver study and three-dimensional analysis. Foot Ankle Int. 2001;22(1):47–50.
14. Snyder J, Owen J, Wayne J, Adelaar R. Plantar pressure and load in cadaver feet after a Weil or Chevron osteotomy. Foot Ankle Int. 2005;26(2):158–65.
15. Maestro M, Besse J-L, Ragusa M, Berthonnaud E. Forefoot morphotype study and planning method for forefoot osteotomy. Foot Ankle Clin. 2003;8(4):695–710.
16. Melamed EA, Schon LC, Myerson MS, Parks BG. Two modifications of the Weil osteotomy: analysis on Sawbone models. Foot Ankle Int. 2002;23(5):400–5.
17. Lau JTC, Stamatis ED, Parks BG, Schon LC. Modifications of the Weil osteotomy have no effect on plantar pressure. Clin Orthop Relat Res. 2004;421:194–8.
18. Pearce CJ, Calder JD. Metatarsalgia: Proximal Metatarsal Osteotomies. Foot Ankle Clin. 2011;16(4):597–608.
19. Derner R, Meyr AJ. Complications and salvage of elective central metatarsal osteotomies. Clin Podiatr Med Surg. 2009;26(1):23–35.
20. Trnka HJ, Muhlbauer M, Zettl R, Myerson MS, Ritschl P. Comparison of the results of the Weil and Helal osteotomies for the treatment of metatarsalgia secondary to dislocation of the lesser metatarsophalangeal joints. Foot Ankle Int. 1999;20(2):72–9.
21. Migues A, Slullitel G, Bilbao F, Carrasco M, Solari G. Floating-toe deformity as a complication of the Weil osteotomy. Foot Ankle Int. 2004;25(9):609–13.
22. Garg R, Thordarson DB, Schrumpf M, Castaneda D. Sliding oblique versus segmental resection osteotomies for lesser metatarsophalangeal joint pathology. Foot Ankle Int. 2008;29(10):1009–14.
23. Doty JF, Coughlin MJ. Metatarsophalangeal joint instability of the lesser toes. J Foot Ankle Surg. 2014;53(4):440–5.
24. Sferra J, Arndt S. The crossover toe and valgus toe deformity. Foot Ankle Clin. 2011;16(4):609–20.
25. Barg A, Courville XF, Nickisch F, Bachus KN, Saltzman CL. Role of collateral ligaments in metatarsophalangeal stability: a cadaver study. Foot Ankle Int. 2012;33(10):877–82.
26. Nery C, Coughlin MJ, Baumfeld D, Raduan FC, Mann TS, Catena F. Prospective evaluation of protocol for surgical treatment of lesser MTP joint plantar plate tears. Foot Ankle Int. 2014;35(9):876–85.
27. Flint WW, Macias DM, Jastifer JR, Doty JF, Hirose CB, Coughlin MJ. Plantar plate repair for lesser metatarsophalangeal joint instability. Foot Ankle Int. 2016;38(3):234–42.
28. Haddad SL, Sabbagh RC, Resch S, Myerson B, Myerson MS. Results of flexor-to-extensor and extensor brevis tendon transfer for correction of the crossover second toe deformity. Foot Ankle Int. 1999;20(12):781–8.
29. Nickisch F, Hodges Davis W. Basilar proximal phalangeal osteotomy (Akinette) for recalcitrant lesser-toe horizontal plane deformities. Tech Foot Ankle Sur. 2008;7(1):41–4.
30. Hodges Davis W, Anderson RB, Thompson FM, Hamilton WG. Proximal phalanx basilar osteotomy for resistant angulation of the lesser toes. Foot Ankle Int. 1997;18:103–4.
31. Boyer ML, DeOrio JK. Transfer of the flexor digitorum longus for the correction of lesser-toe deformities. Foot Ankle Int. 2016;28(4):422–30.
32. Kwon JY, De Asla RJ. The use of flexor to extensor transfers for the correction of the flexible hammer toe deformity. Foot Ankle Clin. 2011;16(4):573–82.
33. Myerson MS, Jung HG. The role of toe flexor-to-extensor transfer in correcting metatarsophalangeal joint instability of the second toe. Foot Ankle Int. 2005;26(9):675–9.

34. Bhatia D, Myerson MS, Curtis MJ, Cunningham BW, Jinnah RH. Anatomical restraints to dislocation of the second metatarsophalangeal joint and assessment of a repair technique. J Bone Joint Surg Am. 1994;76:1371–5.
35. Myers SH, Schon LC. Forefoot tendon transfers. Foot Ankle Clin. 2011;16(3):471–88.
36. Capobianco CM. Surgical treatment approaches to second metatarsophalangeal joint pathology. Clin Podiatr Med Surg. 2012;29(3):443–9.
37. Kilic A, Cepni KS, Aybar A, Polat H, May C, Parmaksizoglu AS. A comparative study between two different surgical techniques in the treatment of late-stage Freiberg's disease. Foot Ankle Surg. 2013;19(4):234–8.
38. Cerrato RA. Freiberg's disease. Foot Ankle Clin. 2011;16(4):647–58.
39. Helix-Giordanino M, Randier E, Frey S, Piclet B. French association of foot s. treatment of Freiberg's disease by Gauthier's dorsal cuneiform osteotomy: retrospective study of 30 cases. Orthop Traumatol Surg Res. 2015;101(6 Suppl):S221–5.
40. Erdil M, Imren Y, Bilsel K, Erzincanli A, Bulbul M, Tuncay I. Joint debridement and metatarsal remodeling in Freiberg's infraction. J Am Podiatr Med Assoc. 2013;103(3):185–90.
41. Xie X, Shi Z, Gu W. Late-stage Freiberg's disease treated with dorsal wedge osteotomy and joint distraction arthroplasty: technique tip. Foot Ankle Int. 2012;33(11):1015–7.
42. Nixon DC, McKean RM, Klein SE, Johnson JE, McCormick JJ. Rheumatoid forefoot reconstruction in the nonrheumatoid patient. Foot Ankle Int. 2017;38(6):605–11.
43. Schade VL. Surgical management of Freiberg's infraction: a systematic review. Foot Ankle Spec. 2015;8(6):498–519.
44. Gauthier G, Elbaz R. Freiberg's infraction: a subchondral bone fatigue fracture. A new surgical treatment. Clin Orthop Relat Res. 1979;(142):93–5.
45. Kim J, Choi WJ, Park YJ, Lee JW. Modified Weil osteotomy for the treatment of Freiberg's disease. Clin Orthop Surg. 2012;4(4):300.
46. Mann RA, Chou LB. Surgical management for intractable metatarsalgia. Foot Ankle Int. 1995;16(6):322–7.
47. Giannini S, Faldini C, Vannini F, Digennaro V, Bevoni R, Luciani D. The minimally invasive osteotomy "S.E.R.I." (simple, effective, rapid, inexpensive) for correction of bunionette deformity. Foot Ankle Int. 2008;29(3):282–6.
48. Bertrand T, Parekh SG. Bunionette deformity: etiology, nonsurgical management, and lateral exostectomy. Foot Ankle Clin. 2011;16(4):679–88.
49. Lee DC, de Cesar Netto C, Staggers JR, Siegel R, Chen R, Bae S-Y, et al. Clinical and radiographic outcomes of the Kramer osteotomy in the treatment of bunionette deformity. Foot Ankle Surg. 2017
50. Baumhauer JF, Digiovanni BF. Osteotomies of the fifth metatarsal. Foot Ankle Clin. 2001;6(3):491–8.
51. Cooper MT, Coughlin MJ. Subcapital oblique osteotomy for correction of bunionette deformity. Foot Ankle Int. 2013;34(10):1376–80.
52. Weitzel S, Trnka HJ, Petroutsas J. Transverse medial slide osteotomy for bunionette deformity: long-term results. Foot Ankle Int. 2007;28(7):794–8.
53. Michels F, Van Der Bauwhede J, Guillo S, Oosterlinck D, de Lavigne C. Percutaneous bunionette correction. Foot Ankle Surg. 2013;19(1):9–14.
54. Magnan B, Samaila E, Merlini M, Bondi M, Mezzari S, Bartolozzi P. Percutaneous distal osteotomy of the fifth metatarsal for correction of bunionette. J Bone Joint Surg Am. 2011;93(22):2116–22.

Part II

Trauma

Revision Surgery for Pilon Fractures

6

Sophia Davis and John Ketz

Introduction

Fractures of the distal tibial plafond are notorious for their poor outcomes even with the most meticulous management. These injuries can occur as a result of lower energy rotational forces or more typically as higher energy mechanisms. There is often substantial articular injury with varying degrees of impaction. Most importantly, this injury pattern represents a significant soft tissue injury, which often dictates the management of pilon fractures. Currently the standard of care is for staged reconstruction, with initial external fixation and definitive surgical stabilization once the soft tissues are healthy [1, 2]. Despite thoughtful consideration when treating these injuries, multiple complications can occur such as nonunion, malunion, infection, avascular necrosis (AVN), and post-traumatic arthritis [3–10].

There are multiple complications that can occur during treatment. Open pilon fractures significantly impact the soft tissue envelope [9]. Proper antibiotic and debridement techniques are needed initially, and then consideration for future planning of fixation is needed. Multiple studies have shown increased risk of infection and nonunion with open pilon fractures [3, 10]. Patient factors also contribute to potential causes of complications. Comorbidities such as diabetes mellitus (DM), peripheral vascular disease (PVD), and chronic steroid use among others may affect the soft tissue and bone healing potential. Careful consideration should be paid not only to the fracture but also to the patient as a whole. Even with ideal management of the fracture in the primary setting, patients still have fair to poor outcomes. The management of complications for pilon fractures is extremely complex and requires significant planning.

S. Davis
Orlando Orthopaedic Center, Orlando, FL, USA

J. Ketz (✉)
Strong Memorial Hospital, University of Rochester, Department of Orthopaedics, Rochester, NY, USA

Pathoanatomy

The reason for poor outcomes for these injuries relates to the mechanism of injury. Pilon fractures are, by definition, impaction injuries of the distal tibial articular surface. This results in immediate injury to the cartilage which cannot be undone. Even with anatomic realignment of the articular surface and restoration of the anatomic axis, there is still the damage done at the time of impact which permanently affects the cartilage. This can lead to avascular necrosis (AVN) of the tibial plafond, and if collapse occurs early, symptomatic post-traumatic arthritis occurs.

Additional causes for poor outcomes relate to anatomic reasons. The metaphyseal-diaphyseal junction of the distal tibia has a poor blood

M. J. Berkowitz et al. (eds.), *Revision Surgery of the Foot and Ankle*,
https://doi.org/10.1007/978-3-030-29969-9_6

supply which puts it at risk for nonunion [11]. The soft tissue injury creates disruption of that blood supply. In addition, surgical dissection causes further disruption, which is why meticulous dissection and careful incision planning is crucial. Additional patient risk factors such as smoking, peripheral vascular disease, or diabetes mellitus can increase the risk of nonunion.

Pilon fractures often have significant comminution involving the articular surface, metaphyseal region, as well as the fibula. While obtaining an anatomical reduction of the articular surface is paramount, the main goal of treating the tibial metaphyseal region and fibula is to restore alignment and rotation [12]. Without this, malunions will occur, and these are more difficult to deal with in the future, particularly in the setting of traumatic arthritis [5, 7]. Malreduction of the fibula can complicate future reduction of the fibula and may inhibit future incisions. As this is often done at the time of external fixation, current recommendations are to let the surgeon who will treat the fracture definitively address the fibula. With respect to the tibial metaphysis, there is often significant medial comminution. Shortening of the medial column of the tibia can lead to varus malunions affecting the mechanical axis.

All of the above are issues that are difficult to treat during the primary surgery. When considering revising a pilon, correcting deformity becomes even harder. As a result, the common response to revising a pilon is ankle fusion or in the case of poor soft tissue coverage, amputation. Options to preserve the ankle joint are supported by few case reports and case series.

Evaluation of the Patient and Reason for Failure

History and Physical Examination

The first step in performing a successful revision pilon is determining why the original procedure failed. Since patient factors are a major cause of failure in pilon fracture fixation, a thorough patient history is important. Knowing the mechanism of the injury as well as whether the fracture was open or closed can give a good picture of the amount of soft tissue damage that occurred at the time of injury. Details on the treatment course are critical, including timing and number of operations, initial external fixation, and known early complications. All of these factors play a role into what type of options exist for reconstruction.

Patient medical and social history is another important and potentially modifiable factor. A history of diabetes and the patients' Hgb A1C, PVD, and controlling an autoimmune condition are all important for maximizing blood supply and healing potential. If the patient has an elevated Hgb A1C (>7), the patient should be referred to endocrinology for tighter glucose control. In a patient with a history of PVD or poor peripheral pulses, a consult with a vascular surgeon could resolve an upstream blockage. While autoimmune disease cannot be cured, the DMARDs used to treat the patient should be noted and held as needed. The patient's social situation is also an important directing factor in the patients care. Nicotine is well-known to cause small vessel constriction and leads to a high nonunion rate. Drug abuse and uncontrolled psychiatric disorders may be considered a contraindication to revision ORIF due to the increased risk of noncompliance and poor outcomes.

There should also be a thorough physical exam noting prior incisions, ankle function, and clinical deformity. Prior incisions should be used for any revision surgery planned, if appropriate, as additional incisions may destroy any remaining blood supply to the soft tissue envelope. A thorough neurovascular exam is performed, including assessment for neuropathy. Range of motion of the ankle, hindfoot, and transverse tarsal joints should be evaluated. Patients with significantly limited motion at the ankle may not benefit from joint-sparing reconstruction. The overall alignment of the limb should be assessed clinically with the patient standing. Alignment in the coronal and sagittal planes should be inspected as well as any limb length discrepancies. Patients with pilon fractures can sometimes have had ipsilateral proximal injuries which may affect alignment distally and should be factored into planning.

Imaging

Weight-bearing ankle and foot radiographs are used to evaluate the overall alignment of the limb and ankle joint as well as the amount of joint space narrowing and arthrosis. If needed, full length tibia and fibula imaging should be ordered to evaluate deformity proximal to the fracture. The mortise should be inspected to evaluate for asymmetry, articular collapse, or sclerosis. Fibular length and reduction can be seen on plain radiography. Residual hardware should be inspected for articular penetration, and if further surgery is considered, removal of the hardware, in particular broken hardware, may present a challenge and will need preoperative planning.

Computed tomography (CT) scan is an extremely useful tool in preoperative planning for revision pilon surgery. It offers a detailed picture of the bony architecture [13]. Alignment can be seen in a three-dimensional orientation. The accuracy of the articular reduction or extent of existing arthrosis can be seen. Mal- or unreduced fragments can be evaluated. Also sclerosis indicative of AVN may be seen in different areas of the plafond. For patients with deformity but a well-preserved articular surface, joint-sparing procedures can be considered. For patients with extensive arthrosis or articular collapse, arthrodesis or ankle replacement may be a better option. Additional information that can be seen on the CT scan includes articular reduction or instability of the syndesmosis. For patients with suspected osteomyelitis, areas of resorption or sequestrum may be identified.

If possible reviewing the initial imaging studies including radiographs and CT imaging is important. This information can provide important bony detail of the initial injury and the quality of the initial reduction. Comparing these to current radiographs can offer information on varus (or valgus) malunion versus collapse and also if there has been collapse or malreduction of the articular surface.

Diagnostic Studies

Aside from imaging, additional diagnostic studies should be performed. As with any revision surgical procedure, a workup of infection should be performed. This includes obtaining a white blood cell count (WBC) with differential, C-reactive protein (CRP), and an erythrocyte sedimentation rate (ESR). Elevated values of any of those laboratory values should be concerning for infection, and this may alter the proposed procedure. Even with normal laboratory values, there can be a subclinical infection. The rate of this can be as high as 20% [14]. Because of this, a bone sample should be sent during the reconstructive procedure. Patient should be counseled about the possibility of encountering infection during the procedure, which may alter the postoperative course.

Surgical Planning/Considerations

A variety of factors should be considered with as part of the preoperative plan. Prior incisions, retained hardware, and residual deformity must be considered when preparing for reconstruction. All of these factors play a role in determining positioning, surgical exposure/incisions, and equipment needs.

Retained Hardware

The presence of retained hardware is an important consideration. The surgeon should determine if all or just some of the hardware needs to be removed. Ideally only the hardware that will be in the way of new hardware or any needed osteotomy should be removed. It is beneficial to know the type of hardware that was used. This can be accomplished through prior operative records or electronic medical records. Obtaining outside records is also important if the procedure was done at another facility. It is important to have the proper screwdriver trays and nail extraction devices. In addition to this, broken screw removal sets and osteotomies are beneficial for difficult to remove hardware.

Patient Positioning

Patient positioning is dependent on what surgical approach(s) will be utilized. Most commonly patients will be placed in a supine position. However, if posterior or posterolateral approaches had been used before with indwelling hardware, a prone position may be useful. However, visualizing the articular surface is difficult in the prone position, and reconstructive procedures/osteotomies may be difficult to complete with the patient in the prone position. At times a prone and then supine positioning is needed. This may require additional time and planning. As an alternative to doing front/back procedures, lateral positioning can be used which allow the surgeon to access the posterolateral and anterior aspect of the lower leg.

Surgical Approaches

During preoperative planning, an approach to correcting the deformity must also be formulated. Due to the nature of the soft tissues in this area, prior trauma to the soft tissue envelope must be considered. If the original injury was an open fracture or a flap needed to be placed, these areas should be avoided. Ideally, the reconstructive procedure should be done through prior approaches whenever possible. However, the surgeon should not compromise exposure by using prior incisions. If a long incision with significant soft tissue stripping was used previously, another extensile incision should be avoided to limit additional soft tissue disruption. Percutaneous techniques may also be beneficial in this scenario, if appropriate.

Use of the anteromedial and anterolateral approaches would be appropriate if these approaches had been used previously [5, 15, 16]. A posterolateral approach is very useful for addressing both the posterior tibia and the fibula through one incision and can be used in combination with another anterior approach.

The author's preferred approach is the anterior approach as it provides the best visualization for the distal tibial metaphysis and articular surface. This approach has typically been described as the plane between EDL and EHL, but in practice the interval between EHL and TA is typically used. By using the latter plane, the neurovascular bundle can be protected under the EHL and retracted laterally. On exposure of the articular surface, the joint can be examined. If the joint is well preserved, this approach allows for osteotomies to be performed in order to restore alignment. If joint salvage is not an option, this approach gives excellent joint visualization for cartilage debridement for fusion and is also a common approach for TAA.

Case Examples

Case 6.1 Infection Case

History

A 29-year-old male sustained a closed, comminuted pilon after falling 7 feet from a ladder. He underwent external fixation for temporary stabilization of the fracture, while the soft tissues healed (Fig. 6.1a). At his initial office visit, he had fracture blisters primarily anterolaterally necessitating delayed fixation. One week after injury, he had initial fixation using a posterolateral approach for initial fixation of the fibula and posterior fixation of the tibia. Ten days after posterior fixation, the patient underwent an anterolateral approach for anterior fixation of the tibia. The medial malleolus was also reduced percutaneously through a small medial incision (Fig. 6.1b). For the next 3 weeks, the patient had continued drainage from his anterior incision and continued pain. Four weeks following stabilization, he was taken to the operating room for serial irrigation and debridement procedures and ultimate hardware removal. Cultures taken at the time of surgery grew methicillin-sensitive *Staph. aureus*. The patient was discharged on oral Keflex. He was then referred for treatment of his infection.

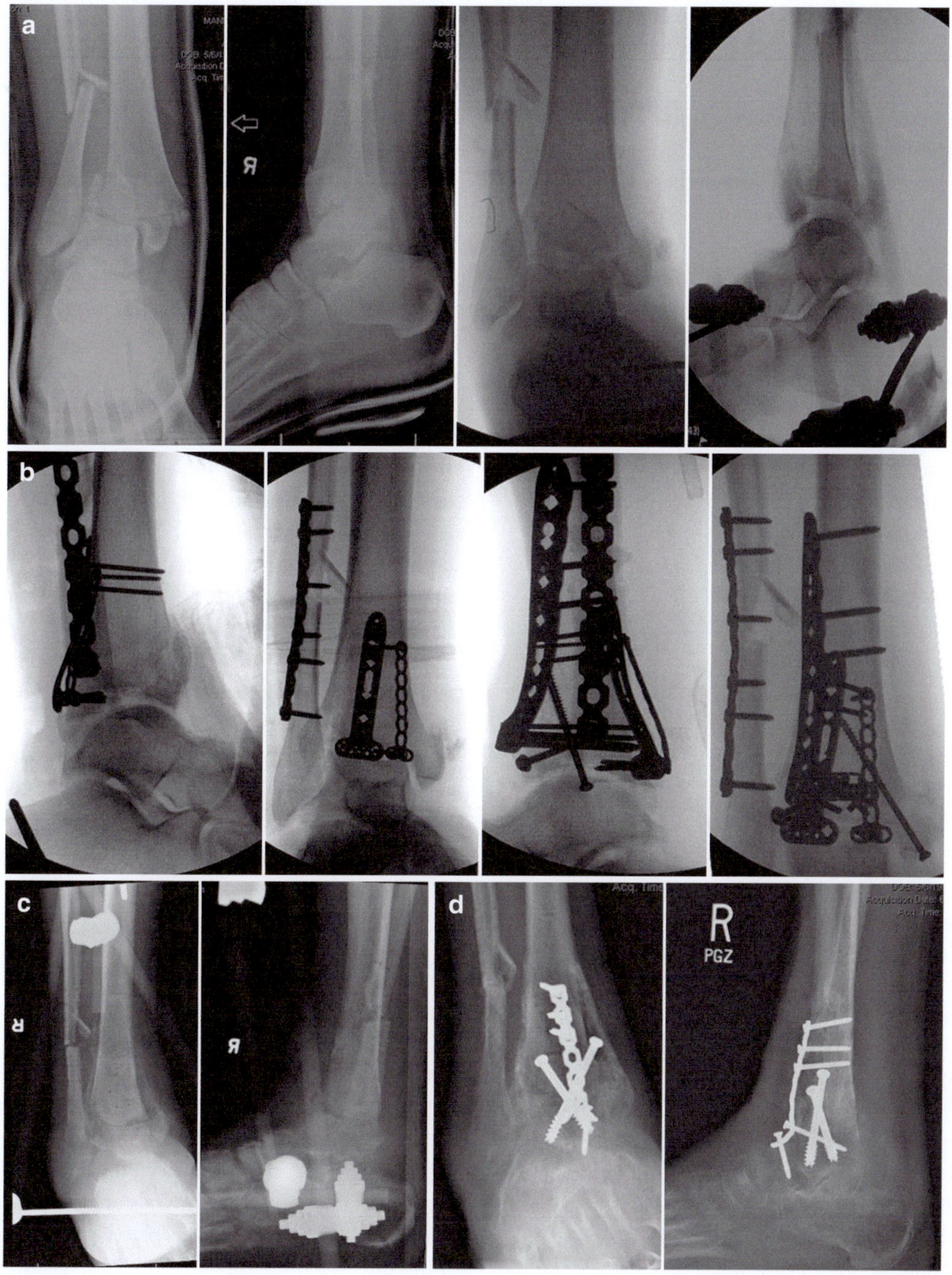

Fig. 6.1 (**a**) AP (left) and lateral (left center) radiographs of a 29-year-old male with a comminuted, closed pilon fracture. AP (right center) and lateral (right) fluoroscopic images following external fixation. (**b**) Lateral (left) and AP (left center) fluoroscopic images of initial posterior fixation of the tibia and fixation of the fibula through a posterolateral approach. Definitive fixation was performed after the soft tissues stabilized through an anterolateral approach. AP (right center) and lateral (right) fluoroscopic images are shown. (**c**) Immediate AP (left) and lateral (right) images were obtained following revision irrigation and debridement and temporary external fixation. (**d**) Following a 6-week antibiotic course, the patient underwent conversion to ankle arthrodesis. AP (left) and lateral (right) radiographs were obtained at 7 months showing a well-healed fracture and arthrodesis

Reasons for Failure

- Delayed recognition of infection/wound issues.
- Delayed and incomplete course of appropriate antibiotics.
- No stabilization of unhealed fracture was performed causing deformity.

Surgical Plan

- Stabilize fracture with external fixator.
- Repeat debridement with bone cultures.
- Removal of external fixator with arthrodesis after completion of antibiotics.

Approach

- Anterolateral ankle approach (previous)
- Percutaneous 7.3 mm lag screws

Implants

- External fixator
- 7.3 mm cannulated screws
- 3.5 mm reconstruction plate with 4.0 mm cortical screws

Pearls and Pitfalls

- The potential for encountering residual deep infection
  - Need intraoperative cultures
- Accounting for bone loss (infection) and post-traumatic cysts
- Need for correction of deformity (anterior translation of the talus)

Surgery

The patient was taken back to the operating room for repeat irrigation and debridement with intraoperative cultures. To provide stability, the patient was then placed into an external fixator (Fig. 6.1c). The patient had a PICC line placed and completed a 6-week course of culture-specific intravenous antibiotics. He was followed weekly in the clinic for evaluation of his soft tissues. One week after cessation of antibiotics, a repeat ESR, CRP, and WBC were obtained and were within normal limits. At this point revision surgical treatment with fusion was planned with repeat intraoperative bone cultures.

Intraoperatively, there were no overt signs of infection. His previous anterolateral ankle wound was used for exposure of the joint. All devascularized bone was removed and the ankle joint prepared for fusion. Autologous iliac crest bone grafting is performed, including bulk grafting for areas of bone loss. Deformity correction was performed and held temporarily with Steinmann pins. Two 7.3 mm cannulated screws were placed percutaneously across the ankle joint. Through the previous anterior ankle wound, a 5 hole, 3.5 mm reconstruction plate was contoured to the anterior joint and affixed to the tibia and talus using 4.0 mm cortical screws. The patient was placed on intravenous antibiotics awaiting final culture results. Cultures ultimately grew MSSA and methicillin-resistant coagulase-negative staphylococcus from his bone cultures. He was kept on intravenous antibiotics for an additional 6 weeks.

Postoperatively, he eventually healed all wounds. After completion of his antibiotics, his inflammatory markers remained within normal limits. He healed with a solid fusion of his ankle joint with good motion at this midfoot and subtalar joints (Fig. 6.1d). He was able to return to work at approximately 6 months following his revision surgery.

Case 6.2 Infection/Immunocompromised

History

A 46-year-old female with a PMH of stroke, lupus, diabetes, and tobacco abuse presented after a high-speed motor vehicle collision with a comminuted, open pilon fracture with a 4 cm anterior wound (Fig. 6.2a). The patient was taken to the OR the same day for formal irrigation and debridement as well as placement of an external fixator (Fig. 6.2b). At the patient's first post-op follow-up visit, she was noted to have erythema and serosanguineous drainage with wound breakdown. The patient was directly admitted to the hospital and started on IV antibiotics. Cultures obtained intraoperatively grew vancomycin-resistant *Enterobacter*. The patient completed the course of antibiotics and had progressive healing of her wound. Two weeks after the initiation of antibiotics, the uniplanar external fixator began to fail with loosening of the pins. At this point the patient was taken to the OR for external fixator removal and placement in a short leg cast. Intraoperatively the external fixator was removed and all pin sites thoroughly debrided. The leg was then stressed, and motion was noted across the fracture sites. The patient was casted for fracture stability. At her first postoperative follow-up, she was noted to have worsening of her wound and deformity, and follow-up CT scan revealed continued nonunion (Fig. 6.2c). She was referred for definitive treatment.

Reasons for Failure

- Multiple medical comorbidities/ immunocompromised.
- Inadequate fracture stabilization/external fixator construct.
- No stabilization of unhealed fracture was performed causing deformity.

Surgical Plan

- Stabilize fracture with external fixator.
- Repeat debridement with bone cultures.
- Staged autologous bone grafting.

Approach

- Anterior ankle approach (previous)
- Percutaneous lateral incision for fibular bone grafting

Implants

- Multiplanar external fixator

Pearls and Pitfalls

- The potential for encountering residual deep infection
  - Need intraoperative cultures
- Need for correction of deformity

Surgery

The patient was taken back to the operating room for irrigation and debridement with repeat bone cultures and placed back into an external fixator. Given the patients multiple comorbidities, it was felt she would benefit from placement into a multiplanar external fixator with a bypass frame to allow for early weight-bearing. A multiplanar fixator was applied, and correction of the deformity was corrected (Fig. 6.2d). Intraoperative bone cultures were negative at that time. She completed her intravenous antibiotic course, and inflammatory markers were negative. The patient was taken back to the operating room for treatment of her impending nonunion. The fracture site was accessed through a small extension of the previous open wound, and the fibrous tissue at the nonunion site was debrided. Then the nonunion site of the fibula was taken down as well at this time through a small incision. Both sites were bone grafted with iliac crest autograft. Final cultures taken from the OR were found to be negative.

Postoperatively, the patient was followed in the clinic. Once the wound was healed, the patient was allowed to bear weight through her fixator. At 5 months following placement of the fixator, A CT scan was obtained that revealed bridging bone across both the fibula and tibia fractures (Fig. 6.2e). The fixator was removed at 6.5 months. Final radiographs were obtained at 12 months which revealed a well-healed, well-aligned fracture (Fig. 6.2f). The patient reported no pain and had returned to work without restrictions.

Case 6.3 Delayed Presentation

History

A 43-year-old migrant worker male presents 2 weeks after injury for definitive fixation of his pilon fracture. He initially sustained his injury after reportedly being tackled while playing soccer (Fig. 6.3a). The patient was placed into a splint and instructed to follow up as an outpatient. He presented back to the ED for management almost 5 weeks from injury. The swelling was amenable to surgery, and the patient had minimal pain. Initial radiographs in his splint revealed significant deformity (Fig. 6.3b). A CT scan was obtained which revealed significant comminution and articular displacement.

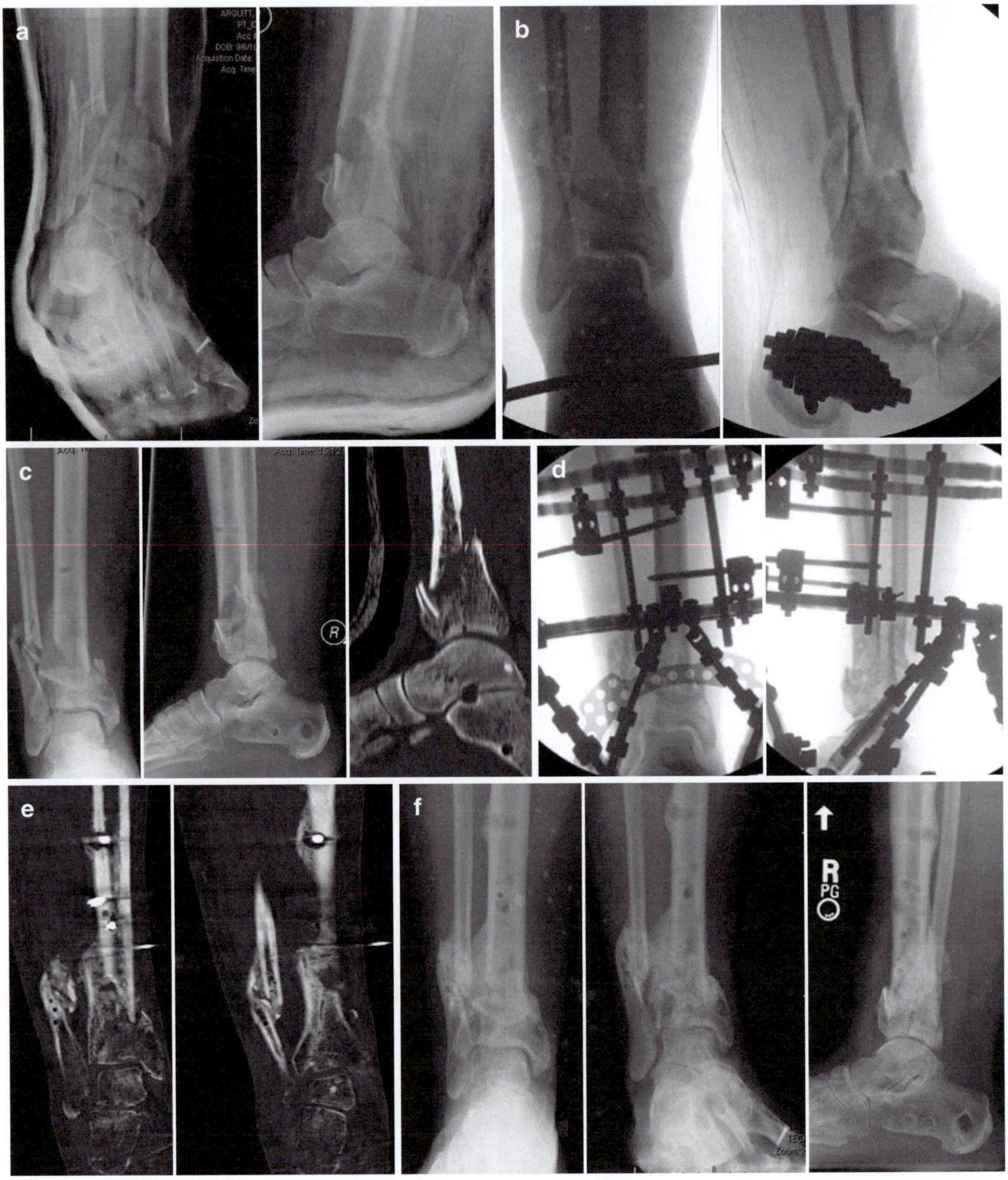

Fig. 6.2 (**a**) AP (left) and lateral (right) images of a 46-year-old female with multiple medical comorbidities who sustained an open comminuted pilon fracture. (**b**) Initial irrigation and debridement and uniplanar external fixation was applied with improved alignment on AP (left) and lateral (right) fluoroscopic imaging. (**c**) The patient had wound dehiscence and loosening of her external fixator that required removal. AP (left) and lateral (center) show a continued nonunion with a large lucency at her calcaneal pin site best seen on the lateral image. A CT scan image (right) reveals persistent fracture lines at the articular surface and metaphysis. (**d**) The patient was placed into a mutiplanar external fixator. AP (left) and lateral (right) fluoroscopic images were obtained following repeat irrigation and debridement and stabilization of the fracture. (**e**) Coronal CT scan images reveal bridging bone at the level of the articular surface and metaphysis of the tibia (left) as well as healing of the fibula fracture (right). (**f**) AP (left), mortise (center), and lateral (right) radiographs were taken at 12 months showing a well-healed, well-aligned pilon fracture with minimal arthritic change

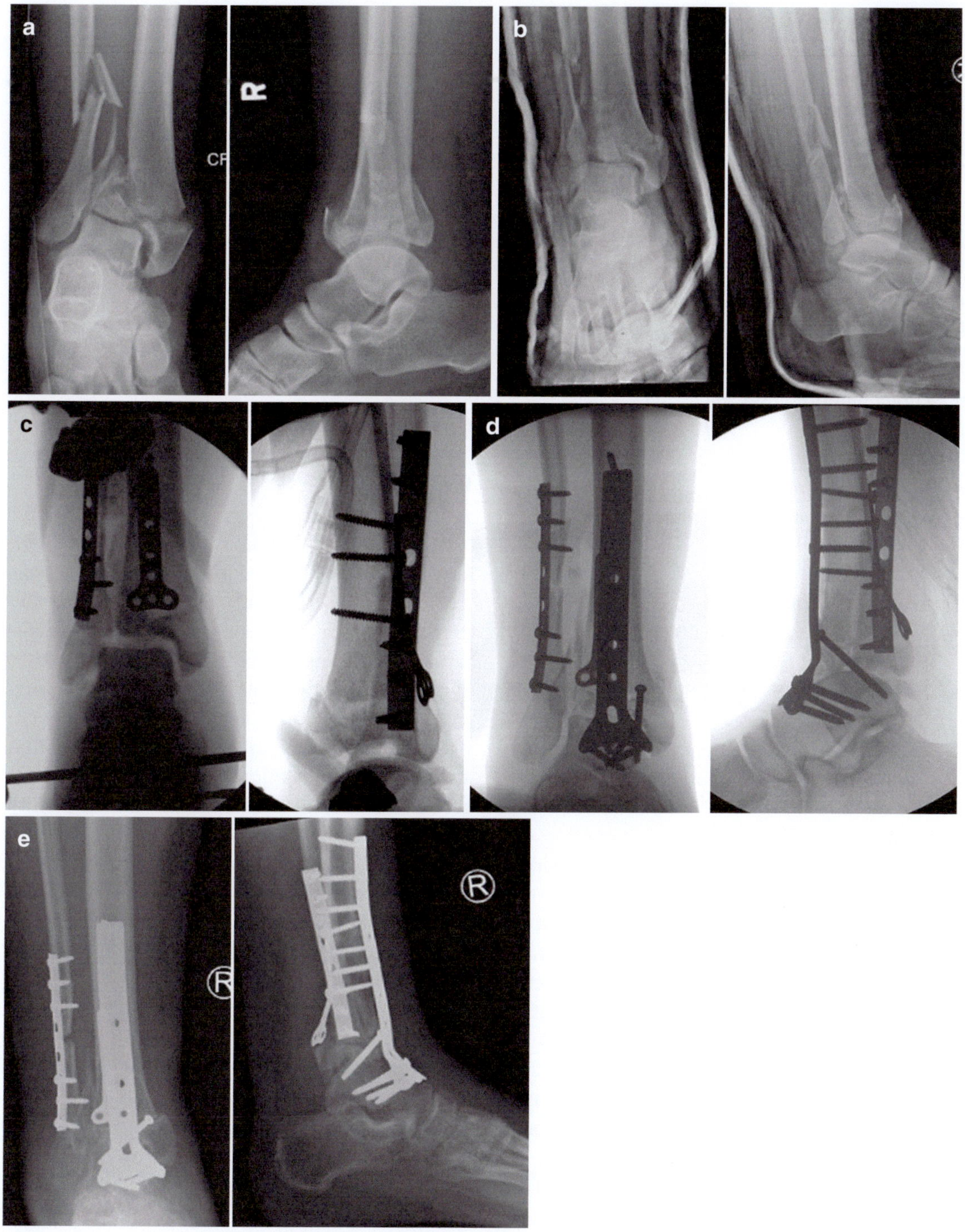

Fig. 6.3 (**a**) AP (right) and lateral (left) radiographs of a 43-year-old migrant worker who injured his leg. (**b**) The patient remained in a splint for 5 weeks following injury. AP (left) and lateral (right) images reveal continued displacement and significant articular comminution. (**c**) The patient was first placed prone and underwent stabilization of the fibula and posterior tibia through a posterolateral approach as seen on AP (left) and lateral (right) fluoroscopic imaging. (**d**) The patient was then placed supine and underwent ORIF with primary fusion through and anterior incision. AP (left) and lateral (right) fluoroscopic images reveal restoration of length and alignment. (**e**) AP (right) and lateral (left) radiographs were obtained at 8 months following surgery showing a healed ankle arthrodesis and fracture

Reasons for Failure

- Delayed presentation
- Inadequate initial fracture reduction
- Partially healed comminuted articular surface

Surgical Plan

- Use an external fixator to regain length.
- Posterior tibial ORIF.
- Anterior tibial ORIF.
- Ankle arthrodesis.

Approach

- Posterolateral
- Direct anterior approach

Implants

- Small fragment implants
- Small fragment "spoon" plate
- 4.0 mm cortical screws

Pearls and Pitfalls

- Need to deal with partially healed displaced fragments
- Have to plan on switching positioning from posterior to anterior
- Plan in place in case bone grafting is needed for the anterior comminution

Surgery

Given the length of time from injury, current deformity, and articular comminution, it was felt he would benefit from ORIF to correct the deformity and primary ankle arthrodesis, as obtaining an anatomic reduction of the articular surface was felt to not be possible. The patient was placed prone on the operating room table, and a posterolateral approach was performed. He had an external fixator placed which was used as a reduction tool. Attention was then turned to the posterior tibia which was reduced and stabilized with a T-shaped buttress plate, and the fibula was stabilized through the same incision (Fig. 6.3c). The patient was then placed supine, and a direct anterior approach was performed to access the joint. Initial reduction of the metaphyseal segment and joint was performed. This was performed with a 4.0 mm screws and temporary K-wire fixation. The articular cartilage was then removed from the comminuted tibia fragments as well as the talar dome. An anterior "spoon" plate was then applied across the joint, and 4.0 mm cortical screws were placed into the tibia and talus (Fig. 6.3d).

Postoperatively, the patient maintained non-weight-bearing precautions for 10 weeks. He then was transitioned to normal shoes. He was lost to follow-up until 8 months from surgery. Radiographs revealed a well-healed fusion (Fig. 6.3e). The patient reported minimal symptoms and had returned to work.

Case 6.4 Malunion

History

A 25-year-old female presents to clinic after a motor vehicle collision 10 weeks prior with an injury to her left ankle (Fig. 6.4a). She was treated with ORIF through a medial incision performed in a different state. She had maintained non-weight-bearing precautions after surgery and had recently began weight-bearing in a fracture boot. Current radiographs were obtained showing an articular malreduction with anterior translation of the talus (Fig. 6.4b). A CT was obtained to evaluate the deformity and fixation (Fig. 6.4c).

Reasons for Failure

- Poor understanding of the fracture pattern
- Incorrect incision used for reduction and stabilization
- Poor articular reduction

Surgical Plan

- Remove previous hardware.
- Tibial osteotomy to find displaced articular fragment.
- Revision fixation using an anterolateral reduction and plating.
- Medial spanning plate.

Approach

- Anterolateral ankle approach
- Percutaneous medial incision (portions of previous medial extensile approach)

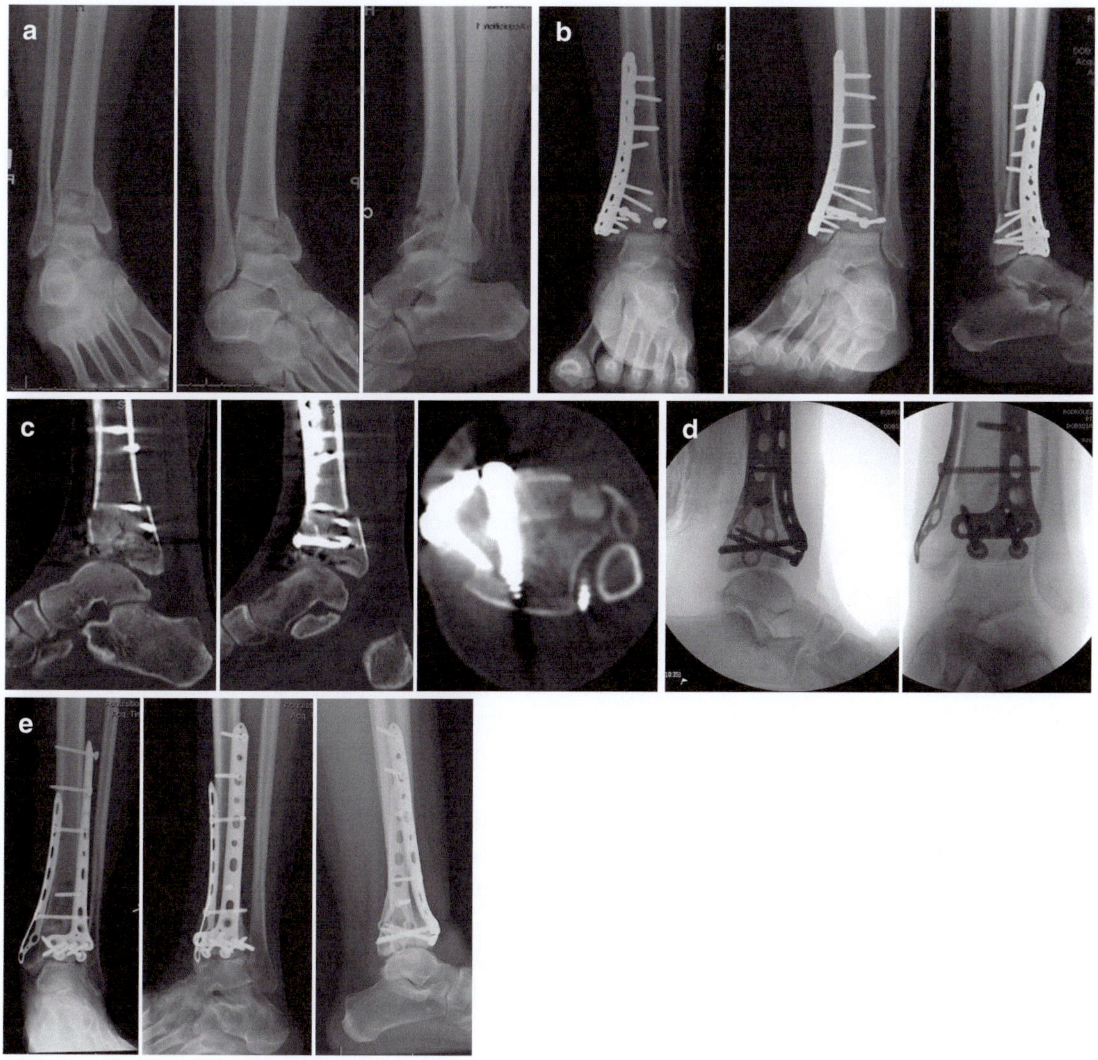

Fig. 6.4 (**a**) AP (left), mortise (center), and lateral (right) radiographs of a 25-year-old female involved in a motor vehicle collision with a comminuted pilon fracture. (**b**) The patient underwent ORIF at an outside facility through a medial approach. AP (left), mortise (center), and lateral (right) radiographs show articular malreduction with anterior translation of the talus best visualized on the lateral radiograph. (**c**) Sagittal CT images (left and center) show anterior translation with impacted articular fragments that remain proximally displaced. The axial image (right) shows no stabilization of the anterolateral articular segments and penetration of the percutaneous anterolateral screw into the syndesmosis. (**d**) The patient was taken back for revision ORIF with osteotomy and articular reconstruction. Lateral (left) and AP (right) fluoroscopic imaging reveals improved articular reduction with reduction of the talus under the plafond. (**e**) AP (right), mortise (center), and lateral (right) X-rays were taken at 2-year follow-up showing minimal arthritic progression

Implants

- Precontoured anterolateral tibial locking plate
- Low profile medial tibial plate
- Small fragment set
- Broken screw removal set (available)

Pearls and Pitfalls

- Need to plan anterolateral incision to maximize skin bridge from prior extensile medial incision
- Careful osteotomy to not affect/damage displaced articular fragment
- Need to address anterior talar translation

Surgery

Given the time from injury and the patient's age and activity level, revision ORIF with revision articular reduction was presented to the patient as well as conversion to fusion. She elected to proceed with revision ORIF. She was taken to the operating room, and the patient's hardware was removed percutaneously using portions of her previous extensile medial incision. An anterolateral incision was created, and dissection was performed to the level of the joint. Osteotomies were used to open the anterior tibial cortex. The large anterolateral fragment was then mobilized and reduced. Reduction of the fragment also helped to reduce the anterior talar translation. With the fragment held with temporary K-wires, a long anterolateral plate was placed using percutaneous techniques and affixed to the tibia. A separate percutaneous medial plate was placed through the previous medial incision (Fig. 6.4d).

Postoperatively, she was kept non-weight-bearing for 10 weeks, with range of motion exercises started at 2 weeks. At follow-up of 26 months, the patient has continued stiffness and discomfort with activities which are limited. She has maintained joint space and has not required conversion to fusion (Fig. 6.4e).

Case 6.5 Nonunion

History

A 47-year-old female with a PMH of significant tobacco use sustained a closed left ankle injury after falling 15 ft. from a ladder (Fig. 6.5a). She was initially taken to the operating room for initial surgical stabilization. She was placed prone, and her posterior tibia and fibula were treated with ORIF through a posterolateral approach (Fig. 6.5b). An external fixator was also placed to maintain the alignment of the anterior tibia. The patient underwent an uncomplicated ORIF at 2 weeks following injury (Fig. 6.5c). She was followed as an outpatient and at 16 months returned to the office with increased pain complaints. Radiographs revealed a failure of the hardware concerning for nonunion (Fig. 6.5d). A follow-up CT was obtained which revealed a healed articular surface with minimal arthritic change and only a metaphyseal nonunion (Fig. 6.5e).

Reasons for Failure

- Smoking
- Combined anterior and posterior approaches
- Poor biological ingrowth

Surgical Plan

- Remove hardware.
- Debridement nonunion site.
- Revision ORIF with anterolateral plate.

Approach

- Anterior ankle approach (previous)
- Iliac crest incision for bone grafting

Implants

- Precontoured anterolateral pilon locking plate
- Small fragment set
- Broken screw removal set (available)

Pearls and Pitfalls

- The potential for encountering residual deep infection
  - Need intraoperative cultures
- Inability to remove hardware
- Need to adequately debride nonunion site
  - Drill into the nonunion to restore intramedullary blood flow
- Bone grafting for atrophic nonunion

Surgery

The patient was felt to benefit from revision ORIF with hardware removal and autologous bone grafting given her atrophic nonunion with bone resorption. Preoperative laboratory workup revealed inflammatory markers were within normal limits. She went to the operating room, and the previous anterior approach was used. First, the hardware was removed, and intraoperative bone cultures were obtained. The metaphyseal portion of the joint was debrided back to healthy bleeding bone. Autologous iliac crest bone graft was then packed into the nonunion site. A long

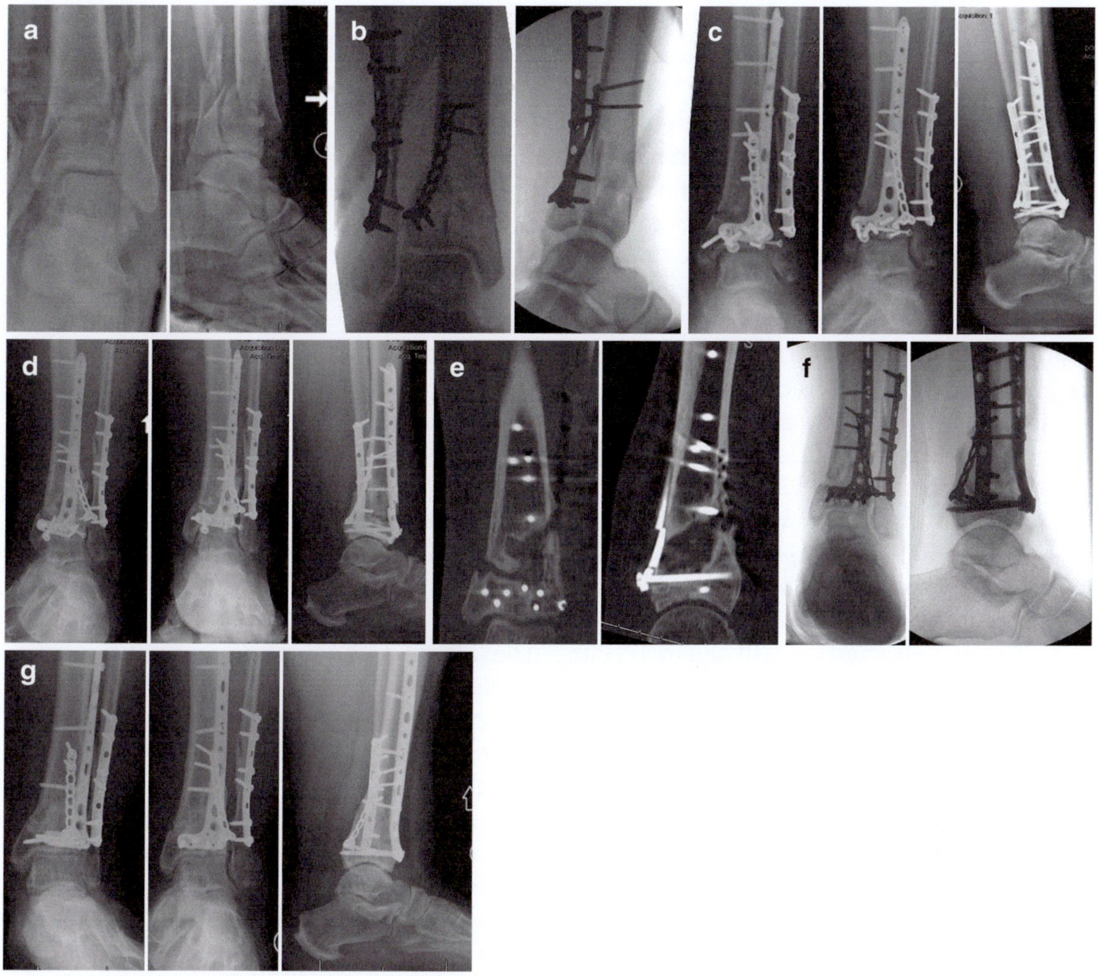

Fig. 6.5 (**a**) AP (left) and lateral (right) radiographs of a 47-year-old female who fell from height. (**b**) Intraoperative AP (right) and lateral (left) fluoroscopic images flowing external fixation with posterior stabilization of the tibia and fibula through a posterolateral incision. (**c**) AP (left), mortise (center), and lateral (right) postoperative radiographs following definitive ORIF at 2 weeks from injury. (**d**) AP (left) and mortise (center) radiographs were obtained at 16 months following surgery showing a persistent fracture line consistent with nonunion. Lateral (right) radiograph shows interval breakage of the anterolateral plate. (**e**) Coronal (left) and sagittal (right) CT reconstruction images reveal a metaphyseal nonunion with bone resorption. The articular surface is well healed with minimal arthritic changes. (**f**) AP (left) and lateral (right) fluoroscopic images following revision plating and autologous iliac crest bone grafting. (**g**) AP (left), mortise (center), and lateral (right) radiographs obtained at 12 months following revision surgery showing consolidation at the nonunion site

anterolateral plate was then placed across the nonunion site and stabilized with locking and nonlocking 3.5 mm screws (Fig. 6.5f).

Postoperatively the patients was placed on non-weight-bearing precautions for 8 weeks and then transitioned back into normal shoewear and activities. Follow-up at 12 months revealed a well-healed nonunion with no activity limitations (Fig. 6.5g).

Case 6.6 Nonunion Metaphyseal and Articular Necrosis

History

A 43-year-old male sustained an open pilon when he fell off a ladder and got his leg caught in the rungs. On physical exam he was noted to have an 8 cm medial wound with exposed bone.

The same day he had a formal debridement in the operating room along with placement of an external fixator and fixation of the fibula through a posterolateral incision (Fig. 6.6a). Four days later, the patient had a repeat irrigation and debridement with fixation of his fibula through a posterolateral approach (Fig. 6.6b). Three weeks later, after his soft tissues had adequately recovered, definitive fixation of the fracture was performed. An anterolateral approach was used for ORIF, given the medial traumatic wound (Fig. 6.6c). The patient had an uncomplicated perioperative course. At 7 months, he reported increased pain. Repeat imaging at that office visit showed intact hardware and alignment with minimal bony healing and arthritic changes at the tibiotalar joint. A CT scan was obtained that showed nonunion at the metaphyseal and articular surface. The articular surface had sclerosis with collapse and extensive post-traumatic arthritis (Fig. 6.6d). Inflammatory workup revealed no evidence of infection.

Reasons for Failure

- Open fracture, soft tissue compromise
- Poor biological ingrowth

Surgical Plan

- Remove indwelling hardware.
- Autologous iliac crest bone grafting.
- Debridement of ankle and metaphyseal nonunion site.
- Revision plating spanning the ankle and nonunion site.

Approach

- Anterolateral ankle approach (previous)
- Percutaneous medial and lateral incisions for lag screws
- Percutaneous approach for medial screw removal

Implants

- 7.3 mm cannulated screws
- Small fragment "spoon" plate
- Small fragment set
- 4.0 mm cortical screws
- Broken screw removal set (available)

Pearls and Pitfalls

- The potential for encountering residual deep infection
  - Need intraoperative cultures
- Accounting for bone loss resorption at nonunion/ankle sites
- Potential issues of hardware removal

Surgery

The patient had a nonunion at the metaphysis as well as early traumatic arthrosis of the ankle joint. Due to this, he was felt to benefit from ankle arthrodesis with open repair of his nonunion with autologous bone grafting. The patient's previous anterolateral incision was used for exposure. The prior hardware was removed including the medial malleolar screw to allow for debridement of the joint. The ankle joint was exposed, and the anterior nonunion fragments were nonviable and necrotic. Intraoperative cultures were sent and were found to be negative. The joint was denuded of the cartilage and any subchondral bone perforated. Tissue from the nonunion site was also sent for intraoperative gram stain and found to be negative for infection. After both areas were prepared, the ankle joint and metaphyseal nonunion was grafted with iliac crest autograft. The ankle was fixed with a medial and lateral 7.3 mm cannulated screw through percutaneous

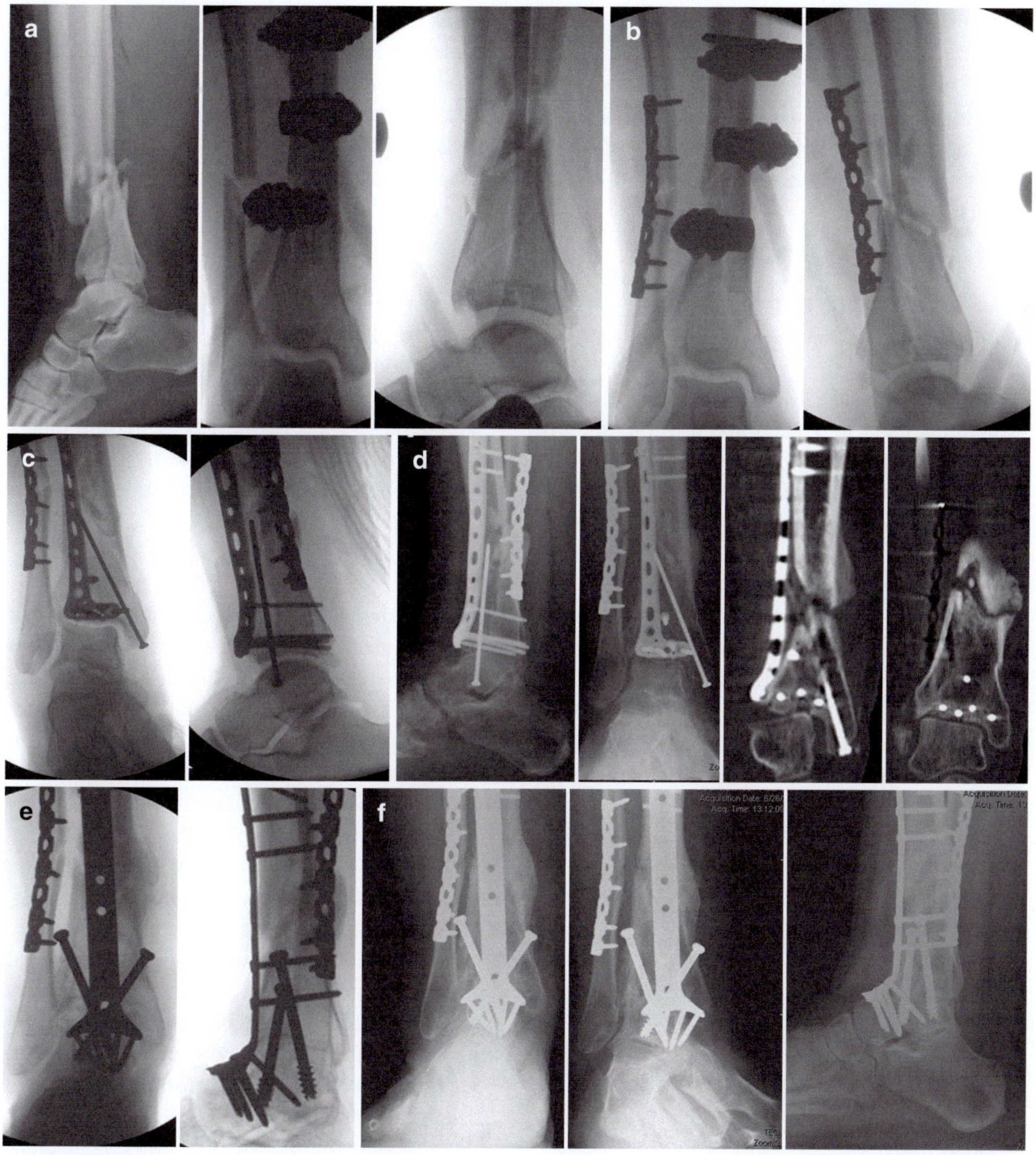

Fig. 6.6 (**a**) Lateral (left) radiograph of a 43-year-old male who fell off of a ladder. AP (center) and lateral (right) fluoroscopic images after irrigation and debridement and placement of an ankle spanning external fixator. (**b**) AP (left) and lateral (right) fluoroscopic images were obtained when the patient was brought back in 2 days for repeat irrigation and debridement and posterolateral plating of his fibula. (**c**) AP (left) and lateral (right) fluoroscopic images following ORIF through a small anterolateral incision performed 3 weeks after injury. (**d**) At 7 months the patient had worsening pain with a persistent fracture line and arthritic changes at the tibiotalar joint seen on lateral (left) and AP (left center) radiographs. Coronal CT images provide further detail of the articular collapse (right center) and a persistent metaphyseal nonunion (right). (**e**) AP (left) and lateral (right) fluoroscopic images following removal of hardware and iliac crest bone grafting and application of a "spoon" plate spanning the ankle joint and nonunion site. (**f**) AP (left), mortise (center), and lateral (right) radiographs obtained at 12 months from surgery show consolidation at the ankle fusion site and metaphyseal nonunion site

incisions. A plate was contoured and placed to cross the nonunion site and ankle joint (Fig. 6.6e).

Postoperatively, the patient had an uncomplicated postoperative course and went on to heal both his fracture and fusion with minimal symptoms (Fig. 6.6f).

Case 6.7 Metaphyseal Malunion

History

A 46-year-old male was involved in a motor vehicle accident and sustained a pilon fracture that was treated with ORIF using an anterolateral approach. The patient had an uncomplicated course and went on to heal his fracture. He had ongoing pain with continued pain, instability, and lateral foot overload. He had previously undergone hardware removal with his initial treating surgeon. He was referred for continued pain. Clinical evaluation revealed cavus foot alignment (Fig. 6.7a). Initial radiographs revealed a varus malunion of his pilon fracture (Fig. 6.7b). Preoperative CT scan revealed a healed fracture with minimal arthritic changes, and preoperative infection workup was negative.

Reasons for Failure

- Poor surgical planning
- Poor initial reduction (varus)

Surgical Plan

- Anterolateral approach to expose distal tibia and fibula
- Open wedge osteotomy of distal tibia
- Potential need for fibular osteotomy
- Autologous tricortical bone grafting
- Surgical stabilization of distal tibia +/− fibula

Approach

- Anterolateral ankle approach (previous)

Implants

- Small fragment metaphyseal locking plate
- Small fragment set

Pearls and Pitfalls

- Need to accurately restore the joint line with the osteotomy
  - K-wires can be used to mark out the osteotomy and can be used to judge correction.
- Need to plan for a fibular osteotomy in case correction cannot be achieved with an isolated tibial osteotomy
- Accounting for structural bone requirements for the opening wedge osteotomy
  - Wait until the joint is corrected to measuring for tricortical graft.

Surgery

The patient went back to the operating room for supramalleolar osteotomy. The patient's previous anterolateral approach was used. K-wires were placed to mark out the osteotomy, and the osteotomy was created using drill holes and osteotomies. To improve mobility of the malunion, the fibula was also osteotomized at the same level using the same incision. A lamina spreader can then be used to open the tibial osteotomy site and correct either the varus or valgus deformity (Fig. 6.7c). The osteotomy site was filled with a tricortical iliac crest autograft. A metaphyseal plate was contoured to the anterolateral tibia and secured above and below the osteotomy site. Following fixation of the tibia, a compression plating technique was performed using a 1/3 tubular plate on the fibula.

Postoperatively, the patient was kept non-weight-bearing for 8 weeks. The patient went on to heal without complications. Final follow-up at 12 months revealed a healed osteotomy with near anatomical alignment and minimal arthritic changes (Fig. 6.7d). The patient also had improved clinical alignment (Fig. 6.7e).

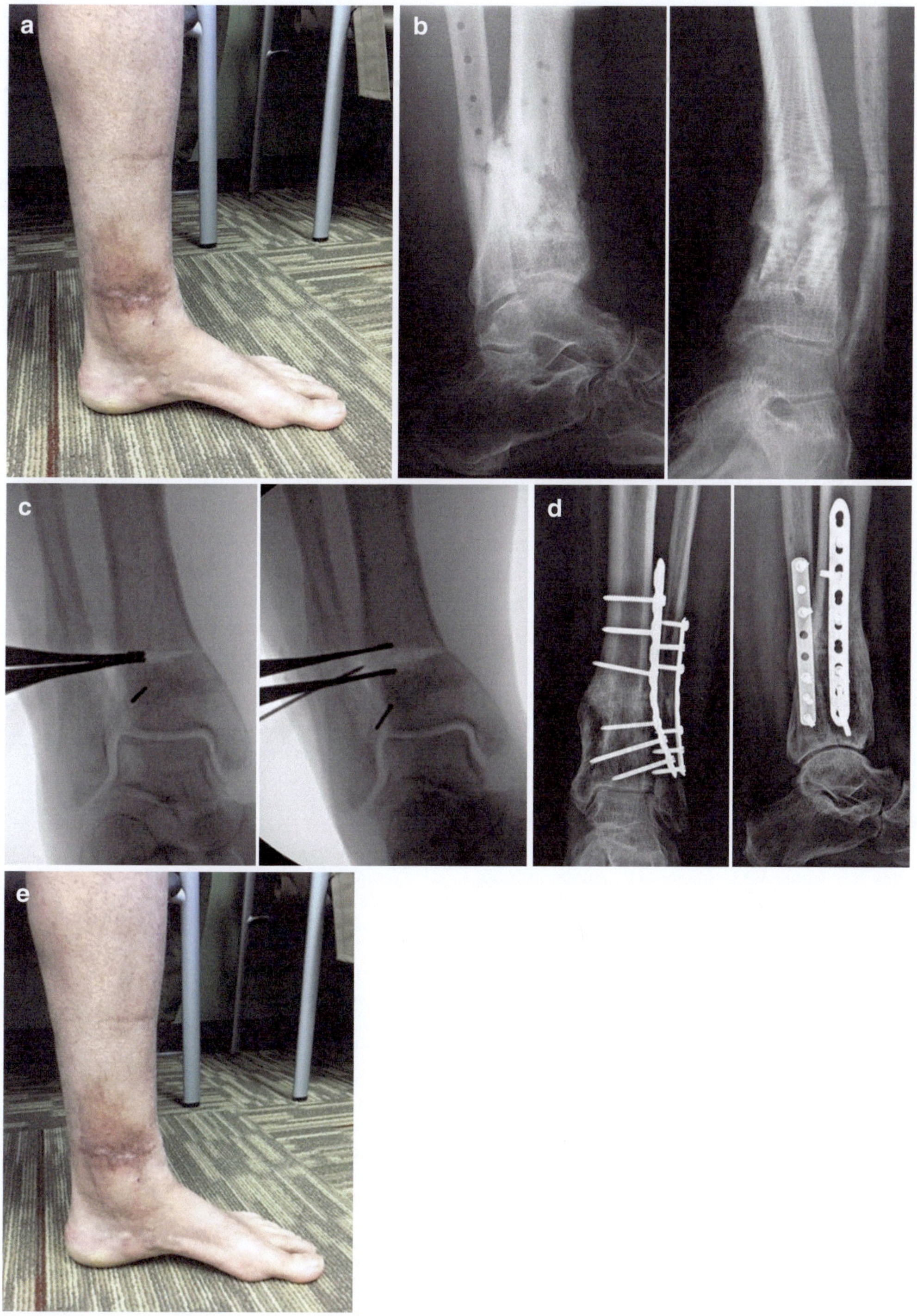

Fig. 6.7 (**a**) Medial standing clinical image of a 46-year-old male who had sustained an open pilon fracture with residual cavus deformity. Image courtesy Michael Swords, DO. (**b**) Weight-bearing lateral (left) and AP (right) radiographs showing a well-healed pilon fracture with varus metaphyseal malunion. The ankle joint remains relatively well preserved. Image courtesy Michael Swords, DO. (**c**) Intraoperative fluoroscopic images that reveal a lateral opening wedge tibial osteotomy (left). Lamina spreaders are then used to correct the deformity bringing the joint surface perpendicular to the long axis of the tibia. Image courtesy Michael Swords, DO. (**d**) At 8 months, AP (left) and lateral (left) radiographs reveal correction of the deformity with preservation of the joint space. Image courtesy Michael Swords, DO. (**e**) Medial standing clinical image showing improvement of the cavus deformity. (Image courtesy Michael Swords, DO)

Summary

Revision surgery for pilon fractures is complicated, and several factors must be taken into account prior to formulating a surgical plan. Patient factors and expectations play a significant role in this. Patients with significant medical comorbidities should understand the potential for complications and wound issues. As with any revision surgery, preoperative infection workup should be performed to plan for the potential of persistent infection. The current condition of the articular cartilage must be taken into account to determine if it is possible to salvage the joint. Once proper preoperative planning has been completed, the surgeon must concentrate on surgical techniques and plan for potential problems during reconstruction. Planning for hardware removal and deformity correction is paramount. The need for bone grafting or orthobiologics should be evaluated on a case-by-case basis. Postoperatively, patients should be followed closely and evaluated for complications.

References

1. Cierny G, Cook WG, Mader JT. Ankle arthrodesis in the presence of ongoing sepsis. Indications, methods, and results. Orthop Clin North Am. 1989;20(4):709–21.
2. Gaulke R, Krettek C. Tibial pilon fractures: avoidance and therapy of complications. Unfallchirurg. 2017;120(8):658–66.
3. Herscovici D Jr, Sanders RW, Infante A, DiPasquale T. Bohler incision: an extensile anterolateral approach to the foot and ankle. J Orthop Trauma. 2000;14(6):429–32.
4. Macnab I, De Haas WG. The role of periosteal blood supply in the healing of fractures of the tibia. Clin Orthop Relat Res. 1974;105:27-33.
5. Marsh JL, Weigel DP, Dirschl DR. Tibial plafond fractures. How do these ankles function over time? J Bone Joint Surg Am. 2003;85(2):287–95.
6. Mast J, Jakob R, Ganz R. Planning and reduction technique in fracture surgery. Berlin: Springer; 1989.
7. McFerran MA, Smith SW, Boulas HJ, Schwartz HS. Complications encountered in the treatment of pilon fractures. J Orthop Trauma. 1992;6(2):195–200.
8. Olszewski D, Streubel PN, Stucken C, Ricci WM, Hoffmann MF, Jones CB, et al. Fate of patients with a "surprise" positive culture after nonunion surgery. J Orthop Trauma. 2016 Jan;30(1):e19–23.
9. Patterson MJ, Cole JD. Two-staged delayed open reduction and internal fixation of severe pilon fractures. J Orthop Trauma. 1999;13(2):85–91.
10. Rosen H. Compression treatment of long bone pseudarthroses. Clin Orthop Relat Res. 1979;138:154–66.
11. Sanders R, Pappas J, Mast J, Helfet D. The salvage of open grade IIIB ankle and talus fractures. J Orthop Trauma. 1992;6(2):201–8.
12. Sarrafian SK. Anatomy of the foot and ankle. Philadelphia: JB Lippincott; 1983.
13. Schatzker J, Tile M. The rationale for operative fracture care. 1st ed. New York: Springer; 1987.
14. Sirkin M, Sanders R, DiPasquale T, Herscovici D Jr. A staged protocol for soft tissue management in the treatment of complex pilon fractures. J Orthop Trauma. 1999 Feb;13(2):78–84.
15. Teeny SM, Wiss DA. Open reduction and internal fixation of tibial plafond fractures. Variables contributing to poor results and complications. Clin Orthop Relat Res. 1993;292:108–17.
16. Tornetta P III, Gorup J. Axial computed tomography of pilon fractures. Clin Orthop Relat Res. 1996;323:273–6.

Revision Surgery of the Malreduced/Malunited Ankle Fracture

7

Michael P. Clare

Key Takeaway Points

- Tibial-foot axis (TFA) is a useful clinical tool to assess rotational alignment of the involved ankle and foot relative to the normal contralateral limb.
- Ankle fracture malunions should generally be taken down through the previous fracture, gently re-creating the original fracture line(s) with osteotomes.
- Restoration of proper fibular length and rotation is critical to restoring stability and symmetry to the ankle mortise and can be performed indirectly with a laminar spreader.
- When involved, the syndesmosis should be reduced in open fashion. A small pointed reduction clamp can be used to correct rotational malalignment of the fibula, followed by provisional K-wire stabilization along the plane of the syndesmosis, prior to definitive implant placement.
- Concomitant medial arthrotomy can be invaluable in assessing the correction of rotational malalignment of the talus.

Introduction

Although rotational ankle fractures may appear seemingly basic and simple, certain unstable fracture patterns may be subtle and potentially problematic if not properly diagnosed and managed. It has long been established that the ankle joint has very limited inherent ability to tolerate even small amounts of asymmetry within the ankle mortise [1]. If left unaddressed, mortise asymmetry often leads to rapid deterioration of the joint and post-traumatic arthritis, presumably due to changes in the surface area of contact [2].

The preeminent goal in the treatment of unstable ankle fractures is to restore the ankle mortise to an anatomic, stable position, in order to maximize function and longevity of the ankle joint. Certain techniques have been developed to address the malunited ankle and syndesmosis as a means of joint preservation, based on AO principles as they relate to basic fracture management. Previous studies have consistently demonstrated with ankle fracture malunions that even in the presence of moderate ankle arthritis, restoration of an anatomic ankle mortise can improve pain, restore function, and preserve the longevity of the ankle joint [3–5].

M. P. Clare (✉)
Florida Orthopaedic Institute, Tampa, FL, USA

M. J. Berkowitz et al. (eds.), *Revision Surgery of the Foot and Ankle*,
https://doi.org/10.1007/978-3-030-29969-9_7

Normal Ankle Alignment/ Radiography

It is essential to thoroughly understand normal, anatomic alignment in order to recognize and manage abnormal, nonanatomic alignment. Rotational alignment of the ankle and foot can be challenging to assess on a plain radiograph of the ankle. The tibial-foot axis (TFA), defined as an imagined straight line extending from the center of the tibial tubercle, along the tibial shaft to the foot, almost always intersects the foot at the 2nd ray (Fig. 7.1). Rarely, the TFA can pass medial to the 2nd ray as a normal variant, as seen with external tibial torsion. The TFA can therefore be used in ankle fracture malunions as a clinical assessment tool, in order to define rotational malalignment in the involved limb relative to normal rotational alignment in the contralateral limb [6].

In the normal radiographic mortise view, the joint space of the ankle mortise is perfectly symmetric medially, laterally, and centrally. The lateral talar body typically aligns with the fibular incisura. The so-called Shenton's line of the ankle extends along the articular surface of the fibula proximally and gently transitions in curvilinear fashion to merge with the articular surface of the lateral tibial plafond. The concavity of the distal tip of the fibula aligns with the inferior margin of lateral talar body, thus resembling a small circular space, the so-called Dime Sign (Fig. 7.2).

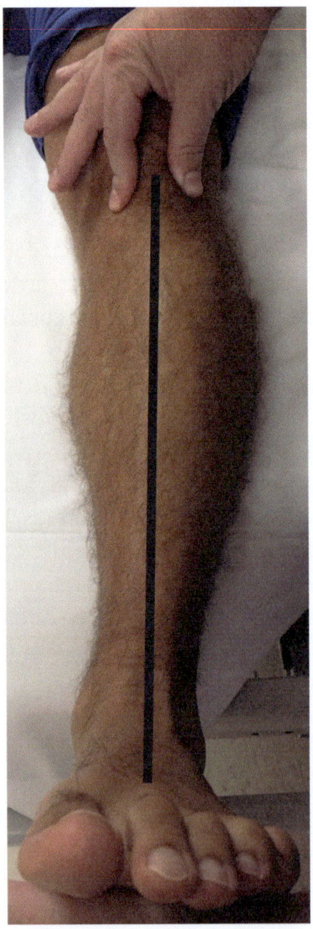

Fig. 7.1 (Normal) Tibial-foot axis. An imagined straight line extending from the center of the tibial tubercle, along the tibial shaft to the foot, almost always intersects the foot at the 2nd ray (black line)

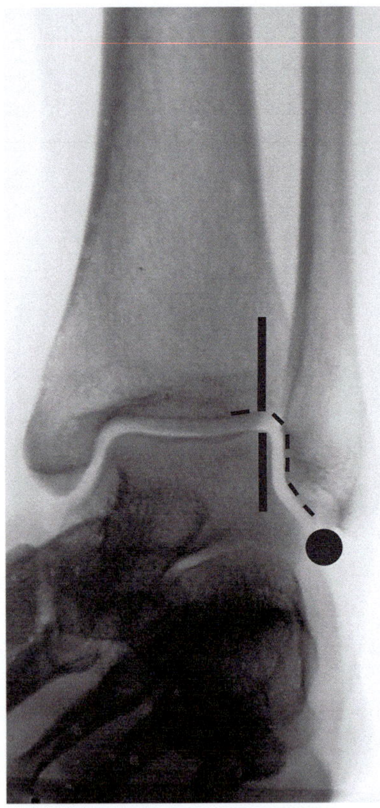

Fig. 7.2 Normal radiographic ankle mortise view. Note the perfectly symmetric joint space medially, laterally, and centrally. The lateral talar body aligns with the fibular incisura (black lines). Shenton's line of the ankle extends along the articular surface of the fibula and gently transitions to merge with the articular surface of the lateral tibial plafond (dashed lines). "Dime Sign": the distal tip of the fibula aligns with the inferior margin of lateral talar body resembling a small circular space (black circle)

Pathoanatomy/Causes for Failure

Supination-External Rotation (S-ER)/ Pronation-External Rotation (P-ER)/ Pronation-Abduction (P-AB)

In these malunion patterns, the fibula almost always heals in a shortened and externally rotated position. With a concomitant medial injury, the talus follows the fibula into a laterally subluxed, externally rotated position, resulting in persistent asymmetry of the ankle mortise. Restoration of proper fibular length and rotation is critical to restoring ankle mortise symmetry and stability.

With more proximal fibular patterns (pronation-external rotation), there may also be malalignment of the syndesmosis. Pronation-abduction patterns may additionally include an element of marginal impaction of the lateral tibial plafond. With involvement of the posterior malleolus, the fragment will similarly heal in a shortened position in accordance to the extent of fibular shortening. With larger posterior malleolar fragments, the talus may sublux posteriorly, resulting in articular incongruity.

Supination-Adduction (S-AD)

These malunions include a transverse fibular fragment of variable size, which may heal in a medially translated position, and a vertical shear pattern through the medial malleolus, which typically heals in a shortened position. The medial fragment may also include marginal impaction of the medial tibial plafond, resulting in varus tilt of the talar body and subsequent deterioration of the medial articular surface.

Evaluation

Clinical evaluation begins with assessment of standing alignment, in which the involved limb is compared to the contralateral limb. The involved limb is evaluated for asymmetry in the coronal, sagittal, and axial planes. Rotational alignment of the involved limb (TFA) is also assessed, with comparison to the contralateral limb [6]. The soft tissue envelope is inspected, noting location of prior incisions or traumatic lacerations and the overall tissue quality in the area. Ankle range of motion is evaluated, comparing the extent of joint stiffness to the contralateral limb. The presence of crepitus with passive motion is also noted.

Radiographic evaluation should include weight-bearing radiographs of the involved ankle and foot. The mortise and lateral views of the ankle are closely assessed for the extent of asymmetry and incongruity, while the remaining views may show secondary deformities related to the chronicity of the ankle malunion. The original fracture pattern should be determined, which is imperative in preoperative planning and surgical decision-making. Particular attention should be directed as to the extent of fibular shortening and/or external rotation; the presence or absence of medial malleolar malalignment or residual widening of the medial clear space; and the presence or absence of posterior malleolar involvement and extent of displacement.

The presence or absence of post-traumatic arthritis should also be assessed, as a determination must be made as to whether or not the ankle joint is salvageable. Joint-sparing osteotomies and reconstruction are contraindicated in the event of severe, end-stage post-traumatic arthritis. In most instances, although some degree of arthritic change may be noted, the joint itself remains salvageable. Comparison weight-bearing views of the contralateral ankle and foot can be invaluable as a means of defining a patient's "normal" alignment.

Computed tomography (CT) scanning is a useful advanced imaging tool and provides essential information regarding the extent of malalignment, detection of marginal impaction, and the extent of arthritic change, where present. CT scans are especially useful in defining the extent of posterior malleolar involvement, where present. The normal contralateral limb can be included in the study, which allows a direct, side-by-side comparison that can be particularly useful in detecting subtle syndesmotic asymmetry.

Surgical Planning/Considerations

Preoperative planning is an essential element of outlining the detailed, structured sequence and the proper execution of a joint-sparing reconstruction. Consideration is given toward the original fracture pattern, indwelling implants, patient positioning, surgical approaches, joint arthrotomy and debridement, need for corrective osteotomy(ies), reduction strategies, and definitive fixation.

Patient Positioning

Other than in the instance of a large posterior malleolar fragment with a chronic posteriorly subluxed ankle joint, most ankle fracture malunions can be addressed from the supine position. A modest bump is placed beneath the ipsilateral hip until the tibial tubercle is perfectly perpendicular to the floor and therefore in line with the ceiling. In this way, the tibial tubercle remains the constant, and the ankle/foot is reduced rotationally relative to the tibial tubercle. The contralateral limb is secured to the radiolucent table to allow bed tilt where necessary.

Surgical Approaches

The fibula is exposed through the previous incision; in the absence of a prior incision, a posterolateral approach is preferred overlying the peroneal tendon sheath proximally and in line with the posterolateral rim of the fibula distally. The superior peroneal retinaculum should be preserved, so as to avoid destabilization of the peroneal tendons. Subperiosteal dissection continues anteriorly to the anterior margin of talofibular joint. Any previous implants are removed, and the bone-implant interface is debrided. In more proximal fibular patterns, the distal syndesmosis should also be visualized and debrided.

The medial malleolus is similarly exposed through the previous incision, and any previous implants are removed; in the absence of a prior incision or prior fracture, an anteromedial incision is preferred to better facilitate an anteromedial arthrotomy and debridement of the medial clear space. Rotational asymmetry of the talus and extent of existing articular cartilage damage should be assessed. In most instances of fibular shortening or external rotation, the talus will similarly be externally rotated relative to the medial malleolus.

Case Examples

Case 7.1

History

- A 19-year-old male/college baseball player
- Twisting injury sliding into 2nd base
- Underwent ORIF elsewhere
- Presents 4 months later with medial ankle pain, ankle rolling inward
- Full ankle motion/TFA medial to 1st ray (Fig. 7.3a)
- Weight-bearing radiographs/CT scan bilateral ankles (Fig. 7.3b–i)

Fig. 7.3 (**a**) Preoperative tibial-foot axis medial to 1st ray, indicating external rotation malunion through syndesmosis. (**b, c**) Weight-bearing radiographs of ankle (**b**) mortise and (**c**) lateral. Fibular length restored. There is subtle widening of medial clear space and asymmetry between lateral talar body and fibular incisura. (**d–f**) Computed tomography scan of involved ankle: coronal (**d**) and axial (**e–f**) cuts. Note subtle widening of medial clear space (white arrow); (**f**) note relative external rotation of fibula to incisura (white arrow). (**g–i**) Computed tomography scans of normal contralateral ankle: coronal (**g**) and axial (**h, i**) cuts. (**j**) Hardware removal of fibula and syndesmosis. Note remnants of syndesmotic screw visualized within syndesmosis (white arrow), indicating external rotation of fibula relative to incisura. (**k**) Anteromedial arthrotomy. Talar body is externally rotated relative to medial malleolus. (**l**) Syndesmosis reduction: pointed reduction clamp used to internally rotate fibula within incisura (white arrow). Provisional stabilization with 2.0 mm K-wire parallel to plane of syndesmosis to prevent anterior-posterior translation of fibula within incisura as pelvic clamp applied. (**m, n**) Revision ORIF syndesmosis: mortise (**m**) and lateral (**n**) views. Symmetry of ankle mortise has been restored. Lateral talar body aligns with incisura. (**o**) Intraoperative tibial-foot axis now in line with 2nd ray. (**p, q**) Final weight-bearing radiographs 2 years post-revision surgery: mortise (**p**) and lateral (**q**) views

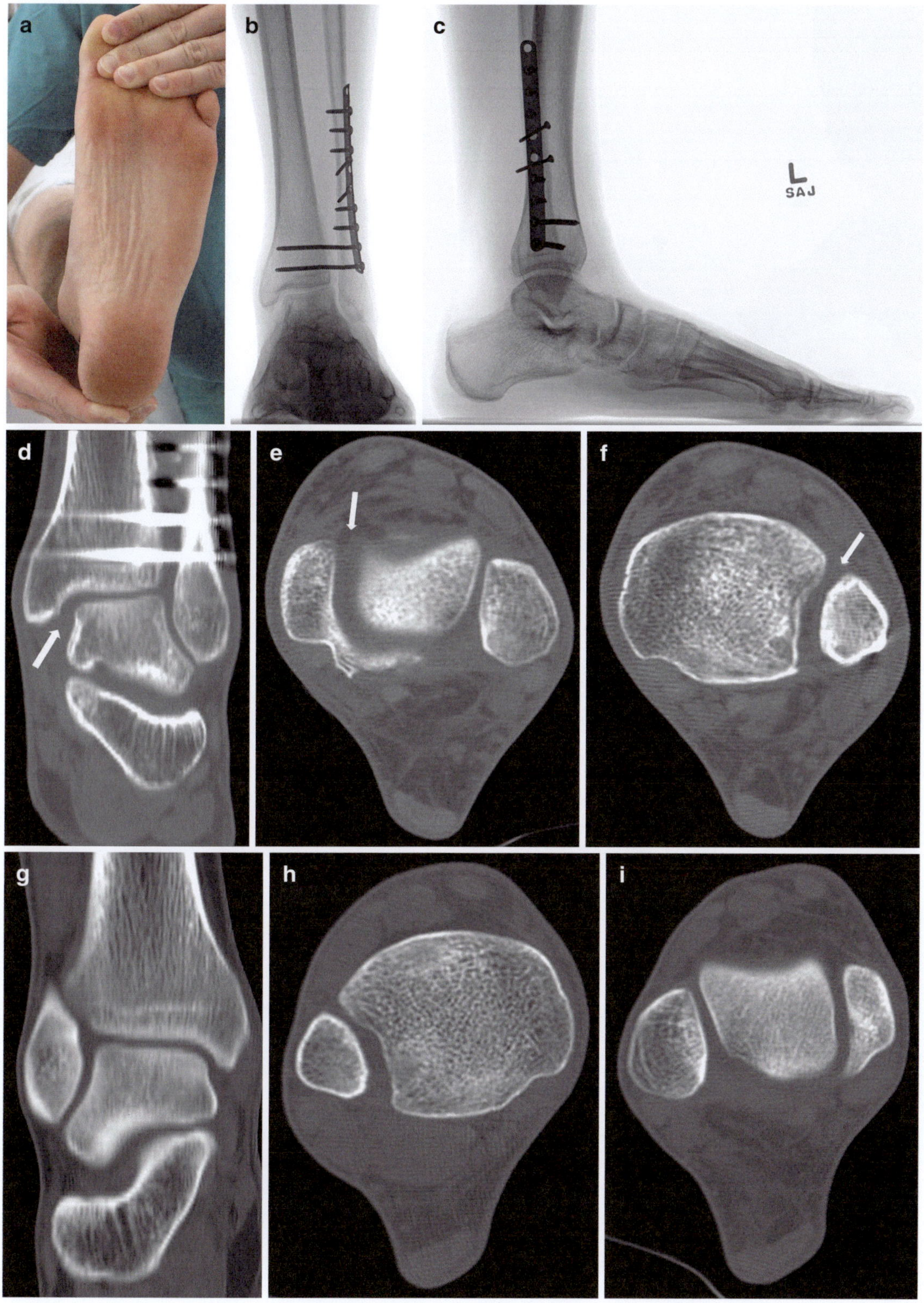
a
b
c
L
SAJ
d
e
f
g
h
i

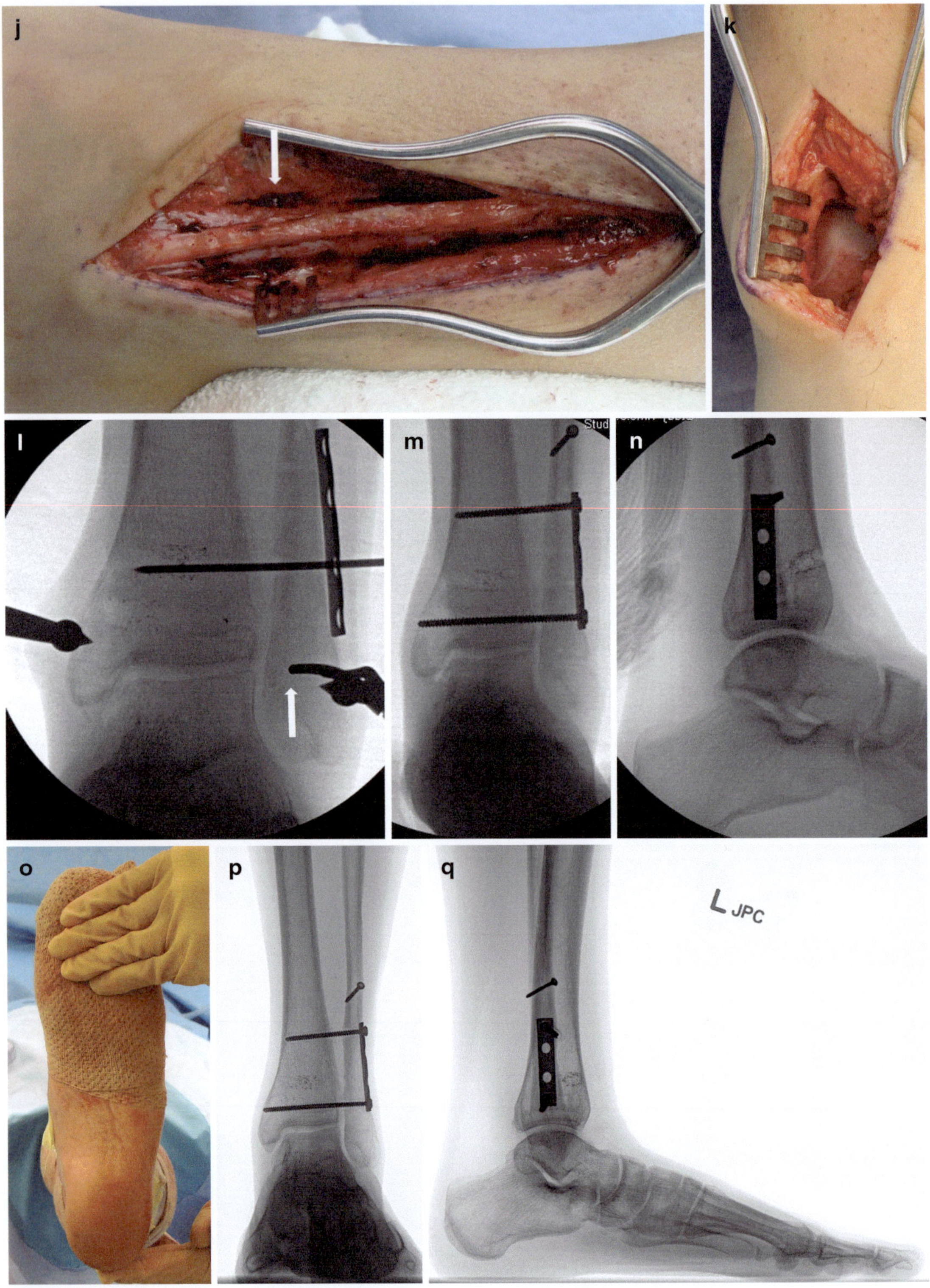

Fig. 7.3 (continued)

Reasons for Failure

- Diagnosis: (P-ER) external rotation malunion of syndesmosis
- Fibular length restored/open reduction of syndesmosis not performed
- Syndesmosis stabilized in relative external rotation

Surgical Plan

- Hardware removal fibula/syndesmosis (Fig. 7.3j)
- Anteromedial arthrotomy/debridement of medial clear space (Fig. 7.3k)
- Open debridement/mobilization of syndesmosis
- Revision ORIF of syndesmosis (Fig. 7.3l–q)

Approach

- Lateral approach to fibula/syndesmosis through prior incision
- Anteromedial arthrotomy

Implants

- Two 3.5 mm quadricortical syndesmosis screws through a 1/3 tubular plate (washer)

Pearls and Pitfalls

- Small fragment point-to-point clamp used to internally rotate fibula relative to incisura (Fig. 7.3l)
- Provisional 2.0 mm K-wire placed parallel to syndesmosis (30 degrees posterolateral to anteromedial) to prevent anterior-posterior translation of fibula within incisura (Fig. 7.3l)
- Pelvic reduction clamp used narrow width of syndesmosis (sliding along plane of K-wire) (Fig. 7.3l)
- Quadricortical screws placed similarly parallel to syndesmosis
- (Fig. 7.3m, n)

Case 7.2

History

- A 67-year-old female/obese
- Twisting injury/ground-level fall
- Underwent ORIF/revision ORIF elsewhere
- Presents 3 months after injury with persistent deformity/pain with weight-bearing
- Radiographs: injury; ORIF; revision ORIF (Fig. 7.4a–f)

Reasons for Failure

- Diagnoses: (P-ER) shortening-external rotation nonunion-malunion of fibula/syndesmosis
- Fibular length still grossly short/mortise grossly malaligned
- Insufficient working length of lateral plate

Surgical Plan

- Hardware removal of fibula/mobilization of fibular nonunion (Fig. 7.4g)
- Anteromedial arthrotomy/debridement of medial clear space
- Indirect restoration of fibular length/rotation (Fig. 7.4h, i)
- Revision ORIF fibula/syndesmosis (Fig. 7.4j–m)

Approach

- Lateral approach to fibula/syndesmosis through prior incision
- Anteromedial arthrotomy

Implants

- Anatomic distal fibular locking plate/multiple locking screws
- Two 3.5 mm quadricortical syndesmosis screws

Pearls and Pitfalls

- Anteromedial arthrotomy critical to assess extent of correction of fibular length/rotation
- Indirect restoration of fibular length/rotation [4]: (Fig. 7.4h, i)
  - Plate secured to distal fragment:
    - Plate must be positioned just anterior to posterolateral rim of distal fragment to simultaneously correct rotation as length restored.
  - Cortical screw (4 mm longer than measured) proximal to plate
  - Laminar spreader placed between cortical screw/proximal tip of plate
  - Proximal fragment provisionally secured with clamp/2.0 mm K-wire

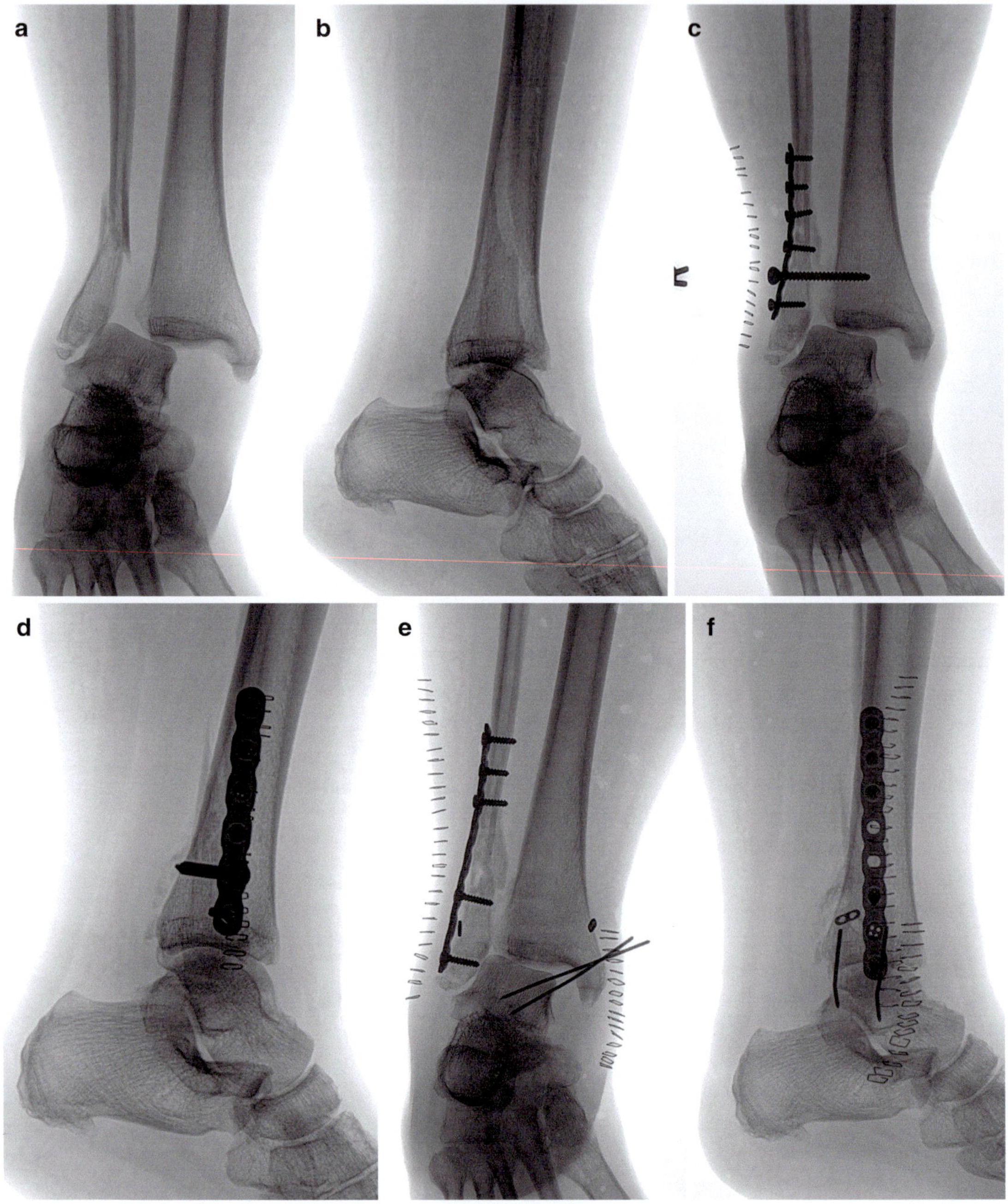

Fig. 7.4 (**a**, **b**) Injury mortise (**a**) and lateral (**b**) radiographs demonstrate a pronation-external rotation trimalleolar-equivalent ankle fracture-dislocation. (**c**, **d**) Initial ORIF elsewhere: mortise (**c**) and lateral (**d**) views. Fibular length not restored; medial clear space still grossly widened; ankle mortise grossly asymmetric; insufficient working length of lateral plate. (**e, f**) Revision ORIF elsewhere: mortise (**e**) and lateral (**f**) views. Fibular length still not restored; medial clear space remains grossly widened; ankle mortise still grossly asymmetric; insufficient working length of lateral plate. (**g**) Mobilization of fibular nonunion. (**h**, **i**) Indirect restoration of fibular length/rotation (different patient): mortise (**h**) and lateral (**i**) views. (**j**, **k**) (2nd) Revision ORIF ankle/syndesmosis: mortise (**j**) and lateral (**k**) views. Fibular length now restored; ankle mortise now stable and symmetric. (**l**, **m**) Final weight-bearing mortise (**l**) and lateral (**m**) radiographs over 1 year post-revision surgery

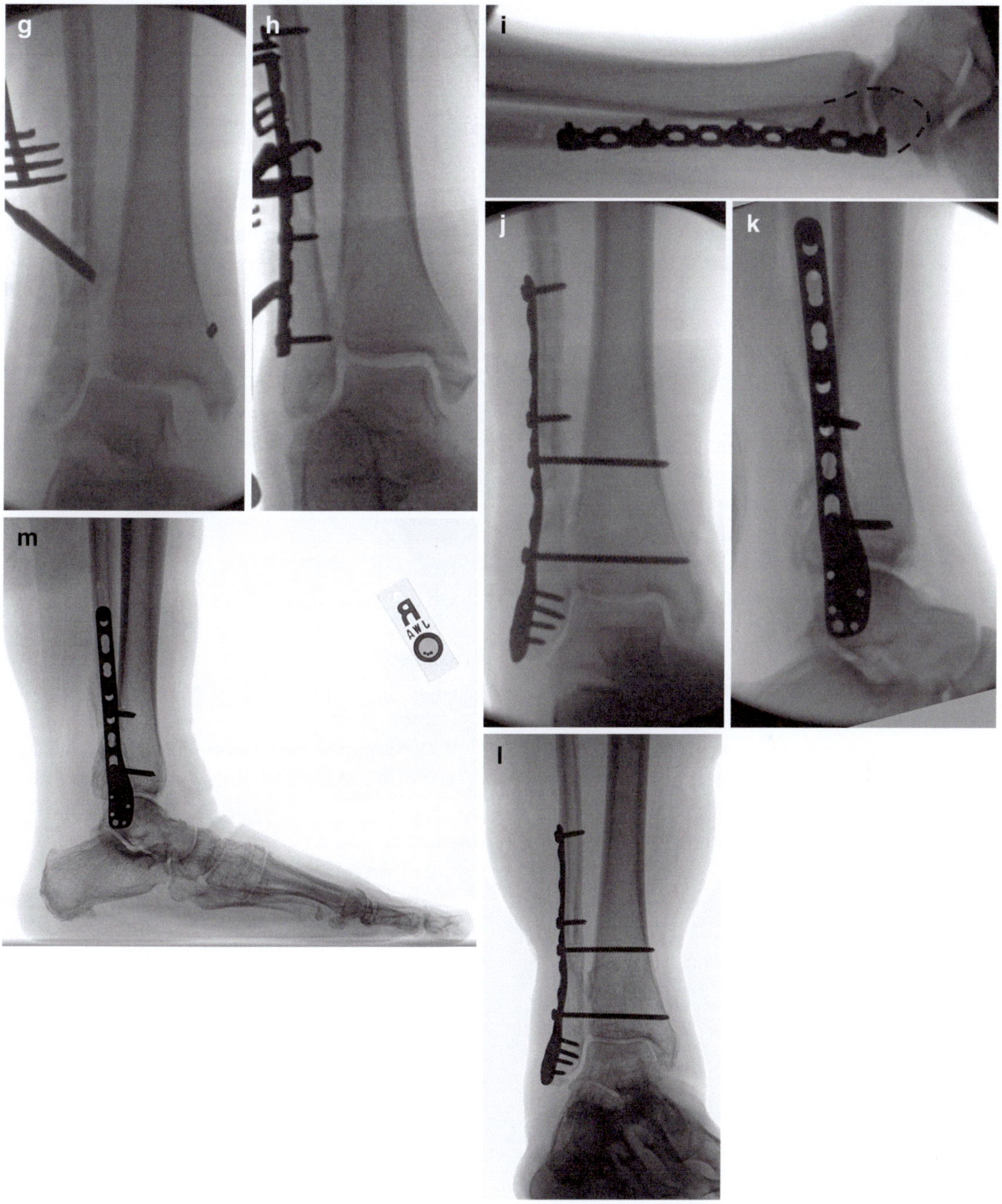

Fig. 7.4 (continued)

Case 7.3

History

- A 78-year-old female/healthy and active
- Twisting injury/ground level fall
- Ankle fracture treated nonoperatively
- Presents 7 months post-injury with poor balance/pain with weight-bearing
- Mild ankle stiffness/tender along ankle joint line
- TFA medial to 1st ray compared to contralateral limb (Fig. 7.5a, b)
- Weight-bearing radiographs (Fig. 7.5c, d)

Reasons for Failure

- Unstable nature of fracture underappreciated
- Chronologic age of patient not necessarily an indication to "undertreat" fracture

Surgical Plan

- Diagnosis: (S-ER) shortening-external rotation malunion fibula/translational malunion medial malleolus
- Medial malleolar malunion takedown/fibular malunion takedown (Fig 7.5e, f)
- Indirect restoration of fibular length/rotation (Fig. 7.5g)
- Revision ORIF ankle (Fig. 7.5h–l)

Approach

- Posterolateral approach to fibula
- Medial approach/anteromedial arthrotomy: medial clear space debridement

Pearls and Pitfalls

- Medial malleolar malunion takedown with osteotomes under fluoroscopy (Fig. 7.5e)
- Fibular malunion takedown: original fracture line re-created with osteotomes under fluoroscopy (Fig. 7.5f)
  - Finesse maneuver: allow osteotome to "find its path"
  - Better facilitates restoration of length/rotation
  - Larger surface area for healing

Case 7.4

History

- A 25-year-old female/western wear model
- Fell from 5 feet while climbing a fence during photo shoot
- Underwent ORIF elsewhere
- Presents 6 months later with medial ankle pain, frequent rolling episodes
- Near full ankle motion/TFA medial to 1st ray (Fig. 7.6a, b)
- Weight-bearing radiographs/CT scan (Fig. 7.6c–h)

Reasons for Failure

- Diagnoses: (1) shortening-varus-medial impaction (S-AD) malunion; (2) external rotation fibular malunion
- Vertical shear fracture line not opened
- Shortening/medial impaction not recognized
- Distal fibula likely (iatrogenically) externally rotated during plate application

Surgical Plan

- Hardware removal of fibula/takedown of fibular malunion (Fig. 7.6i)
- Hardware removal of distal tibia/takedown of vertical shear malunion (Fig. 7.6j, k)
- Intra-articular osteotomy/disimpaction of medial tibial plafond (Fig. 7.6l–n)
- Backfill defect with adjacent cancellous autograft
- Revision ORIF medial distal tibia/revision ORIF fibula (Fig. 7.6o–v)

Approach

- Medial and lateral approaches through prior incision lines
- Anteromedial arthrotomy/articular surface and original fracture line visualized

Implants

- Small fragment T-plate medially
- Cortical lag screws distally as rafter support to disimpacted area
- Single cortical screw laterally (transverse, length-stable pattern)

Pearls and Pitfalls

- Anteromedial arthrotomy essential to expose articular surface
- Original fracture line visualized and confirmed under fluoroscopy
- Posterior tibial tendon exposed and protected during takedown of original fracture line perform disimpaction ~1 cm proximal to joint surface to preserve bone attached to articular surface/gently lever downward with osteotome/backfill defect with adjacent cancellous bone/provisional K-wires to support disimpacted area (Fig. 7.6l–n)

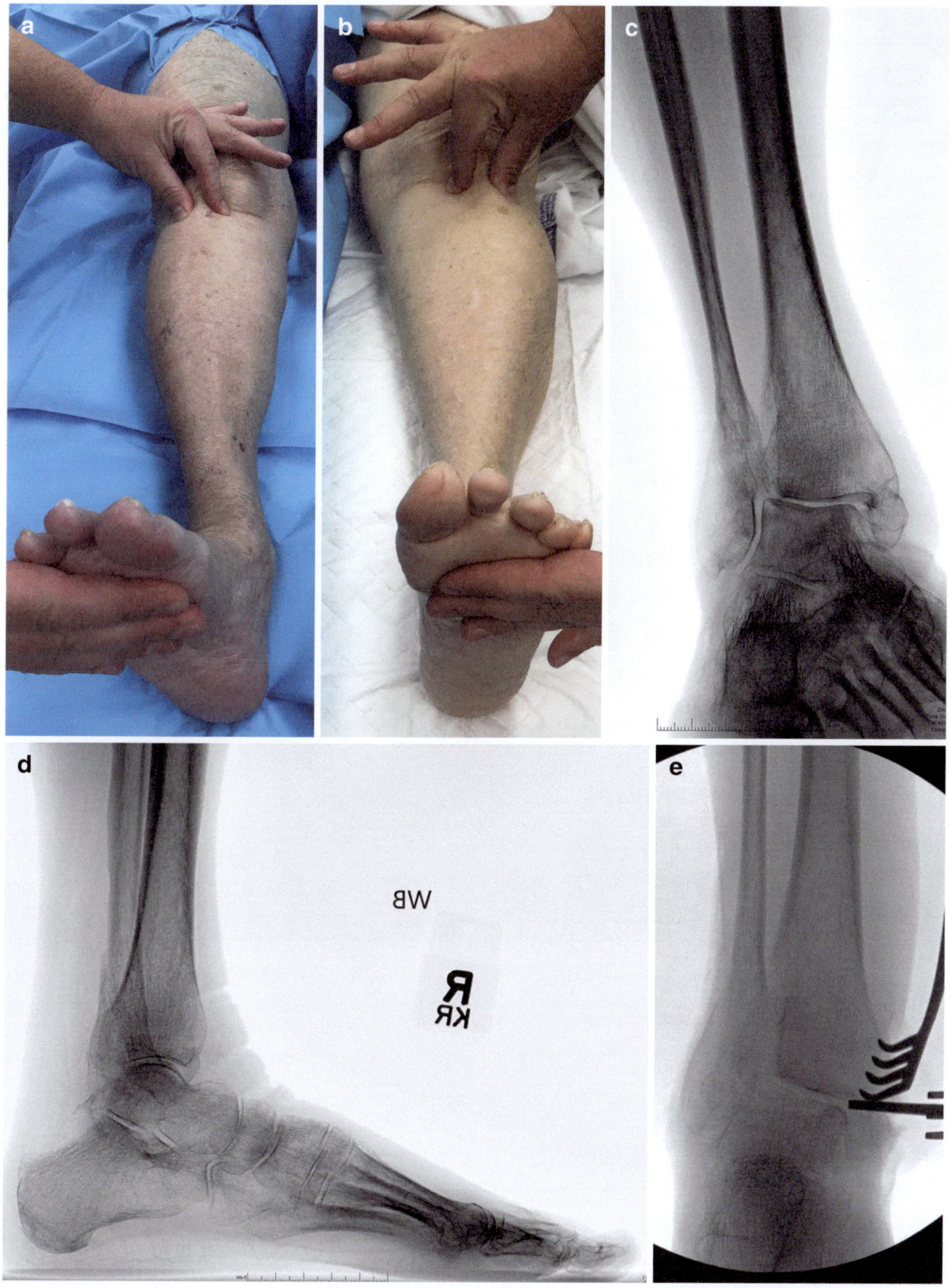

Fig. 7.5 (**a**, **b**) Preoperative tibial-foot axis (**a**) medial to 1st ray on involved limb; (**b**) aligned with 2nd ray on contralateral limb. (**c**, **d**) Weight-bearing mortise (**c**) and lateral (**d**) radiographs of ankle. Note fibular shortenening, lateral translation of talus, and overall asymmetry of ankle mortise. Lateral talar body not aligned with incisura suggesting rotational malalignment. (**e**, **f**) Medial malleolar malunion (**e**) and fibular malunion (**f**) takedown. Original fracture lines are gently re-created with osteotomes (dashed line). (**g**) Indirect restoration of fibular length/rotation. (**h**, **i**) Revision ORIF: mortise (**h**) and lateral (**i**) views. Fibular length and mortise symmetry restored. Lateral talar body aligns with incisura. (**j**) Intraoperative tibial-foot axis now aligns with 2nd ray. (**k**, **l**) Final weight-bearing mortise (**k**) and lateral (**l**) radiographs 6 months post-revision surgery

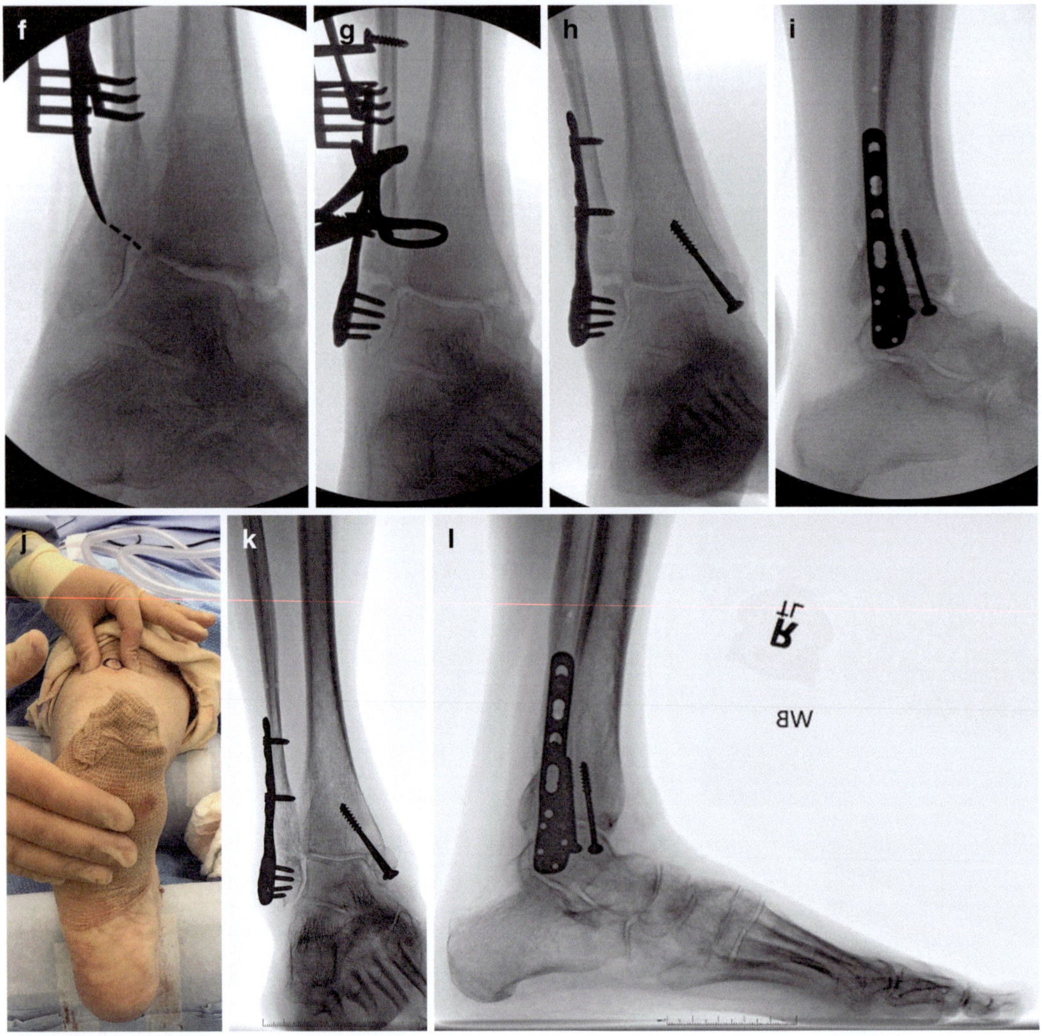

Fig. 7.5 (continued)

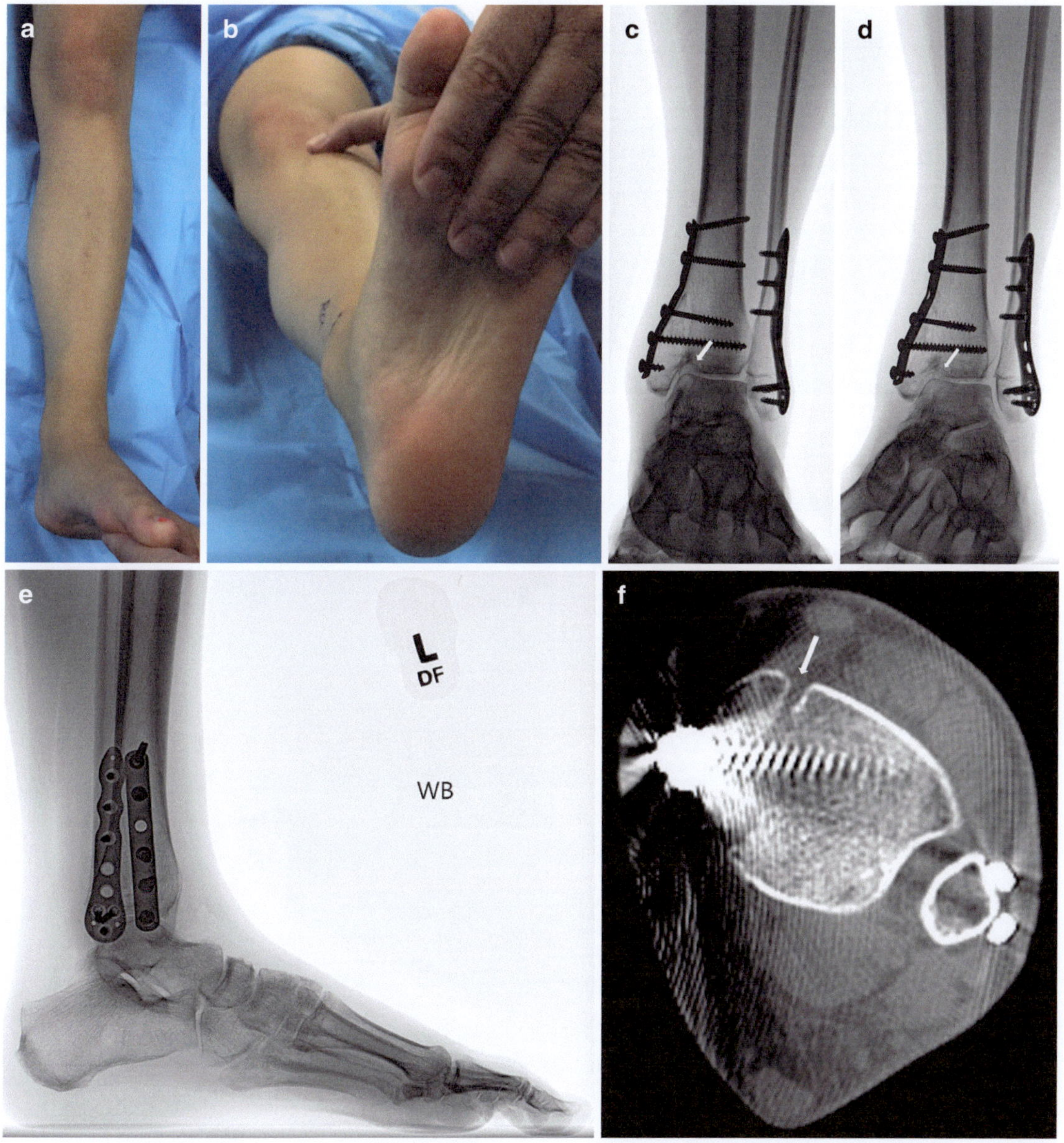

Figs 7.6 (**a**, **b**) Preoperative tibial-foot axis medial to 1st ray, indicating external rotation malunion through prior fibula fracture. (**c–e**) Weight-bearing A/P (**c**), mortise (**d**), and lateral (**e**) radiographs of involved ankle. Note residual impaction of medial tibial plafond (white arrow). (**f–h**) Computed tomography scan of involved ankle: axial (**f**), sagittal (**g**), and coronal (**h**) cuts. The vertical shear fracture line is fixed in relative external rotation (white arrow), suggesting that the fracture site was never exposed. Orientation of fixation is non-perpendicular to plane of fracture line. Also note residual impaction of medial tibial plafond ((**g**): black arrows/(**h**): white arrow). (**i**) Fibular malunion takedown. Note relative external rotation of distal fragment (white arrow), producing external rotation malunion of fibula. (**j**, **k**) Distal tibial malunion takedown. Note impaction of medial tibial plafond (white arrow). (**l–n**) Disimpaction of medial tibial plafond. The osteotomy is performed approximately 1 cm proximal to joint line to preserve bone attached to articular surface (**1**). Defect is backfilled with adjacent cancellous autograft. Provisional 2.0 mm K-wires are placed above disimpacted bone for rafter support (**m**, **n**). (**o–q**) Reduction and revision ORIF. Mortise view demonstrating provisional reduction (**o**); mortise (**p**) and lateral (**q**) views following revision ORIF. Articular congruity has been restored. (**r**, **s**) Intraoperative tibial-foot axis now in line with 2nd ray. (**t–v**) Final weight-bearing A/P (**t**), mortise (**u**), and lateral (**v**) radiographs 1 year post-revision surgery

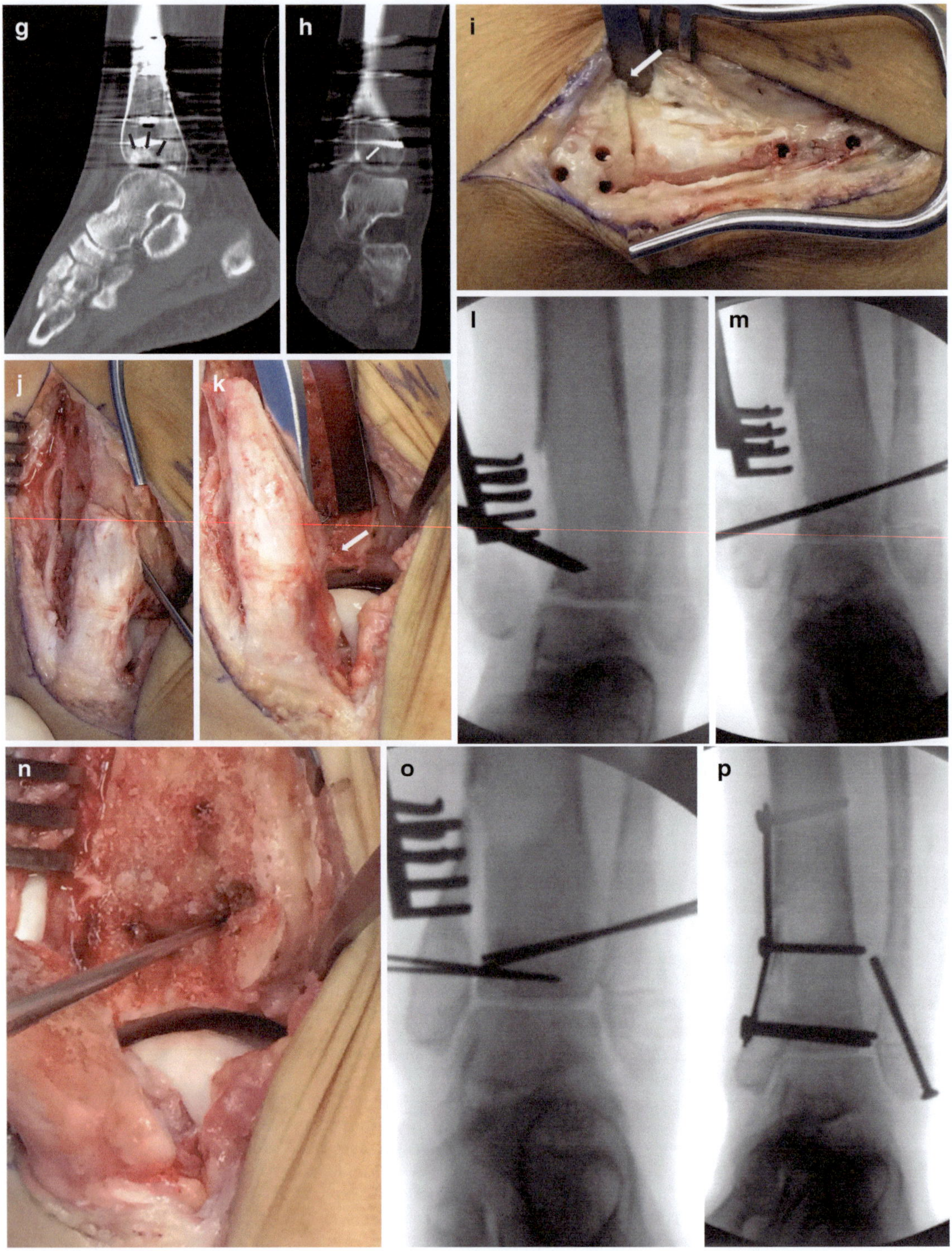

Fig. 7.6 (continued)

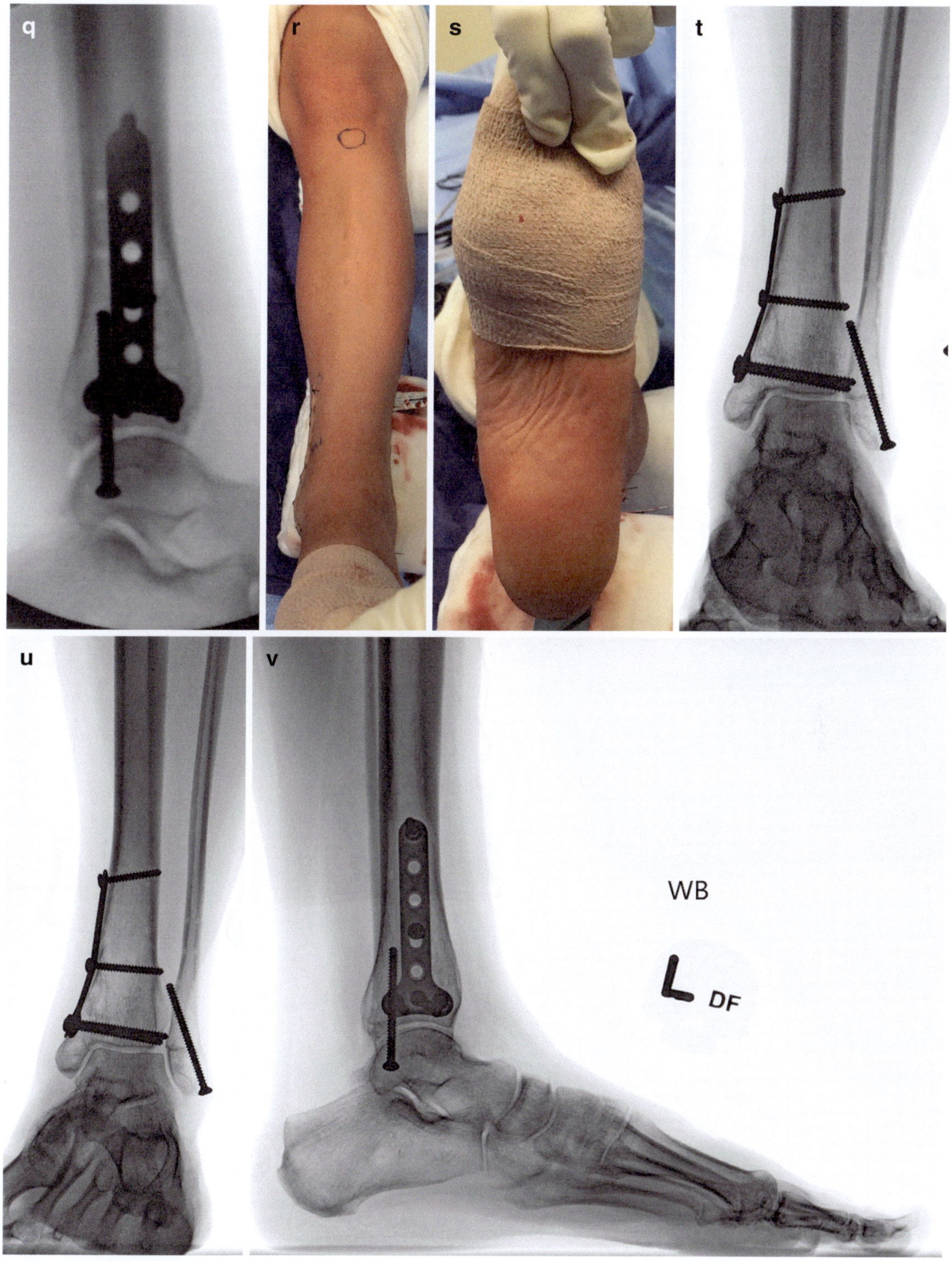

Fig. 7.6 (continued)

References

1. Ramsey PL, Hamilton W. Changes in tibiotalar area of contact caused by lateral talar shift. J Bone Joint Surg Am. 1976;58(3):356–7.
2. Thordarson DB, Motamed S, Hedman T, Ebramzadeh E, Bakshian S. The effect of fibular malreduction on contact pressures in an ankle fracture malunion model. J Bone Joint Surg Am. 1997;79(12):1809–15.
3. Reidsma II, Nolte PA, Marti RK, Raaymakers EL. Treatment of malunited fractures of the ankle: a long-term follow-up of reconstructive surgery. J Bone Joint Surg Br. 2010;92(1):66–70.
4. Weber BG, Simpson LA. Corrective lengthening osteotomy of the fibula. Clin Orthop Relat Res. 1985;(199):61–7.
5. Weber BG. Trauma of the ankle joint and of its neighborhood. In: Weber BG, editor. AO masters' cases: minimax fracture fixation. New York, NY: Thieme; 2004. p. 101–37.
6. Clare MP. unpublished data.

8 Revision Surgery After Failed Calcaneal ORIF

Michael P. Clare

> **Key Takeaway Points**
> - When properly performed, ORIF is best.
> - Some calcaneal malunions, particularly fracture-dislocation variants and those patterns with limited posterior facet involvement, can be taken down through the original fracture pattern with osteotomes and reconstructed, thereby preserving subtalar motion.
> - With most calcaneal malunions, the subtalar joint is not salvageable and is therefore sacrificed as part of the reconstructive salvage.

Introduction

Displaced intra-articular fractures of the calcaneus are among the most challenging fractures for the orthopedic surgeon. These fractures are typically the result of a fall from height or motor vehicle collision. Fracture patterns in the calcaneus are generally three-dimensionally complex, yet relatively predictable. Although the calcaneus itself has abundant vascularity, the limited surrounding soft tissue envelope can be particularly problematic.

The preeminent goal in the treatment of displaced intra-articular calcaneal fractures is to restore the posterior facet articular surface, as well as calcaneal height, length, and overall morphology, in order to maximize function and longevity of the subtalar joint. When properly performed by an experienced surgeon, ORIF offers by far the best opportunity for a successful long-term outcome, even in the instance of post-traumatic arthritis requiring late subtalar arthrodesis [1–4].

In the instance of a failed ORIF, certain malunions are amenable to take down and reconstruction with subtalar joint preservation. In many instances, the extent of post-traumatic arthritis is such that the subtalar joint is not salvageable and must therefore be sacrificed as part of the reconstructive salvage.

Normal Radiography of the Calcaneus

It is essential to thoroughly understand normal, anatomic alignment in order to recognize and manage abnormal, non-anatomic alignment. In the normal radiographic lateral view, the posterior facet articular surface sits superior to the calcaneal tuberosity, indicative of normal calcaneal height, and is reflected in the tuber angle of

M. P. Clare (✉)
Florida Orthopaedic Institute, Tampa, FL, USA

M. J. Berkowitz et al. (eds.), *Revision Surgery of the Foot and Ankle*,
https://doi.org/10.1007/978-3-030-29969-9_8

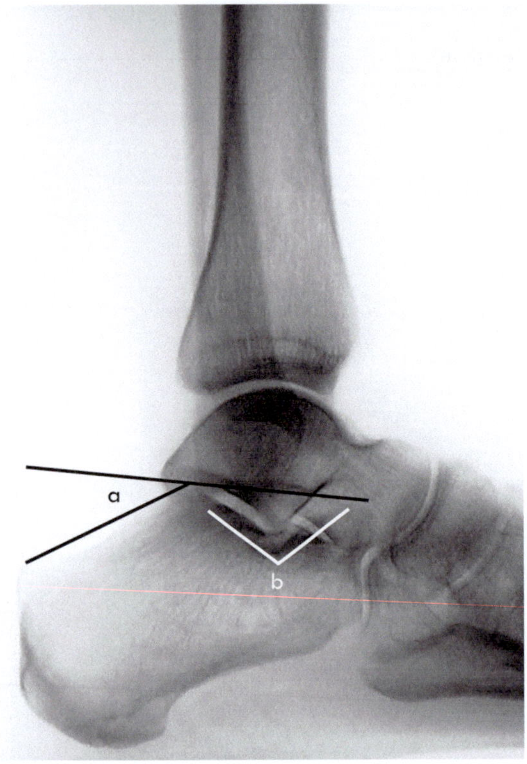

Fig. 8.1 Normal lateral radiographic view. Tuber angle of Böhler (**a**): angle formed by confluence of line from superior edge of tuberosity to superior-most edge of posterior facet and line from superior-most edge of posterior facet to superior edge of anterior process (black lines). Crucial angle of Gissane (**b**): angle formed by line parallel to posterior facet and line parallel to anterior process (white lines)

Böhler (Fig. 8.1). The posterior facet angles gently downward and merges with the anterior process of the calcaneus, as defined by the crucial angle of Gissane (Fig. 8.1). This confluence lies distinctly inferior to the tarsal canal and middle facet and accommodates the lateral process of the talus to facilitate subtalar motion.

Pathoanatomy/Causes for Failure

In most instances, a calcaneal malunion is the result of a lack of understanding of the three-dimensional fracture pattern on the part of the treating surgeon. The vast majority of displaced intra-articular calcaneal fractures can be categorized as joint depression type, tongue type, or fracture-dislocation variant type patterns. Each pattern requires distinct reduction maneuvers to proper restore alignment, such that if the treating surgeon does not thoroughly comprehend the orientation of the fracture pattern, a poor result is imminent.

In almost all calcaneal malunions, there is residual loss of calcaneal height and length, with concomitant relative widening from lateral wall expansion, which may impinge against the distal fibula or impede normal peroneal tendon function. The resulting misshape causes relative flattening of the longitudinal orientation of the talus, which secondarily decreases ankle dorsiflexion. Residual intra-articular step off within the posterior facet often results in a stiff, painful hindfoot, with rapid deterioration of the joint surface and post-traumatic arthritis [5].

In some instances, particularly the "far lateral" fracture patterns (Sanders type 2A joint depression-type or split tongue-type, or fracture-dislocation variant), the extent of intra-articular involvement is limited, such that the subtalar joint can often be preserved. These same patterns, however, can include disruption of the superior peroneal retinaculum and peroneal tendon dislocation.

Evaluation

Clinical evaluation begins with assessment of standing alignment, in which the involved limb is compared to the contralateral limb. The involved limb is evaluated for asymmetry in the coronal, sagittal, and axial planes. The soft tissue envelope is inspected, noting location and status of prior incisions and the overall tissue quality in the area. Ankle and hindfoot range of motion is evaluated, comparing the extent of joint stiffness to the contralateral limb.

Radiographic evaluation should include weight-bearing radiographs of the involved ankle and foot, as well as axial and Brodén views. The lateral view is closely assessed for the extent of loss of calcaneal height and relative secondary flattening of the talus, as well as congruity or incongruity of the crucial angle of Gissane. The lateral view will also distinguish between a joint depression-type and a tongue-type pattern. The axial view is evaluated for residual shortening through the primary fracture line and any residual coronal plane deformity of the tuberosity (typically varus) relative to the remainder of the calcaneal body. The mortise view of the ankle and Brodén views are assessed for the extent of intra-articular step-off, potential salvageability of the subtalar joint, and to delineate a fracture-dislocation variant pattern. The remaining views of the foot are evaluated for extent of lateral wall expansion, extension into the calcaneocuboid joint, and any secondary deformities related to the chronicity of the calcaneal malunion. The original fracture pattern should be determined, which is imperative in preoperative planning and surgical decision-making.

The presence or absence of post-traumatic arthritis should also be assessed in order to determine the salvageability of the subtalar joint. Joint-sparing osteotomies are contraindicated in the presence of severe, end-stage post-traumatic arthritis; hindfoot reconstruction combined with arthrodesis of the subtalar joint is often employed in these instances. Comparison weight-bearing views of the contralateral ankle and foot can be invaluable as a means of defining a patient's "normal" alignment.

Computed tomography (CT) scanning is a critical advanced imaging tool in the evaluation and management of the calcaneal malunion. The scan provides invaluable information regarding the original fracture pattern, extent of loss of calcaneal height and length, degree of overall three-dimensional malalignment, and the extent of post-traumatic arthritic change, where present.

Surgical Planning/Considerations

Preoperative planning is an essential element of outlining the detailed, structured sequence and the proper execution of a joint-sparing reconstruction. Consideration is given toward the original fracture pattern, indwelling implants, patient positioning, surgical approaches, joint arthrotomy and debridement, need for corrective osteotomy(ies), reduction strategies, and definitive fixation.

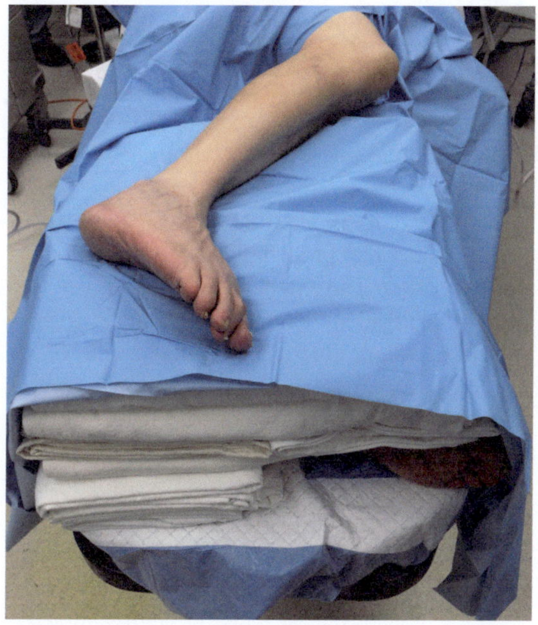

Fig. 8.2 Lateral decubitus position

Patient Positioning

Calcaneal malunions are generally best addressed from the lateral decubitus position on a beanbag. The lower extremities are arranged in a scissor-like configuration: the nonsurgical limb is extended at the knee, directed away from the eventual surgical field; the surgical limb flexed at the knee and angled toward the near corner of the operating table. An operating platform is created with blankets and secured to the radiolucent table, such that the surgical limb is oriented parallel to the floor (Fig. 8.2).

Surgical Approaches

Extensile Lateral Approach

Because of the complex pathoanatomy associated with calcaneal malunions, the extensile lateral approach is most commonly utilized. Soft tissue complications following the surgical management of calcaneal fractures remain a major source of morbidity, such that careful attention to detail with respect to placement of the incision and gentle handling of the soft tissues are of paramount importance.

In the event of a prior, properly performed extensile lateral approach, the same surgical incision is utilized. The extensile lateral incision may also be used in the event of a prior sinus tarsi approach. Alternatively, if the soft tissue envelope is especially scarred and non-mobile, and if calcaneal height is markedly off, the original extensile lateral approach may be used for implant removal (and/or lateral wall exostectomy), and staged reconstruction completed using only the vertical limb of the incision (Gallie approach) [6].

The extensile lateral incision begins approximately 2 cm proximal to the tip of the lateral malleolus, immediately lateral to the Achilles tendon and thus posterior to the sural nerve and the lateral calcaneal artery, and the vertical limb extends toward the plantar foot. The horizontal limb continues at the junction of the skin of the lateral foot and the heel pad and extends to the base of the fifth metatarsal, with a gentle curve connecting the two limbs of the incision (Fig. 8.3). Dissection is specifically taken "straight to the bone" at the level of the calcaneal tuberosity proximally, avoiding any beveling of the skin, and continues to the midpoint of the horizontal limb.

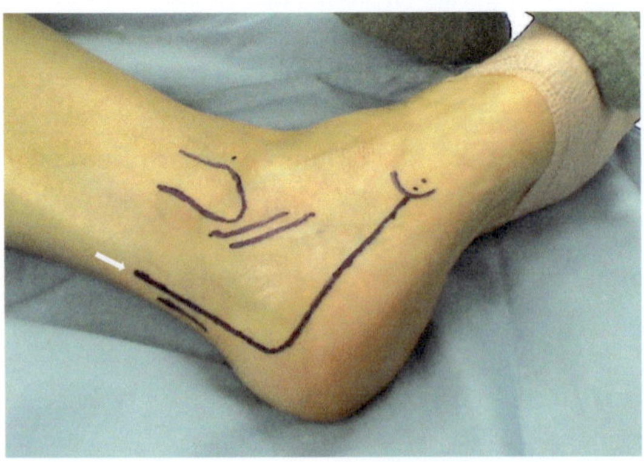

Fig. 8.3 Incision for extensile lateral approach. Note proximity of vertical limb, immediately adjacent to Achilles tendon, and therefore posterior to lateral calcaneal artery and sural nerve (white arrow)

A full-thickness, subperiosteal flap is raised, beginning at the apex of the incision. The use of retractors is avoided until a sizable subperiosteal flap is developed, which prevents separation of the skin from the underlying subcutaneous tissue. The peroneal tendons are exposed only at the level of the peroneal tubercle, and a periosteal elevator is used to gently mobilize the flap distally to the calcaneocuboid joint. Thus, the peroneal tendons, the sural nerve, and the lateral calcaneal artery are contained entirely within the flap, and devascularization of the lateral skin is minimized.

Deep dissection continues to the sinus tarsi dorsally, anterior process and calcaneocuboid joint distally, and the superior-most portion of the calcaneal tuberosity proximally for "backside" access to the posterior facet. Using a "no touch" technique, three 1.6 mm Kirschner wires (K-wires) are placed for retraction of the subperiosteal flap: One into the fibula as the peroneal tendons are slightly subluxated anterior to the lateral malleolus, a second wire in the talar neck, and a third wire in the cuboid as the peroneal tendons are levered away from the anterolateral calcaneus with a periosteal elevator. A fourth wire may be placed in the talar body posteriorly for additional exposure of the posterior facet articular surface.

Following procedure completion, the full-thickness flap is closed over a deep drain with deep No. 0 absorbable sutures placed in interrupted fashion starting at the proximal and distal ends and progressing toward the apex of the incision. The sutures are hand-tied sequentially in similar fashion to eliminate tension at the apex of the incision. The skin layer is closed with 3-0 monofilament suture using the modified Allgöwer-Donati technique.

Posterolateral Approach to Fibula for Superior Peroneal Retinaculum Reconstruction

In the event of dislocating peroneal tendons, and following extensile lateral closure, a small (<3 cm) incision is made along the posterolateral edge of the lateral malleolus, which should provide sufficient skin bridge to the vertical limb of

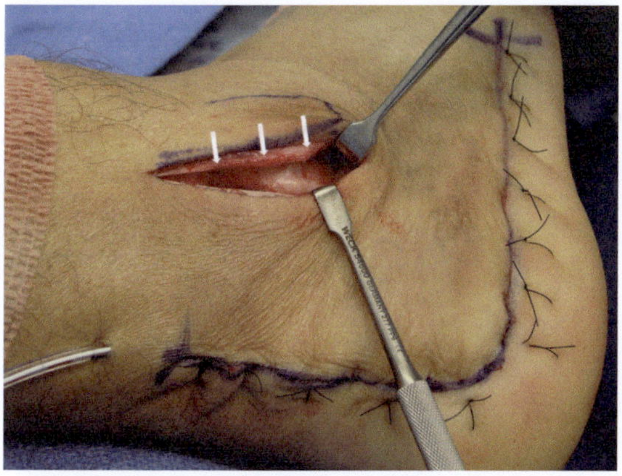

Fig. 8.4 Posterolateral approach to fibula for Superior Peroneal Retinaculum repair. Note preservation of retinacular tissue for later closure (white arrows)

the extensile lateral incision. The peroneal sheath is incised, preserving sufficient retinacular tissue for later closure and avoiding iatrogenic damage to the dislocated peroneal tendons (Fig. 8.4) [7].

Case Examples

Case 8.1

History

- A 21-year-old female/healthy/non-smoker/fall from 10 feet 4 months prior
- Diagnosed with calcaneus fracture/treated elsewhere with closed reduction and casting
- Presents with locked subtalar joint/still unable to bear weight due to pain
- Radiographs/CT scan (Fig. 8.5a–f)

Reasons for Failure

- Diagnosis: (unrecognized) calcaneal fracture-dislocation variant malunion
- Tuberosity fragment remains attached to superolateral articular fragment/driven into talofibular joint: locks subtalar joint
- Associated with fibular avulsion fracture/dislocated peroneal tendons

Surgical Plan

- Young age/majority of posterior facet articular surface preserved
- Malunion takedown: modified Romash osteotomy
- Joint preservation/ORIF calcaneus (Fig. 8.5g–k)

Approach

- Extensile lateral approach

Implants

- Anatomic locking calcaneal plate/3.5 mm cortical and locking screws

Pearls and Pitfalls

- Romash osteotomy originally described from anterior to posterior through primary fracture line of joint depression malunion patterns/combined with subtalar arthrodesis [8]
- Modified Romash osteotomy: posterior to anterior along original fracture-dislocation line
  - Visualize entry point and path of osteotome directly.
  - Allow osteotome to "find its path" along original fracture line (Fig. 8.5l, m).
  - Confirm on axial fluoro views (Fig. 8.5n–p).
  - Schanz pin in tuberosity facilitates control of tuberosity fragment.

Case 8.2

History

- A 51-year-old male/fell from height 6 months prior
- Worker's compensation injury/treated non-operatively elsewhere
- Presents with persistent lateral hindfoot pain/unable to return to work
- Tender in lateral subfibular region/peroneal tendons chronically dislocated
- Weight-bearing radiographs: (Fig. 8.6a–c)
- CT scan: (Fig. 8.6d–g)

Reasons for Failure

- Diagnosis: Sanders type I calcaneal malunion/dislocated peroneal tendons
- Unrecognized dislocated peroneal tendons

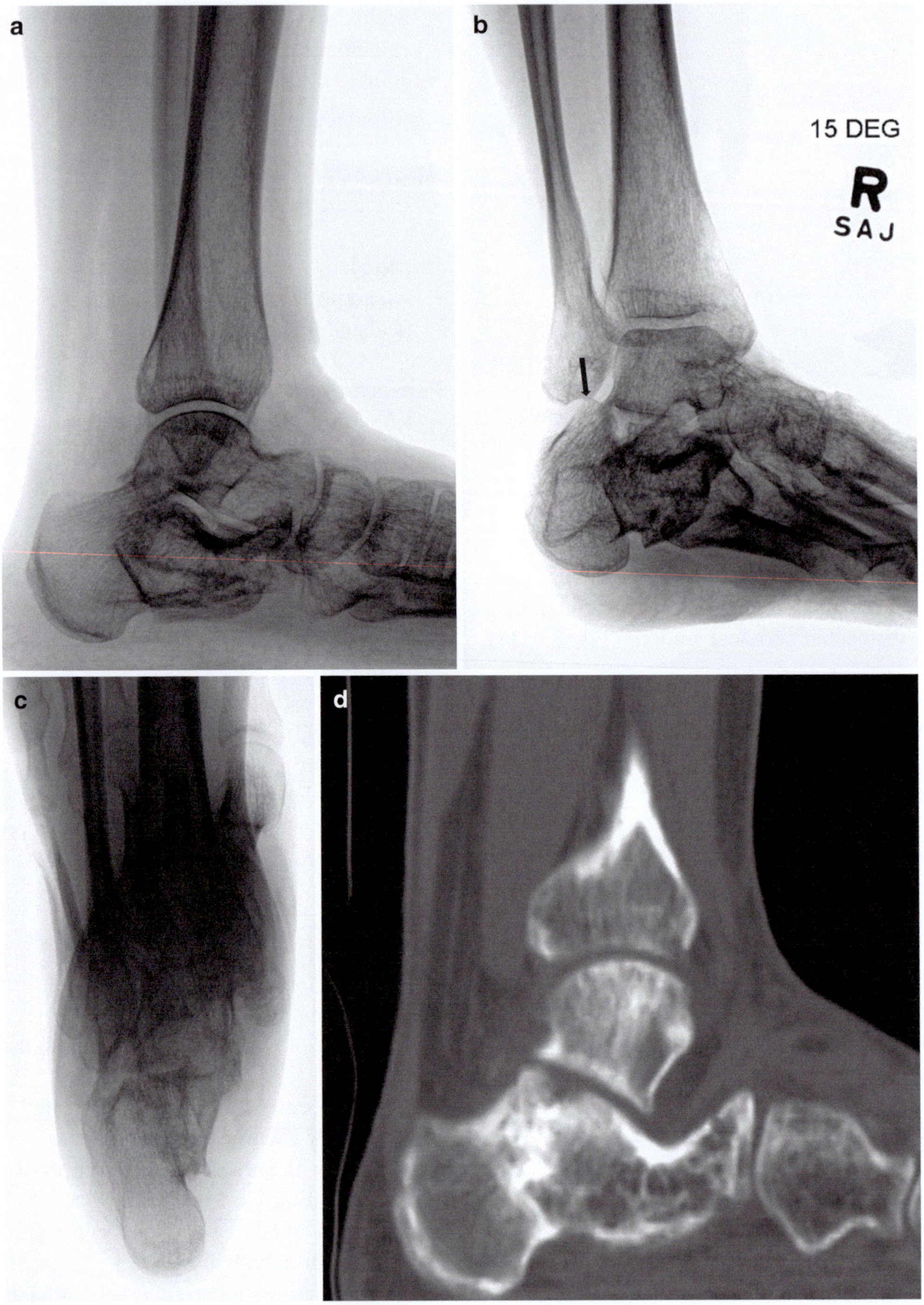

Fig. 8.5 (**a**–**c**) Weight-bearing lateral (**a**), Broden (**b**), and axial (**c**) radiographs of ankle and foot. Note chronically dislocated tuberosity fragment (with attached superolateral articular fragment) (black arrow). (**d**–**f**) Computed tomography scan of involved hindfoot. (**d**) sagittal view; (**e, f**): coronal views. (**g, h**) Provisional intra-operative reduction: (**g**) fluoroscopic Broden view. Note posterior facet reduction (white arrow); (**h**): fluoroscopic axial view. Note calcaneal height/length has been restored (black arrow). (**i**–**k**) Final weight-bearing (**i**) lateral, (**j**) Broden, and (**k**) axial radiographs 9 months post-surgery. Note posterior facet reduction (white arrow); calcaneal height/length has been restored (black arrow). (**l, m**) Intra-operative views of modified Romash osteotomy. (**n**–**p**) Intra-operative fluoroscopic views of modified Romash osteotomy

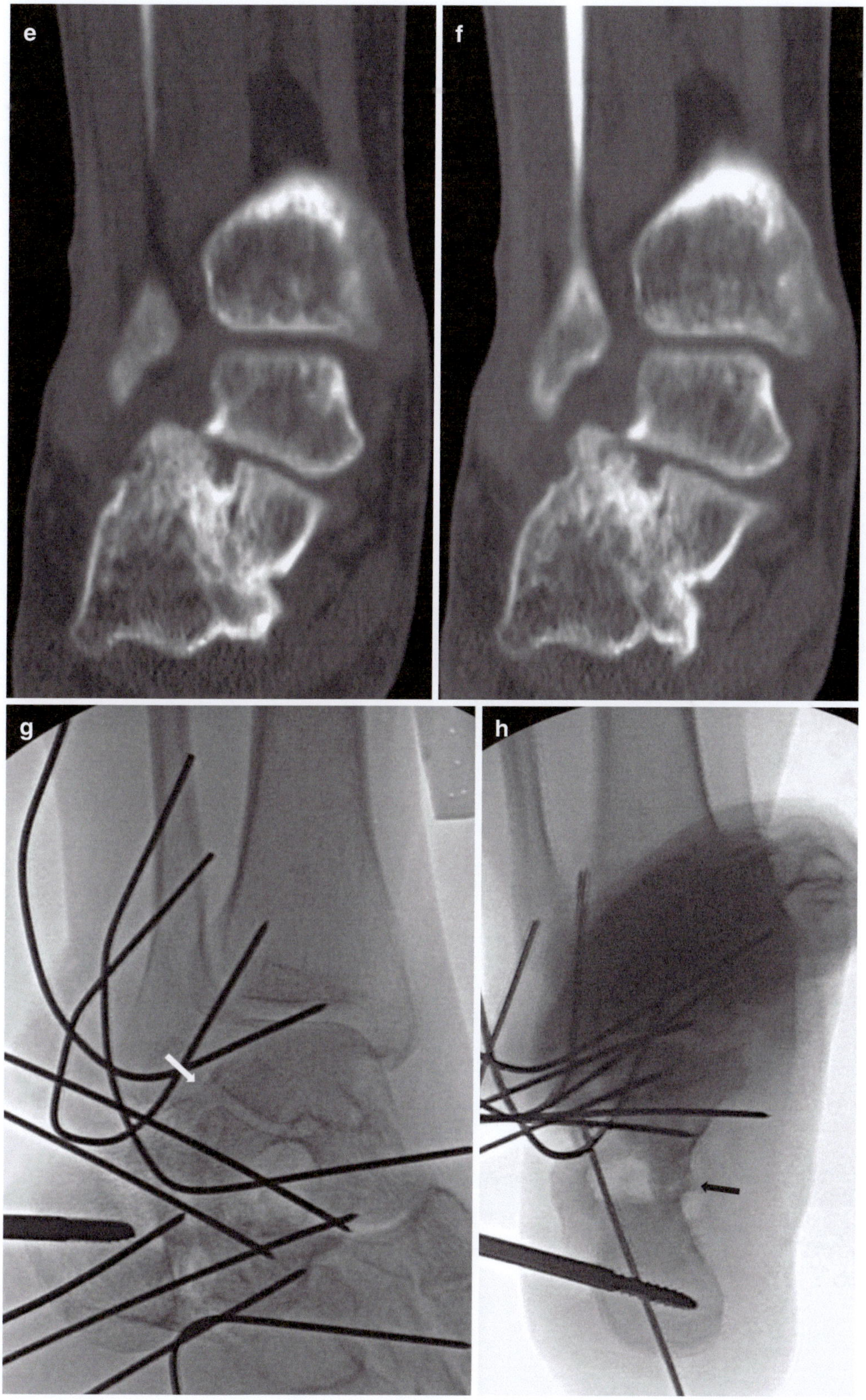

Fig. 8.5 (continued)

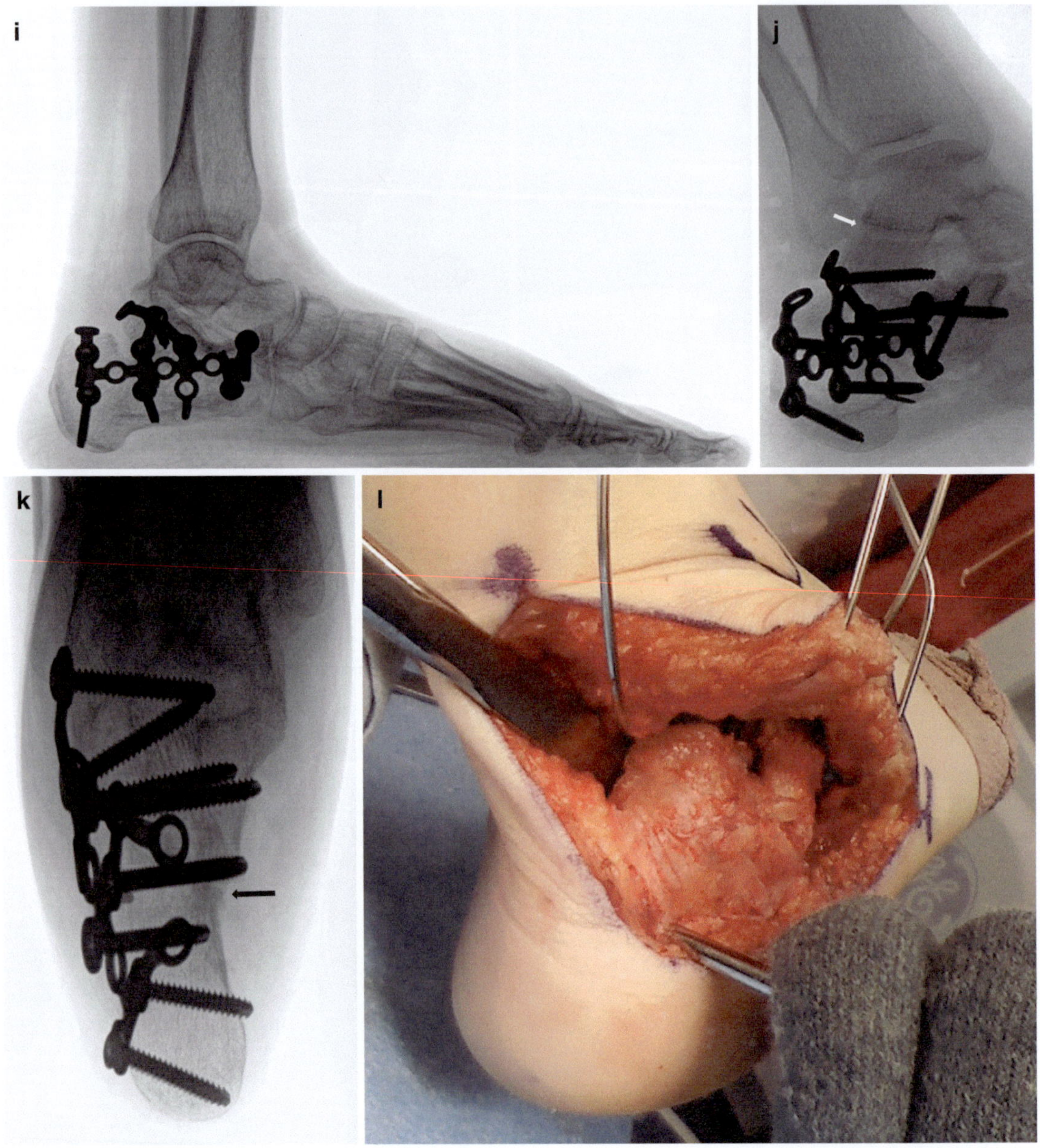

Fig. 8.5 (continued)

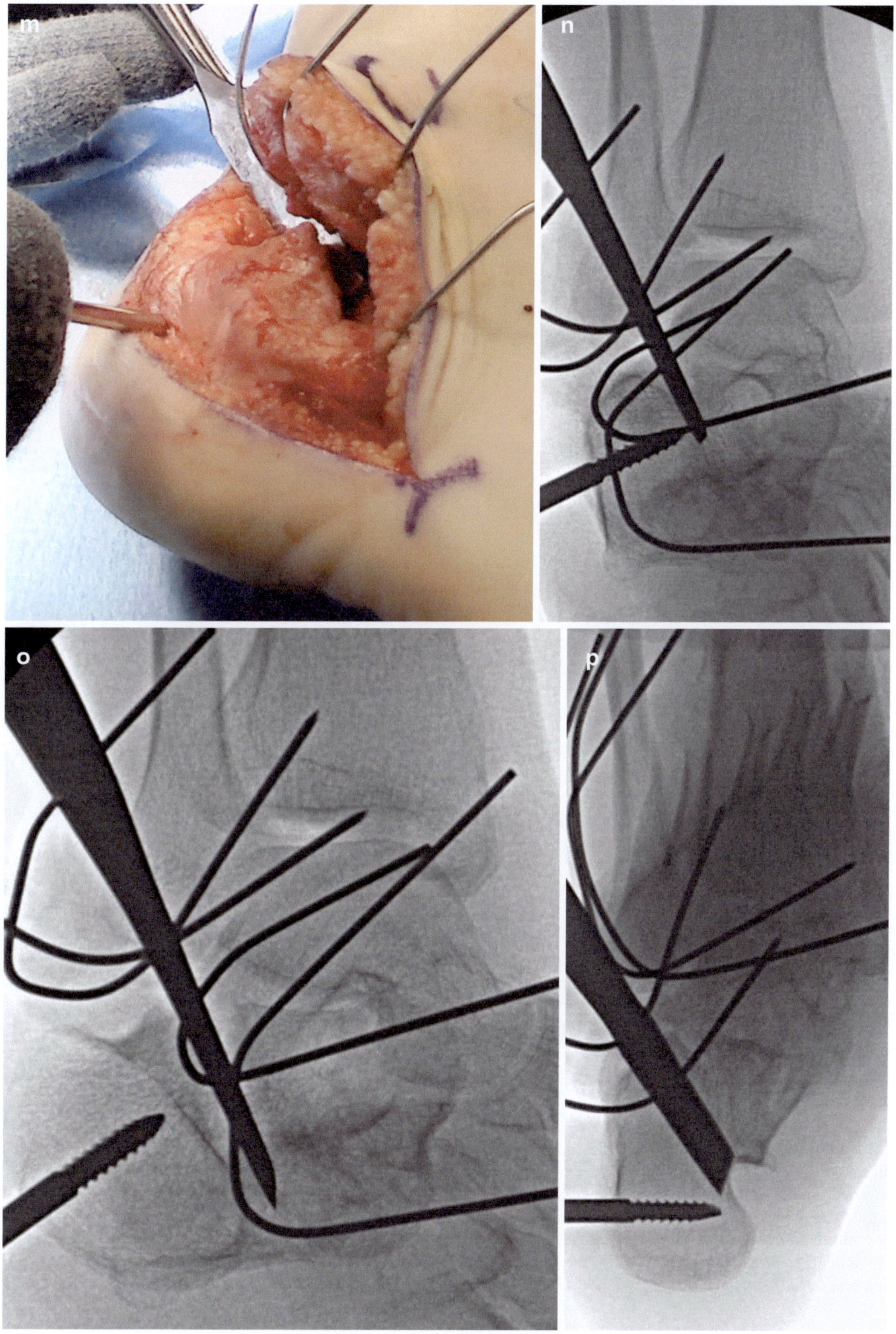

Fig. 8.5 (continued)

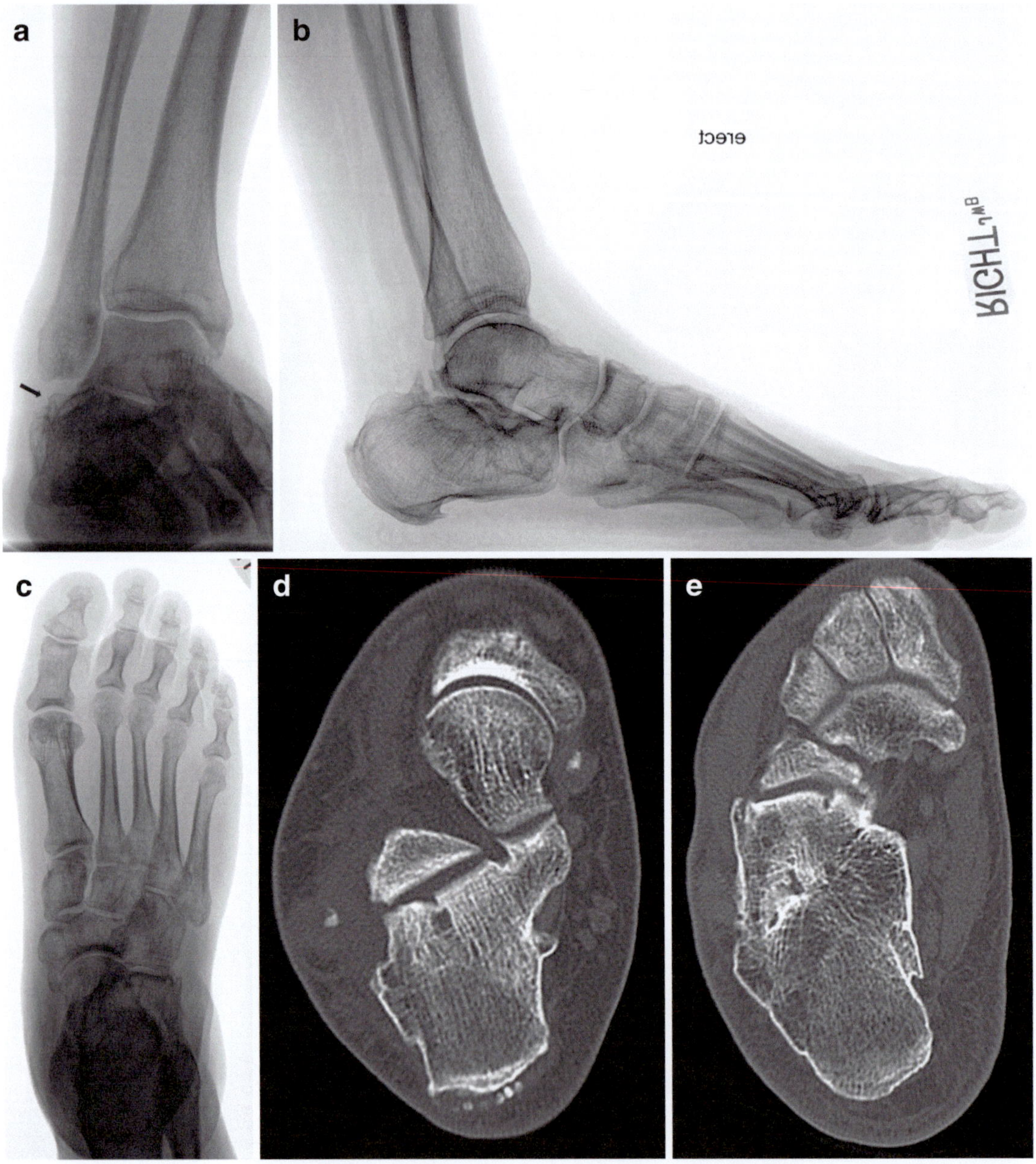

Fig. 8.6 (**a–c**) Weight-bearing (**a**) mortise, (**b**) lateral, and (**c**) A/P foot radiographs demonstrating Sanders type 1 calcaneal malunion. Note minimal loss of calcaneal height, minimal articular involvement, and residual lateral wall exostosis producing subfibular impingement (black arrow). (**d–g**) CT scan of Sanders 1 calcaneal malunion. (**d, e**): axial views; (**f**): coronal view; (**g**): sagittal view. Note minimal loss of calcaneal height, minimal articular involvement, and residual lateral wall exostosis producing subfibular impingement (white arrow). (**h–j**) Final weight-bearing (**h**) lateral, (**i**) Broden, and (**j**) axial radiographs 6 months post-surgery. Note decompression of lateral subfibular area (black arrow). (**k, l**) Lateral wall exostectomy. Note prominence of lateral wall before (**k**) and after (**l**) exostectomy (Different patient). (**m, n**) Superior Peroneal Retinaculum reconstruction. (**m**) sutures from suture anchors passed in horizontal mattress configuration to eliminate false pouch; (**n**) sutures tied, restoring checkrein along posterolateral rim of fibula

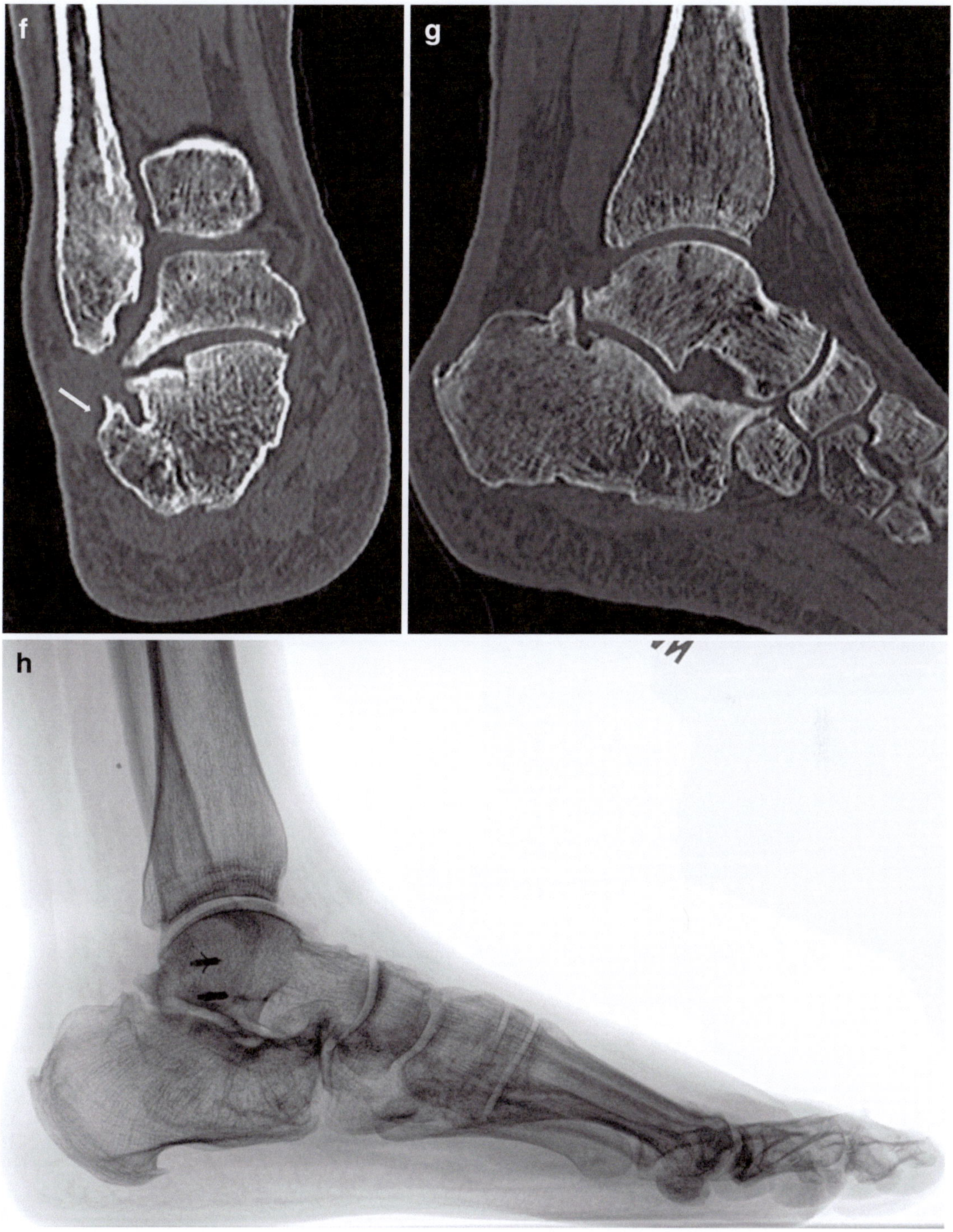

Fig 8.6 (continued)

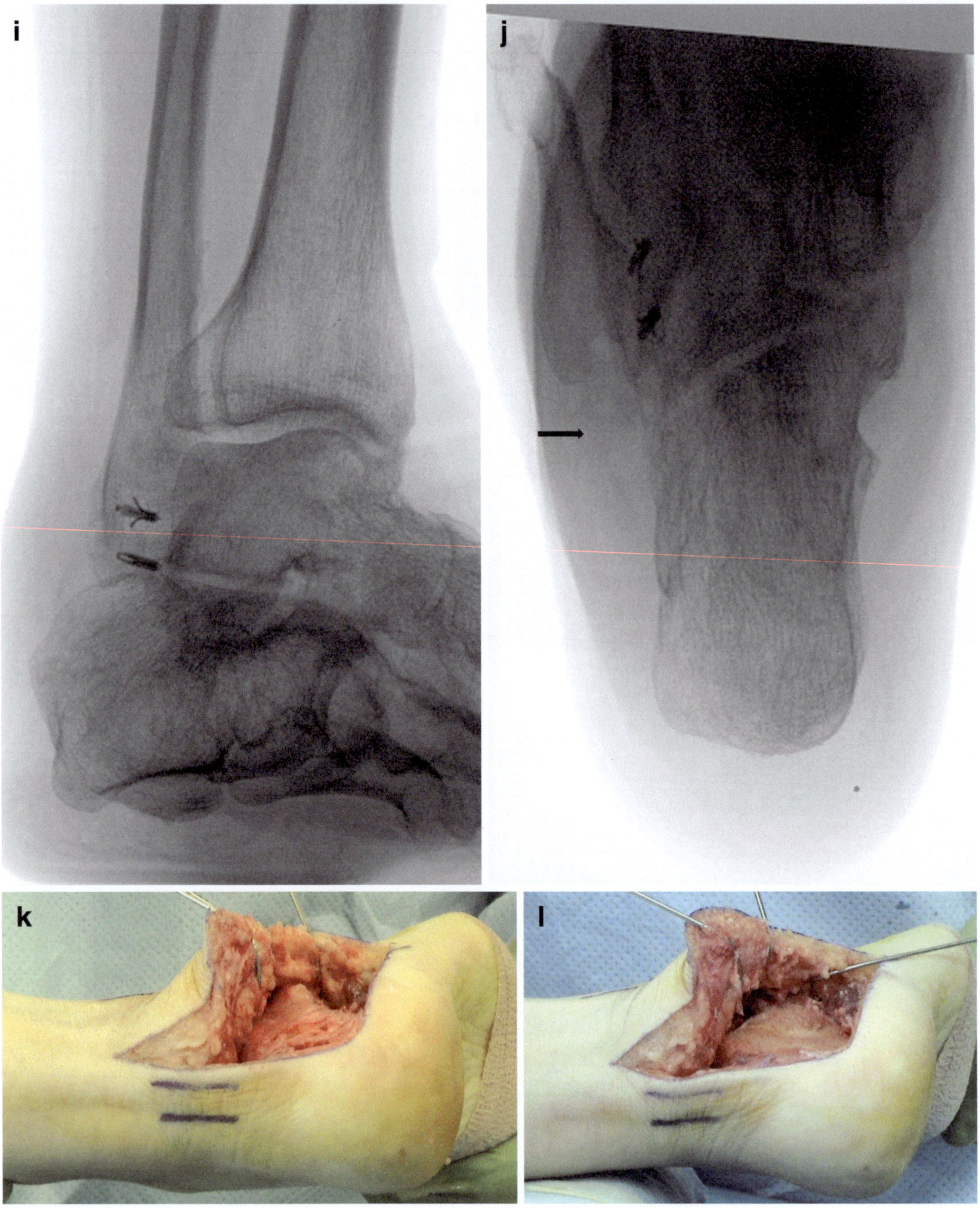

Fig. 8.6 (continued)

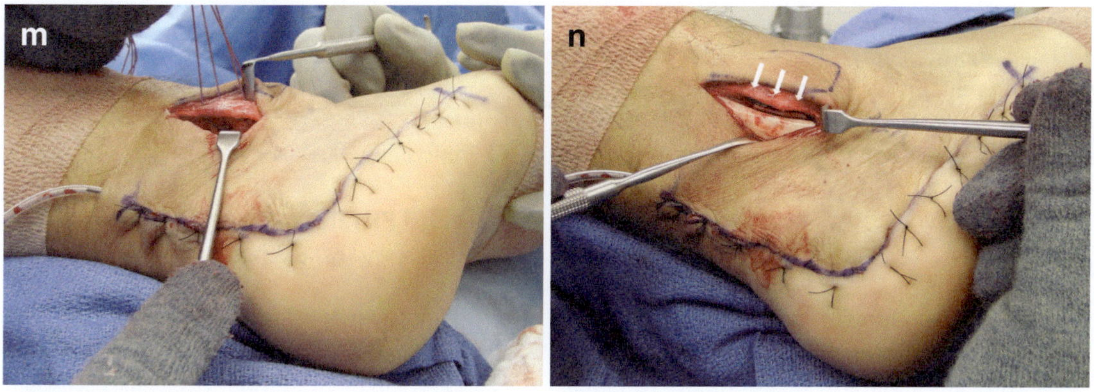

Fig. 8.6 (continued)

- Minimal posterior facet involvement/minimal loss of calcaneal height
- (+) Lateral subfibular impingement

Surgical Plan

- Lateral wall exostectomy with A-O osteotomy saw
- Superior Peroneal Retinaculum reconstruction (Fig. 8.6h–j)

Approach

- Extensile lateral approach (lateral wall exostectomy)
- Posterolateral approach to fibula (SPR reconstruction)

Implants

- Suture anchors

Pearls and Pitfalls

- Lateral wall exostectomy (Fig. 8.6k, l)
  - Retractor placed at crucial angle of Gissane to protect lateral process of talus
  - Exostectomy includes articular margin of minimal, involved portion of articular surface/blade angled to preserve more bone plantarly than dorsally
  - Exostectomy completed with large osteotome at calcaneocuboid joint
- Superior Peroneal Retinaculum reconstruction (Fig. 8.6m, n)
  - Identify false pouch anterior to peroneal rim/mobilize SPR sleeve
  - Prepare bony surface of lateral fibula immediately anterior to posterolateral rim
  - Assess peroneal tendons for intra-substance tears or surrounding tenosynovitis
  - Two suture anchors placed within peroneal rim
  - Sutures passed as anterior as possible into SPR sleeve in horizontal mattress configuration to facilitate elimination of false pouch
  - Peroneal tendons held reduced/sutures tied down restoring checkrein along posterolateral rim
  - Peroneal sheath closure/can be imbricated where necessary

Case 8.3

History

- A 28-year-old female/former aspiring model/1 ppd. smoker
- High speed MVC/calcaneal fracture treated by ORIF
  - Significant comminution in body/poor bone quality
- Lost to follow-up: presents 5 years later with pain with weight-bearing
- Stiff hindfoot/minimal subtalar motion/tender at sinus tarsi and subfibular area
- Weight-bearing radiographs (Fig. 8.7a–c)

Reasons for Failure

- High energy nature of fracture pattern/extent of comminution/poor bone quality
- Lack of suitable anatomic locking plate (to maintain calcaneal height during healing)

Surgical Plan

- Diagnosis: Sanders type II calcaneal malunion/post-traumatic subtalar arthritis
- Hardware removal/lateral wall debridement
- Subtalar joint mobilization/preparation
- Tricortical allograft bone block subtalar arthrodesis (Fig. 8.7d–f)

Approach

- Extensile lateral approach

Implants

- 7.3 mm cannulated screws

Pearls and Pitfalls

- Mobilization of ankylosed/arthritic subtalar joint
  - Start with #15 blade along posterior and lateral margins of joint.
  - Then small osteotome (used as periosteal elevator) to define orientation of joint.

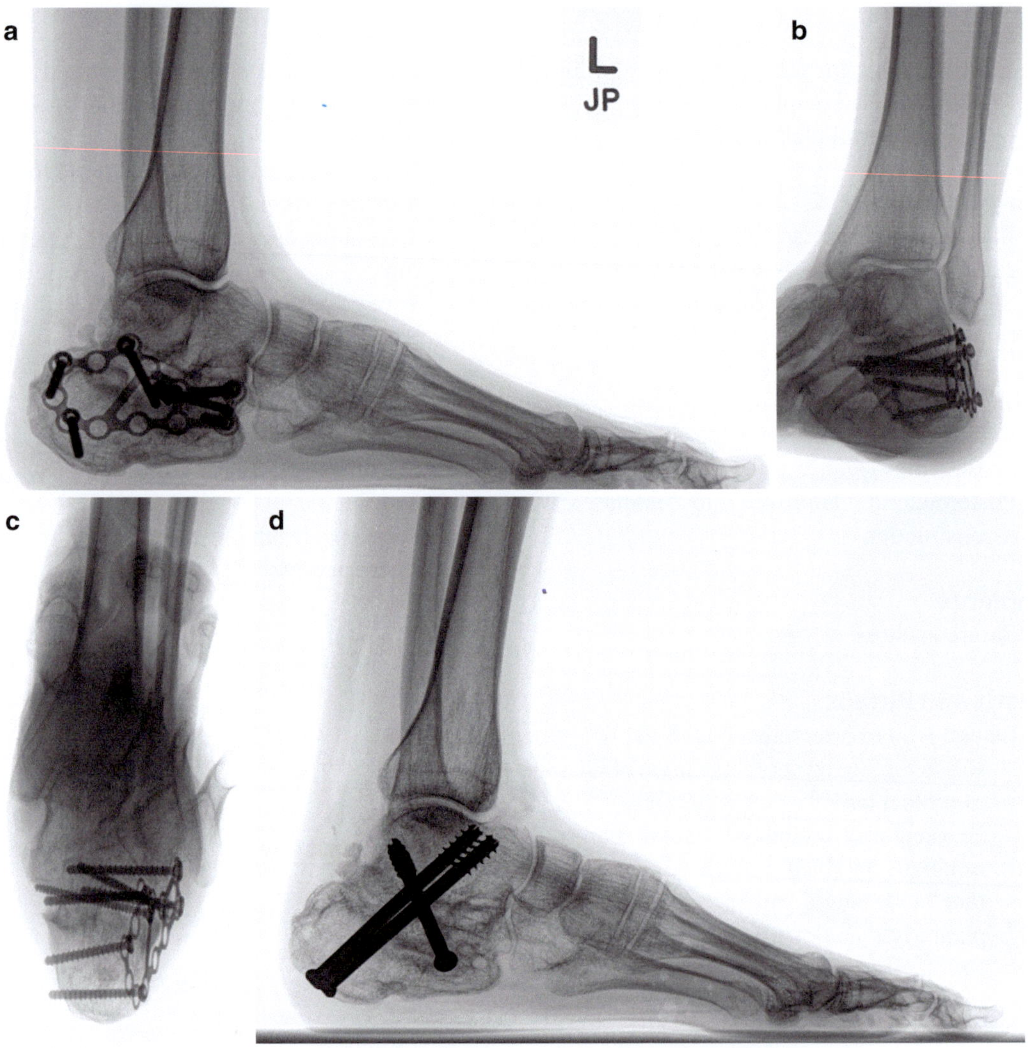

Fig. 8.7 (**a**–**c**) Weight-bearing (**a**) lateral, (**b**) Broden, and (**c**) axial views showing Sanders type II calcaneal malunion with severe loss of calcaneal height, but no coronal plane deformity. (**d**–**f**) Final weight-bearing (**d**) lateral, (**e**) mortise, and (**f**) A/P foot views 9 months post-surgery. (**g**) Subtalar mobilization/distraction. Laminar spreader is placed in posterior portion of posterior facet, as medial as possible to symmetrically distract joint. (**h**) Intra-operative fluoroscopic lateral view showing subtalar bone block arthrodesis with tricortical allograft (black arrow)

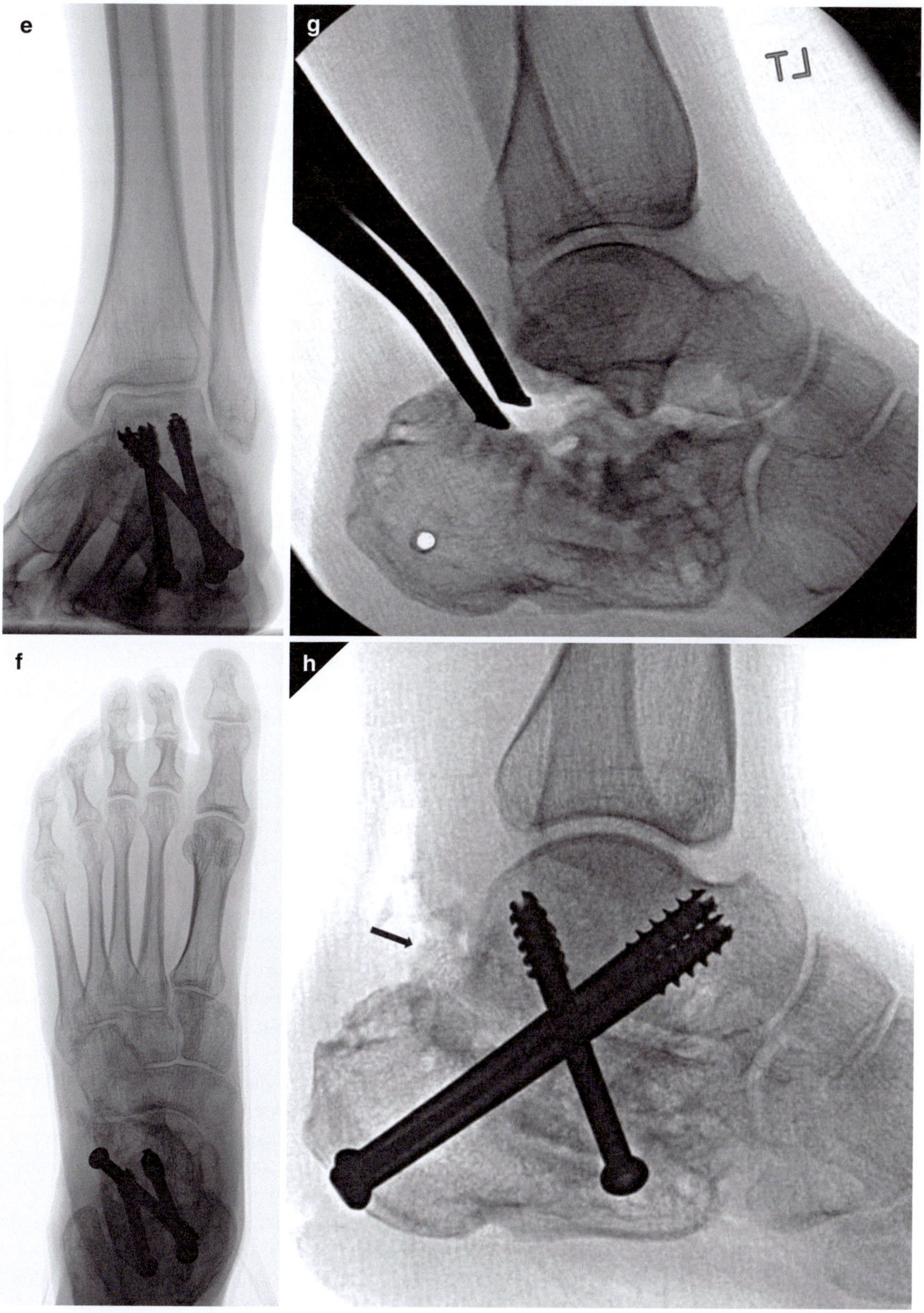

Fig. 8.7 (continued)

   - Then laminar spreader from posterior portion of posterior facet/as medial as possible to symmetrically distract joint (Fig. 8.7g).
   - Measure amount of joint distraction/shape bone block accordingly (Fig. 8.7h).

Case 8.4

History

- A 68-year-old male/multiple medical problems
- Type 2 diabetes/COPD/current non-smoker but 50-pack year smoking history
- Fell 8 feet from ladder 1 year prior/diagnosed with calcaneus fracture
- Treated with ORIF elsewhere: complicated by wound breakdown/apparent infection
- 3 months post-surgery: underwent incision and drainage/hardware removal/attempted subtalar arthrodesis elsewhere
- Continued wound drainage: 5 months later underwent repeat incision and drainage/hardware removal elsewhere
- Presents with persistent intermittent drainage/pain with weight-bearing
- Severe valgus-external rotation deformity through hindfoot
- Very stiff hindfoot/minimal hindfoot motion/intact ankle motion
- Small pinpoint lateral wound/prominent bone underlying wound
- Scarred, adherent lateral soft tissue envelope
- No recent fevers, chills, or constitutional signs/no major shifts in blood glucose levels
- Intact sensation to light touch
- Intra-operative fluoroscopic views of initial ORIF (Fig. 8.8a, b) and attempted subtalar arthrodesis (Fig. 8.8c)
- Weight-bearing radiographs (Fig. 8.8d–h)
- CT scan (Fig. 8.8i–n)

Reasons for Failure

- Diagnoses

1. Calcaneal fracture-dislocation variant malunion
2. Post-traumatic subtalar arthritis/arthrodesis (in situ) nonunion
3. Chronic wound infection/underlying bone prominence

- Fracture-dislocation pattern unrecognized/poor fracture reduction
- Poorly performed extensile lateral incision contributing to wound breakdown
- Poorly performed subtalar arthrodesis in situ

Surgical Plan

- Incision and drainage/lateral wall exostectomy
  - Immobilization/po antibiotics until lateral wound fully sealed
- Staged open tendo-Achilles lengthening/peroneal tendon fractional lengthening/modified Romash osteotomy/revision subtalar arthrodesis (Fig. 8.8o–r)

Approach

- Gallie approach (vertical limb of extensile lateral incision)

Implants

- 4.0 mm cancellous lag screws for osteotomy
- 6.5 mm headless compression screws for revision arthrodesis

Pearls and Pitfalls

- Gallie approach utilized due to scarred, adherent lateral soft tissue envelope
- Tendo-Achilles lengthening/peroneal tendon fractional lengthening utilized due to severe chronic deformity to eliminate deforming force/facilitate soft tissue balancing
- Posterior facet articular surface prepared
  - Sharp periosteal elevator to remove remaining cartilage/preserve subchondral plate
  - Subchondral plate drilled with 2.5 mm drill bit to stimulate vascular ingrowth
- Modified Romash osteotomy: posterior to anterior along original fracture-dislocation line
  - Visualize entry point and path of osteotome directly.
  - Allow osteotome to "find its path" along original fracture line.
  - Confirm on axial fluoro views (Fig. 8.8s, t).

- Laminar spreader used to assist restoration of calcaneal height.
- Osteotomy provisionally stabilized with 2.0 mm K-wires (Fig. 8.8u, v).
- Definitive fixation with 4.0 mm cancellous lag screws (Fig. 8.8w, x).

- Subtalar joint reduced to neutral-neutral position (coronal/axial planes)
  - Previous severe valgus-external rotation deformity corrected
- Definitive fixation of subtalar arthrodesis with 6.5 mm headless compression screws

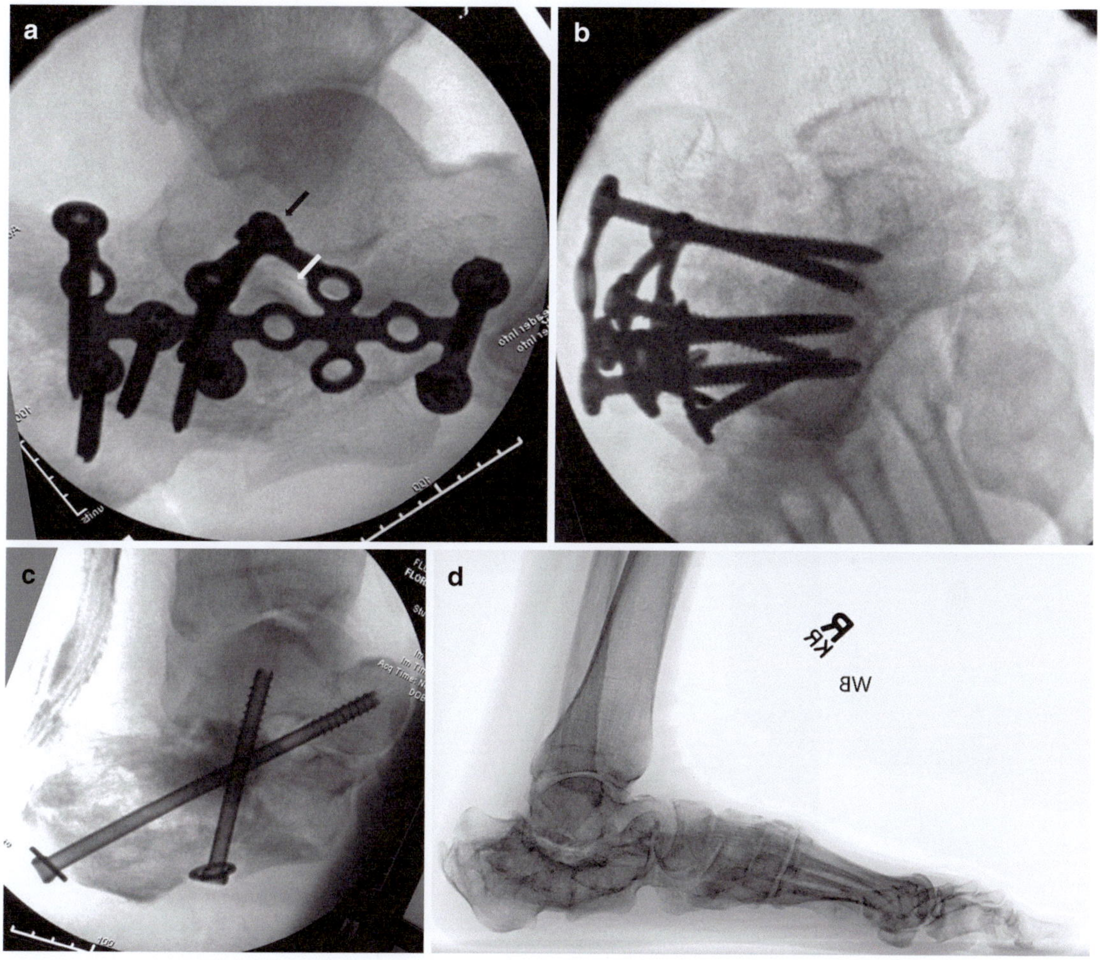

Fig. 8.8 (**a**–**c**) Intra-operative fluoroscopic views of (**a**, **b**) initial ORIF and (**c**) attempted subtalar arthrodesis. (**a**) Note overlap of plate and posterior facet articular surface (black and white arrows). (**b**) Note lack of discernable bony landmarks suggesting poor fracture reduction. (**d**–**h**) Weight-bearing (**d**) lateral, (**e**) mortise, (**f**) Broden, (**g**) A/P foot, and (**h**) axial views. Note persistent dislocation of tuberosity fragment (black arrows) and resultant severe valgus, external rotation deformity. (**i**–**n**) CT scan. (**i**, **j**) Coronal, (**k**) axial, (**l**, **m**) sagittal, and (**n**) 3-D reconstruction views. (**i**) Note invaginated, adherent lateral soft tissue envelope (white arrow). (**k**–**n**) note chronic dislocation of tuberosity fragment abutting distal fibula (black arrows). (**o**–**r**) Final weight-bearing (**o**) lateral, (**p**) mortise, (**q**) A/P foot, and (**r**) axial views 1 year post-surgery. One of the cancellous lag screws was removed at 8 months post-surgery. (**s**, **t**) Intra-operative fluoroscopic (**s**) Broden and (**t**) axial views showing modified Romash osteotomy. Osteotome is allowed to "find its' path" along original fracture line. Laminar spreader is used to assist in restoration of calcaneal height. (**u**, **v**) Intra-operative fluoroscopic (**u**) lateral and (**v**) axial views following provisional stabilization of modified Romash osteotomy. Chronic dislocation of tuberosity fragment has been reduced, and calcaneal height and length restored. (**w**, **x**) Intra-operative fluoroscopic (**w**) lateral and (**x**) axial views following definitive stabilization of modified Romash osteotomy. Terminally threaded guide pins (for large headless compression screws) have been placed

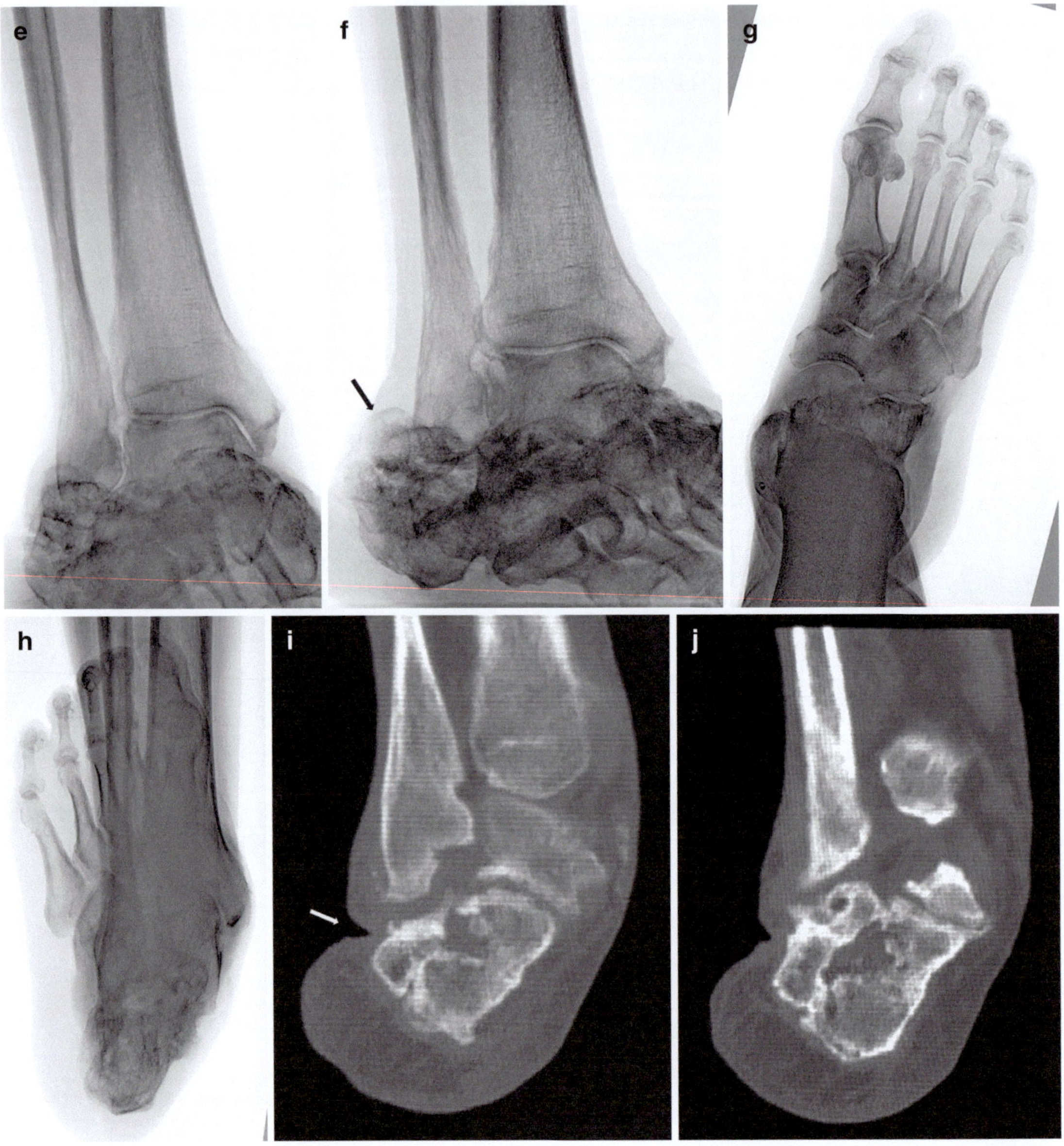

Fig. 8.8 (continued)

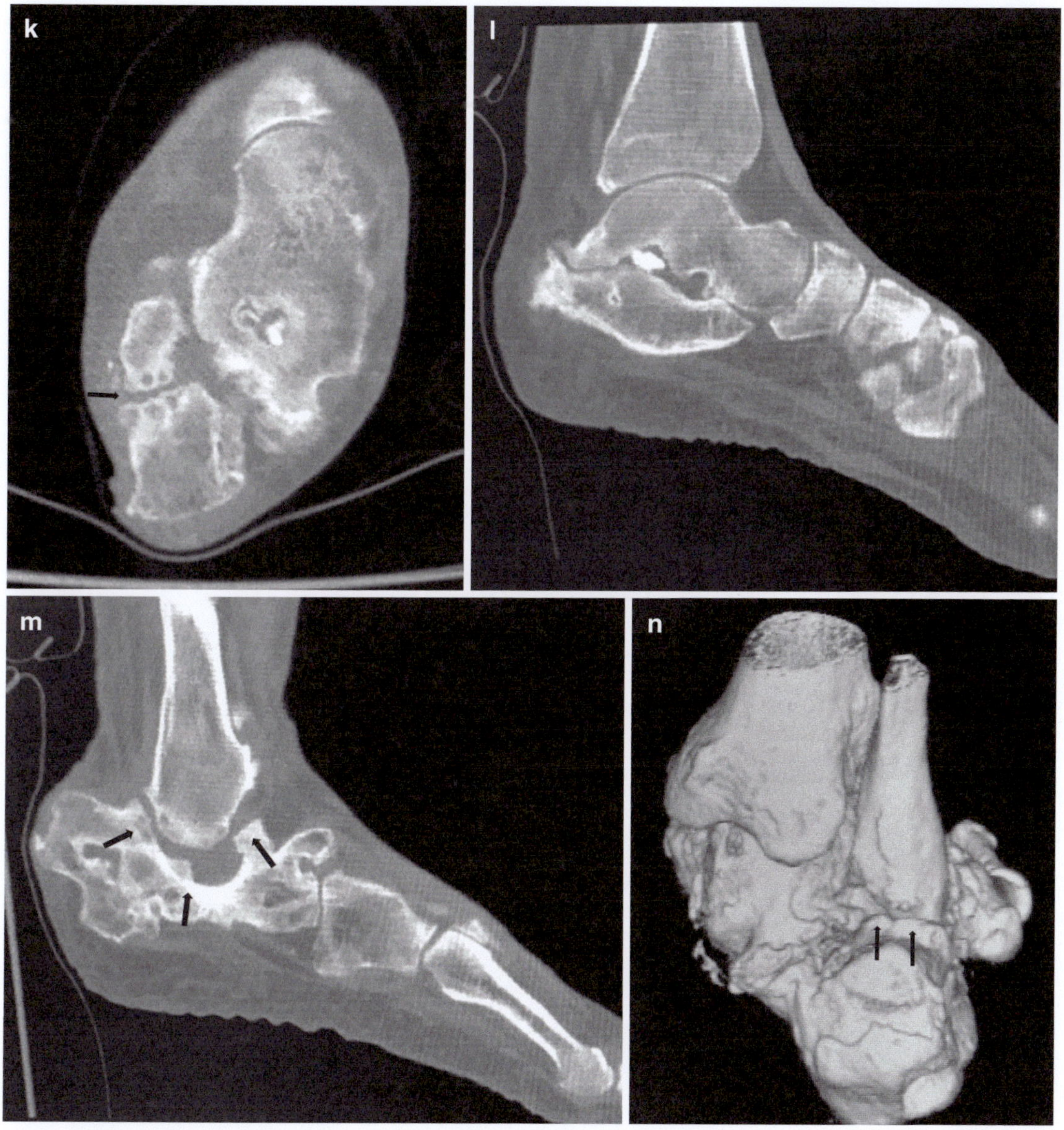

Fig. 8.8 (continued)

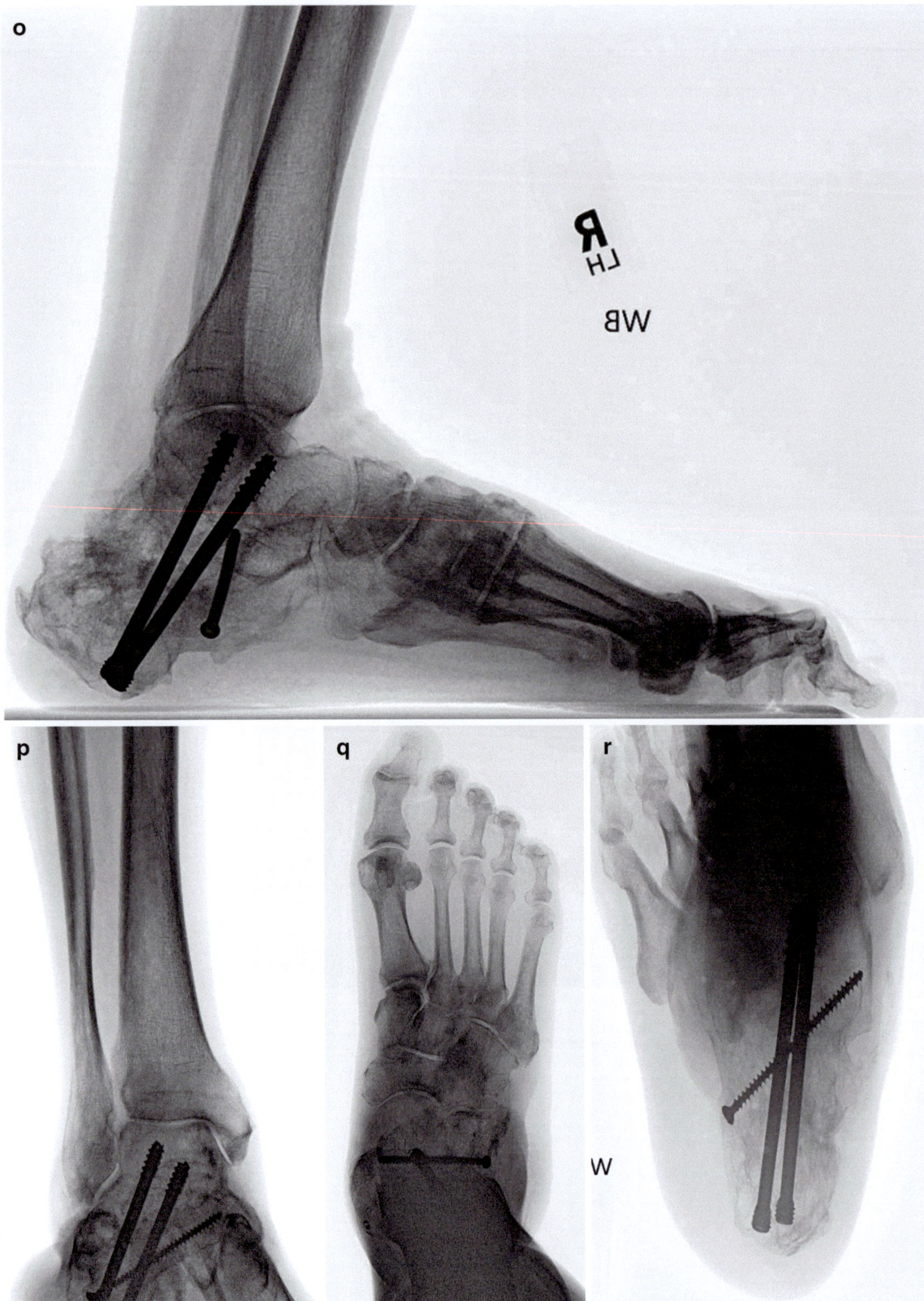

Fig. 8.8 (continued)

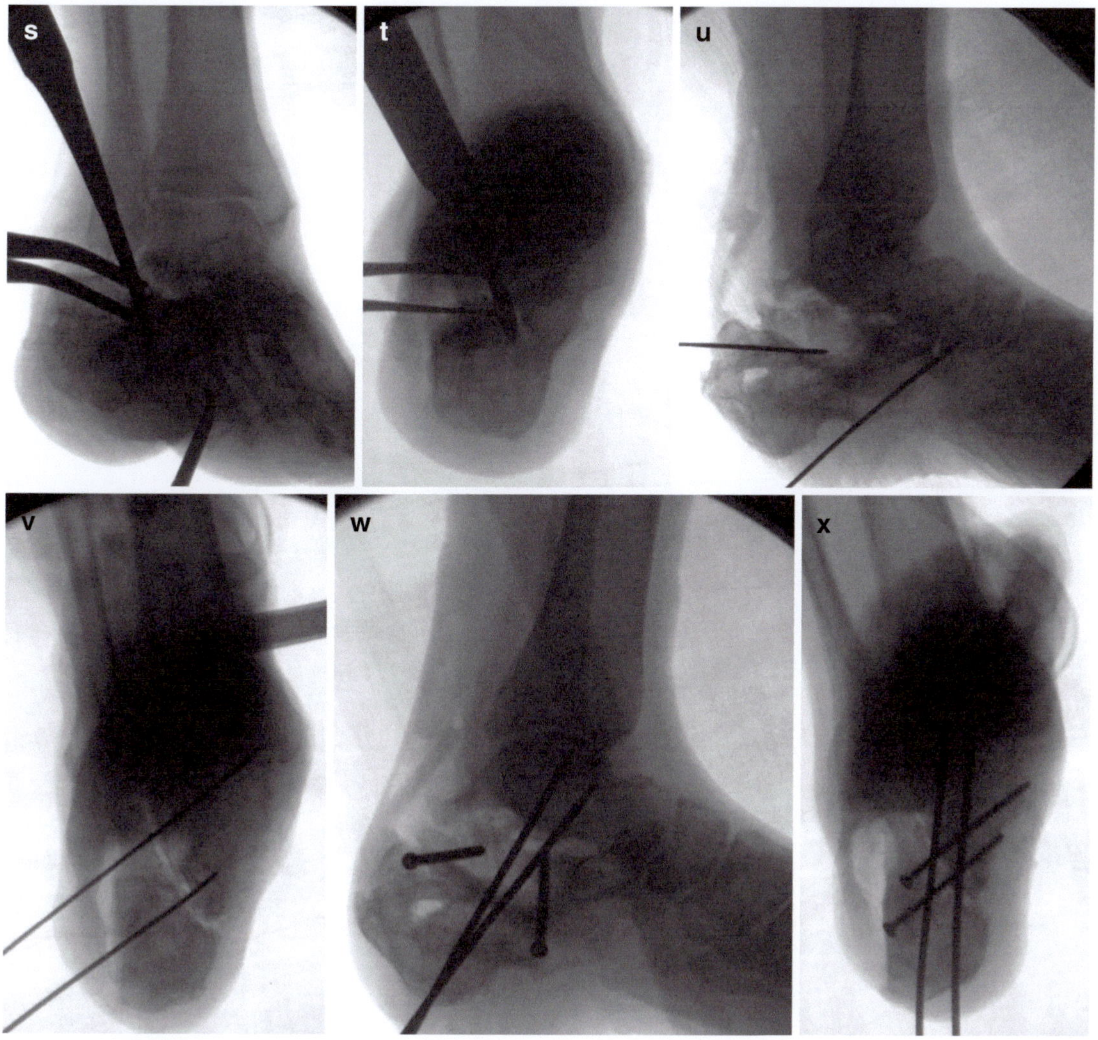

Fig. 8.8 (continued)

References

1. Sanders R, Fortin P, DiPasquale T, Walling A. Operative treatment in 120 displaced intraarticular calcaneal fractures: results using a prognostic computed to-mography scan classification. Clin Orthop Relat Res. 1993;(290):87-95.
2. Sanders R. Displaced intra-articular fractures of the calcaneus. J Bone Joint Surg Am. 2000;82(2): 225–50.
3. Barei DP, Bellabarba C, Sangeorzan BJ, Benirschke SK. Fractures of the calcaneus. Orthop Clin North Am. 2002;33(1):263–85.
4. Radnay CS, Clare MP, Sanders RW. Subtalar fusion after displaced intra-articular calcaneal fractures: does initial operative treatment matter? J Bone Joint Surg Am. 2009;91(3):541–6.
5. Clare MP, Lee WE III, Sanders RW. Intermediate to long-term results of a treatment protocol for calcaneal fracture malunions. J Bone Joint Surg Am. 2005;87(5):963–73.
6. Carr JB, Hansen ST, Benirschke SK. Subtalar distraction bone block fusion for late complications of os calcis fractures. Foot Ankle. 1988;9(2):81–6.
7. Clare MP. Acute and chronic peroneal tendon dislocations. Tech Foot Ankle Surg. 2009;8:112–8.
8. Romash MM. Reconstructive osteotomy of the calcaneus with subtalar arthrodesis for malunited calcaneal fractures. Clin Orthop Relat Res. 1993;(290):157–67.

9 Corrective Osteotomy for Talar Neck Malunions

Stefan Rammelt and Elisabeth Manke

Key Takeaway Points

- Integrity of the talus and its joint is essential for global foot function.
- Malalignment of the talar neck leads to three-dimensional foot deformity and asymmetric loading of the joints.
- Talar neck osteotomy aims at restoring the three-dimensional alignment of the ankle, hindfoot, and midfoot.
- Joint-preserving osteotomy is possible in reliable patients with good bone stock and preserved cartilage.
- Partial avascular necrosis of the talar body without collapse does not preclude joint-preserving correction.

Introduction

The talus and its joints are essential for foot function. Almost 60% of its surface is covered by cartilage and there are no muscular attachments. The talus serves as a so-called bony meniscus between the lower leg and foot and contributes to the ankle, subtalar, and talonavicular joints. Not only does each individual articulation need to be congruent, but the three-dimensional relationship of each joint to the others is important for proper ankle and hindfoot function. Malunion at the talar neck disrupts the three-dimensional alignment and thus leads to global foot dysfunction and complex deformity.

Causes for Failure

Malunions and nonunions at the talar neck frequently result from inadequate reduction and fixation, or non-operative treatment of displaced talar neck fractures, and invariably lead to poor results [1–7].

In fractures of the talar neck, medial comminution is often seen, probably due to the impaction forces exerted by the sustentaculum tali, which acts as a lever (hypomochlion) at the time of injury. Reasons for medial shortening and subsequent varus malalignment include:

- Non-operative management
- Inadequate reduction because of limited surgical exposure
- Inadequate fixation with the use of K-wires or medial lag screws
- Loss of reduction after overdrilling the wires for cannulated screws.

S. Rammelt (✉) · E. Manke
University Hospital Carl Gustav Carus at TU Dresden, University Center of Orthopaedics and Traumatology, Dresden, Germany

M. J. Berkowitz et al. (eds.), *Revision Surgery of the Foot and Ankle*,
https://doi.org/10.1007/978-3-030-29969-9_9

Consequences of Malalignment

Even though the apex of the deformity is extra-articular, malalignment of the talar neck directly affects joint function. Experimental varus deformity of the talar neck has led to a significant decrease of subtalar motion resulting in an inability to evert the foot, internal rotation of the hindfoot, and adduction of the forefoot [8]. A direct correlation of the degree of varus malalignment and change in subtalar motion and foot position was observed. Furthermore, varus malalignment of the hindfoot decreases the mobility of the mid-tarsal joints and compromises the physiological reciprocal relationship between the hindfoot and forefoot [8].

Incomplete reduction of talar neck fractures also frequently leads to a step-off at the talar neck and dorsal displacement of the talar body, resulting in limited dorsiflexion at the ankle joint [2, 8] Even if the fracture does not extend into the tibiotalar joint, declination of the talar body secondary to subtalar dislocation leads to incongruity in the ankle joint with loss of dorsiflexion.

The incidence of nonunion after fractures of the talar neck is reported between 0% and 10% [3–5]. Sanders et al. reported that secondary reconstructive procedures after malunited talar neck fractures are needed in 24% of patients after 1 year, 32% after 2 years, 38% after 5 years, and 48% after 10 years [9, 10].

Talar neck fractures may be accompanied by peripheral talar fractures. Therefore, malunion or nonunion of the lateral or posterior talar process may be present concurrently as many of these fractures are often not diagnosed acutely. They regularly lead to painful nonunions and a rapid progression to subtalar arthritis [11–15]. Mills and Horne noted a 60% nonunion rate after lateral process fractures treated non-operatively [16]. Nonunions of the lateral process have to be discriminated from a symptomatic accessory ossicle (talus secundarius). Posterior process malunions potentially lead to damage in both the ankle and subtalar joints [11, 15, 17]. Nonunions of the posterior process have to be discriminated from a loose os trigonum or rare anatomic variants like talus bipartitus [18].

Malaligned, prominent bony fragments or osteophytes may lead to impingement of the posterior tibial tendons, tarsal tunnel, or sinus tarsi syndrome [19].

Post-traumatic Arthritis

Biomechanical investigations on cadaver specimens with pressure-sensitive film have shown that simulated malalignment of only 2 mm at the talar neck results in significant load redistribution between the posterior, medial, and anterior facets of the subtalar joint [8]. Besides joint incongruity, the impact during the initial injury producing chondrocyte death and comminution of the joint surfaces may lead to post-traumatic arthritis. The rates of post-traumatic arthritis after central talar fractures provided in the literature vary considerably from 16% to 100% and appear to increase over time. In a report of Vallier et al. in 38% of 26 cases AVN developed [20]. Of these patients, 65% showed post-traumatic arthritis in tibiotalar joints, 34% suffered subtalar arthritis [20, 21]. But only about one-third of patients with radiographic signs of arthritis eventually become clinically symptomatic with the need for a secondary arthrodesis [7].

Avascular Necrosis (AVN)

Because a substantial part of the blood supply to the talar body enters the talus at the talar neck via the sinus tarsi and canalis tarsi arteries, avascular necrosis (AVN) of the talar body is a specific complication after talar neck fractures. The initial amount of dislocation has an impact on the risk of AVN and there appears to be a correlation between fracture classification and the occurrence of AVN after talar neck and body fractures although the reported rates differ considerably in the literature [7, 22]. AVN is usually diagnosed 4–6 months after the injury by a radiopaque appearance of the talar body on plain radiographs. The necrotic zone is best visualized on MRI.

While the timing of definite fixation does not appear to affect the rates of AVN [20, 22, 23], emergent reduction of dislocation protects the blood supply to both the talus and the soft tissues after the injury [7, 10, 20, 24]. When performing magnetic resonance imaging (MRI) on all displaced talar neck and body fractures, some areas of reduced blood supply will be found in virtually all cases [25].

For the management of talar fractures and its complications, it is important to distinguish between partial AVN, which affects less than one-third of the talar body or total AVN that almost invariably results in a collapse of the talar body [19]. Only total AVN of the talar body with eventual collapses of the talar dome becomes clinically relevant [6, 20, 26]. In case of partial AVN, the necrotic areas of the talar body are gradually replaced by creeping substitution bone remodeling over a course of 2–3 years. From the largest patient cohort on talar fractures that has been reported in the literature back in 1983, Schuind et al. have calculated that within 2 years after a talar fracture, complete revascularization of the talus takes place in 21%, asymptomatic AVN persists in 42%, and collapse of the talar dome occurs in 37% of cases [5]. It appears from more recent studies that these historic rates could be lowered considerably by a more aggressive approach with early, stable internal fixation and functional after treatment [7]. Overall, the prevalence of AVN after talar neck fractures in the literature ranges from 0% to 24% after Hawkins type I, from 0% to 50% after Hawkins type II, and from 33% to 100% after Hawkins types III and IV [7]. Open talar neck and body fractures appear to have an increased risk of AVN [20, 23]. The latter may also lead to the most dreaded complication after talar fracture, i.e., septic necrosis of the talar body.

Evaluation and Assessment

Patients with talar malunions and nonunions have to be evaluated clinically with respect to pain, gross deformity, soft tissue conditions, callosities, neurovascular status, range of motion and stability in the ankle, subtalar, and talonavicular joints. The whole leg is examined while walking and standing and the formerly uninjured side serves as an internal control. Shoes and insoles that are regularly worn by the patient provide valuable information about chronic eccentric loading of the foot. Important patient-related factors to be considered are activity level, professional demands, comorbidities (above all osteoporosis, diabetes, and any neurovascular deficits), substance abuse, and inability to comply with the postoperative protocol.

Radiographic assessment of the overall alignment and stability includes bilateral weight-bearing anteroposterior, dorsoplantar and lateral radiographs of the foot and ankle (Fig. 9.1), and a hindfoot alignment view. Computed tomographic (CT) scanning is mandatory for planning the correction (Fig. 9.2). It reveals the exact three-dimensional outline of the malunited fragments and joint incongruities as well as the extent of arthritis and bony union. Magnetic resonance imaging (MRI) is used to determine the presence and extent of AVN, osteochondral defects, and associated soft tissue pathologies like tendon impingement (Fig. 9.3). Ongoing infection should be ruled out with routine leukocyte counts and C-reactive protein serum levels.

Because malalignment of the talar body and its joints will invariably cause pain around the ankle and hindfoot, it may be difficult to assess if radiologic evidence of post-traumatic arthritis is clinically relevant. Diagnostic injections with anesthetics or Technetium bone scanning can be of help. However, the final decision to reconstruct or fuse one or more joints around the talus will frequently be made during reconstructive surgery by visually assessing and directly probing the cartilage quality. Both treatment options – fusion and joint reconstruction – must be discussed with the patient prior to surgery.

Preoperative Planning

When a patient with a talar neck malunion is identified, an attempt should be made to operate

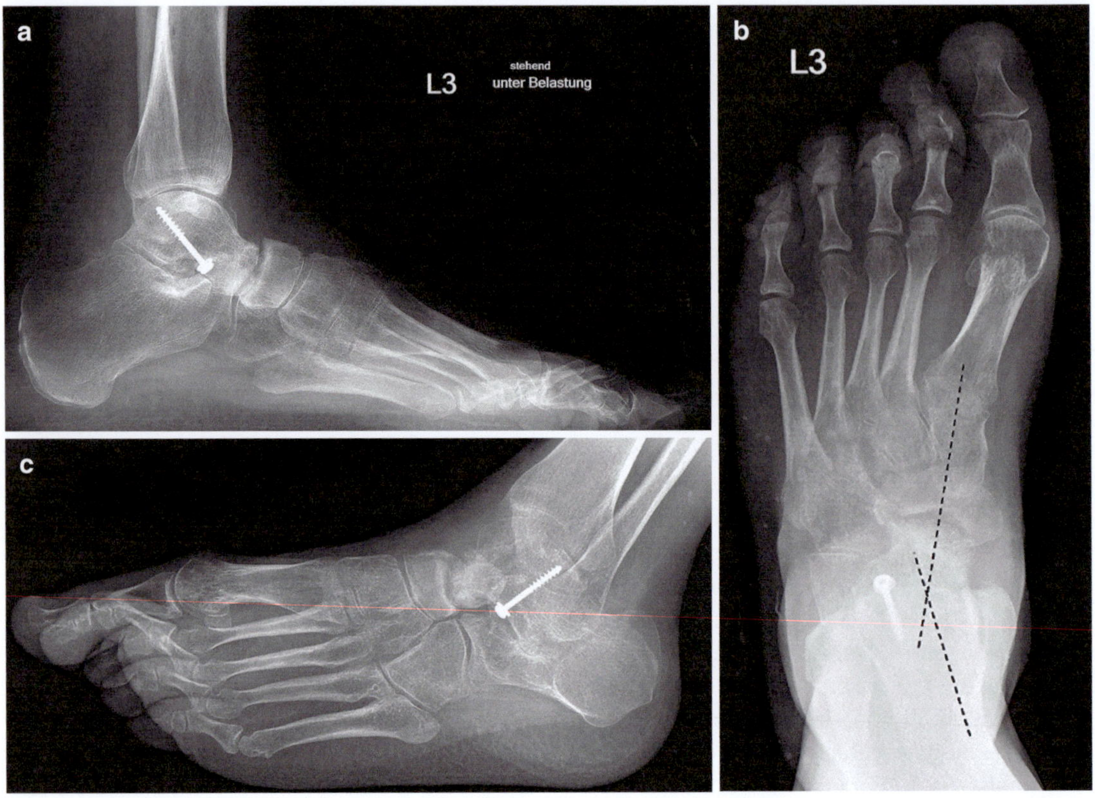

Fig. 9.1 (**a**) Standing lateral radiograph of a 32-year-old male patient 9 months after open reduction and internal fixation of a displaced talar neck fracture with one screw from lateral and two screws from medial which have been removed 6 months after surgery because of talonavicular joint irritation. Overall there is a varus deformity of the hindfoot, incongruity at the talonavicular joint, and the medial facet of the subtalar joint while the posterior facet of the subtalar joint appears congruent but to be tilted in varus. (**b**) The standing dorsoplantar radiograph (with the tube tilted 30 degrees toward the toes) shows varus malalignment of the talar neck resulting in forefoot adduction ("C-foot"). (**c**) The 45° oblique view shows the talar head fragment tilted downwards with the convex joint surface facing the straight anterior and medial facets of the subtalar joint

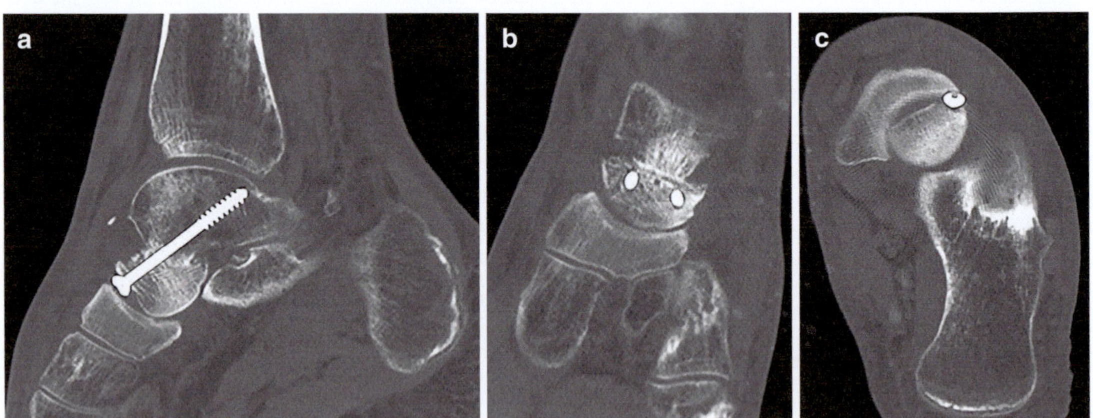

Fig. 9.2 (**a**) Sagittal, (**b**) coronal, and (**c**) axial CT scans of same patient as in Fig. 9.1, 6 months after the injury with the two medial screws still in place, showing a malrotation of the talar head fragment of about 50° due to the solid malunion at the talar neck

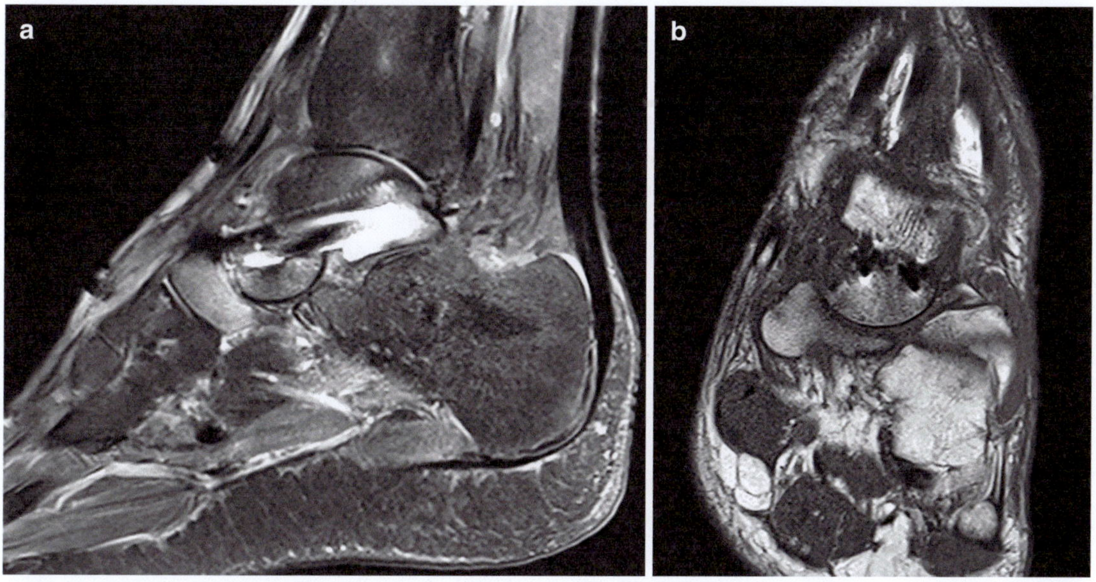

Fig. 9.3 (**a**, **b**) MRI of the same patient as in Figs. 9.1 and 9.2 6 months after the injury shows a full cartilage cover at the convex joint surface of malrotated talar head and no signs of AVN, i.e., a type I deformity amenable to a joint-preserving osteotomy

Table 9.1 Classification of post-traumatic deformities after talar fractures (modified from Zwipp & Rammelt [19])

		Treatment options	
Type	Features	Active, reliable patient, no symptomatic arthritis	Noncompliant patient, comorbidities, arthritis
I	Malunion and/or joint displacement	Osteotomy, secondary reconstruction, and internal fixation with joint preservation	Corrective fusion of the affected joint(s)
II	Nonunion with displacement		
III	Types I/II with partial AVN		
IV	Types I/II with complete AVN	Necrectomy, (vascularized) bone grafting, corrective fusion	
V	Types I/II with septic AVN	Radical debridement(s), bone grafting, corrective fusion	

AVN is considered to be "partial," if less than one-third of the talar body is involved, and "complete" if more than one-third of the talar body is affected leading to talar collapse

early, as arthritis will usually develop rapidly. Consequently, the reconstruction planning for talar body malunions and nonunions is based on the presence of post-traumatic arthritis and the extent of AVN. The decision is also influenced by other important factors like bone quality and patient compliance. The following classification [6, 19] is an easy-to-use guideline for treatment (Table 9.1).

Joint-preserving corrections are aimed at regaining a maximum of function while correcting the deformity and reducing pain. They might be considered in the absence of manifest arthritis and with no or only partial AVN of the talar body (Type I–III deformities) in selected cases of active, compliant patients.

- Typically, the patient with complete osteonecrosis and collapse of the talar body (type IV deformity) is treated with excision of necrotic bone, autologous bone grafting, and realignment and fusion of the affected joint or joints.
- In the presence of osteomyelitis (type V deformity), repeated débridement of infected and necrotic bone almost invariably leads to subtotal talectomy. In staged procedures, tibiocalcaneal or tibiotalocalcaneal fusion is obtained.

The talar head and the talonavicular joint are preserved whenever possible.

Malunions and nonunions of the lateral or posterior process can be salvaged at an early stage by complete excision of the malunited fragments and joint revision [17, 27]. If severe arthritis of the subtalar joint is present already, in situ fusion is the treatment of choice [15].

In patients with limited dorsiflexion secondary to dorsal displacement, resection of a dorsal talar beak at the ankle or an osteophyte at the talonavicular joint may lead to improved function.

Relevant comorbidities such as poorly controlled diabetes mellitus, stage IIb peripheral vascular disease, or systemic immune deficiency are seen as contraindications. The same holds for non-compliant patients, above all those with substance abuse.

Surgical Technique

Surgical Approaches and Patient Positioning

Anatomical correction of malunited fractures of the talar neck is generally carried out via the same surgical approaches that are used in acute fractures [7, 20, 23]. Pre-existing scars from previous surgery are only used if deemed adequate, which will only rarely be the case in malunions.

- To obtain adequate exposure of the talar neck, ankle, and subtalar joint, dual approaches are necessary in most instances. A medial approach is used to gain access to the medial aspect of the talar neck and head, running from the medial malleolus to the navicular tuberosity [6, 28]. An anterolateral approach is used to access the subtalar joint and lateral process from lateral [7]. The patient is placed in a supine position with a bump placed beneath the ipsilateral hip to place the foot in a neutral position. The lower leg is draped free so that the foot can be rotated internally and externally.
- If the malunion extends into the talar body, a femoral distractor with Schanz screws placed into the tibia and the calcaneus is helpful to gain adequate overview over the ankle and subtalar joint surfaces. A posterolateral or posteromedial approach is needed in cases of malunions or nonunions of the posterior process and the posterior part of the talar body [7, 17]. For these approaches, the patient is placed in a prone position.

Surgical Procedure

To access the talar neck from medially, an incision is carried out from the medial malleolus to the tuberosity of the navicular. The capsule is entered above the tibialis posterior tendon. The lateral aspect of the talar neck and subtalar joint are accessed via an anterolateral (sinus tarsi) or oblique (Ducroquet-Ollier) approach.

The amount and quality of the cartilage at the ankle, subtalar, and talonavicular joints is assessed by thorough inspection and probing of all accessible parts (Fig. 9.4). The final decision on joint-preserving osteotomy versus is made at this point. Smaller cartilaginous lesions may be treated with curettage and drilling or microfracturing. Loose, nonviable fragments are excised. If a full-thickness cartilage defect is present at the weight-bearing area, the affected joint is fused after correction of the deformity. Fibrous intra- and extra-articular

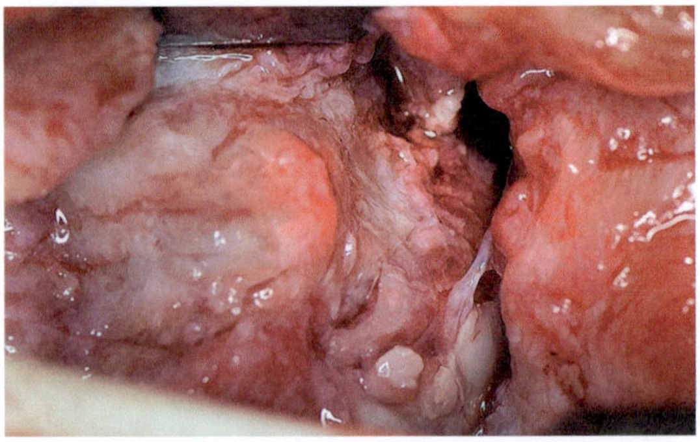

Fig. 9.4 Medial approach to the talar neck and head showing the tilted surface of the latter facing the subtalar instead of the talonavicular joint but displaying a complete cartilage cover (Same patient as in Figs. 9.1, 9.2, and 9.3, 10 months after the original injury)

adhesions around the talus are released and tenolysis of the peroneal tendons is performed as needed. A collinear foot distractor is most useful to access all parts of the talonavicular joint (Fig. 9.5).

The original fracture lines, as assessed preoperatively with CT imaging, are exposed from medial and lateral. Care is taken to not compromise the blood supply to the talar body. Therefore, preparation on the medial side should not extend behind the sustentaculum tali in order not to injure the deltoid branches from the tibialis posterior artery. Laterally, preparation should be strictly confined to the lateral aspect of the talar neck and the lateral process of the talus. Preparation on the superior aspect of the sinus and canalis tarsi should be avoided.

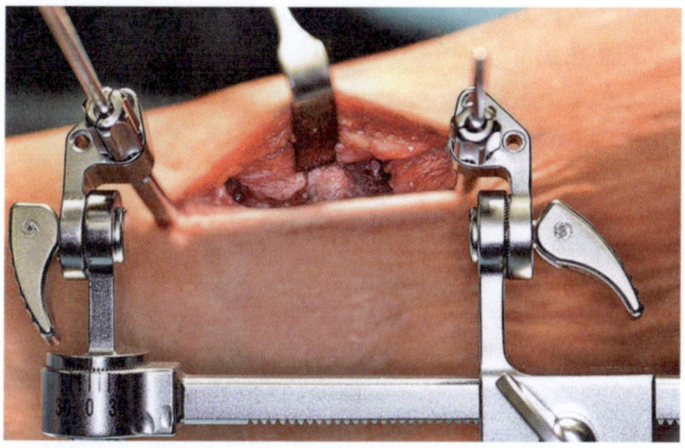

Fig. 9.5 A collinear foot distractor is applied from medial with Steinmann pins placed into the talar body and navicular in order to access all parts of the talonavicular joint. (Same patient as in Figs. 9.1, 9.2, 9.3, and 9.4)

In cases of solid malunion, an osteotomy is carried out stepwise and carefully along the former fracture plane with small osteotomes (Fig. 9.6). The viability of the talar body after performing the osteotomy is checked with the tourniquet released. Avascular areas of the talar body may be subjected to curettage and subchondral drilling to enhance bone regeneration. If the fracture is not yet completely united, the fragments are cautiously mobilized with a sharp elevator or osteotome. Manifest non-unions (Type II deformities) are treated with complete resection of the fibrous pseudarthrosis and underlying sclerotic bone until viable cancellous bone becomes visible. The resulting defect is then filled with bone graft to avoid shortening or axial deviation [6].

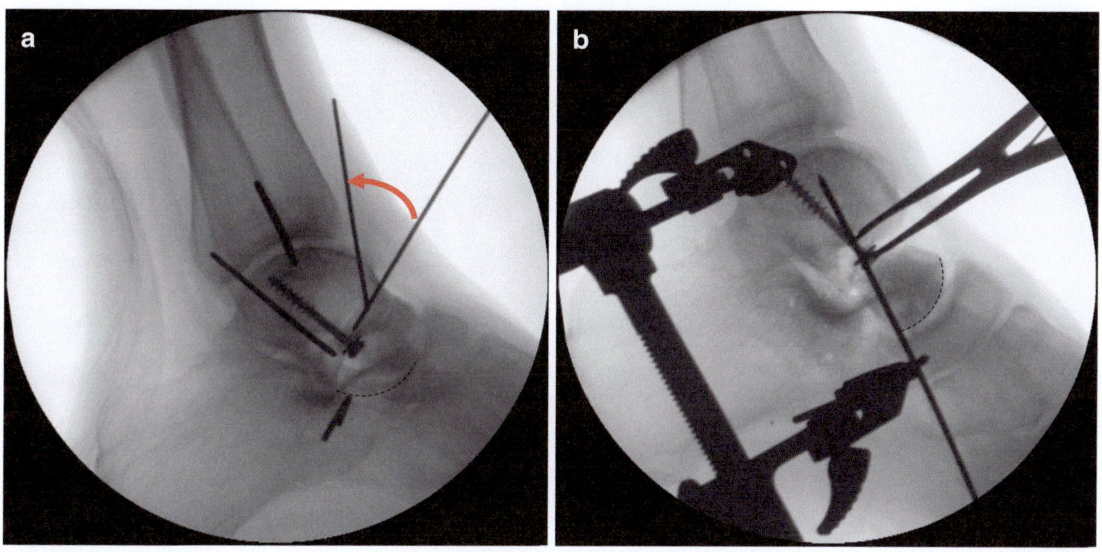

Fig. 9.6 Lateral fluorosopic view (**a**) before and (**b**) after the osteotomy of the talar neck with derotation of the talar head fragment and interposition of a tricortical graft from the iliac crest from medial in order to correct varus malalignment. The dotted line depicts the joint surface of the talar head. The K-wires in (**a**) mark the site of the former fracture and thus osteotomy at the talar neck. (Same patient as in Figs. 9.1, 9.2, 9.3, 9.4, and 9.5)

The typical varus deformity of the talar neck is corrected with an extra-articular osteotomy and interposition of a corticocancellous bone graft from medial. The fragments can be manipulated with K-wires that are used as joy sticks rather than direct clamping to avoid damage to the joint surfaces or further fragmentation. Anatomic realignment of the talar neck, the ankle, and subtalar joints is assessed visually through the bilateral approaches (Fig. 9.7). After temporary fixation with K-wires, axial realignment is controlled fluoroscopically (Fig. 9.6b).

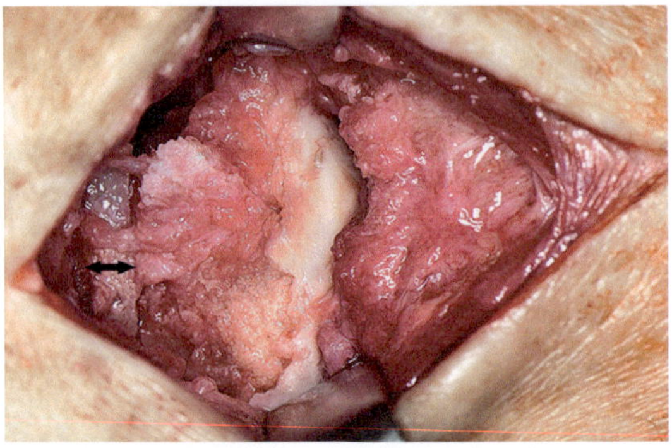

Fig. 9.7 Intraoperative view from medial showing the correct position of the now derotated talar head with the joint surface facing the navicular. The double arrow depicts the corticocancellous bone graft from the iliac crest. (Same patient as in Figs. 9.1, 9.2, 9.3, 9.4, 9.5, and 9.6)

After anatomical reduction has been obtained, fragment fixation is typically achieved with 3.5 millimeter small fragment screws. Alternatively, a mini-fragment plate is applied from medially or bilateral plates (Fig. 9.8) are used to bridge a former comminution zone or stabilize a relatively small talar head fragment [6].

Pearls

- Careful patient selection
- Meticulous preoperative planning
- Bilateral approaches for adequate exposure and control of reduction
- Careful, step-wise osteotomy along the former fracture

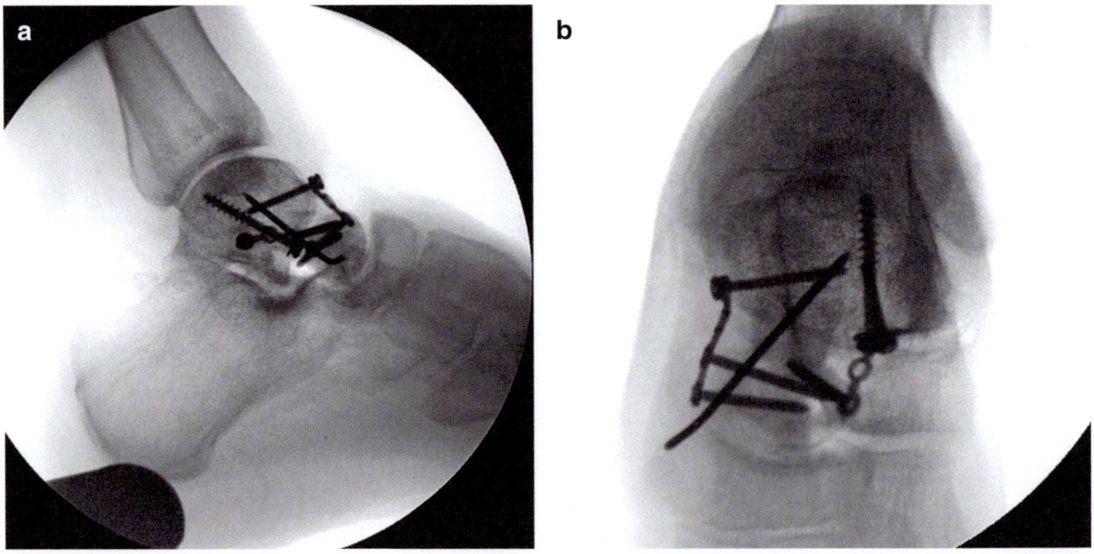

Fig. 9.8 Postoperative fluoroscopic images showing anatomic alignment of the talar neck and head and fixation with bilateral minifragment (2.4 mm) interlocking plates. The lateral screw was left in place. An axial additional K-wire was introduced in a retrograde manner and left in place for 6 weeks. (Same patient as in Figs. 9.1, 9.2, 9.3, 9.4, 9.5, 9.6, and 9.7)

- Bone grafting after resection of a pseudoarthrosis or necrotic bone
- Individually tailored aftertreatment with early range of motion

Pitfalls

- Conversion to corrective fusion for patients with inadequate cartilage cover
- Avoid dissection of the deltoid ligament and upper aspect of the sinus tarsi in order to preserve the blood supply to the talar body
- No prolonged offloading with partial AVN

Immediate Postoperative Care, Rehabilitation, and Recovery

Aftertreatment aims at early motion of the ankle, subtalar, and mid-tarsal joints. Only in rare cases with relatively small juxtaarticular fragments, temporary joint transfixation with a K-wire may be useful for 6 weeks.

Immediately after surgery, the foot and ankle is immobilized in a short leg splint with elevation and non-weight-bearing. Physical therapy with active and passive range of motion exercises of the ankle and hindfoot joints usually starts at the second postoperative day, in order to maintain motion and prevent recurrence of adhesions. At 4–7 days a walking cast, special boot, or walker is fitted, which is usually applied for 6 weeks. Patients are mobilized on two crutches with partial weight-bearing of 15–20 kg for about 10–12 weeks postoperatively. After union has been confirmed with weight-bearing radiographs (Fig. 9.9), weight-bearing is increased progressively over 1–2 weeks until full weight-bearing is achieved.

The presence of a pre-existing partial AVN should not prolong the period of partial weight-

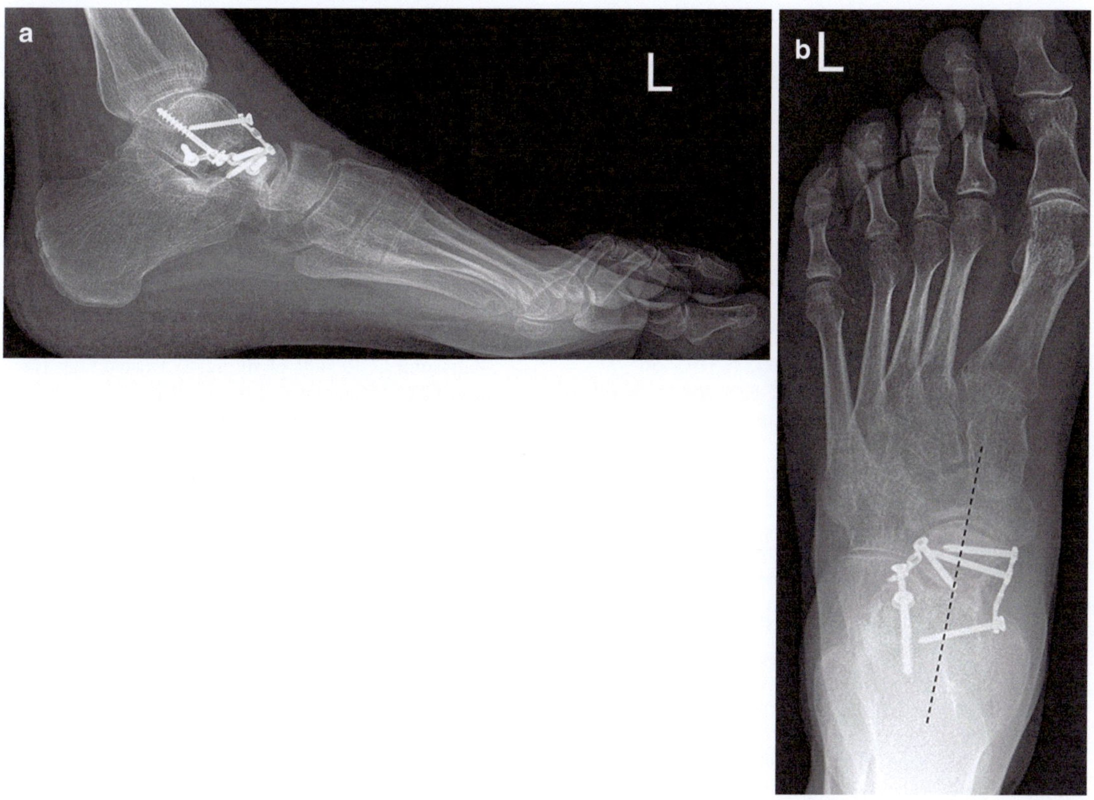

Fig. 9.9 Standing (**a**) lateral and (**b**) dorsoplantar radiographs showing anatomic alignment of the talar neck and solid bony union at the site of the osteotomy with incorporation of the graft. (Same patient as in Figs. 9.1, 9.2, 9.3, 9.4, 9.5, 9.6, 9.7, and 9.8, 6 months after the correction)

bearing and does not appear to influence the functional result of corrective surgery [6]. In a series of 22 joint-preserving corrections of talar malunions and nonunions, among them 12 talar neck malunions, we have observed neither development nor progression of AVN [29]. In 12 of 20 patients (60%) that were followed for a mean of 5 years, progression of arthritis has been noted. However, late fusion of the ankle, subtalar, or talonavicular joint was necessary in only three patients between 1.5 and 8 years after correction [29]. These results have been echoed recently by other authors [30–33] and in a later follow-up of our series with the patients being followed up to 21 years [34].

In summary, corrective osteotomy after malunited talar neck fractures or nonunions at that site leads to a considerable functional improvement in properly selected patients with adequate bone stock and without symptomatic arthritis or total AVN of the talus with collapse of the talar dome. Furthermore, patients should be reliable, free of infection, and the cartilage should appear viable under direct intra-operative inspection. Late in situ fusion in case of progressive arthritis still remains a salvage option on a well aligned talus.

References

1. Hawkins LG. Fractures of the neck of the talus. J Bone Joint Surg Am. 1970;52:991–1002.
2. Canale ST, Kelly FB Jr. Fractures of the neck of the talus. J Bone Joint Surg Am. 1978;60:143–56.
3. Lorentzen JE, Christensen SB, Krogsoe O, Sneppen O. Fractures of the neck of the talus. Acta Orthop Scand. 1977;48:115–20.
4. Peterson L, Goldie IF, Irstam L. Fracture of the neck of the talus. A clinical study. Acta Orthop Scand. 1977;48:696–706.
5. Schuind F, Andrianne Y, Burny F, Donkerwolcke M, Saric O. Fractures et luxations de l'astragale. Revue de 359 cas. Acta Orthop Belg. 1983;49(6):652–89.
6. Rammelt S, Winkler J, Heineck J, Zwipp H. Anatomical reconstruction of malunited talus fractures: a prospective study of 10 patients followed for 4 years. Acta Orthop. 2005;76(4):588–96.
7. Rammelt S, Zwipp H. Talar neck and body fractures. Injury. 2009;40(2):120–35.
8. Daniels TR, Smith JW, Ross TI. Varus malalignment of the talar neck. Its effect on the position of the foot and on subtalar motion. J Bone Joint Surg Am. 1996;78:1559–67.
9. Sanders DW, Busam M, Hattwick E, et al. Functional outcomes following displaced talar neck fractures. J Orthop Trauma. 2004;18(5):265–70.
10. Jordan RK, Bafna KR, Liu J, Ebraheim NA. Complications of talar neck fractures by Hawkins classification: a systematic review. J Foot Ankle Surg. 2017;56(4):817–21.
11. Sneppen O, Christensen SB, Krogsoe O, Lorentzen J. Fracture of the body of the talus. Acta Orthop Scand. 1977;48:317–24.
12. Heckman JD, McLean MR. Fractures of the lateral process of the talus. Clin Orthop. 1985;199:108–13.
13. Nyska M, Howard CB, Matan Y, Cohen D, Peyser A, Garti A, et al. Fracture of the posterior body of the talus--the hidden fracture. Arch Orthop Trauma Surg. 1998;117(1–2):114–7.
14. Bibbo C, Anderson RB, Davis WH. Injury characteristics and the clinical outcome of subtalar dislocations: a clinical and radiographic analysis of 25 cases. Foot Ankle Int. 2003;24(2):158–63.
15. Rammelt S, Winkler J, Grass R, Zwipp H. Reconstruction after talar fractures. Foot Ankle Clin. 2006;11(1):61–84, viii.
16. Mills HJ, Horne G. Fractures of the lateral process of the talus. Aust N Z J Surg. 1987;57(9):643–6.
17. Giuffrida AY, Lin SS, Abidi N, Berberian W, Berkman A, Behrens FF. Pseudo os trigonum sign: missed posteromedial talar facet fracture. Foot Ankle Int. 2003;24(8):642–9.
18. Rammelt S, Zwipp H, Prescher A. Talus bipartitus: a rare skeletal variation. J Bone Joint Surg Am. 2011;93:e21 (1–9.
19. Zwipp H, Rammelt S. Posttraumatic deformity correction at the foot [in German]. Zbl Chir. 2003;128:218–26.
20. Vallier HA, Nork SE, Benirschke SK, Sangeorzan BJ. Surgical treatment of talar body fractures. J Bone Joint Surg Am. 2003;85-A(9):1716–24.
21. Yeganeh A, Alaee A, Bodduhi B, Behkam-rad A, Shahoseini G. Results of surgically treated talar fractures. Chin J Traumatol. 2013;16:361–4.
22. Rammelt S, Zwipp H. Corrective arthrodeses and osteotomies for post-traumatic hindfoot malalignment: indications, techniques, results. Int Orthop. 2013;37(9):1707–17.
23. Lindvall E, Haidukewych G, DiPasquale T, Herscovici D Jr, Sanders R. Open reduction and stable fixation of isolated, displaced talar neck and body fractures. J Bone Joint Surg Am. 2004;86-A(10):2229–34.
24. Stake IK, Madsen JE, Hvaal K, Johnsen E, Husebye EE. Surgically treated talar fractures. A retrospective study of 50 patients. Foot Ankle Surg. 2016;22(2):85–90. https://doi.org/10.1016/j.fas.2015.05.005. Epub 2015 May 16.
25. Schwarz N, Eschberger J, Kramer J, Posch E. Radiologic and histologic observations in central talus fractures [in German]. Unfallchirurg. 1997;100:449–56.

26. Adelaar RS, Madrian JR. Avascular necrosis of the talus. Orthop Clin North Am. 2004;35(3):383–95, xi.
27. Langer P, Nickisch F, Spenciner D, Fleming B, DiGiovanni CW. In vitro evaluation of the effect lateral process talar excision on ankle and subtalar joint stability. Foot Ankle Int. 2007;28(1):78–83.
28. Cronier P, Talha A, Massin P. Central talar fractures--therapeutic considerations. Injury. 2004;35 Suppl 2:SB10–22.
29. Rammelt S, Zwipp H. Secondary correction of talar fractures: asking for trouble? Foot Ankle Int. 2012;33(4):359–62.
30. Huang PJ, Cheng YM. Delayed surgical treatment for neglected or mal-reduced talar fractures. Int Orthop. 2005;29(5):326–9.
31. Yu GR, Li B, Yang YF, Zhou JQ, Zhu XZ, Huang YG, et al. Surgical treatment of malunited or nonunited talus fractures [in Chinese]. Zhonghua Wai Ke Za Zhi. 2010;48(9):658–61.
32. Suter T, Barg A, Knupp M, Henninger H, Hintermann B. Surgical technique: talar neck osteotomy to lengthen the medial column after a malunited talar neck fracture. Clin Orthop Relat Res. 2013;471:1356–64.
33. Chen G, Hu M, Xu Y, Zhen YH, Hong Y, Xu XY. Joint-preserving surgery for talar malunions or nonuions. Orthop Surg. 2017;9(1):34.
34. Zwipp H, Gavlik M, Rammelt S. Secondary anatomical reconstruction of malunited central talus fractures [in German]. Unfallchirurg. 2014;117(9):767–75.

Failed Lisfranc ORIF

10

Brandon Levy and Andrew K. Sands

Introduction

Lisfranc injuries typically are injuries to the tarsometatarsal joint complex, specifically between the medial cuneiform and base of the second metatarsal. There are many variations also involving fractures of the base of the metatarsals, intercuneiform ligament disruptions, and cuneiform fractures. In general then, a "Lisfranc" injury may be considered any injury, whether bony or ligamentous, in the region from the naviculocuneiform joint through the intertarsal and tarsimetatarsal area, extending distal to the base of the metatarsals. Injuries proximal to this involving the navicular and talo-navicular as well as cuboid and calcaneo-cuboid areas are Chopart injuries. Injuries can range in severity and may be purely ligamentous or contain fractures and/or joint disruptions.

Injuries to the Lisfranc region may be due to direct high energy mechanisms, sometimes with vascular injury, or due to axial loads applied to a plantarflexed forefoot.

Injuries are often overlooked by initial assessing providers and can be mistakenly labeled a foot "sprain."

Timely initial diagnosis does not necessarily improve outcome and in fact, delay may lead to better surgical results. Accurate diagnosis of a Lisfranc-type injury is made by a thorough physical examination with high suspicion for Lisfranc injury and radiographic imaging. Most often the diagnosis can be made using simple inexpensive means. Expensive imaging is not needed in most instances of Lisfranc injury.

We will review our methods and discuss why and how treatments sometimes fail.

Diagnosis

A keen understanding of the Lisfranc joint and mechanisms of injury are important when correctly diagnosing a Lisfranc injury. At initial presentation to an emergency room, these injuries may be misdiagnosed as a foot "sprain" by an untrained eye.

B. Levy (✉)
Kingsbrook Jewish Medical Center, Division of Orthopedic Surgery, Brooklyn, NY, USA

A. K. Sands
Weill Cornell Medical College, New York Presbyterian – Lower Manhattan Hospital, Department of Orthopedic Surgery, New York, NY, USA

M. J. Berkowitz et al. (eds.), *Revision Surgery of the Foot and Ankle*, https://doi.org/10.1007/978-3-030-29969-9_10

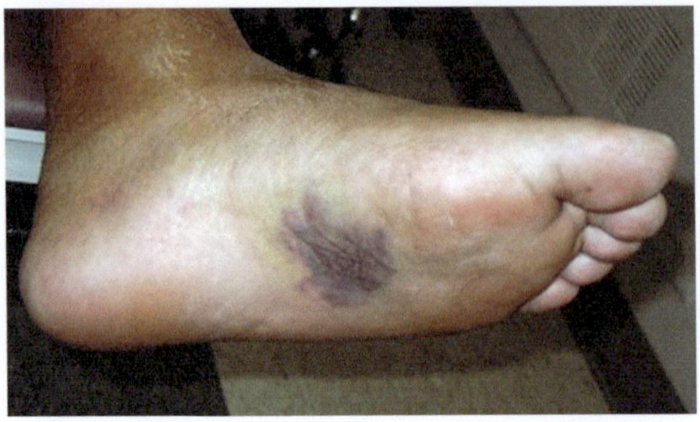

Fig. 10.1 Clinical picture of a foot demonstrating plantar ecchymosis

At initial inspection, plantar ecchymosis might be seen, which is a strong indication of a Lisfranc type injury. Soft tissue swelling is also present and should be evaluated to identify possible presence of associated foot compartment syndrome (Fig. 10.1).

Patients may describe extreme pain that seemingly exceeds what might be expected from a common "sprain." They report feelings of severe pain with nausea and an inability to bear weight.

A thorough physical examination may be difficult to perform due to the patient's pain. A gentle examination can be performed but if the pain is too severe, there are other modalities of evaluation described below.

Weight-bearing X-rays are often diagnostic but, as previously described, can be difficult to obtain due to pain. Every effort should be made to have the patient stand on the X-ray plate for imaging as full weight-bearing images are often diagnostic. Any degree of weight-bearing is better than non-weight-bearing images. Contralateral images might also be obtained for comparison. If weight-bearing radiographs are not initially obtained at the time of injury or if there is a question as to whether there is an injury, the patient can have weight-bearing images at the time of their first visit in the office which should be within 1–2 weeks (Figs. 10.2, 10.3, and 10.4).

At the time of injury, it is acceptable to place the patient in a non-weight-bearing splint until clinic follow up.

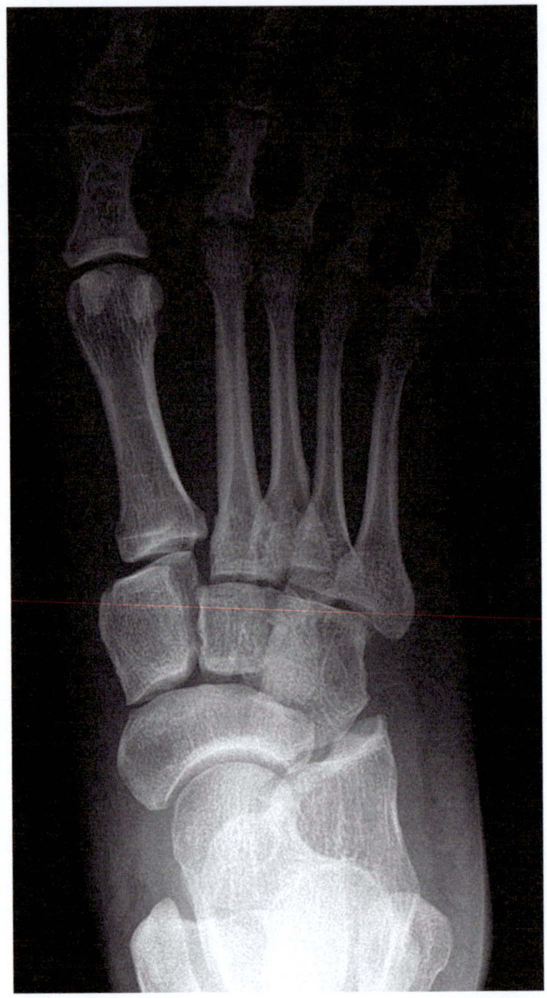

Fig. 10.2 Weight-bearing AP view of the foot demonstrating the lateral displacement of the first and second TMT joints

Physical Exam

The physical exam begins with thorough inspection and palpation of the affected foot. These injuries are commonly associated with plantar foot ecchymosis. It is important to note any visible bony deformities or, less commonly, open wounds. There will typically be dorsal foot swelling and tenderness to palpation over the tarsometatarsal joint.

An instability test can be performed by grasping the metatarsal heads and applying force while

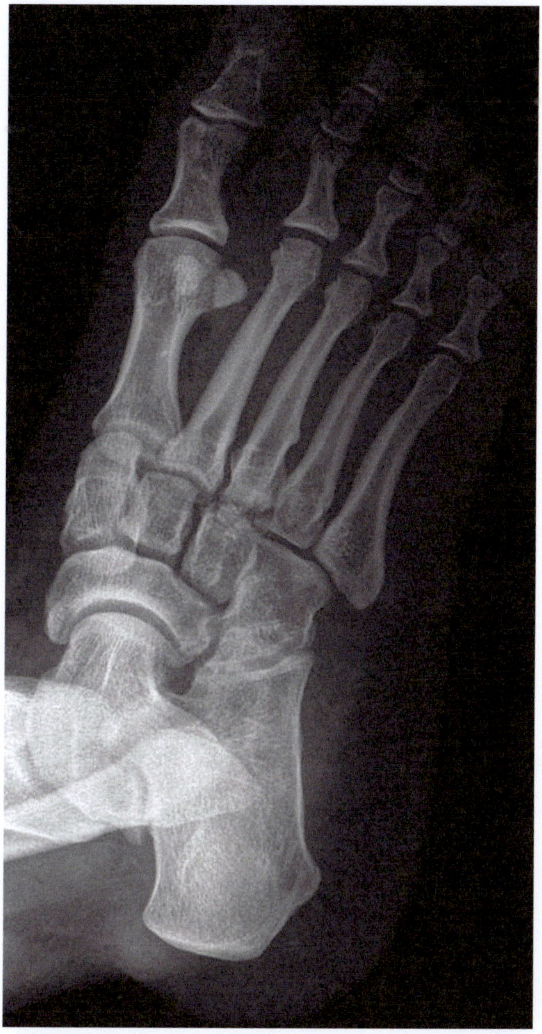

Fig. 10.3 30-degree oblique view of the foot demonstrating lateral displacement of third metatarsal on lateral cuneiform

the other hand palpates the tarsometatarsal joint. While holding the heel firmly, varus and valgus manipulation by the other hand can elicit pain and gross instability. If the pain is severe, it may not be possible to elicit a gross midfoot instability. If physical exam is too painful, an ankle block or use of propofol in the ER can be used to allow manipulation, with radiographic or mini-fluoro images showing the gross instability (Fig. 10.5).

Less obvious entities including avulsion fractures can be seen on CT scan. This is important to evaluate, as properly selected treatment is dictated by pathology (Fig. 10.6).

Inspect and palpate the lower limb musculature to check for compartment syndrome.

It is also important to perform a Silverskiold exam to test for equinus contracture. If there is a

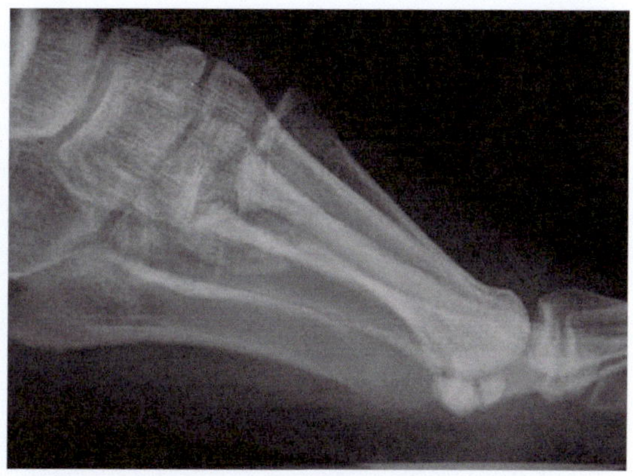

Fig. 10.4 Lateral view of the foot demonstrating dorsal displacement of the metatarsals

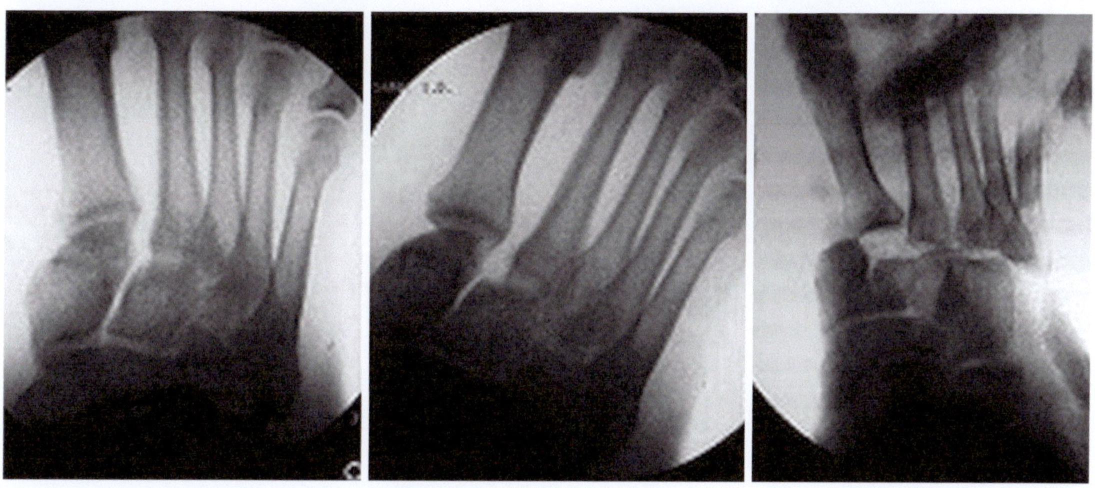

Fig. 10.5 Instability test demonstrating displacement of the Lisfranc joint

contracture, it must be addressed. This will be discussed further in the treatment section.

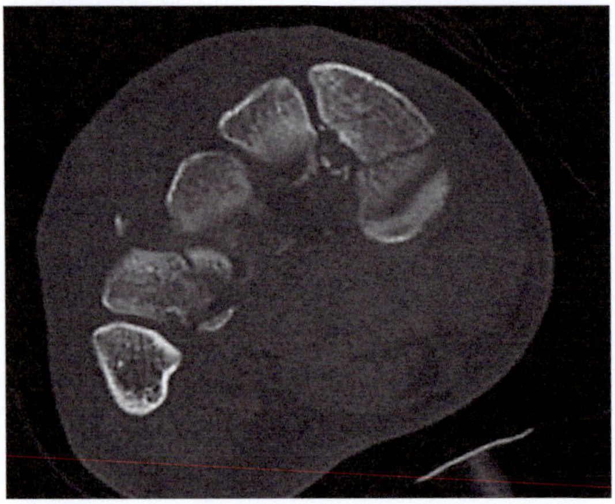

Fig. 10.6 Axial CT scan of the foot demonstrating multiple metatarsal fractures

Technique for Fixation

Approach

The goal for reconstruction is to restore anatomy and function. Pre-op planning is an important tool that can help decide on an appropriate surgical approach, choice of implant, and order of operation. Our surgical approach entails a dorsal double parallel and medial mini incision. The medial incision will give you access to the first tarsometatarsal and medial second tarsometatarsal joint, and the lateral incision will give you access to the lateral second and third tarsometatarsal joint. It is important to work back and forth between the two dorsal incisions, seen in Fig. 10.7a, b, and to not undermine the middle flap. This will help to protect the dorsal flap from damage and necrosis.

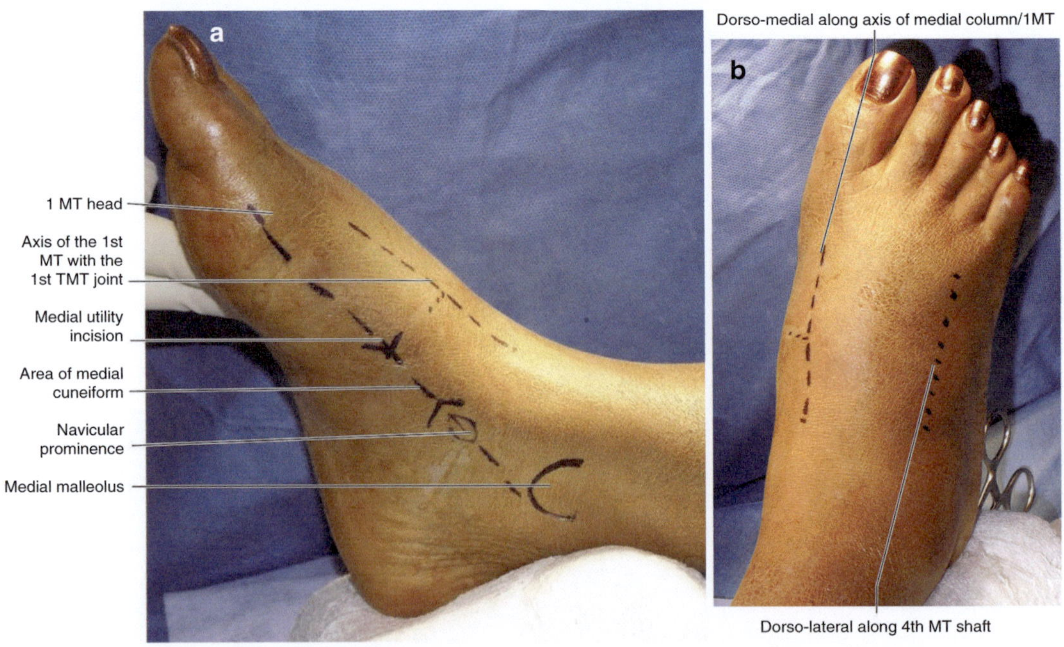

Fig. 10.7 (a, b) Clinical pictures of right foot demonstrating anatomic landmarks and surgical incisions. (Reprinted from Sands and Swords, © 2018, with permission from Elsevier)

Helpful Hardware/Implants

It is important to gather all appropriate hardware and implants prior to surgery so that there are no intraoperative delays retrieving hardware. Reduction clamps are a vital tool that can be used initially to stabilize the bony structures (Fig. 10.8).

It is important to have multiple drills, ranging from sizes 2.0, 2.5, 2.7, 3.5, and 4.0, as well as smooth 1.6 and 2.0 K-wires. Longer drills are better used by allowing the chuck to be located more distally. If a short bit is used, the chuck, when spinning, can hit the dorsal skin and toes. A wide array of hand instruments, including elevators and pics, should be used to help free up bony margins and maintain appropriate alignment prior to fixation (Fig. 10.9).

There is a wide variety of implants available for fixation but we prefer a 4.0, fully threaded solid screw. This screw provides a low-profile head, a larger shaft compared to 2.7 and 3.5 screws, a 1.25 thread pitch, and a self-tapping tip (Fig. 10.10).

Surgical Tips and Tricks

It is not enough to have the appropriate approach and surgical implants. Proper techniques for fixation are vital for successful outcomes. A pocket hole is used to prevent dorsal cortical breakout as the screw head engages bone. It is important to start the screw at least 2 cm from the joint in order to create a long lever arm (Fig. 10.11).

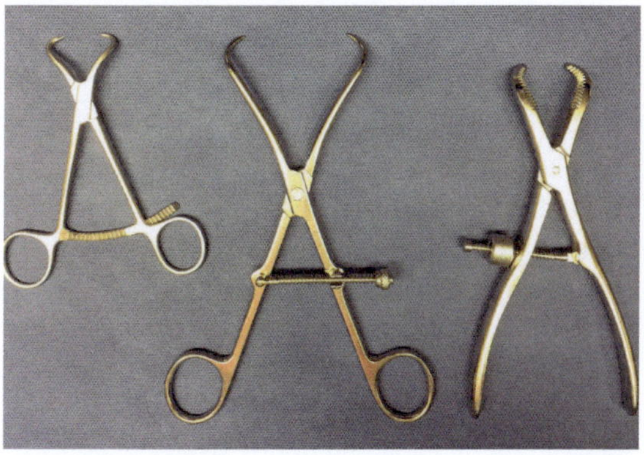

Fig. 10.8 Synthes point-to-point reduction clamps used in the dorsal double parallel approach

Drill techniques can vary and are important to consider in different pathology. A gliding hole and lag technique should be used for tarsometatarsal compression. When compression is not wanted across the joint, be sure to drill straight through

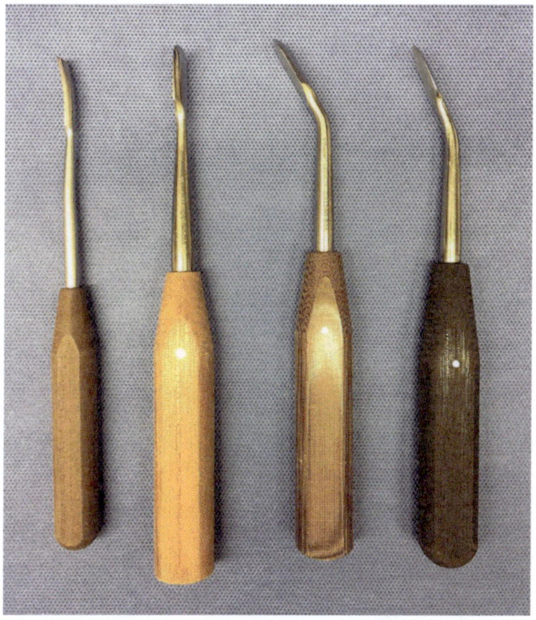

Fig. 10.9 Synthes hand instruments

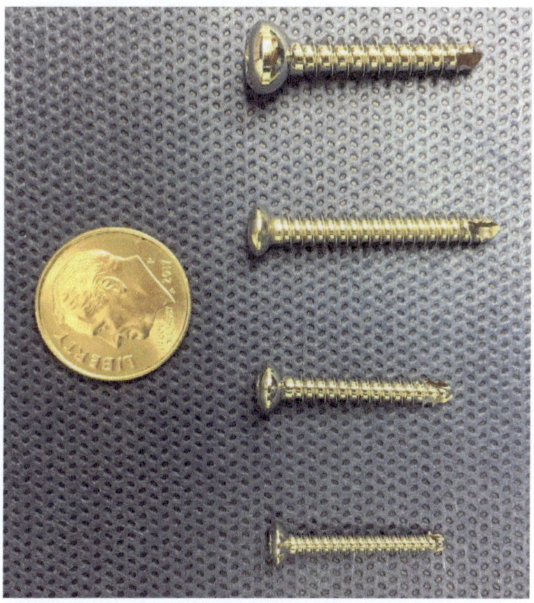

Fig. 10.10 Synthes screws sized from top to bottom, 4.5 mm, 4.0 mm, 3.5 mm, 2.7 mm

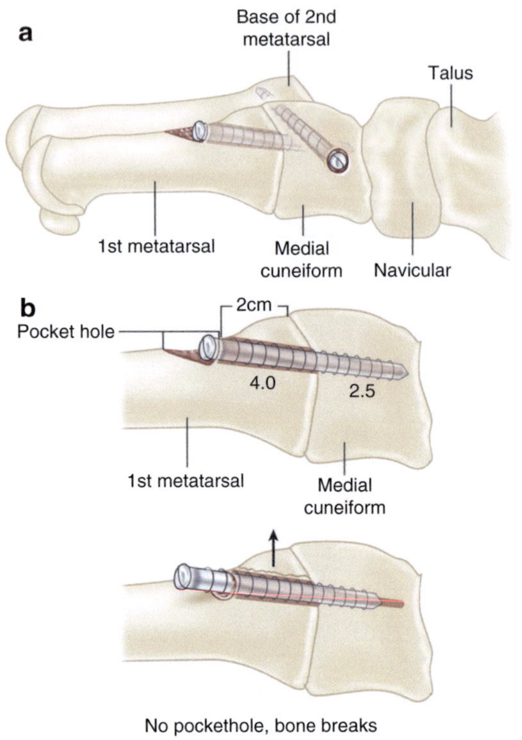

Fig. 10.11 Picture of pocket hole technique. (Reprinted from Sands and Swords, © 2018, with permission from Elsevier)

and avoid a lag technique. As mentioned above, longer screws placed farther from the joint create better leverage. For a fusion of a pure ligamentous injury, proper joint prep leads to increased fusion rates—denuding the area, drilling the subchondral bone, and creating a symmetric joint space—and shear strain relief bone grafting is critical for good fusion outcome. For an open reduction and internal fixation, perfect anatomic reduction is the most important concept.

The order of operation is also important to take in to account. This will be further described later in the chapter, but if an intertarsal injury is found, this should be addressed first.

Open Reduction Internal Fixation

For a fracture-dislocation of the Lisfranc joint, we prefer the dual dorsal parallel and mini medial incision. The medial incision is cheated a bit medial. Deeper dissection follows the interval between the EHL and EHB. These tendons are retracted with a self retaining retractor and a blue pen marker can be used to identify the capsule and periosteum for closure. However, these structures are often disrupted by mechanism of injury.

Step 1

If there is no intertarsal injury, as in this case, we initially pay attention to fixing the second tarsometatarsal joint. Using the medial dorsal incision, closely inspect the medal base of the second metatarsal and clean the corner to remove any soft tissue or loose fragments, taking care to not destroy the sharp corner where the base of the second MT fits into the keystone area. Then, reduce the base of second metatarsal into the corner and hold with a point-to-point reduction clamp that is placed in the mini medial and lateral dorsal incisions. Using the medial incision, a 4.0 drill hole is made through the medial cuneiform and then a 2.5 drill through the base of the second metatarsal under fluoroscopic guidance. Insertion of the 4.0 screw will lag and reduce the base of the second metatarsal into the corner, in optimal position. Alternatively, the lag screw can be paced from the base of the second MT through the dorsolateral incision into the medial cuneiform (Fig. 10.12).

Step 2

Next, we focus on the first tarsometatarsal joint. Through the dorsal medial incision, we can visualize the joint, directly reduce, and provisionally hold with smooth k-wires. A long 2.5 mm drill bit is then passed from distal to proximal through the first tarsometatarsal joint. A 4.0 solid screw is then inserted (Fig. 10.13a, b).

Step 3

Through the dorsolateral incision, attention is turned to the third metatarsal base. A point-to-point reduction clamp is placed with the tips in the medial incision and dorsolateral incision. Again, note that access to the lateral base of the second metatarsal and third metatarsal base is through the dorsolateral incision and not by overly aggressive dissection and lateral pulling through the dorsomedial incision, as it causes soft tissue damage to

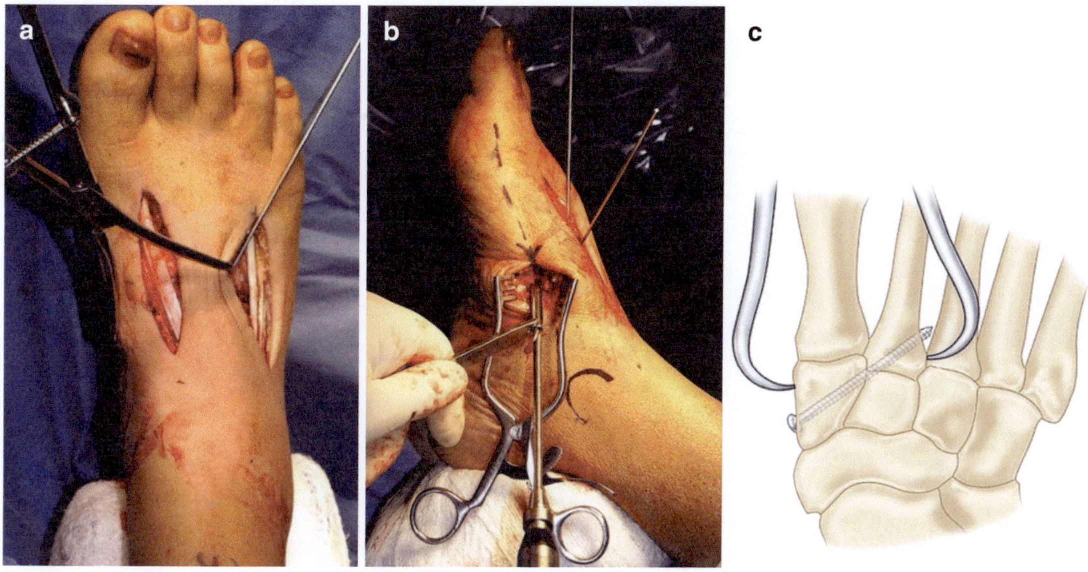

Fig. 10.12 Reduction of the second TMT joint. (Reprinted from Sands and Swords, © 2018, with permission from Elsevier)

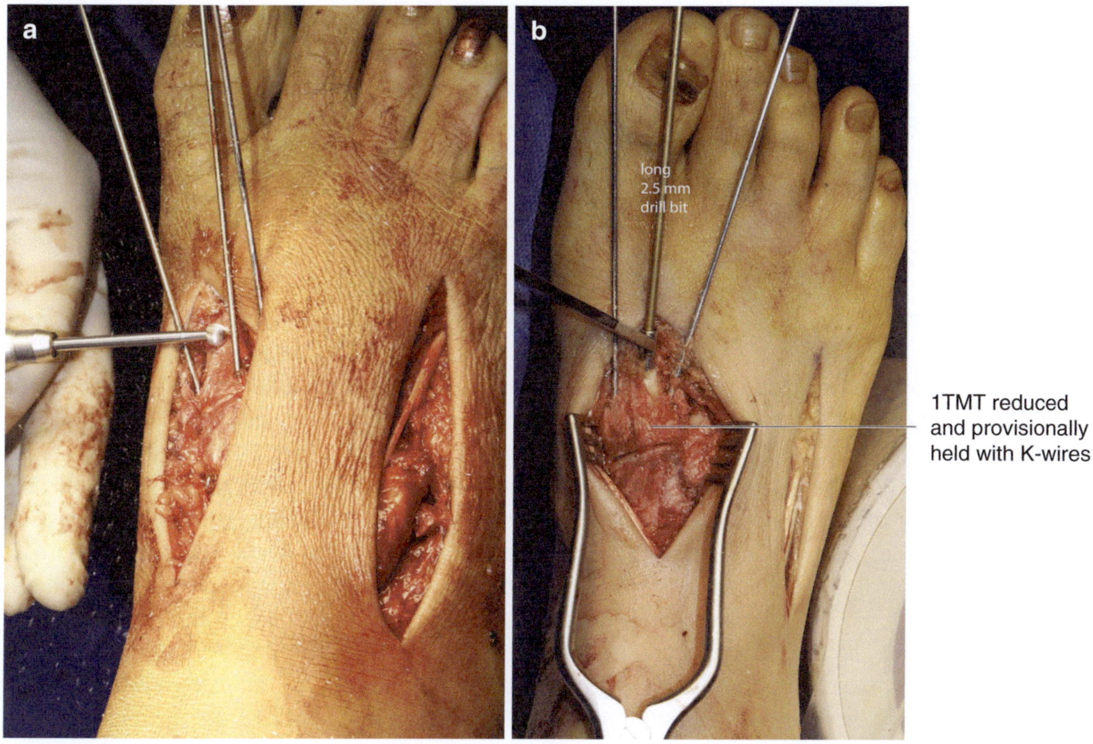

Fig. 10.13 (**a**, **b**) Fixation of the first TMT joint. (Reprinted from Sands and Swords, © 2018, with permission from Elsevier)

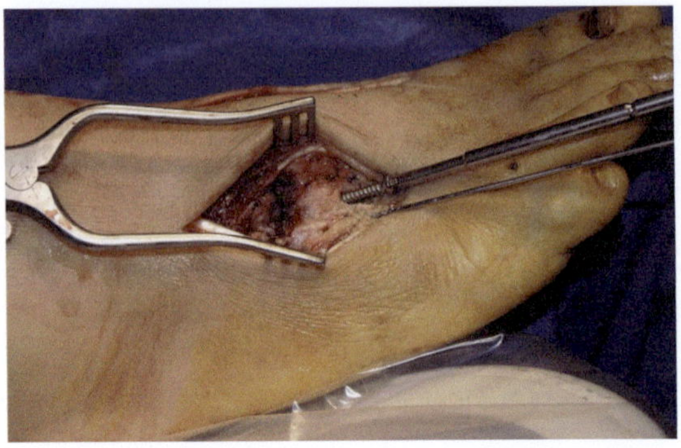

Fig. 10.14 Fixation of the base of the third MT. (Reprinted from Sands and Swords, © 2018, with permission from Elsevier)

the bridge and may injure the vascular bundle which is within the flap. Again using a 4.0/2.5 drill combination with a pocket hole on the dorsal base of the third metatarsal, a lag screw is placed from the base of the third metatarsal into the lateral or intermediate cuneiform (Fig. 10.14).

Step 4

The fourth and fifth tarsometatarsal joints often reduce with the more medial reduction. As such, K-wires can be placed from 4/5 metatarsal base into the cuboid under fluoroscopic guidance. More rigid implants can fail and lead to poor outcomes (Fig. 10.15).

Intertarsal Instability

Intertarsal instability can be concomitantly seen with Lisfranc injuries. If this is the case, the goal is to fix the intertarsal instability first. This reduction is initially achieved by placing smooth K-wires (1.6–2.0 mm) from medial to lateral across the unstable joints. Often these injuries are corrected under fluoroscopic indirect reduction. If the injury is more severe and direct reduction is needed, the medial and dorsomedial incision can be extended proximally. Lag technique can be used as these are non-essential non-mobile joints, and, so, stiffness does not lead to loss of function. Screws should be placed after the tarsometatarsal screws have been placed as smaller screws are often needed to stabilize intertarsal injuries. 2.7 or 3.5 screws can be used

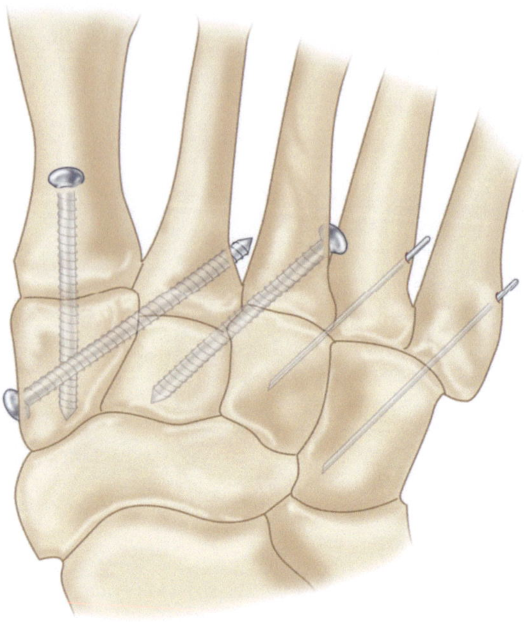

Fig. 10.15 Fixation of the fourth and fifth TMT joint. (Reprinted from Sands and Swords, © 2018, with permission from Elsevier)

transversely if insertion among the criss-cross screw pattern is difficult.

Base of Metatarsal Fracture

Frequently associated with Lisfranc joint disruption are injuries sustained to the base of the second metatarsal. These fragments can be provisionally held in position and reduced with small K-wires coming in perpendicular to the metatarsal shaft. Further, ORIF with screws of all tarsometatarsal joints takes place. Often, the LF ligament, which is attached to the plantar base of the second metatarsal avulses, leading to a triangular plantar fragment. During the reduction, the base of the second metatarsal can be moved a bit lateral and any debris and soft tissue from the inter-fragmentary area is removed. Since the fragment is rigidly held by the ligament and the injury is the avulsion and displacement of the base of the second metatarsal, then reducing this to the intact plantar ligament fragment leads to reduction of the fracture. Fixation of the base of the second metatarsal to the medial cuneiform leads to reduction of the plantar fragment and bone-to-bone healing. As such, it is unnecessary to perform direct ORIF of the plantar fragment.

If there is a more complex fracture on the base of the second and/or third metatarsal, then a spanning plate can be used from the MT shaft onto the cuneiforms.

Equinus Contracture

As part of the initial physical exam, all patients should be examined for equinus contractures. Testing of the uninjured side can suggest that the contracture exists on the injured side as well. This is especially important in purely ligamentous injuries. If not addressed, this can lead to breakdown of the repair. Gastrocnemius release is often needed and is the first step in order of operations. Through a small medial incision at the level of the musculotendinous junction, a speculum can be inserted to visualize the full medial to lateral extent of the fascial plane across the muscle belly. This allows easy visualization and access to releasing the fascial layer.

Why Does It Fail?

Failure of treating Lisfranc injuries can be due to multiple modalities. These include misdiagnosis, intraoperative shortcomings, patient-specific variables, and improper postoperative care. Failure can also be seen in patients who choose to be treated non-operatively.

Intraoperative Shortcomings and Improper Implants

Proper implants and appropriate surgical technique are important for successful outcomes in Lisfranc injuries. What is most cost effective might not be the best option and sometimes it may be necessary to have more than one manner of fixation across the joint. A keen knowledge of the anatomy is important for being able to use implants appropriately, by recognizing that there is a forefoot long bone torsional rotation moment versus a mid-foot bending moment.

In the following case, not only do we see the use of unnecessary and expensive constructs, but we see implant failure due to improper screw placement and lack of appropriate reduction.

Case 10.1

This is a 55-year-old man who suffered a twisting injury to his foot. He was seen at a local ER and sent to a local allied health provider who took him for surgery. Injury films show a stress test indicating a purely ligamentous Lisfranc injury. The allied health provider initially placed the patient in an external fixator, followed by a second surgery placing two cannulated screws. The patient came to our clinic 3 months after surgery with continued pain. The initial technique and implants for fusion was inadequate. We took the patient to the OR for a mid-foot fusion and total Achilles lengthening (Figs. 10.16a, b, 10.17a, b, and 10.18).

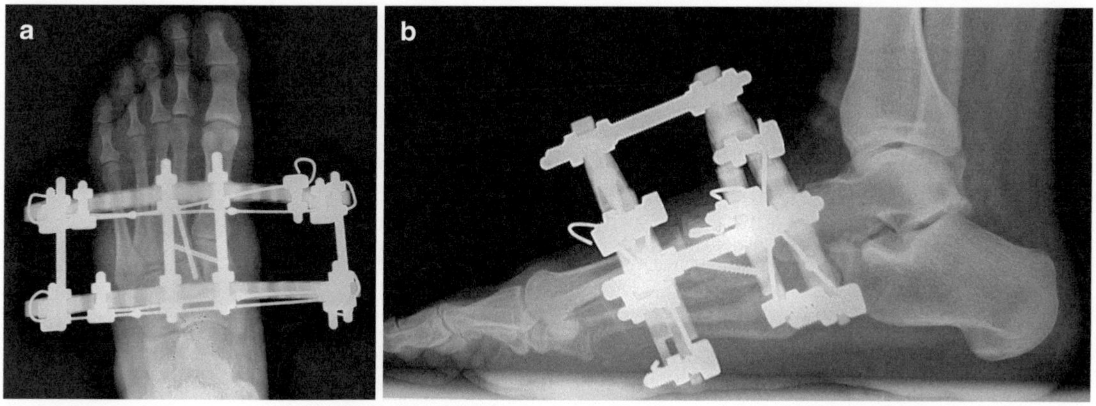

Fig. 10.16 (**a**) AP and (**b**) Lateral X-Ray of left foot showing placement of an external fixator

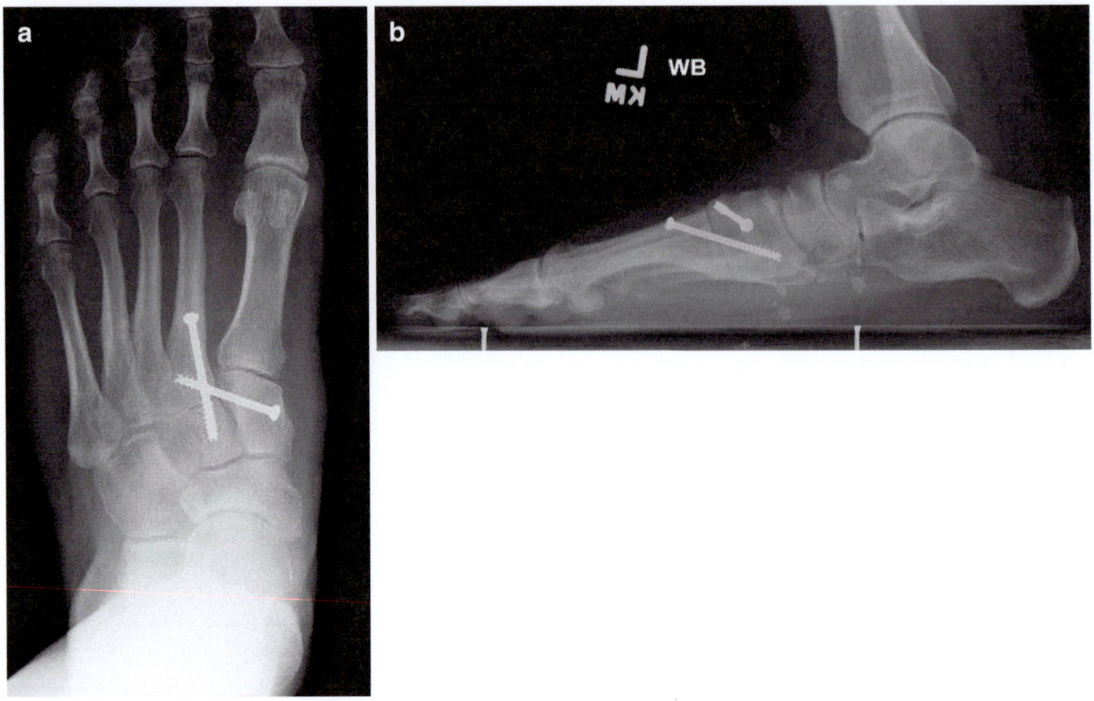

Fig. 10.17 (**a**) AP and (**b**) lateral X-ray of left foot 3 months post-op, demonstrating a non-reduced joint space and improper screw placement

Misdiagnosis

A misdiagnosis in the ED, commonly classified as a "sprained foot" can lead to continued pain and limitations in a missed Lisfranc injury. Similarly, Lisfranc injuries can be improperly treated with closed reduction.

Failure to recognize the injury pattern can lead to improper treatment. For example, in a purely ligamentous injury, treatment with immediate fusion does better than ORIF. Access to advanced imaging may help identify injuries missed on initial evaluation, including plantar avulsion fractures. Occasionally, however, a correct diagnosis of a Lisfranc injury is made, but the severity of the injury is not appreciated and treated improperly. In the following case, we have a patient with a grossly unstable Lisfranc injury. The patient was initially treated improperly, by the provider failing to identify the associated intertarsal injury. We took the patient to the operating room for open reduction and internal fixation through a medial approach and insertion of a mesh plate (Figs. 10.19, 10.20, 10.21, and 10.22).

Subtle injuries can often be overlooked in high performing athletes, and their foot injuries should be thoroughly worked up. Failure to identify these injuries and initiate appropriate treatment can lead to loss of a career in sports (Figs. 10.23a, b, and 10.24).

Cost

There are a variety of implants that can be used to treat a Lisfranc injury, and it is important to understand relevant cost disparities between them. One should not always choose the cheapest option. For example, using screws plus a plate versus only using screws in a husky individual.

Comorbidities

Unrecognized diabetes mellitus and charcot arthropathy. Charcot mid foot often presents as an acute injury but really is a gradual process, and failure to recognize this can lead to improper

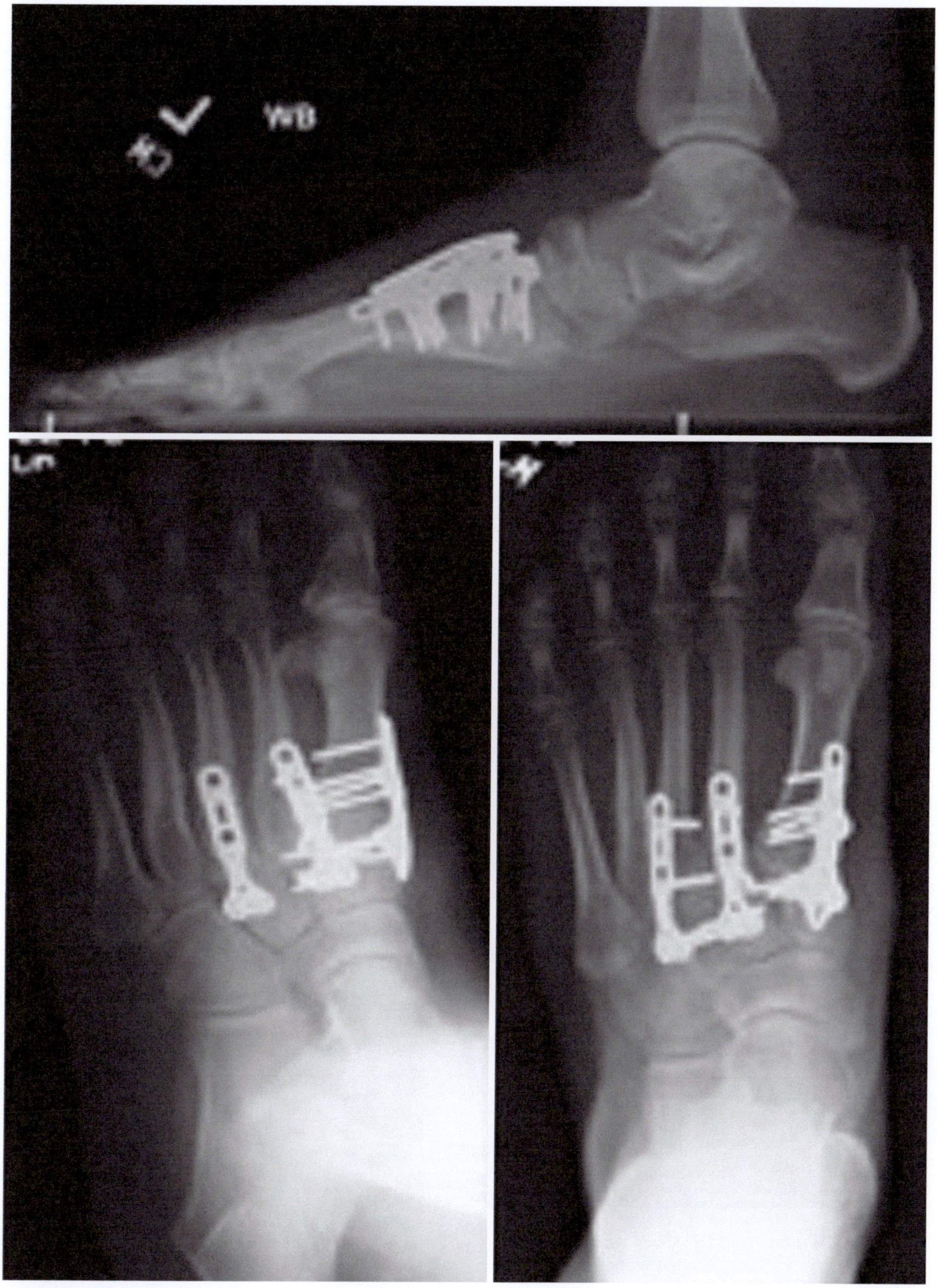

Fig. 10.18 Three views of the left foot 6 months after hardware removal and subsequent midfoot fusion and calf gastrocnemius release

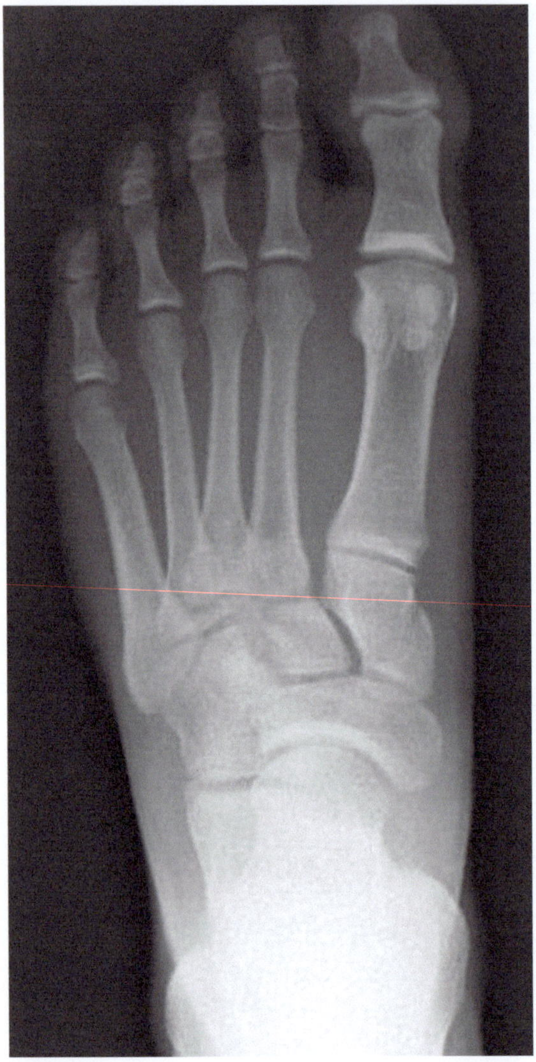

Fig. 10.19 Pre-operative injury film of left foot showing first and second intertarsal widening and medial cuneiform abnormality

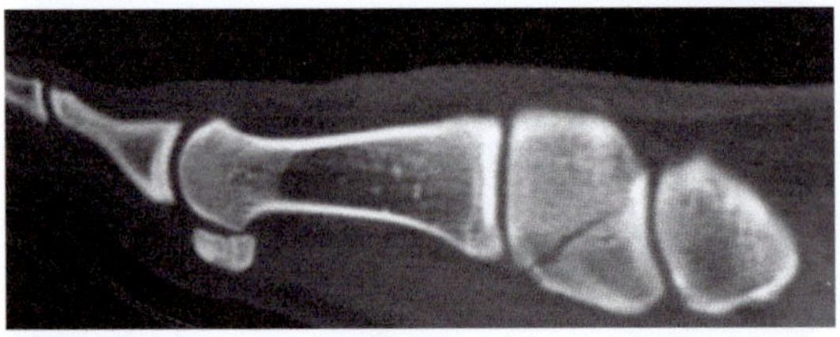

Fig. 10.20 CT scan of left foot showing a minimally displaced fracture at the base of the medial cuneiform

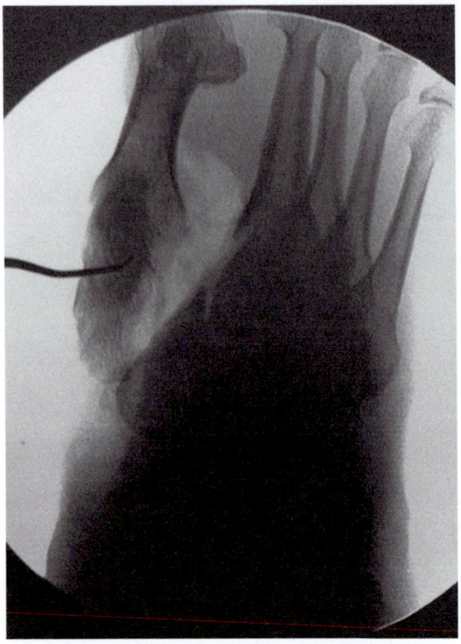

Fig. 10.21 Intraoperative fluoroscopy showing intertarsal instability

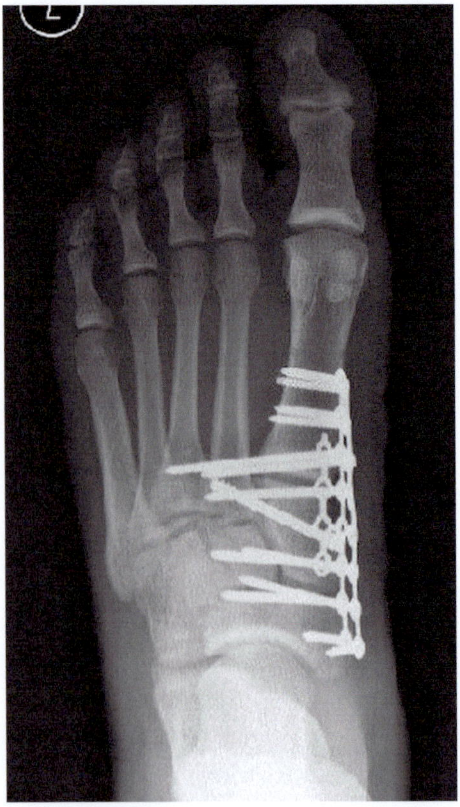

Fig. 10.22 AP left foot with plate in place

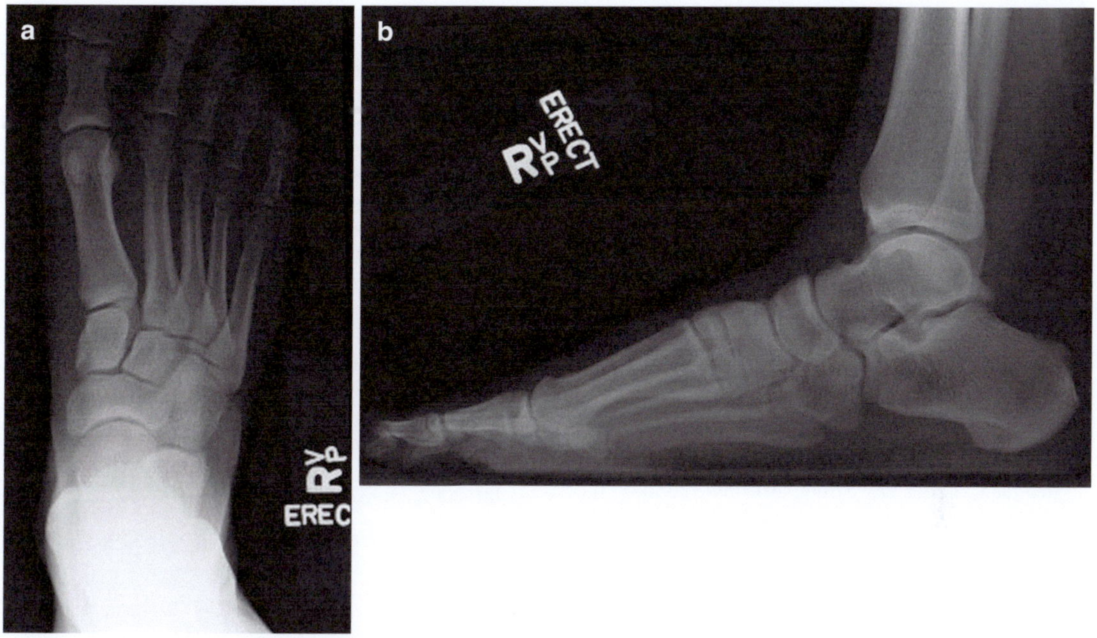

Fig. 10.23 (**a**) AP and (**b**) lateral weight-bearing radiographs of an athlete who suffered an on-field right foot injury. No apparent injury is identified on initial imaging

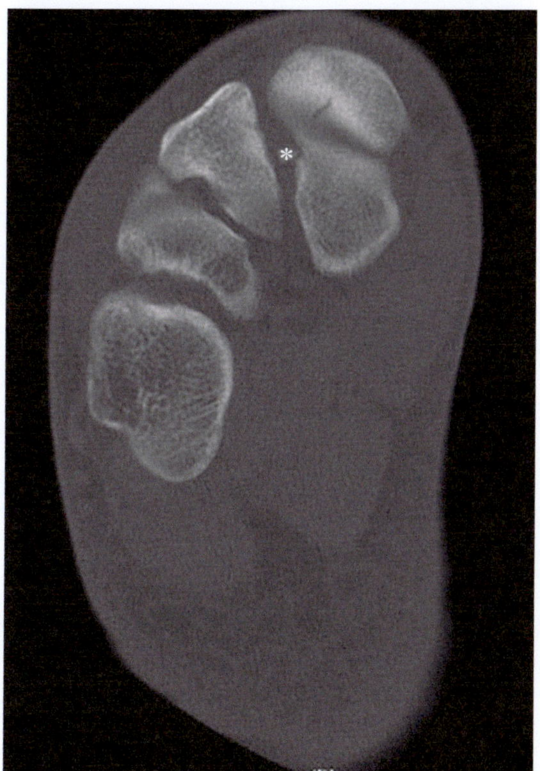

Fig. 10.24 CT scan of right foot showing a fleck of bone in the Lisfranc joint

treatment with an ORIF versus a more appropriate extensive fusion. It is important to recognize that these cases require a longer period of non-weight-bearing compared to patients without this comorbidity. Metabolic bone disease (renal failure) patients might be best treated non-operatively for the fact that operative techniques most likely will fail.

Postoperative Care

Postoperative care starts intraoperatively by applying a three sided, fluffy splint covered with an ace wrap. The patient will return to clinic in 2 weeks for wound inspection and evaluation of soft tissue swelling. The patient will be non-weight-bearing for 6 weeks with crutches; then transitioned to six more weeks in a cane with a CAM boot or short leg cast. The advantage of a CAM boot is that it allows wound care and gentle active range of motion at the ankle joint. As each injury behaves independently, it has been shown that fractures heal faster than pure ligamentous injuries and might be able to advance to weight-bearing sooner in the postoperative course. At 3 months, transition to a cushioned shoe or molded insert and begin physical therapy, focusing on gait training, range of motion exercises, and lower extremity rehabilitation. Delay weight-bearing to 3 months for patient with charcot arthropathy or metabolic bone disease.

Suggested Readings

1. Aronow MS. Treatment of the missed Lisfranc injury. Foot Ankle Clin. 2006;11(1):127–42.
2. Crates JM, Barber FA, Sanders EJ. Subtle Lisfranc subluxation: results of operative and nonoperative treatment. J Foot Ankle Surg. 2015;54(3):350–5.
3. Kuo RS, Tejwani NC, DiGiovanni CW, Benirschke SK, Hansen ST, Sangeorzan BJ. Outcome after open reduction and internal fixation of Lisfranc joint injuries. J Bone Joint Surg. 2000;82(11):1609–18.
4. Ly TV, Coetzee JC. Treatment of primarily ligamentous Lisfranc joint injuries: primary arthrodesis compared with open reduction and internal fixation. J Bone Joint Surg. 2006;88(3):514–20.
5. Sands AK, Swords MP. Procedure 22: Open reduction and internal fixation of Lisfranc/tarsometatarsal injuries. In: Operative techniques: Foot and Ankle surgery: Elsevier Health Sciences; 2017. p. 172–9.
6. Sangeorzan BJ, Veith RG, Hansen ST Jr. Salvage of Lisfranc's tarsometatarsal joint by arthrodesis. J Foot Ankle Surg. 1990;10:193–200.
7. Teng AL, Pinzur MS, Lomasney L, Mahoney L, Havey R. Functional outcome following anatomic restoration of tarsal-metatarsal fracture dislocation. Foot Ankle Int. 2002;23:922–6.

Part III

Sports

Revision Surgery for 5th Metatarsal Fractures

11

Taylor N. Cabe, Sydney C. Karnovsky, and Mark C. Drakos

Key Takeaway Points

- 5th metatarsal fractures are difficult to treat as they occur in a watershed area and an area that experiences high amounts of stress during activity.
- Common causes for re-fracture can be premature return to activity or inappropriate screw length or placement with the initial procedure.
- Comorbidities such as a cavovarus foot must also be addressed in order to achieve a lasting repair and prevent re-fracture.
- Due to the curvature of the 5th metatarsal but the necessity to use a straight screw in fixation, care should be taken in selecting screw size, and, typically, shorter screws should be used to prevent bowing and plantar and lateral gapping in the repair.

Introduction

Fractures of the 5th metatarsal (MT) occurring at the proximal fifth metatarsal metaphysis were first described in 1902 by Sir Robert Jones and are commonly referred to as Jones fractures [1, 2]. The fracture itself generally occurs at the junction of the proximal metaphysis and diaphysis approximately 2 cm distal of the most proximal portion of the tuberosity [1]. Jones fractures pose a difficult problem to physicians as they occur in a watershed area (low blood supply) making healing difficult and often quite prolonged [3]. Bony union typically occurs after approximately 3 months in fractures treated operatively [4]. Healing rates following nonoperative treatment vary depending on the severity of delayed healing or nonunion at the fracture site [5]. In patients who do unfortunately experience an acute re-fracture, re-fracture occurs on average 5–6 months following screw fixation, and healing occurs approximately 3 months following revision surgery [6].

There are a variety of factors that predispose patients to Jones fractures, though there is no consensus across existing reports. Some authors have argued that people with a high arch are more predisposed to Jones fractures, while others have found this to be a nonsignificant factor [3, 7]. It has also been found that people with an adducted foot are more at risk for Jones fractures [8].

Jones fractures can be treated both operatively and nonoperatively. Generally, operative treatment leads to a faster recovery and lower rates of re-fracture and is recommended in the athletic population [8]. There are numerous different operative techniques that exist, including intramedullary screw fixation, autogenous inlay bone graft, the use of a

T. N. Cabe · S. C. Karnovsky · M. C. Drakos (✉)
Hospital for Special Surgery, Foot and Ankle Service, New York, NY, USA
e-mail: drakosm@hss.edu

M. J. Berkowitz et al. (eds.), *Revision Surgery of the Foot and Ankle*,
https://doi.org/10.1007/978-3-030-29969-9_11

small plate, as well as a tension band [4, 8, 9] . Intramedullary screws are most commonly accepted, though many surgeons use screws of different lengths and widths [2, 10]. DeLee et al., Mindrebo et al., and Kavenaugh et al. all recommended using a 4.5 mm malleolar screw though other authors have advocated the use of bigger screws, such as Nunley who supported the use of a 6.5 mm screw [2, 8, 11, 12, 13]. Furthermore, long screws have historically been used with the "high and inside" technique, but more recently the use of shorter screws has been advocated, due to the curvature of the bone and inability of a long screw to follow the exact shape of the bone [14].

When treated operatively, the majority of Jones fractures heal without any complications. However, re-fracture has been reported to occur in 4–12% of athletes [9]. The predicted reasons for re-fracture include the use of inappropriate lengths and diameters for screws, screws placed incorrectly, as well as premature return to activity before complete radiographic and symptomatic healing is clear [6]. In cases where re-fracture occurs, revision procedures typically include removal of the existing hardware, debridement of the fracture site, if needed, and revision fixation with a more appropriate intramedullary screw along with possible addition of a biological adjuvant, such as bone marrow aspirate, to the bone graft to encourage healing [15].

When a patient is suspected to have a re-fractured 5th MT fracture, the first step is to obtain standard AP, lateral, and oblique foot radiographs and assess for fracture. If fracture is present, the decision to proceed with either operative or nonoperative treatment must be made. If further assessment is needed, a computed tomography (CT) scan may be ordered to further assess the injured area for chronicity and sclerosis. If there is a re-fracture present, operative intervention is recommended.

Case Examples

Case 11.1

History

- A 25-year-old male, presented with right foot pain, specifically continued soreness, 9 months status post Jones fracture ORIF at an outside facility.
  – Initially rolled his foot playing basketball and had immediate pain necessitating the initial ORIF
- Radiographs suggest possible nonunion (Fig. 11.1)
- CT is ordered to further investigate healing and shows that the fracture is healing (Fig. 11.2).
- Two months after CT is reviewed, patient has persistent pain and felt another pop.
- Patient came into the office, and radiographs showed re-fracture of his 5th MT and persistent nonunion.
- Revision surgery was indicated to remove the original screw and put a more appropriately sized screw in.

Surgical Plan

Positioning

- Place the patient in a supine position.

Obtaining Bone Marrow Aspirate from the Iliac Crest

- The hip was approached, and a Jamshidi needle was inserted into the superior iliac crest (approximately 2–3 cm posterior to the ASIS).
- 60 cc of bone marrow aspirate withdrawn.
- The needle was removed from the hip in addition to three sleeves of iliac crest bone graft and bone marrow aspirate spun down to 3 cc.

Approaching the 5th Metatarsal

- The proximal 5th MT was identified and a 2 cm incision was made (Fig. 11.3).
- Dissection was carried out to the level of the 5th MT with attention made to protect the anterior branch of the sural nerve as well as the peroneal tendon.
- The existing screw was removed (Fig. 11.4).
- A guide wire was used in this area and drilled with a 3.2 mm drill reaming around the site of the fracture.
- It was then tapped with a 4.5, 5.5, and 6.5 tap (Fig. 11.5).
- The fracture site was then exposed through a second incision.

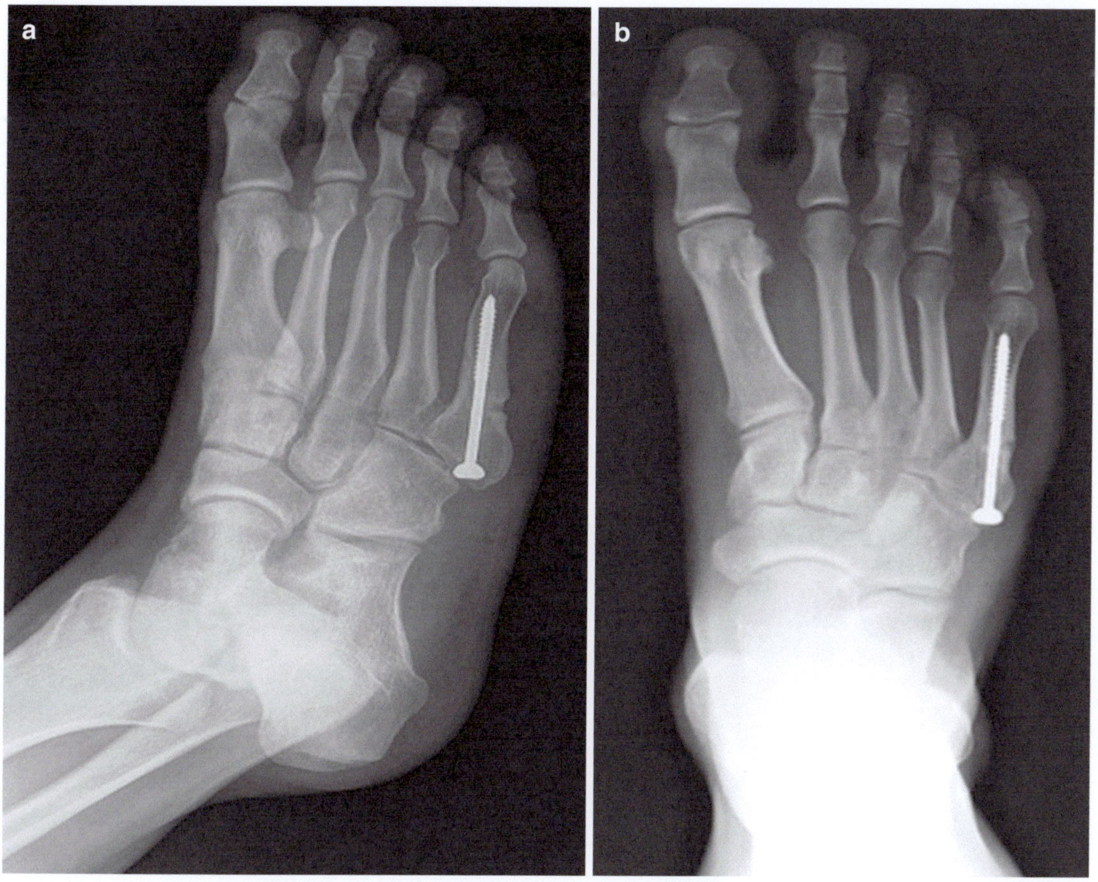

Fig. 11.1 (**a**, **b**) Initial preoperative X-ray images for the **Case 11.1** patient suggesting a potential nonunion of the initial 5th MT repair

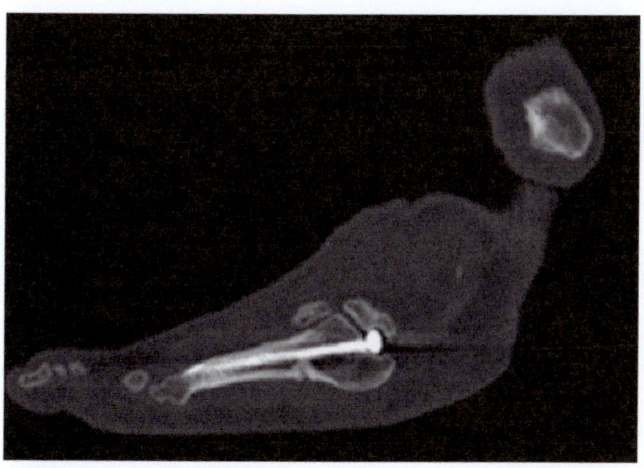

Fig. 11.2 CT imaging prior to revision surgery for the **Case 11.1** patient which appears to show persistent lucency

- All callous fibrous tissue was removed and this exposed a gap plantarly.
- Bone graft from the iliac crest harvest was used to graft the site of the gap (Fig. 11.6).
- A 6.5 by 40 mm 5th MT screw was then inserted (Fig. 11.7).

Closing

- The patient was placed in a non-weight-bearing splint for 2 weeks.

Postoperative Course

- After the splint was removed, the patient was placed into a controlled ankle movement (CAM) walker boot and instructed to remain non-weight-bearing.
- After 4 weeks in the CAM walker boot, the patient was allowed to progress to partial weight-bearing. He was allowed to start with 50 pounds and advance 25–50 pounds per week, as guided by his physical therapist. Radiographs were obtained to assess healing (Fig. 11.8).

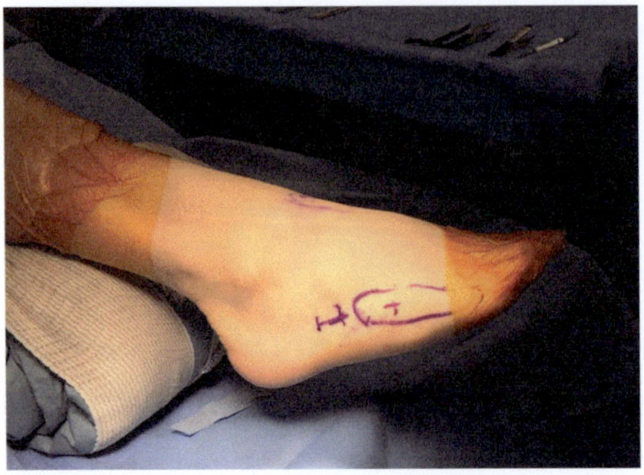

Fig. 11.3 The proximal 5th MT is identified, and an approximately 2 cm incision site is marked

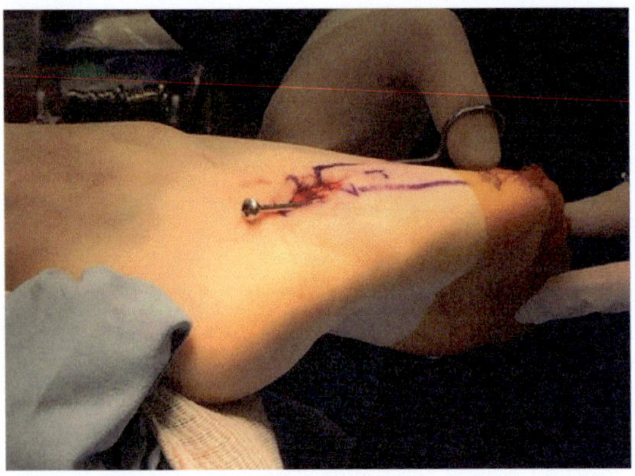

Fig. 11.4 The screw from the original repair is removed

- At 3 months postoperatively, the patient was instructed to begin wearing sneakers and continue strengthening and stretching in physical therapy. Radiographs were obtained to assess healing.
- Five-month postoperative radiographs show bridging of the fracture (Fig. 11.9).

Implants

- 40 × 6.5 mm screw

Pearls and Pitfalls

- The previous screw was too long, straightening the bone and creating persistent planter and lateral gap due to distraction, ultimately leading to the need for revision surgery.

Case 11.2

History

- A 71-year-old female presented with a 6-month history of right foot pain. She initially fell and twisted her foot and had a Jones fracture which was treated with ORIF at an outside facility. She complained of persistent pain in the foot.
  - Radiographs showed a persistent fracture (Fig. 11.10).

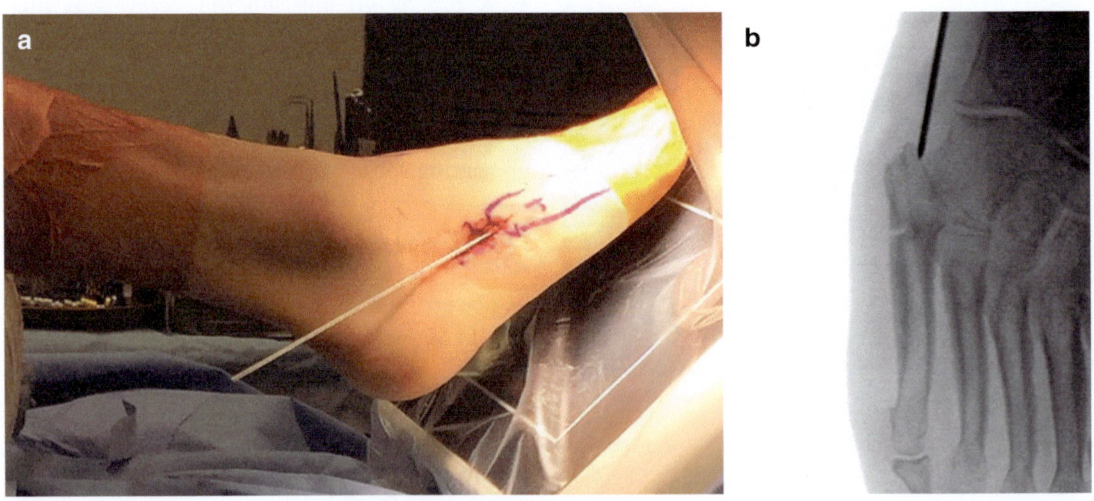

Fig. 11.5 A guide wire is advanced along the fracture site being careful to aim down the middle of the canal of the 5th MT (**a**). Fluoroscopy is used intraoperatively to confirm positioning of the guide wire (**b**) as well as other components of the repair. The fracture site is reamed (**c**) and tapped (**d**) to encourage healing and prepare for screw placement. Screw size is estimated, again, using fluoroscopy (**e**)

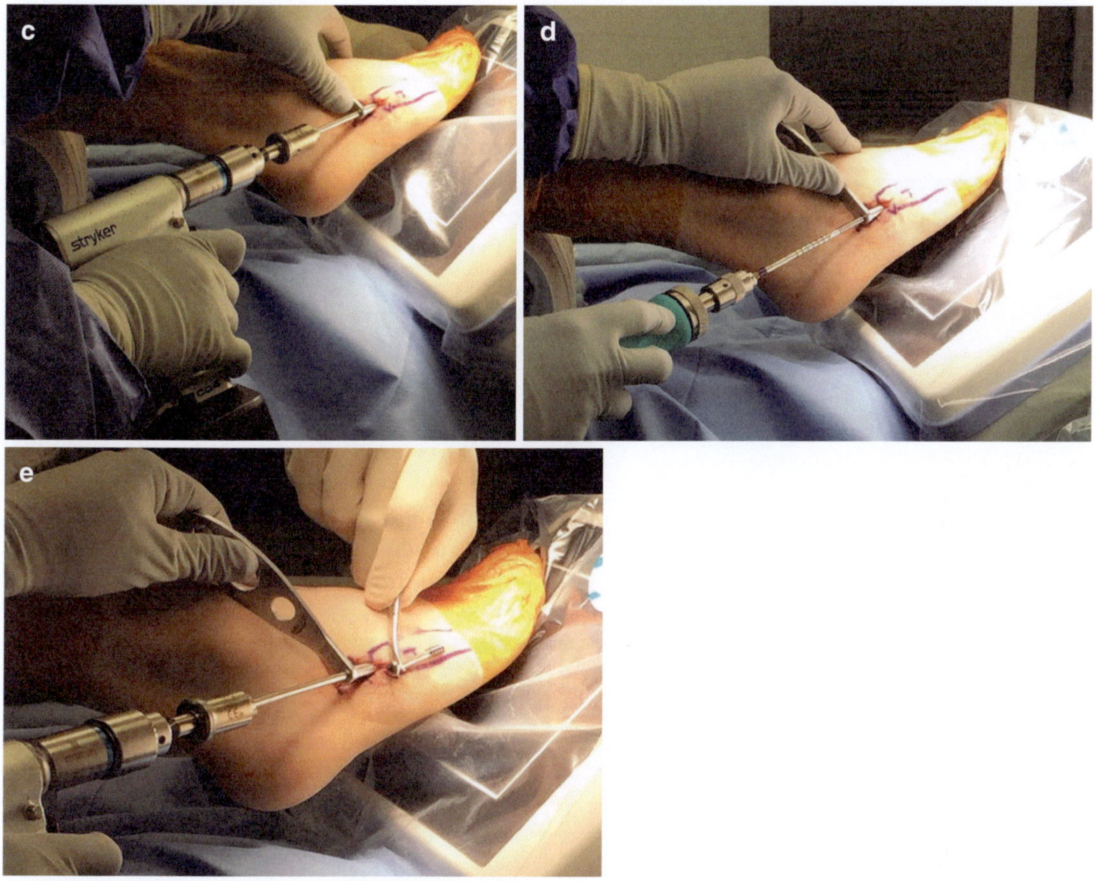

Fig. 11.5 (continued)

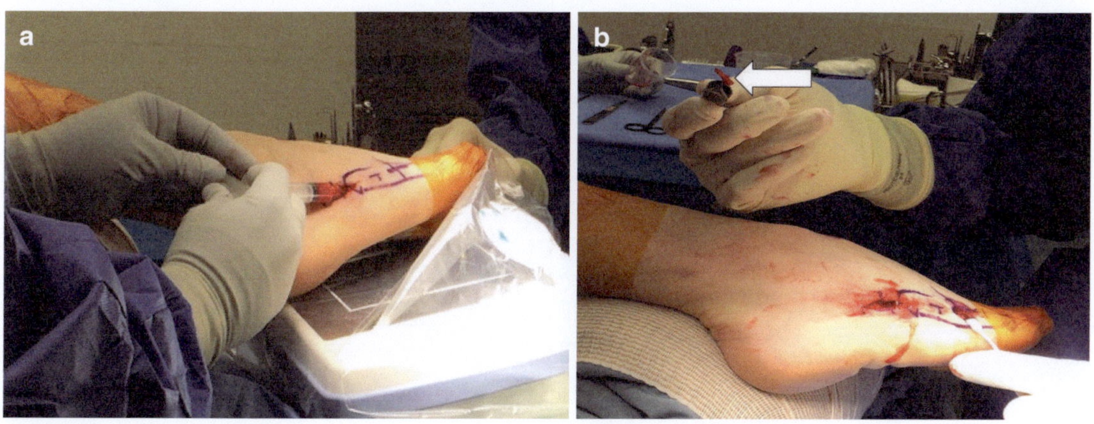

Fig. 11.6 (**a**, **b**) Bone marrow aspirate and bone graft (indicated by the arrow) taken from the iliac crest are prepared and placed at the fracture site

– CT shows persistent fracture as well as malpositioned hardware in the 5th MT (Fig. 11.11).

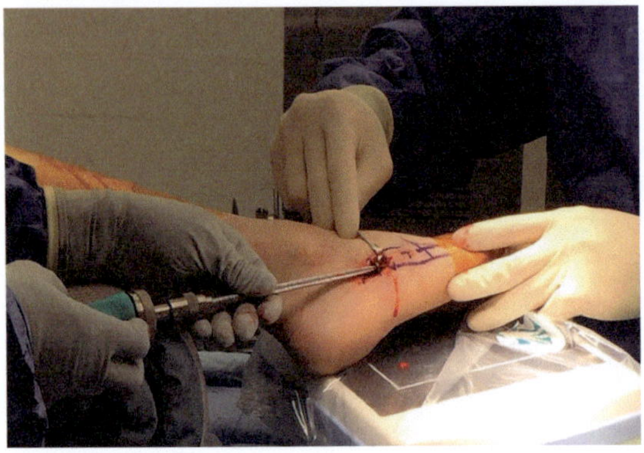

Fig. 11.7 The 5th MT screw is placed along the fracture site

- Revision surgery was indicated to remove the original screw and put a more appropriately sized screw in.

Surgical Plan

Positioning

- Place the patient in a supine position.

Obtaining Bone Marrow Aspirate from the Iliac Crest

- The hip was approached and a Jamshidi needle was inserted into the superior iliac crest (approximately 2–3 cm posterior to the ASIS).
- 60cc of bone marrow aspirate was withdrawn and spun down to a concentration of 3cc in addition to three sleeves of iliac crest bone graft.

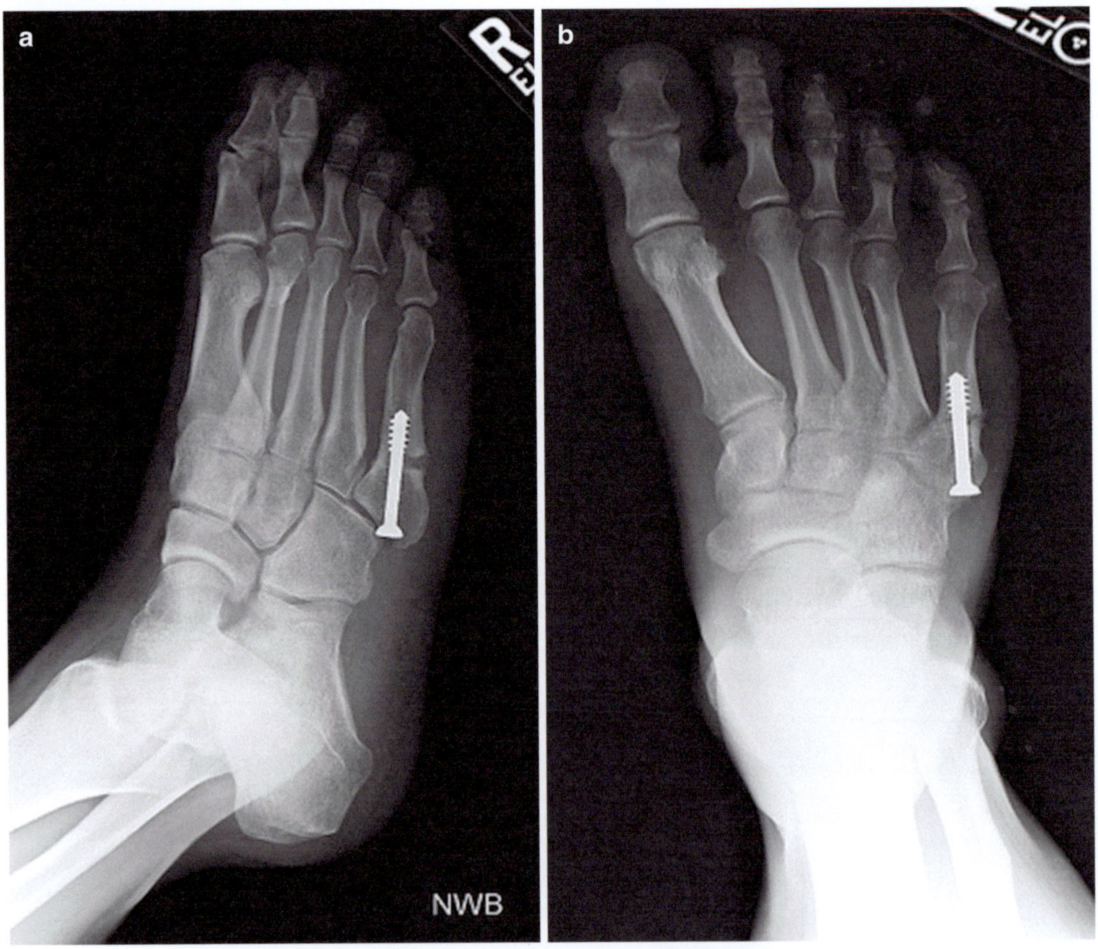

Fig. 11.8 (**a**, **b**) Standard 6-week postoperative X-ray images show healing progress for **Case 11.1** patient

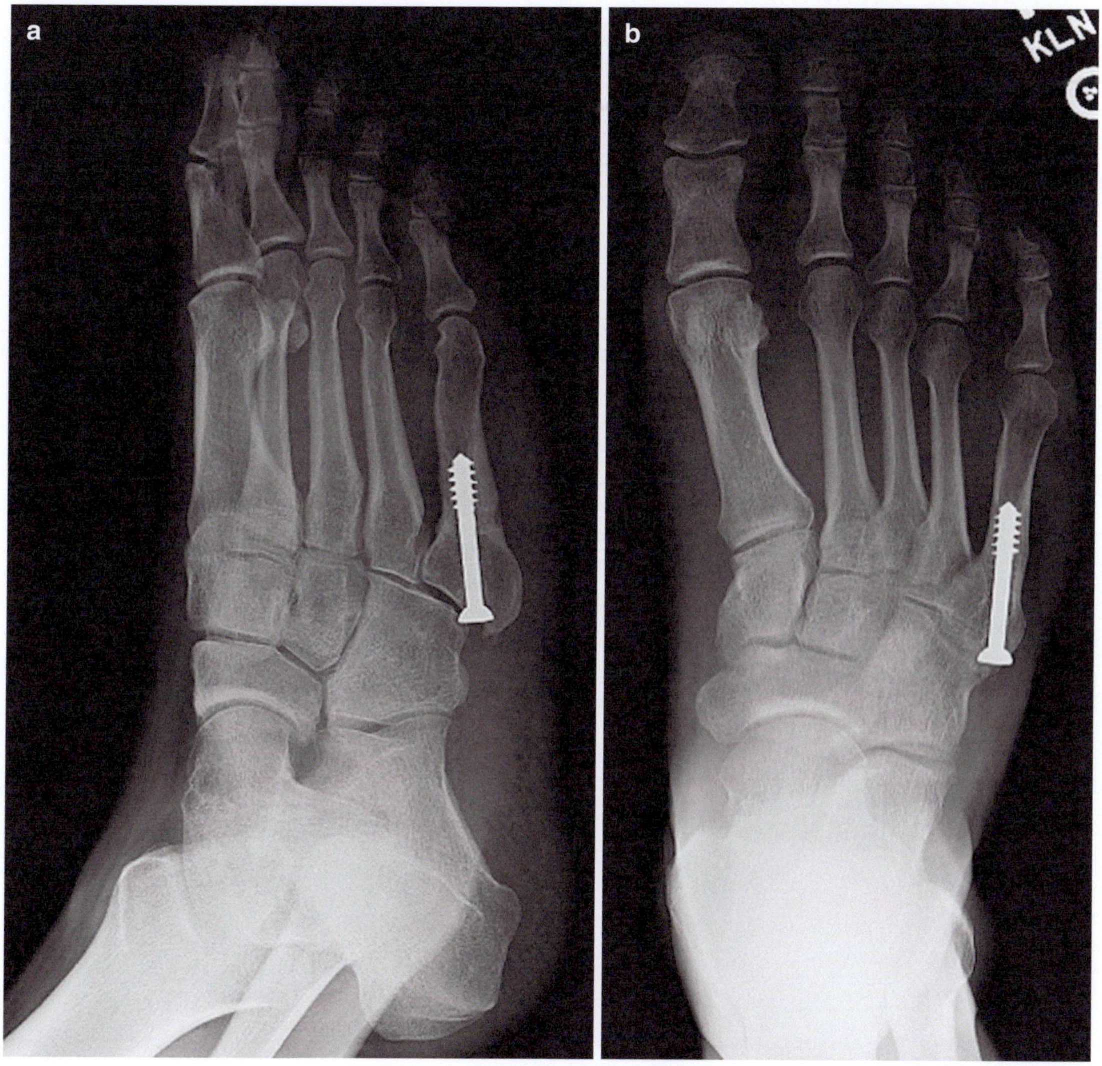

Fig. 11.9 (**a**, **b**) Five months postoperative X-rays indicate proper screw alignment and healing for **Case 11.1** patient

Approaching the 5th Metatarsal

- The proximal 5th MT was identified, and a 1 cm incision was made over the patient's prior incision.
- Dissection was carried out to the level of the 5th MT and the previous screw.
- The screw was noted to be irritating the peroneus brevis tendon.
- The screw was removed.
- A new incision was then made 1 cm proximal to the base of the 5th MT, and dissection was carried out to the base of the 5th MT.
- A guide wire was then placed in the center-center position, and we drilled with a 3.2 drill bit. The drill was put on reverse and reamed back over the base of the 5th MT.
- It was then tapped with a 4.5, 5.5, and 6.5.
- A 6.5 × 40 mm screw was measured.
- A third incision was made over the fracture site, and dissection was carried out to the fracture site.
- The edges were curetted and this exposed a small defect.
- Bone graft from the iliac crest harvest was used to graft the site of the gap.
- A 6.5 × 40 mm 5th MT screw was then inserted.

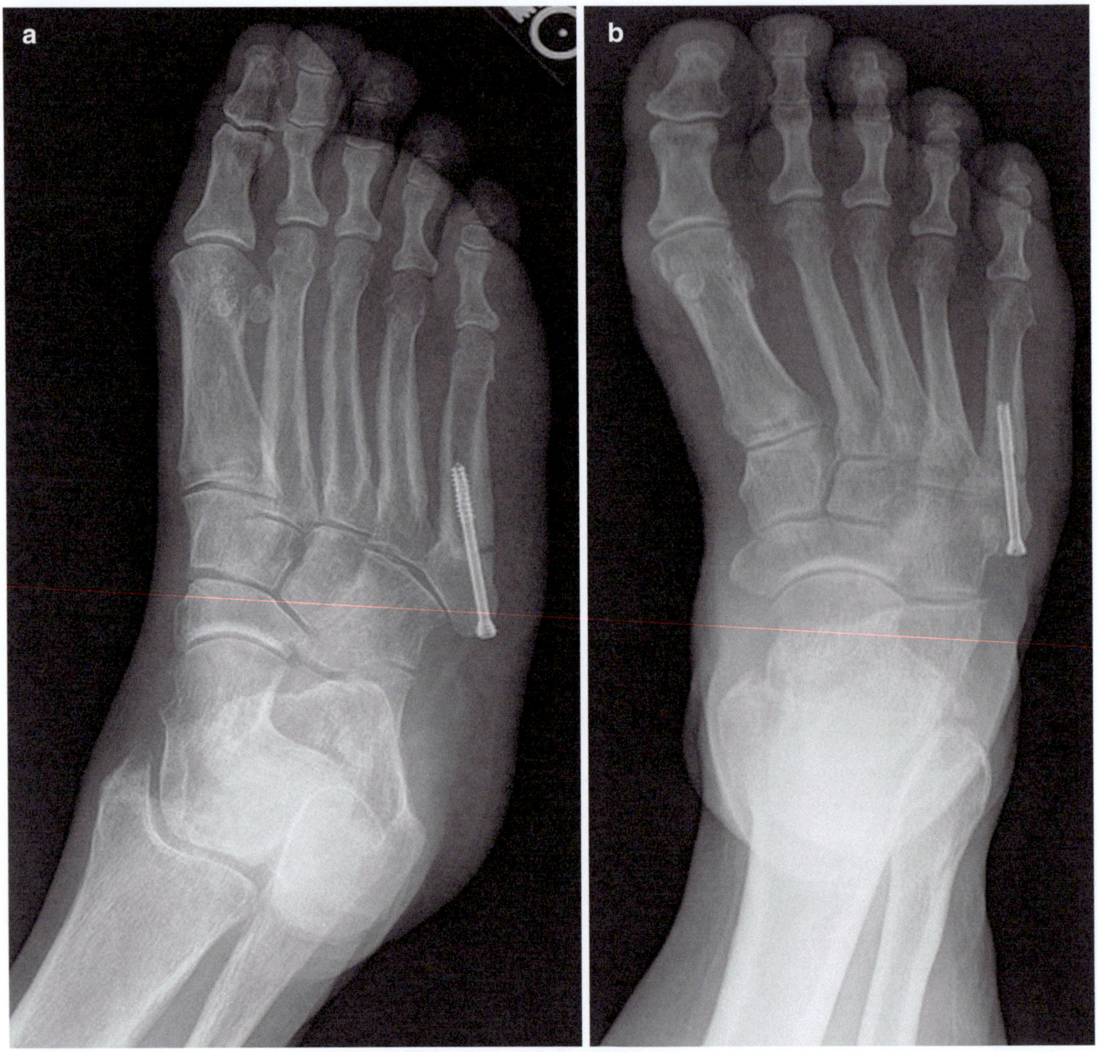

Fig. 11.10 (**a**, **b**) Preoperative X-ray images show a persistent fracture despite repair in the **Case 11.2** patient

Closing

- The patient was placed in a non-weight-bearing splint for 2 weeks.

Postoperative Course

- After the splint was removed, the patient was placed into a cast for 4 weeks and remained non-weight-bearing.
- After 4 weeks in the cast, the patient was transitioned into a CAM walker boot and allowed to progress to partial weight-bearing. She started with 50 pounds and advanced 25–50 pounds per week, as guided by her physical therapist. New radiographs were obtained to assess healing over time (Fig. 11.12).
- At 3 months postoperatively, the patient was instructed to begin wearing sneakers and continue strengthening and stretching in physical therapy.

Implants

- 40 × 6.5 mm screw

Pearls and Pitfalls

- The previous screw was too small and, in a nonideal location, placed bicortically as opposed to perpendicular to the fracture to achieve a better reduction.

Case 11.3

History

- A 57-year-old male, presented with 2 years of consistent right foot pain. He initially jammed his foot 2 years prior to presenting to us.
  - This was initially treated at an outside facility with a foot reconstruction (16 months prior to presenting to us).
  - Radiographs showed an acute on chronic 5th MT stress fracture in the setting of a cavovarus foot (Fig. 11.13).

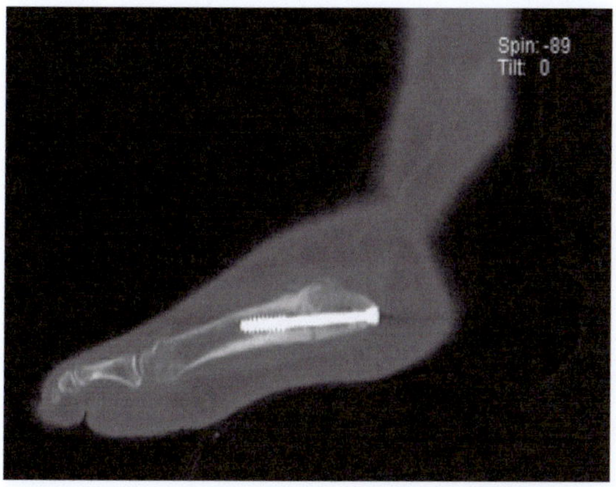

Fig. 11.11 Preoperative CT for **Case 11.2** patient indicates a persistent fracture as well as improperly positioned hardware. Note screw alignment is not perpendicular to the fracture

  - MRI revealed a peroneus longus to brevis transfer that appeared to be intact.
- Surgery was indicated to perform an ORIF. Patient was advised that in order to avoid repeating the calcaneal osteotomy, he would have to wear an orthotic postoperatively.
  - ORIF done – used plate instead of screw because of the distracted fracture (from the 4.5 tap) (Fig. 11.14)
    - Cast at 2 weeks
    - Boot at 8 weeks
    - Sneaker at 3 months
    - Did well for 1 year
  - A 1-year post-op patient had a re-fracture in the setting of a cavovarus foot (Fig. 11.15).
  - Revision ORIF indicated with cavovarus foot reconstruction, lateralizing calcaneal osteotomy, first ray dorsiflexion osteotomy, and fifth metatarsal ORIF of nonunion.

Surgical Plan

Positioning

- Patient was placed in a supine position.

Obtaining Bone Marrow Aspirate from the Iliac Crest

- The hip was approached, and a Jamidi needle was inserted into the superior iliac crest (approximately 2–3 cm posterior to the ASIS).
- 50cc of bone marrow aspirate was withdrawn.

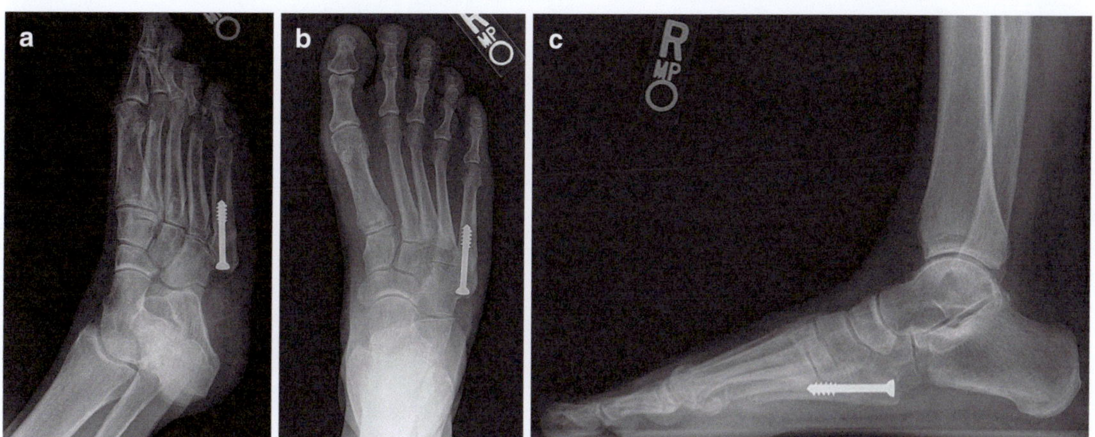

Fig. 11.12 (**a–c**) X-ray images taken 9 months postoperatively show healing progress for **Case 11.2** patient

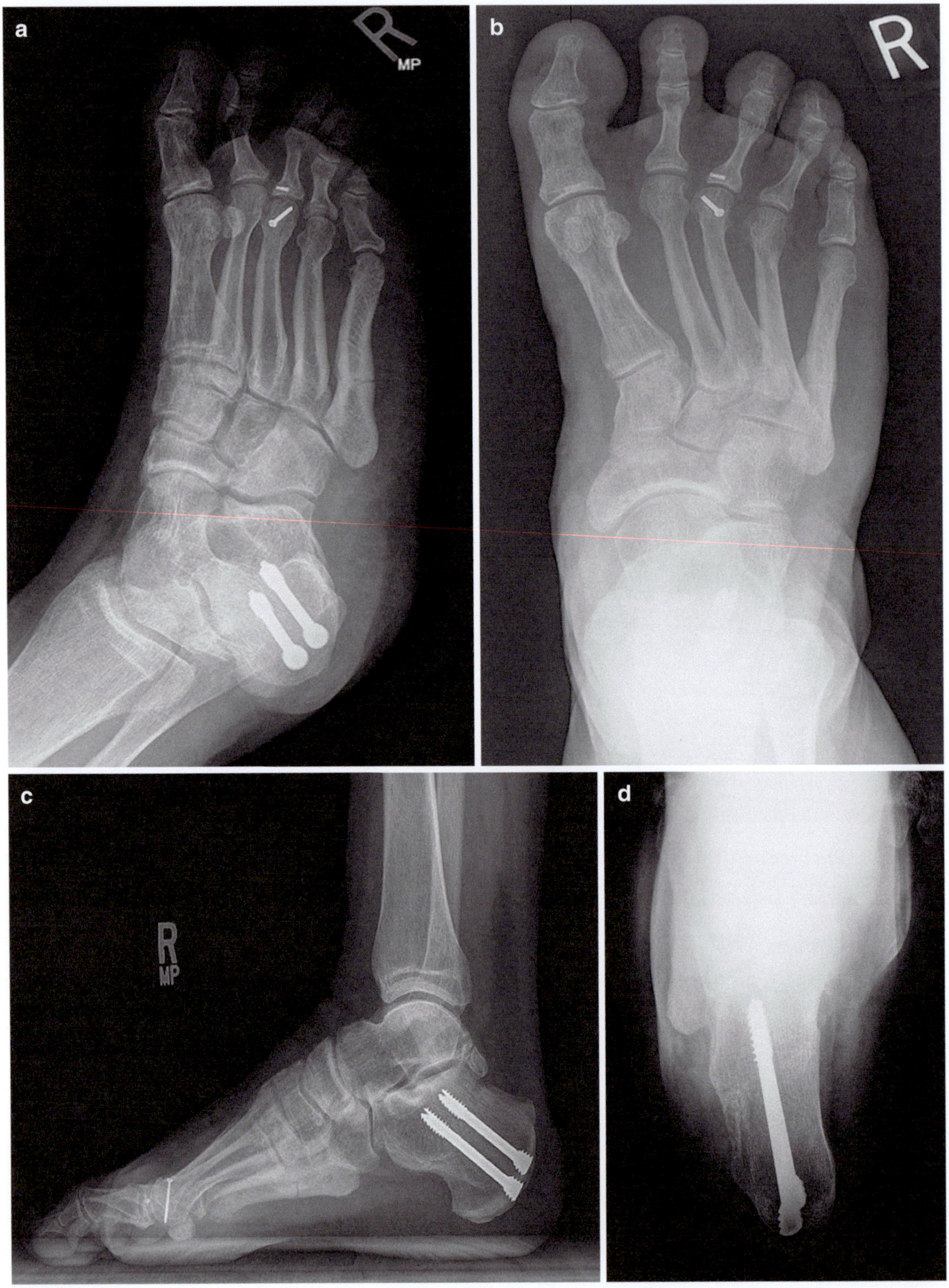

Fig. 11.13 (**a–d**) Preoperative X-ray images for **Case 11.3** patient showing a 5th MT fracture in the setting of a cavovarus foot

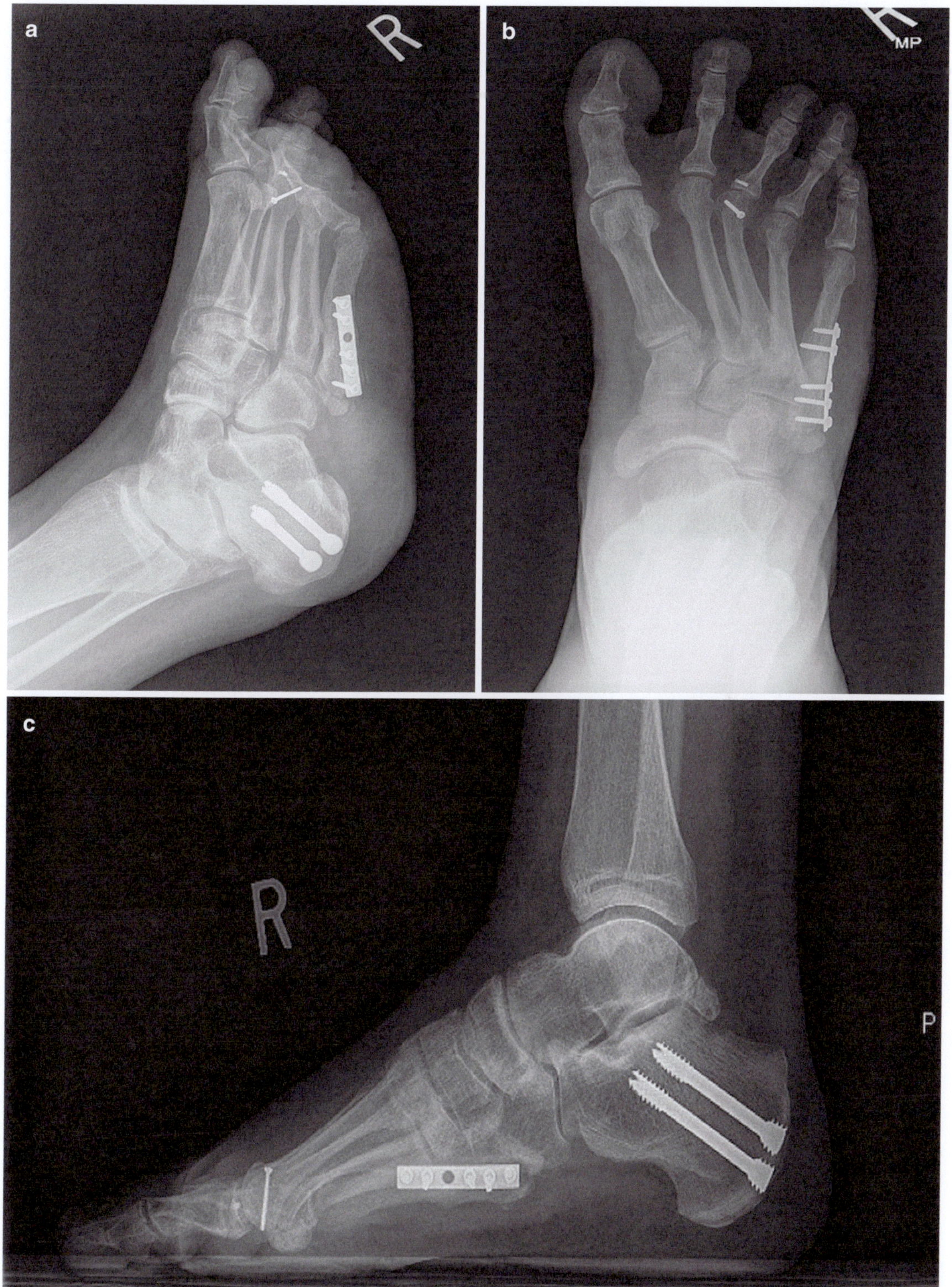

Fig. 11.14 (**a–c**) Postoperative X-rays following initial procedure to repair the 5th MT fracture in **Case 11.3** patient

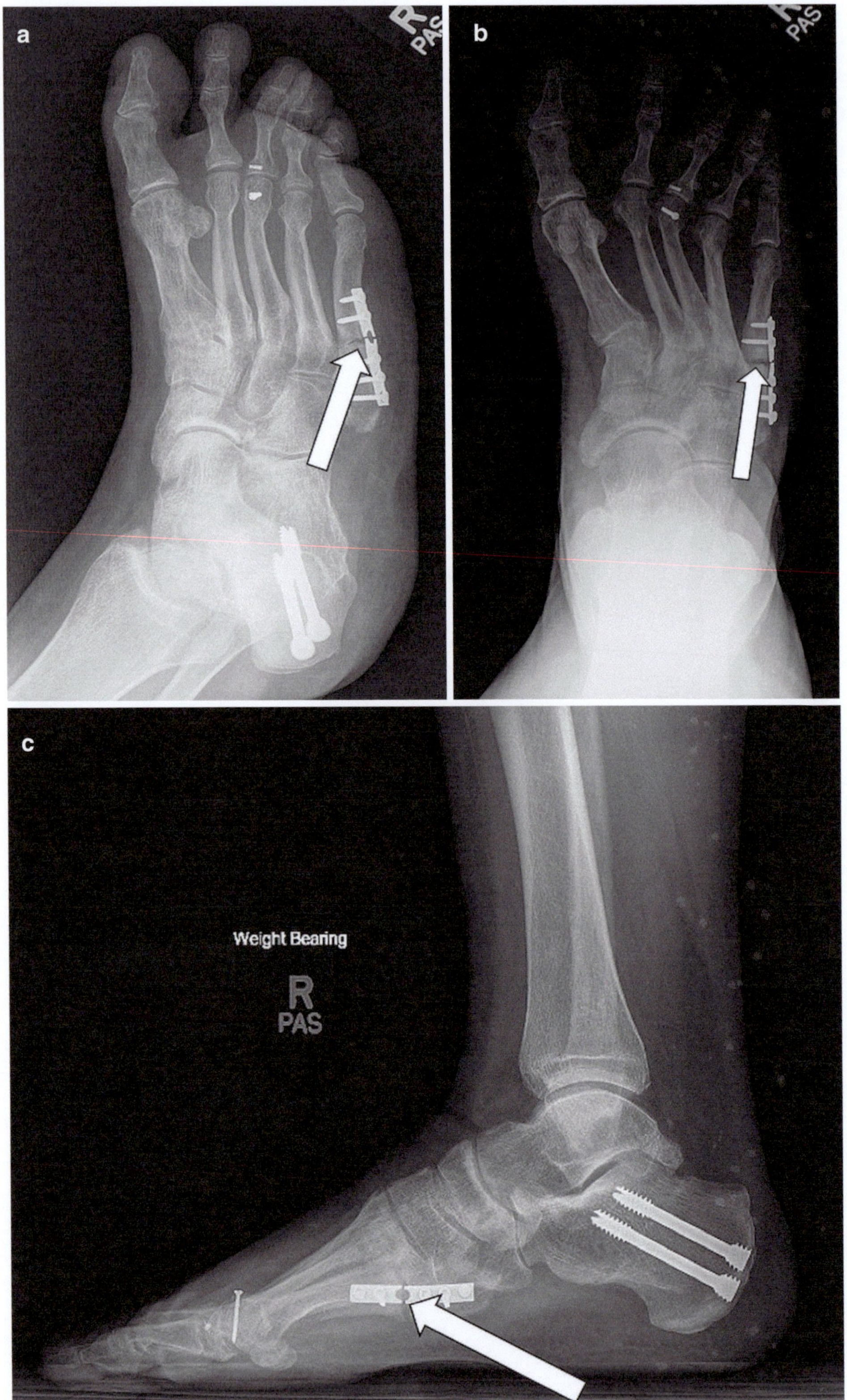

Fig. 11.15 (**a–c**) X-ray images showing re-fracture of the 5th MT in **Case 11.3** patient following initial repair. The re-fracture site is indicated by arrows in each view

- The needle was removed from the hip.
- The bone marrow aspirate was sent for concentration.

Hardware Removal

- Two small percutaneous incisions were made over the patients heel, and two pins were placed through cannulated crews to remove the patient's screws.

Calcaneal Osteotomy

- A 5 cm incision was made over the posterior aspect of the patient's heel.
- Retractors were placed dorsally and plantarly.
- A lateralizing Malerba type osteotomy was then performed.
- The heel was shifted 7–8 mm laterally.
- Two 6.5 screws were placed through the heel making excellent compression across the osteotomy site.
- At this point, bone graft was taken from the heel for use in the 5th MT.

Approaching the 5th Metatarsal

- The proximal 5th MT was identified, and a 1 cm incision was made over the patient's prior incision.
- Dissection was carried out to the level of the 5th MT and the broken plate.
- The plate and screws were all removed.
- The patient had some motion at the nonunion site.
- A guide wire was then placed in the center-center position.
- We then crossed the fracture line and drilled and reamed it.
- It was then tapped with a 4.5 and 5.5 tap. It measured 5.5 mm × 55 mm.
- The nonunion site was prepared and curetted, and then the bone graft from the calcaneus was placed at the nonunion site.
- The site was prepped, and then a 5.5 × 55 mm screw was inserted.

First Ray Dorsiflexion Osteotomy

- A 3 cm incision was made over the first MT.
- A dorsal closing wedge osteotomy was performed with a 2 mm wedge of bone dorsally.
- A wedge was then performed to elevate the first ray 10 degrees.
- A 9 × 11 staple was then placed across the osteotomy.

Closing

- The patient was placed in a non-weight-bearing splint for 2 weeks.

Postoperative Course

- After the splint was removed, the patient was placed into a cast for 4 weeks and remained non-weight-bearing.
- After 4 weeks in the cast, the patient was transitioned into a CAM walker boot and allowed to progress to partial weight-bearing. She started with 50 pounds and advanced 25–50 pounds per week, as guided by her physical therapist. New radiographs were obtained over time to assess healing (Fig. 11.16).
- At 3 months postoperatively, the patient was instructed to begin wearing sneakers and continue strengthening and stretching in physical therapy.

Implants

- 55 mm × 5.5 mm screw
- Two 6.5 screws
- One 10 × 11 speed stable

Pearls and Pitfalls

- Needed revision calcaneal osteotomy and 1st ray plantarflexion osteotomy to address deformity.
- The plate alone in first ORIF was not enough due to deformity of the foot.

Summary

A great deal of debate exists about the ideal management of Jones fractures. While there is a general consensus that young, athletic patients looking to return to sports as quickly as possible are indicated for operative management, there is a lack of consensus about the ideal screw length and diameter that should be used for ORIF of Jones fractures. Furthermore, there are few

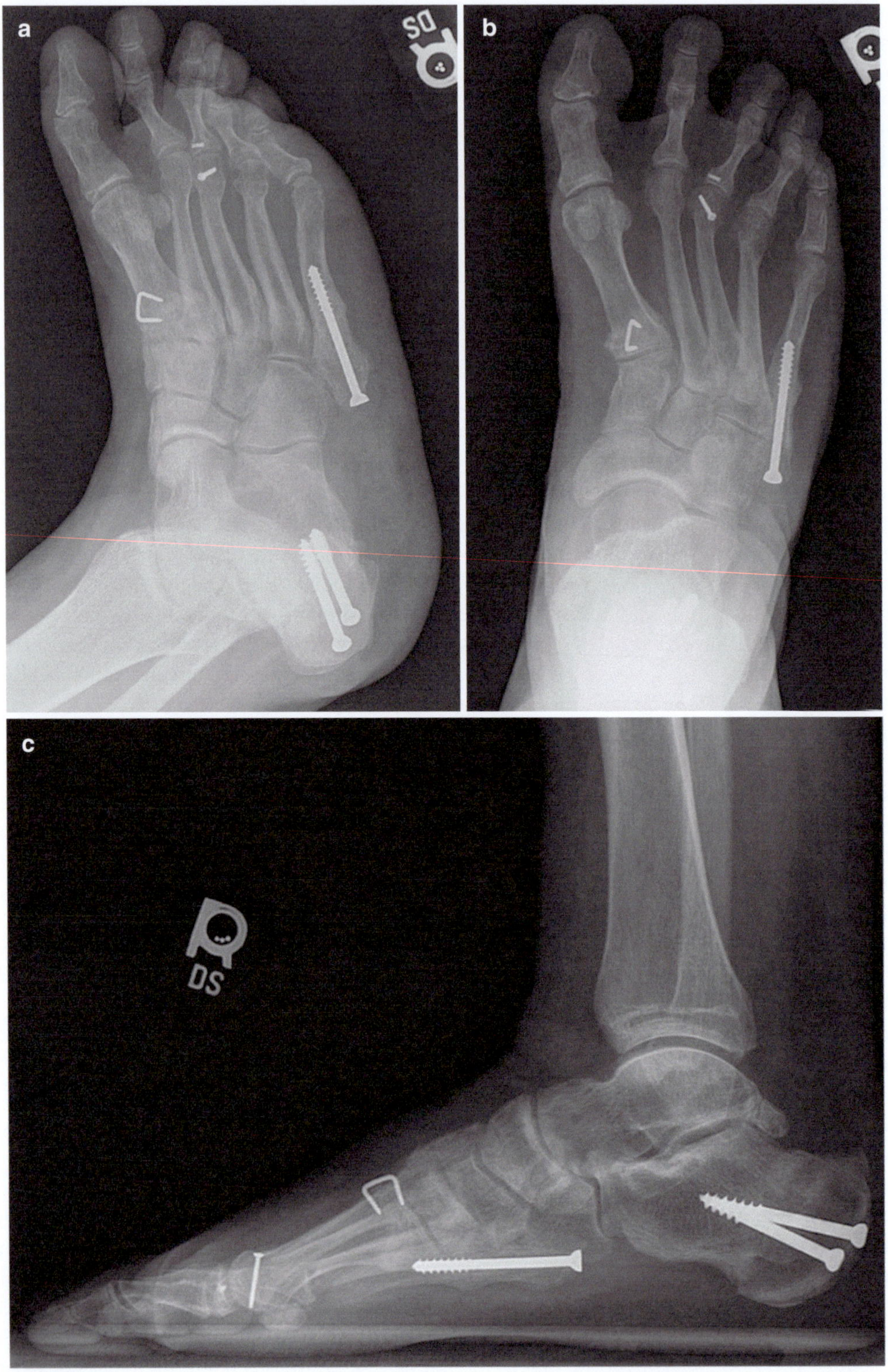

Fig. 11.16 (**a–c**) Postoperative X-ray images taken 5 months out show healing progress for **Case 11.3** patient following revision surgery to repair the 5th MT and cavovarus foot reconstruction

reports that specifically address the placement of the screw into the intramedullary canal, which can be difficult due to the curved nature of the canal but a straight screw [14]. In our experience, re-fracture can be the result of an inappropriately sized or malpositioned screw. Furthermore, re-fracture can occur, in part, due to underlying foot deformities that may need to be corrected in order to alleviate the risk of re-fracture. In cases of re-fracture, we have had success with revision ORIF in which we first remove the original screw and then insert a more appropriately sized screw with the addition of bone marrow aspirate from the iliac crest and bone grafting, if needed. Nevertheless, 5th MT revision can be a technically challenging procedure due to vitamin D deficiencies, low blood flow, impact of any type of cavovarus deformity, and high-impact activities such as basketball.

References

1. Low K, Noblin JD, Browne JE, Barnthouse CD, Scott AR. Jones fractures in the elite football player. J Surg Orthop Adv. 2004;13:156–60.
2. Nunley JA. Jones Fracture Technique: Tech. Foot Ankle Surg. 2002;1:131–7.
3. Hetsroni I, Nyska M, Ben-Sira D, Mann G, Segal O, Maoz G, et al. Analysis of foot structure in athletes sustaining proximal fifth metatarsal stress fracture. Foot Ankle Int. 2010;31:203–11.
4. Hulkko A, Orava S, Nikula P. Stress fracture of the fifth metatarsal in athletes. Ann Chir Gynaecol. 1985;74:233–8.
5. Torg JS, Balduini FC, Zelko RR, Pavlov H, Peff TC, Das M. Fractures of the base of the fifth metatarsal distal to the tuberosity. Classification and guidelines for non-surgical and surgical management. J Bone Joint Surg Am. 1984;66:209–14.
6. Larson CM, Almekinders LC, Taft TN, Garrett WE. Intramedullary screw fixation of Jones fractures. Analysis of failure. Am J Sports Med. 2002;30:55–60.
7. Lee KT, Kim KC, Park YU, Kim TW, Lee YK. Radiographic evaluation of foot structure following fifth metatarsal stress fracture. Foot Ankle Int. 2011;32:796–801.
8. Kavanaugh JH, Brower TD, Mann RV. The Jones fracture revisited. J Bone Joint Surg Am. 1978;60:776–82.
9. Lareau CR, Hsu AR, Anderson RB. Return to play in National Football league players after operative Jones fracture treatment. Foot Ankle Int. 2016;37:8–16.
10. Furia JP, Juliano PJ, Wade AM, Schaden W, Mittermayr R. Shock wave therapy compared with intramedullary screw fixation for nonunion of proximal fifth metatarsal metaphyseal-diaphyseal fractures. J Bone Joint Surg Am. 2010;92:846–54.
11. Wright RW, Fischer DA, Shively RA, Heidt RS, Nuber GW. Refracture of proximal fifth metatarsal (Jones) fracture after intramedullary screw fixation in athletes. Am J Sports Med. 2000;28:732–6.
12. DeLee JC, Evans JP, Julian J. Stress fracture of the fifth metatarsal. Am J Sports Med. 1983;11:349–53.
13. Mindrebo N, Shelbourne KD, Van Meter CD, Rettig AC. Outpatient percutaneous screw fixation of the acute Jones fracture. Am J Sports Med. 1993;21:720–3.
14. Watson GI, Karnovsky SC, Konin G, Drakos MC. Optimal starting point for fifth metatarsal zone II fractures: a cadaveric study. Foot Ankle Int. 2017;38:802. https://doi.org/10.1177/1071100717702688.
15. Hunt KJ, Anderson RB. Treatment of Jones fracture nonunions and refractures in the elite athlete. Am J Sports Med. 2011;39:1948–54.

Failed OCL Talus/Revision OLT

12

Karim Boukhemis, Eric Giza, and Christopher D. Kreulen

Key Takeaway Points

- Must define reasons the previous treatments failed and to correct any underlying deformity that may have led to the treatment failure.
- Thorough imaging modalities are necessary to fully prepare for any revision surgery.
- Lesion size must be determine because this can affect surgical options.
- Must remove any loose or unstable cartilage to a stable rim prior to any further treatments.

Introduction

Osteochondral lesions of the talus (OLT) represent 4% of cartilage lesions in the body [1]. These lesions often require multiple surgeries to improve patient's quality of life. The etiology of the OLTs is still being elucidated, with known causes such as acute trauma, ankle sprains or fractures, repetitive stress [2, 3], local ischemia [4, 5], and even genetic causes with identical lesions found in twins [6]. The pathogenesis can involve direct trauma to the talar articular cartilage which can lead to subchondral edema and eventually cystic changes. The other mechanism in cases of nontraumatic OLTs involves subchondral bone injury or avascular event which precipitates softening of the overlying cartilage and eventual separation of the fragment [7]. These defects continue to challenge surgeons treating patients with this pathology. While short-term treatment results of osteochondral lesions are satisfactory, the long-term results continue to disappoint with patients having recurrence of symptoms. Many patients also undergo surgery with the expectation of returning to their sport. Many of the outcome scores fail to capture the "return to sport" in this patient group with the SF-36 or AOFAS scores [8, 9]. However, when sporting activity has been specifically studied, the return to sport shows lower levels of activity achieved [10, 11]. One study shows hope using a modified scoring system but only short-term follow-up (48 months) and still with only 72% returning to their pre-injury sport [12].

Treatment modalities vary depending on the location and type of lesion. Zengerink [3] performed a systematic review which shows success rates of 85% for bone marrow stimulation (BMS), 87% for osteoarticular transfer system (OATS), 76% for autologous chondrocyte implantation (ACI), and 88% for retrograde filling. The ongoing challenge of OLT surgical intervention is to

K. Boukhemis (✉) · E. Giza · C. D. Kreulen
University of California at Davis, Department of Orthopaedics, Sacramento, CA, USA

M. J. Berkowitz et al. (eds.), *Revision Surgery of the Foot and Ankle*,
https://doi.org/10.1007/978-3-030-29969-9_12

improve return to activity and reduce the rate of failure. The causes for failure can be multifactorial, ranging from poor biology, patient compliance issues, poor surgical technique, and improper surgical planning and execution. Initial treatment has mainly been bone marrow stimulation (microfracture), but long-term results never held up. In one long-term study looking at OLTs, 19 patients had greater than 5-year follow-up, 32% were worse, 47% remained unchanged, and only 18% improved. This questions whether long-term results of microfracture last [13].

Nonetheless, bone marrow stimulation is the treatment of choice for lesions less than 1.5cm^2; however there have been recent studies that have shown improved outcomes using allograft cartilage extracellular matrix (ECM) in lesions of 1.5cm^2 or less [14]. The resulting cartilage that forms after bone marrow stimulation is fibrocartilage. Fibrocartilage works as a patch to stabilize the subchondral bone, but it also progressively degenerates from type II collagen with an increase in type I collagen [15, 16]. Without the use of adjuvants, BMS alone may be a cause for revision. Numerous authors have shown the benefits to using platelet-rich plasma (PRP) or bone marrow aspirate concentrate (BMAC) as an adjunct to BMS [17–20]. Kruger et al. found that PRP increases chondrogenesis, collagen type II depositions, and inhibition of IL-1Beta and TNF-alpha [21]. The process also induces hemarthrosis which increases matrix metalloproteinase MMP-2 and MMP-9 production by synoviocytes [17]. The inflammatory process along with the mesenchymal cells from the BMS leads to fibrocartilage formation.

Another cause of failure can be the medial malleolar osteotomy site used in open OLT procedures. Kim et al. studied 52 ankles that underwent second look of OATS [18]. At 1 year they showed that a cause of failure in OCL was medial mal-osteotomy site from malreduction. If the cartilage surface of the tibial plafond was not anatomic, then the patients had worse outcomes. 13 of the 52 ankles had a malreduced osteotomy site, and clinical results were worse at follow-up based on VAS and AOFAS scores. They found no association between number of plugs and outcomes. Additionally, 15 ankles had impingement in the anterior process, and synovitis was observed as common finding on second-look arthroscopy.

Undiagnosed kissing lesions were a cause for failure 5% of 104 ankles [19]. Often these lesions were missed secondary to failed systematically performed ankle arthroscopy after finding the talar lesions. Another study showed 16/146 ankles presented with opposing bone lesions after arthroscopy that wasn't present on initial imaging [22].

Instability is an additional cause of failure in OLT surgery. Lee et al. performed a study comparing patients with OLT and instability and those without instability. Those with instability were more likely to have concomitant tibia lesions, had inferior outcomes, and decrease return to sport in comparison to those without instability [14]. In an effort to improve the functional results of surgery on these defects, various newer surgical strategies have evolved. Arthroscopic treatment is considered a better alternative than the invasiveness of open treatment, unless the open treatment provides a clear advantage.

Outside of large osteochondral autograft or allograft, treatment has focused on the stimulation of the bone or cartilage healing using scaffolds or biologics within the defect. Broadly these have focused on either cartilage regeneration, bone regeneration, or a combination of both. However there have been few publications to date that demonstrate the effectiveness of these treatments, which can also be expensive to use.

The size of the lesion can be an indication of initial treatment failure. Buda et al performed study in lesions >1.5 cm^2 and looked at 40 patients, 20 ACI and 20 BMDCT (bone marrow-derived cell transplantation)- FU to 48 months 69% return to sport with all professional athletes returning, ACI 11% at lower level and 27% with BMDT. ACI had three failures, and BMDCT had one failure. All cases were readdressed with BMDCT procedure. The advantage being it is a one surgery process. At follow-up 85% BMDCT and 75% ACI had hyaline-like tissue on MRI [21]. Another study showed OLTs had a 80%

failure rate in ankles treated larger than 150 mm^2 and only a 10% failure rate in lesions less than 150 mm^2 [23]. Cuttica studied 130 patients who underwent BMS. They found 2 lesions over 1.5 cm and 110 less than 1.5 cm^2. For large OCD over 1.5 cm, microfracture does not work as well. They also combined contained vs uncontained lesions, 113 contained and 17 uncontained. The odds of a poor outcome increase by 1.42 [24]. Uncontained lesions are considered a poor prognostic indicator for debridement and could represent an additional reason for failure [24]. 9/20 patients underwent second-look arthroscopy after microfracture with all lesions less than 1.5 cm. showed incomplete healing, and 40% had abnormal ICRS repair grades of III. Regardless of second-look findings, 90% had good AOFAS outcomes of over 80; however this was only 12 months after surgery [25].

Evaluation and Assessment

Plain radiographs are always the initial step in obtaining imaging studies. Standard weight-bearing films may not show posterior lesions, and a view of the ankle fully plantar flexed can help show those lesions. Some authors also recommend a 4 cm heel-rise view [19]. Plain radiographs are a starting point, but most of lesions will need an MRI for further clarification. In one study plain radiographs missed 41% of lesions [19].

CT can be used to look for cystic changes or examine the bony structure more closely. They should not be used in isolation and are not the best test for finding chondral lesions of the talus. One study showed helical CT scan missed 5/22 OLTs. Of those lesions 2/5 were Grade 1 lesions, 2/5 Anderson Grade 2 A, and 1/5 was arthritic [19].

MRI is the imaging modality of choice for OLTs. In a comparison study of MRI, CT, and diagnostic arthroscopy, MRI found 25/26 OLT [19]. Along with showing cartilage lesions, they also show bone marrow edema. MRI can also be used to evaluate previous cartilage repairs. Knee studies have shown that using coronal and sagittal high-resolution proton density and STIR imaging can provide qualitative assessment of cartilage lesions and repair [26]. In the situation of evaluating an OLT for a possible revisions surgery, it is recommended to order both a CT and MRI for a thorough assessment of the bony and cartilage components of the lesion.

Diagnostic arthroscopy is another option for revision evaluation and may be part of a staged revision to debride and fully assess the OLT repair that is causing the patient pain. In the same comparison study, arthroscopy found 29/27 lesions with two false positives on the talus. However, on the tibia 4/8 lesions were missed [26].

Treatment Options

Debridement

The goals of debridement are to remove the delaminated cartilage, remove the loose bone, and stimulate the repair of both the cartilage and bone by the migration of stem cells into the defect. The potential pain generators within the joint that can be addressed with debridement include loose fragments, unstable cartilage, and unstable bone causing increased intraosseous pressure; changes in ph may stimulate bone pain fibers. Van Dijk has proposed that the likely source of pain is from the subchondral bone and the likely mechanical and nociceptive properties from joint fluid [27]. Arthroscopic debridement will be reduced pain in the short term, and activity levels will increase. In the longer term, degenerative change may be prevented, and activity levels should be maintained.

Through debridement, the loose fragments are removed, and the peripheral articular cartilage is cleaned back to stable cartilage. With limited clinical data demonstrating the benefit of cartilage or bone replacement into the defect, debridement still remains the primary treatment option for many surgeons. Debridement may favor smaller defects (2–4 mm diameter), but fibrocartilage coverage of the defect is the end result, leaving other surgeons looking to improve this outcome with their index surgery on an OLT.

The knee literature on debridement cannot be extrapolated to the ankle as the cartilage thickness is different (1.2 mm vs 2.2 at the knee). The ankle is more congruent and has higher joint and fluid forces. The loads are spread over a wide area, and the cartilage deformation is minimal. Microfracture (the penetration of the subchondral bone and restoration of blood supply) is of use if the subchondral bone is intact. The microfracture awl is used to penetrate at 3–4 mm intervals. This allows mesenchymal stem cells to penetrate the joint and the production of type 11 collagen. Type 1 collagen may replace type 11 in time, and fibrocartilage repair may ensue.

A systematic review by Zengerink et al. reviewed 52 studies from between 1966 and 2006 [3]. These included 7 nonoperative series, 35 debridement papers, 9 OATS, 4 ACI, 3 retrograde drilling, and 2 trans-malleolar drilling. Note that these treatment groups may not be equivalent for all pathologies. Within the main treatment groups, the success rate of OATS was 87%, BMS was 85%, and ACI was 76%. They concluded that all were effective treatment strategies.

Choi et al. (2009) demonstrated that lesion size is a poor predictor of outcome: In a 120 ankles undergoing debridement, those that were over 150 mm^2 had a 10.5% failure rate defined by conversion to OATS, while 80% failed if the lesion was over 150 mm^2 [23]. Additionally, Scranton et al. (2006) noted that large cysts were also a poor predictor of outcome for debridement [28].

Cartilage and Cartilage Substitutes

Autologous osteochondral transplantation (AOT), allograft cartilage extracellular matrix, and allograft juvenile cartilage are all treatment modalities for OCL of the talus. They are often used for lesions that are not amenable to microfracture or debridement alone. In a systematic review in 2017, only 33 patients in 4 studies fulfilled the criteria for determination of outcome. The mean follow-up was 14.3 months with one revision surgery being performed. The authors recommended larger studies with longer follow-up before any conclusions could be made [29]. One study prospectively followed patients after implantation of juvenile cartilage. The lesions were from 10 to 15 mm in size, so no graft was in the large category. The results were on par with debridement alone [30]. As stated earlier in the chapter, there has been recent studies that have shown improved outcomes using allograft cartilage extracellular matrix (ECM) in lesions of 1.5cm^2 or less [14]. There may be a role for juvenile cartilage/ECM for midsize defects, and its use appears to be safe, but more follow-up is required to determine how it performs against debridement alone as to whether it is cost-effective compared to debridement.

Osteochondral autograft and allograft is another subcategory that has evolved. Autologous osteochondral transplantation (AOT) is an osteochondral replacement technique performed by inserting a cylindrical osteochondral graft, typically harvested from a non-weight-bearing portion of the ipsilateral knee into the prepared site of the defect on the talus. The goal of this procedure is to reproduce similar mechanical, structural, and biochemical properties of the native hyaline articular cartilage. It is traditionally accepted that large lesion (>150 mm^2 in size or >15 mm in diameter) or failed previous bone marrow stimulation (BMS) is indicated for AOT [23, 31, 32]. Recently the optimal indication size has been challenged, and it is now believed that 10.4 mm or 107.4 mm^2 or greater is suitable for AOT grafts [33]. When a lesion size is even larger, two or more grafts may be required [32].

Biological adjuvants, including platelet-rich plasma or bone marrow aspirate concentrate, (BMAC) are added to help improve cartilage repair. In a systematic review in 2010, 87% of patients obtained good to excellent outcomes in a series of 243 patients [3]. A recent case series of 85 patients improved the mean foot and ankle outcome score (FAOS) from 50 to 81 at mean 47.2 months follow-up, and the mean MOCART score was 85.8 postoperatively at mean 24.8 months follow-up [34]. In the athletic population, Fraser et al. reported that AOFAS scores were improved to 89.4 at final follow-up of 24 months and found that 90% of professional athletes and 87% of recreational athletes had return to pre-injury sports activity [35]. Other studies showed that 63–95% athletes can return to full sports activity following this procedure [11, 32, 36]. Although short- and midterm outcomes are favorable, no study has demonstrated the long-term outcomes of AOT.

While the reported clinical outcomes do not show significant deterioration over time, there are some concerns of both mechanical and biological factors. In a mechanical study, Fansa et al. [37] showed that a 1.0 mm of graft protrusion increased the contact pressure on the graft surface almost sevenfold, and a range of 1 mm sunk to 0.4 mm proud is acceptable to partially restore the contact mechanics of the ankle, highlighting the need for accurate placement of the graft. The character of the cartilage is inherently different between the knee and ankle significantly in shearing durability, friction, and energy dissipation [38]. In addition, the use of osteotomy carries the potential risk of mal/nonunion at the site of osteotomy. Lamb et al. [39] reported that 94% of patients were asymptomatic at the site of medial malleolar osteotomy and almost all had satisfactory healing and fixation with fibrocartilaginous tissue evident on MRI evaluation. Cyst formation following this procedure has been reported in up to 75% of patients [40, 41]. However, the clinical influence of cyst formation around the grafts was not found to be significant at a mean follow-up of 15 months, while increasing age was related to increased cyst prevalence [41]. On the other hand, previous failed bone marrow stimulation has negatively influenced clinical outcome following AOT. Secondary AOT after previous failed microfracture has shown worse functional outcomes compared with primary AOT [42]. Finally, MMP-8 (neutrophil collagenase) is present in knee cartilage, which is not typically seen in ankle cartilage [43]. This cytokine is one of the key enzymes in the pathogenesis of osteoarthritis, producing a catabolic response, and may contribute to graft failure.

Donor-site morbidity is also a concern. Several studies have shown that 2–50% of patients have knee symptoms following AOT [32, 40, 44, 45]. More recent studies, however, have reported a low incidence with good functional outcomes. In a retrospective case series of 39 patients, donor-site morbidity was present in 5% of patients, and Lysholm knee scores were at 99.4 at mean 42 months follow-up [46].

AOT provides good functional outcomes in the short-term and midterm follow-up. It does not appear to deteriorate significantly over time when the graft is properly placed in the most congruent position. Concerns of osteotomy and donor-site knee pain still remain, but their incidence remains low.

Role of BMAC

A study has assessed the addition of PRP to the defect. In this study patients either underwent debridement alone or debridement and the addition of PRP. At an average of 16 months, the patients undergoing debridement plus PRP treatment demonstrated better outcomes [47]. Gormeli [48] compared PRP versus HA after debridement and showed a benefit to PRP. PRP injection within the ankle joint has also been advocated. Studies comparing PRP to HA and to saline have demonstrated that PRP injection was more beneficial than control [49].

Bone marrow aspirate has also been used in single-stage debridements [50]. In this study 64 patients underwent debridement and addition of bone marrow aspirate on a collagen scaffold. Results were followed for 54 months. The AOFAS score improved, but no clear comparison or benefit over isolated debridement is clearly demonstrated. A systematic review outlined four studies performed to date with no clear benefit to BMAC over debridement alone [51]. One small study (22 patients) demonstrated a potential benefit to MACI over BMAC [52]. A recent study of 140 athletes defined the outcome after arthroscopic debridement and bone marrow derived cell transplantation. All the patients had the cells harvested from the iliac crest, condensed and loaded on a scaffold, and then implanted. The results were reported at 48 months. Seventy-two percent were able to participate in their sport at 48 months after surgery. One failure with repeat surgery was noted [12].

Overall this technique has gained popularity with initial studies. It may be more applicable to treating these defects for revision purposes in the future, but further studies will be needed to verify consistent benefits.

Associated Ankle Instability

Ankle instability may negatively affect the outcome of the osteochondral defect. Recurrent instability may further damage the injured cartilage. Lee et al. looked at the outcome of combined procedures for the treatment of osteochondral defects with ankle instability. This showed a benefit to the combined procedure with a final follow-up score in 16 patients of 91 on AOFAS scores. In their study they compared patients with chronic lateral ankle instability and OLTs with those without instability. Those with instability had a higher rate of failure and a lower return to sport [8, 20].

Bone Marrow Lesions

A more recent treatment recommended for lesions with minimal cartilage involvement is the treatment of bone marrow lesions with calcium phosphate cement. In this surgery a lesion with intact or almost intact articular cartilage is treated with liquid calcium phosphate injected into the bone, with the intent that the edema fluid within the bone is displaced by the calcium phosphate and stabilizes the bone marrow lesion. In time, the bone graft substitute will be replaced by regular bone. To date there are no publications on outcomes in the ankle, and the literature from the knee is case reports [53] and one case series [54] that shows early promise with this technique.

Cases

Case 12.1

History

A 17-year-old female presented to clinic who had an inversion injury to her left ankle when she was 13 years old. She had pain and swelling at that time, but it slowly subsided, but pain did not. She had continued difficulty, did not have any episodes of giving or instability, but does get occasional swelling with activities such as basketball, volleyball, etc. Patient previously had a microfracture and initially did well in the early time period. The pain and dysfunction, however, returned to her prior to surgery levels, and she described her pain as deep and achy. Roughly pain score is 8/10 with activity. Ice and elevation did help intermittently. She previously had two ankle scopes as well including the microfracture. Other than a slight effusion and some medial talar neck pain with palpation, her clinical exam was essentially normal. Advanced imaging revealed a possible unstable cartilage cap with underlying bony edema.

Reasons for Failure

- Failed microfracture secondary to unstable fibrocartilage cap. Grade 4 lesion measuring 12 × 8 mm

Surgical Plan

The patient had exhausted all nonoperative modalities as well as previously failed microfracture. She is young and active, and therefore the plan was to move forward with juvenile cartilage allograft via an arthroscopic approach.

Approach

Patient was placed supine with leg holder to aid in ankle arthroscopy. Previously used medial and lateral portals were reestablished. Inspection of the joint was performed, as well as debridement of all scar tissue. The osteochondral lesion was found and curetted of all unstable fibrocartilage to a stable rim. Microfracture was performed into the subchondral bone. After active bleeding was visualized, the ankle joint was dried out as much as possible in preparation for the allograft and slight traction was attached. Juvenile allograft cartilage was then placed within the OCD lesion. The allograft cartilage was flattened out to cover the entire lesion, but care was taken to not be higher than the natural cartilage rim. Fibrin glue was used to secure the allograft in place within the defect. Care was taken to rid the joint of any loose bodies. The fibrin glue is allowed to solidify, and the joint was inspected one last time. Portals were closed using 3-0 nylon suing a horizontal mattress technique.

Implants

- Juvenile allograft cartilage – DeNovo (Zimmer-Biomet; Warsaw, IN)
- Fibrin glue – Tisseel (Abbott Laboratories; Baxter Healthcare Corporation)

Pearls and Pitfalls

- It is key to debride back the previous fibrocartilage cap to a stable cartilage rim prior to DeNovo implantation.
- Important not to allow DeNovo to exceed the cartilage rim.
- Allow fibrin glue to adhere prior to placing the ankle through range of motion.
- Recommend using two packets of DeNovo if the defect measures more than 1.5 cm^2 (Figs. 12.1, 12.2, 12.3, 12.4, 12.5, 12.6, 12.7, 12.8, 12.9, and 12.10).

Case 12.2

History

A 39-year-old male with an ankle talus defect that occurred after playing basketball. He underwent arthroscopy 4 months after his injury and a

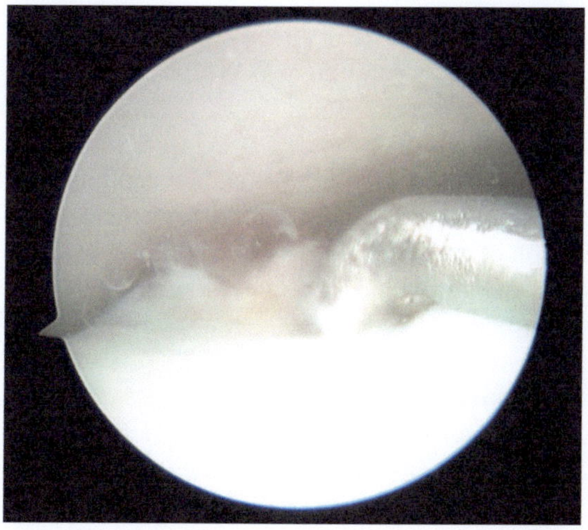

Fig. 12.1 Initial probing of OCD from original surgery

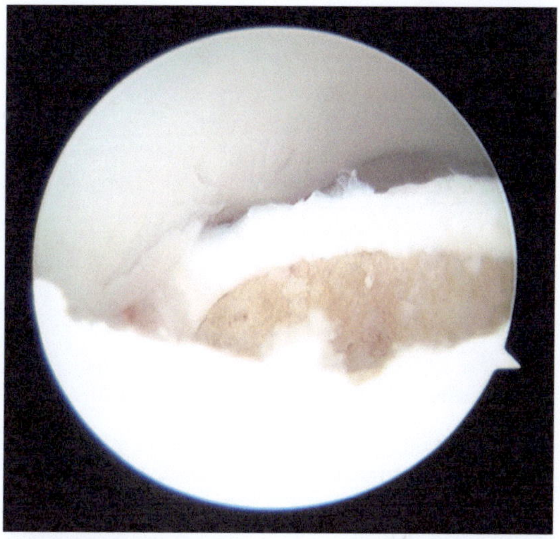

Fig. 12.2 s/p Curettage of defect with the subchondral bone exposed

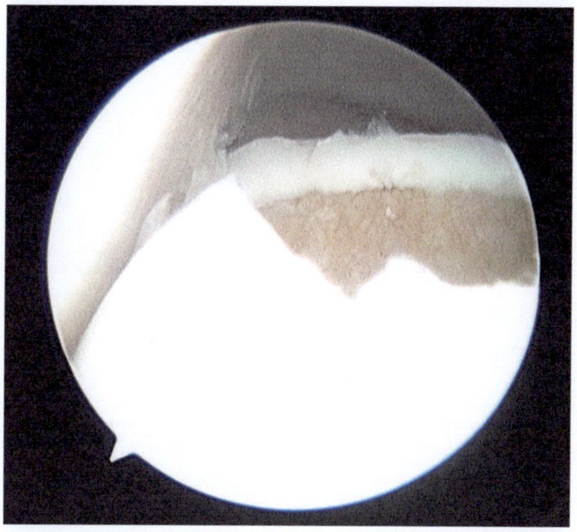

Fig. 12.3 s/p Curettage of defect (additional view of stable rim)

microfracture, and debridement was performed on the OLT. Patient did not have significant relief from his pain and underwent an OATS procedure with a graft from the left knee 6 months later. He continued to have pain despite both of these procedures. He also described his pain actually getting worse. Patient was incapable of running and could only walk about three city blocks before his ankle started throbbing and aching. He rated his pain at a 6/10 on a daily basis and worse with increased activity. He was unable to remain active despite conservative and operative measures.

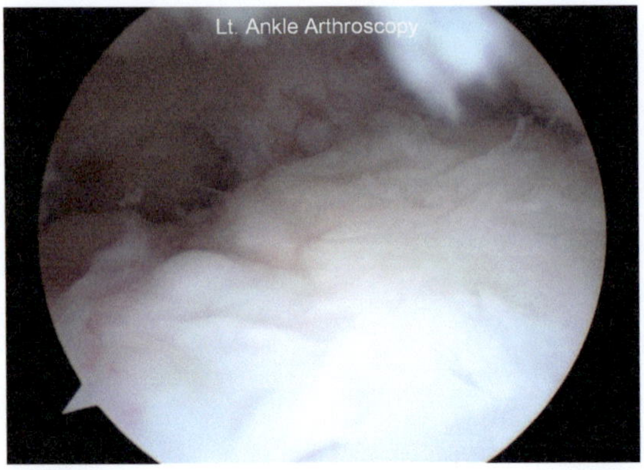

Fig. 12.4 Initial arthroscopic evaluation of cartilage defect after microfracture with unorganized fibrocartilage

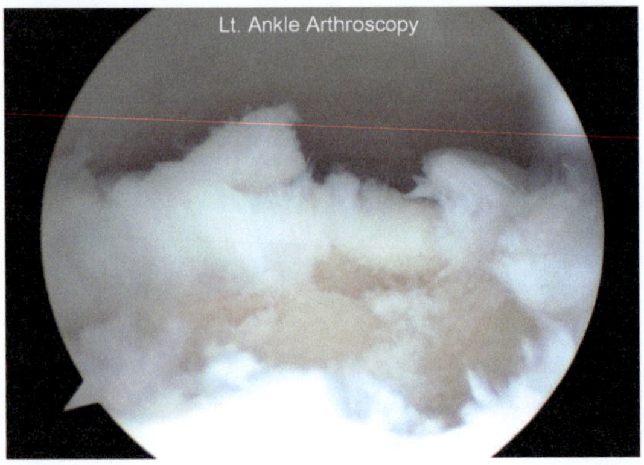

Fig. 12.5 Curettage of the fibrocartilage down to the subchondral bone

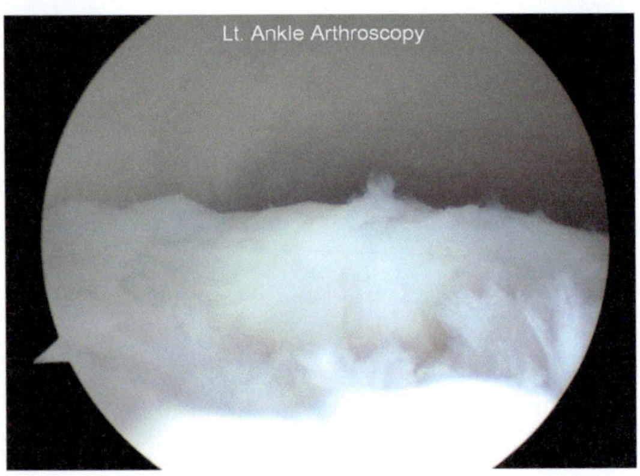

Fig. 12.6 Additional view of debridement of unstable fibrocartilage

Other than some medial talar neck tenderness and mild effusion, the patient's exam is normal. After obtaining further imaging, including radio-

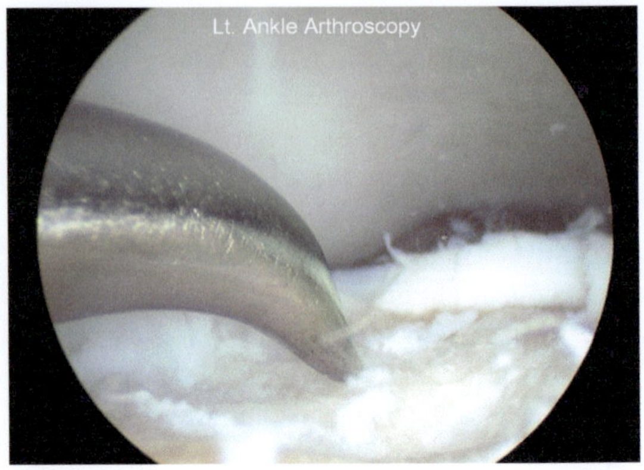

Fig. 12.7 Microfracture of the subchondral bone

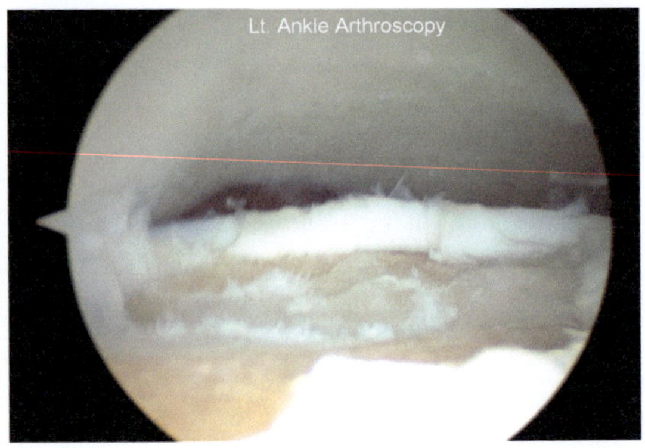

Fig. 12.8 Completion of microfracture and curettage to stable rim

graphs, CT scan, and MRI, it appeared that the OATS plug had some irregularity and dissociation of the articular surface underneath.

Reason for Failure

- Failed incorporation of OATS plug

Surgical Plan

Plan was discussed with the patient and included repeat ankle arthroscopy with debridement, evaluation of cartilage plug, removal of unstable portion of plug, and juvenile allograft cartilage placement as needed.

Approach

Patient was placed supine with leg holder to aid in ankle arthroscopy. Previous medial and lateral portals were again established. Evaluation of the ankle joint and debridement of any scar tissue

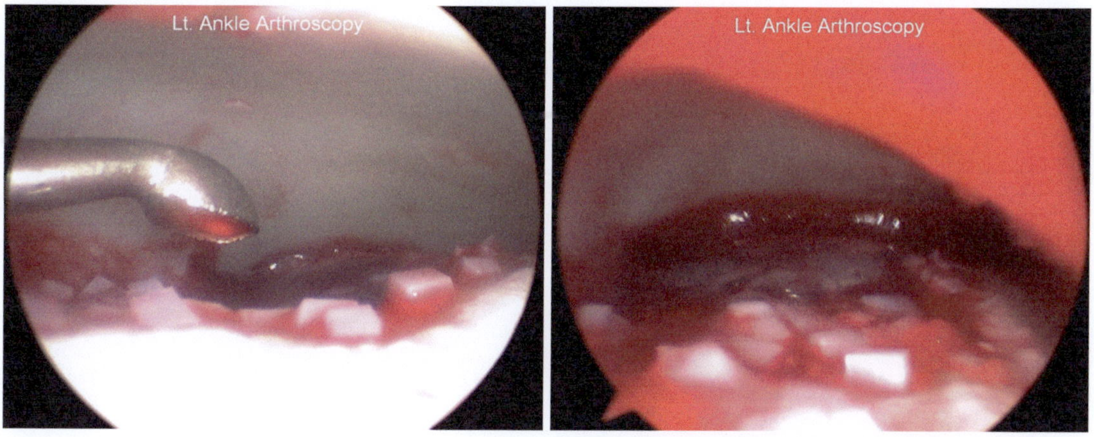

Figs. 12.9 and 12.10 Placement of DeNovo with fibrin glue over top

were performed. Inspection of the previous OATS revealed unstable plug with delamination of the osteochondral border. The unstable lesion was curetted out and brought to a stable rim. The overall size was 18 × 10 mm with a depth of approximately 6 mm requiring calcaneus bone autograft. The ankle was dried to the best of our ability; prior to this it was evaluated for any residual loose bodies. Juvenile allograft cartilage was prepared and introduced into the lesion. The defect was filled, but did not exceed the height of the rim. Fibrin glue was used to hold the allograft in place.

Implants

- Juvenile allograft cartilage – DeNovo (Zimmer-Biomet; Warsaw, IN)
- Fibrin glue – Tisseel (Abbott Laboratories; Baxter Healthcare Corporation)
- Calcaneus autograft

Pearls and Pitfalls

- It is key to debride back the previous fibrocartilage cap to a stable cartilage rim prior to DeNovo implantation.
- Important not to allow DeNovo to exceed the cartilage rim.
- Allow fibrin glue to adhere prior to placing the ankle through range of motion.
- Recommend using two packets of DeNovo if the defect measures more than 1.5cm^2 (Figs. 12.11, 12.12, 12.13, 12.14, 12.15, 12.16, 12.17, 12.18, 12.19, 12.20, and 12.21).

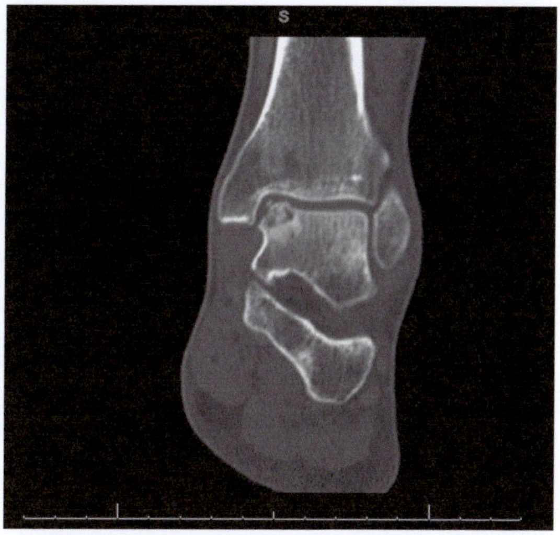

Fig. 12.11 Coronal CT of talar defect

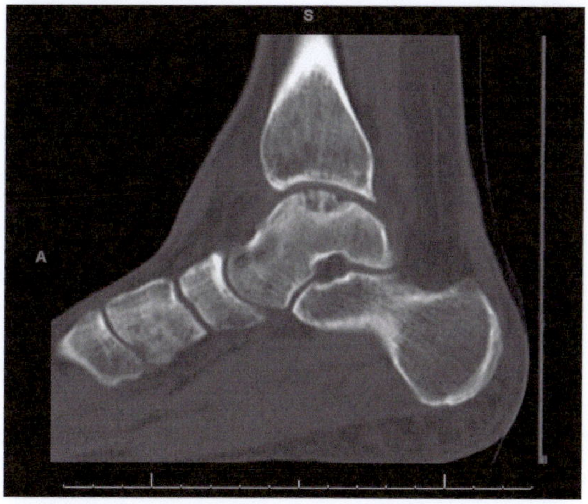

Fig. 12.12 Sagittal image of talar defect

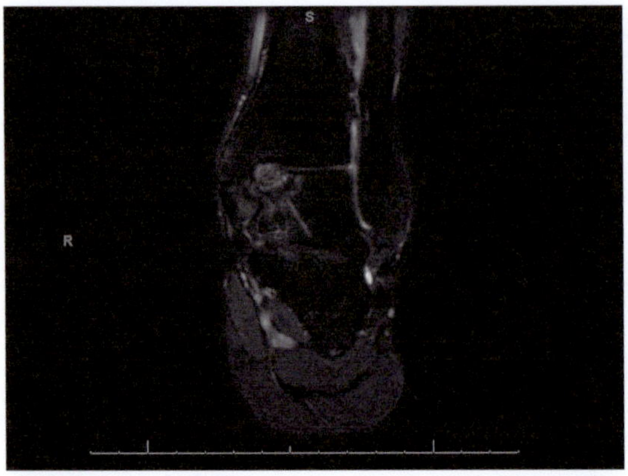

Fig. 12.13 Coronal T2 MRI of talar defect

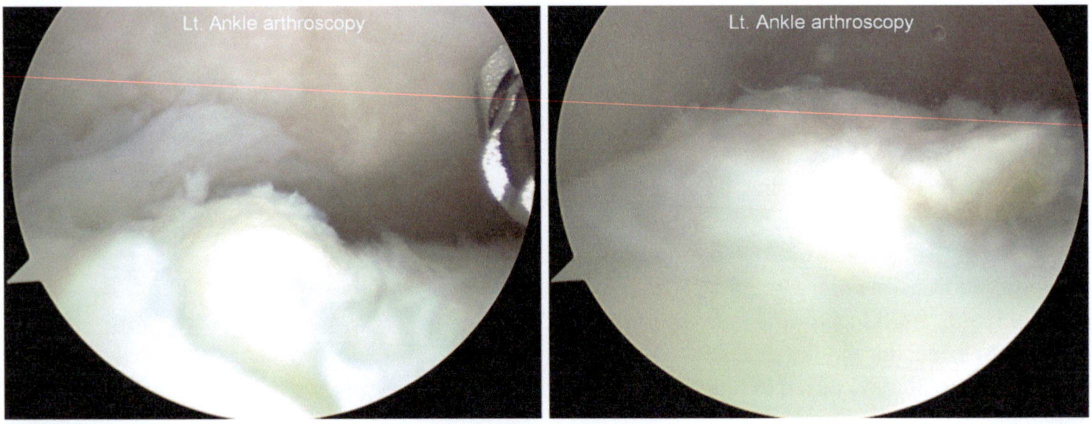

Figs. 12.14 and 12.15 Initial evaluation of OCD lesion and fibrocartilage cap

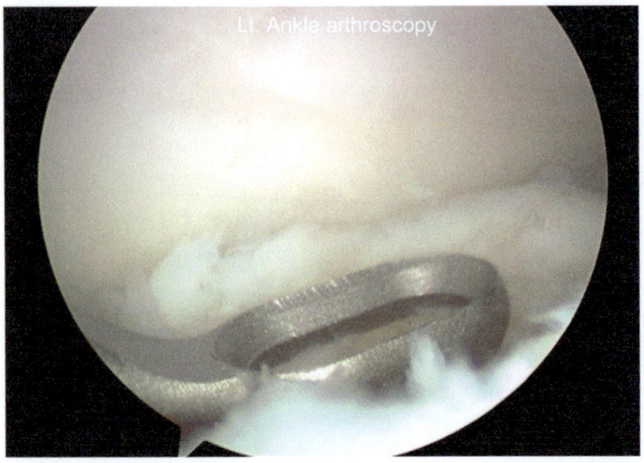

Fig. 12.16 Defect size after curettage

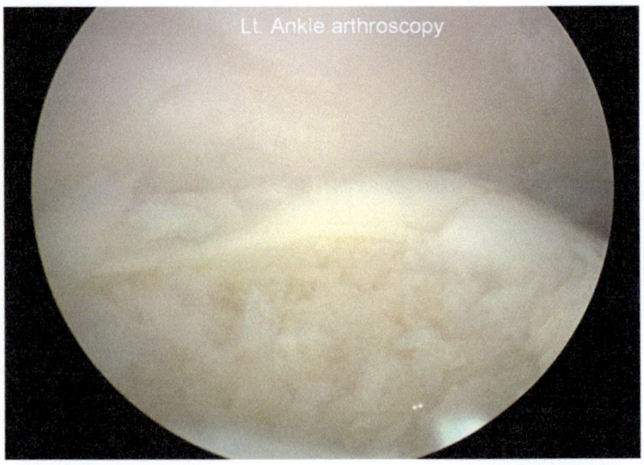

Fig. 12.17 Curettage of lesion down to subchondral bone

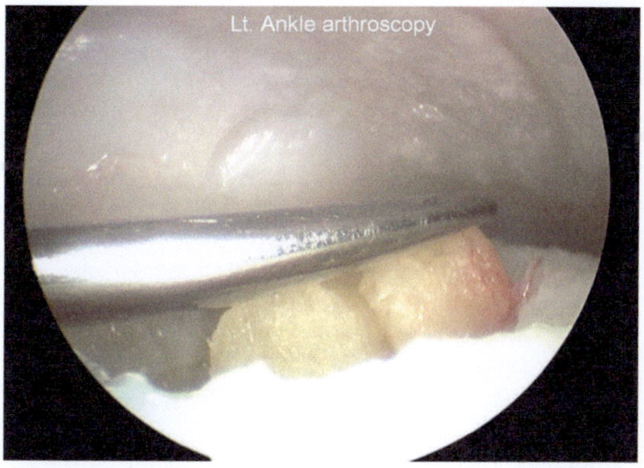

Fig. 12.18 Bone grafting of the lesion with spatula

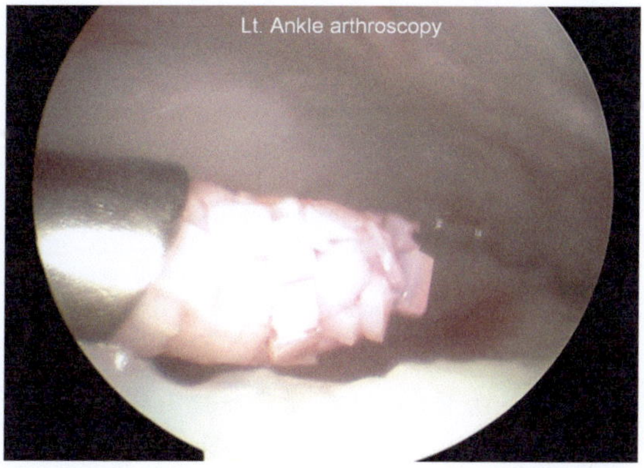

Fig. 12.19 DeNovo articular cartilage placement within the defect

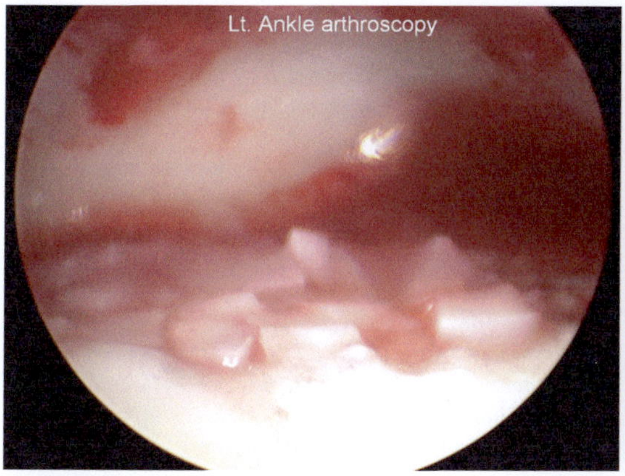

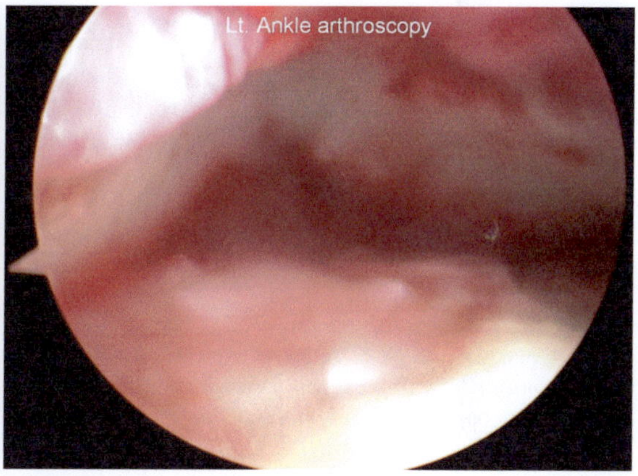

Figs. 12.20 and 12.21 DeNovo placed within the defect with fibrin glue holding it in place

References

1. Alexander A, Lichtman D. Surgical treatment of transchondral talar-dome fractures (osteochondritis dissecans). Long-term follow-up. J Bone Joint Surg Am. 1980;62(4):646–52.
2. O'loughlin PF, Heyworth BE, Kennedy JG. Current concepts in the diagnosis and treatment of osteochondral lesions of the ankle. Am J Sports Med. 2010;38(2):392–404.
3. Zengerink M, Struijs PA, Tol JL, van Dijk CN. Treatment of osteochondral lesions of the talus: a systematic review. Knee Surg Sports Traumatol Arthrosc. 2010;18:238–46.
4. Tol JL, Struijs PAA, Bossuyt PMM, Verhagen RAW, Van Dijk CN. Treatment strategies in osteochondral defects of the talar dome: a systematic review. Foot Ankle Int. 2000;21(2):119–26.
5. VanNini F, CaVallO M, BalDaSSarrI M, CaStagnini F, Olivieri A, Ferranti E, et al. Treatment of juvenile osteochondritis dissecans of the talus: current concepts review. Joints. 2014;2(4):188.
6. Hammett RB, Saxby TS. Osteochondral lesion of the talus in homozygous twins—the question of heredity. Foot Ankle Surg. 2010;16(3):e55–6.
7. Berndt AL, Harty M. Transchondral fractures (osteochondritis dissecans) of the talus. J Bone Joint Surg Am. 1959;41(6):988–1020.
8. van Eekeren IC, Reilingh ML, van Dijk CN. Rehabilitation and return-to-sports activity after debridement and bone marrow stimulation of osteochondral talar defects. Sports Med. 2012;42:857–70.
9. Pinsker E, Inrig T, Daniels TR, Warmington K, Beaton DE. Symptom resolution and patient-perceived recovery following ankle arthroplasty and arthrodesis. Foot Ankle Int. 2016;37:1269–76.

10. van Eekeren IC, van Bergen CJ, Sierevelt IN, Reilingh ML, van Dijk CN. Return to sports after arthroscopic debridement and bone marrow stimulation of osteochondral talar defects: a 5- to 24-year follow-up study. Knee Surg Sports Traumatol Arthrosc. 2016;24:1311–5.
11. Paul J, Sagstetter M, Lammle L, et al. Sports activity after osteochondral transplantation of the talus. Am J Sports Med. 2012;40:870–4.
12. Vannini F, Cavallo M, Ramponi L, et al. Return to sports after bone marrow-derived cell transplantation for osteochondral lesions of the talus. Cartilage. 2017;8:80–7.
13. Ferkel RD, Zanotti RM, Komenda GA, Sgaglione NA, Cheng MS, Applegate GR, et al. Arthroscopic treatment of chronic osteochondral lesions of the talus: long-term results. Am J Sports Med. 2008;36(9):1750–62.
14. Ahmad J, Maltenfort M. Arthroscopic treatment of osteochondral lesions of the talus with allograft cartilage matrix. Foot Ankle Int. 2017;38(8):855–62.
15. Murawski CD, Foo LF, Kennedy JG. A review of arthroscopic bone marrow stimulation techniques of the talus: the good, the bad, and the causes for concern. Cole BJ, Kercher JS, editors. Cartilage. 2010;1(2):137–44.
16. Tang QO, Shakib K, Heliotis M, Tsiridis E, Mantalaris A, Ripamonti U, et al. TGF-β3: a potential biological therapy for enhancing chondrogenesis. Expert Opin Biol Ther. 2009;9(6):689–701.
17. Smyth NA. Establishing proof of concept: platelet-rich plasma and bone marrow aspirate concentrate may improve cartilage repair following surgical treatment for osteochondral lesions of the talus. World J Orthop. 2012;3(7):101.
18. Kim YS, Park EH, Kim YC, Koh YG, Lee JW. Factors associated with the clinical outcomes of the osteochondral autograft transfer system in osteochondral lesions of the talus. Am J Sports Med. 2012;40(12):2709–19.
19. Verhagen RAW, Maas M, Dijkgraaf MGW, Tol JL, Krips R, van Dijk CN. Prospective study on diagnostic strategies in osteochondral lesions of the talus. J Bone Joint Surg Br. 2005;87(1):41–6.
20. Lee M, Kwon JW, Choi WJ, Lee JW. Comparison of outcomes for osteochondral lesions of the talus with and without chronic lateral ankle instability. Foot Ankle Int. 2015;36(9):1050–7.
21. Buda R, Vannini F, Castagnini F, Cavallo M, Ruffilli A, Ramponi L, et al. Regenerative treatment in osteochondral lesions of the talus: autologous chondrocyte implantation versus one-step bone marrow derived cells transplantation. Int Orthop. 2015;39(5):893–900.
22. Sijbrandij ES, van Gils AP, Louwerens JW, de Lange EE. Posttraumatic subchondral bone contusions and fractures of the talotibial joint: occurrence of "kissing" lesions. AJR Am J Roentgenol. 2000;175(6):1707–10.
23. Choi WJ, Park KK, Kim BS, Lee JW. Osteochondral lesion of the talus: is there a critical defect size for poor outcome? Am J Sports Med. 2009;37:1974–80.
24. Cuttica DJ, Smith WB, Hyer CF, Philbin TM, Berlet GC. Osteochondral lesions of the talus: predictors of clinical outcome. Foot Ankle Int. 2011;32:1045–51.
25. Lee K-B, Bai L-B, Yoon T-R, Jung S-T, Seon J-K. Second-look arthroscopic findings and clinical outcomes after microfracture for osteochondral lesions of the talus. Am J Sports Med. 2009;37(1_suppl):63S–70S.
26. Brown WE, Potter HG, Marx RG, Wickiewicz TL, Warren RF. Magnetic resonance imaging appearance of cartilage repair in the knee. Clin Orthop. 2004;422:214–23.
27. van Dijk CN, Reilingh ML, Zengerink M, van Bergen CJ. Osteochondral defects in the ankle: why painful? Knee Surg Sports Traumatol Arthrosc. 2010;18:570–80.
28. Scranton PEJ, Frey CC, Feder KS. Outcome of osteochondral autograft transplantation for type-V cystic osteochondral lesions of the talus. J Bone Joint Surg Br. 2006;88:614–9.
29. Saltzman BM, Lin J, Lee S. Particulated juvenile articular cartilage allograft transplantation for osteochondral talar lesions. Cartilage. 2017;8:61–72.
30. Coetzee JC, Giza E, Schon LC, et al. Treatment of osteochondral lesions of the talus with particulated juvenile cartilage. Foot Ankle Int. 2013; 34:1205–11.
31. Chuckpaiwong B, Berkson EM, Theodore GH. Microfracture for osteochondral lesions of the ankle: outcome analysis and outcome predictors of 105 cases. Arthroscopy. 2008;24:106–12.
32. Kennedy JG, Murawski CD. The treatment of osteochondral lesions of the talus with autologous osteochondral transplantation and bone marrow aspirate concentrate: surgical technique. Cartilage. 2011;2:327–36.
33. Ramponi L, Yasui Y, Murawski CD, et al. Lesion size is a predictor of clinical outcomes after bone marrow stimulation for osteochondral lesions of the talus: a systematic review. Am J Sports Med. 2017;45(7):1698–705.
34. Flynn S, Ross KA, Hannon CP, et al. Autologous osteochondral transplantation for osteochondral lesions of the talus. Foot Ankle Int. 2016;37:363–72.
35. Fraser EJ, Harris MC, Prado MP, Kennedy JG. Autologous osteochondral transplantation for osteochondral lesions of the talus in an athletic population. Knee Surg Sports Traumatol Arthrosc. 2016;24:1272–9.
36. Hangody L, Dobos J, Balo E, Panics G, Hangody LR, Berkes I. Clinical experiences with autologous osteochondral mosaicplasty in an athletic population: a 17-year prospective multicenter study. Am J Sports Med. 2010;38:1125–33.
37. Fansa AM, Murawski CD, Imhauser CW, Nguyen JT, Kennedy JG. Autologous osteochondral transplantation of the talus partially restores contact mechanics of the ankle joint. Am J Sports Med. 2011;39:2457–65.

38. Henak CR, Ross KA, Bonnevie ED, et al. Human talar and femoral cartilage have distinct mechanical properties near the articular surface. J Biomech. 2016;49:3320–7.
39. Lamb J, Murawski CD, Deyer TW, Kennedy JG. Chevron-type medial malleolar osteotomy: a functional, radiographic and quantitative T2-mapping MRI analysis. Knee Surg Sports Traumatol Arthrosc. 2013;21:1283–8.
40. Valderrabano V, Leumann A, Rasch H, Egelhof T, Hintermann B, Pagenstert G. Knee-to-ankle mosaicplasty for the treatment of osteochondral lesions of the ankle joint. Am J Sports Med. 2009;37:105S–11S.
41. Savage-Elliott I, Smyth NA, Deyer TW, et al. Magnetic resonance imaging evidence of postoperative cyst formation does not appear to affect clinical outcomes after autologous osteochondral transplantation of the talus. Arthroscopy. 2016;32:1846–54.
42. Ross AW, Murawski CD, Fraser EJ, et al. Autologous osteochondral transplantation for osteochondral lesions of the talus: does previous bone marrow stimulation negatively affect clinical outcome? Arthroscopy. 2016;32:1377–83.
43. Chubinskaya S, Huch K, Mikecz K, et al. Chondrocyte matrix metalloproteinase-8: up-regulation of neutrophil collagenase by interleukin-1 beta in human cartilage from knee and ankle joints. Lab Investig. 1996;74:232–40.
44. Reddy S, Pedowitz DI, Parekh SG, Sennett BJ, Okereke E. The morbidity associated with osteochondral harvest from asymptomatic knees for the treatment of osteochondral lesions of the talus. Am J Sports Med. 2007;35:80–5.
45. LaPrade RF, Botker JC. Donor-site morbidity after osteochondral autograft transfer procedures. Arthroscopy. 2004;20:e69–73.
46. Fraser EJ, Savage-Elliott I, Yasui Y, et al. Clinical and MRI donor site outcomes following autologous osteochondral transplantation for talar osteochondral lesions. Foot Ankle Int. 2016;37:968–76.
47. Guney A, Akar M, Karaman I, Oner M, Guney B. Clinical outcomes of platelet rich plasma (PRP) as an adjunct to microfracture surgery in osteochondral lesions of the talus. Knee Surg Sports Traumatol Arthrosc. 2015;23:2384–9.
48. Gormeli G, Karakaplan M, Gormeli CA, Sarikaya B, Elmali N, Ersoy Y. Clinical effects of platelet-rich plasma and hyaluronic acid as an additional therapy for talar osteochondral lesions treated with microfracture surgery: a prospective randomized clinical trial. Foot Ankle Int. 2015;36:891–900.
49. Jazzo SF, Scribner D, Shay S, Kim KM. Patient-reported outcomes following platelet-rich plasma injections in treating osteochondral lesions of the talus: a critically appraised topic. J Sport Rehabil. 2018;27(2):177–84.
50. Buda R, Vannini F, Cavallo M, et al. One-step bone marrow-derived cell transplantation in talarosteochondral lesions: mid-term results. Joints. 2013;1:102–7.
51. Chahla J, Cinque ME, Shon JM, et al. Bone marrow aspirate concentrate for the treatment of osteochondral lesions of the talus: a systematic review of outcomes. J Exp Orthop. 2016;3:33.
52. Desando G, Bartolotti I, Vannini F, et al. Repair potential of matrix-induced bone marrow aspirate concentrate and matrix-induced autologous chondrocyte implantation for talar osteochondral repair: patterns of some catabolic, inflammatory, and pain mediators. Cartilage. 2017;8:50–60.
53. Abrams GD, Alentorn-Geli E, Harris JD, Cole BJ. Treatment of a lateral tibial plateau osteochondritis dissecans lesion with subchondral injection of calcium phosphate. Arthrosc Tech. 2013;2:e271–4.
54. Cohen SB, Sharkey PF. Subchondroplasty for treating bone marrow lesions. J Knee Surg. 2016;29:555–63.

Revision Surgery for Lateral Ankle Instability

13

Taylor N. Cabe, Sydney C. Karnovsky, and Mark C. Drakos

Key Takeaway Points

- Traditional Brostrom-Gould repair may not be an ideal repair for chronic lateral ankle instability in all patients. Specifically, patients with confounding factors such as higher physical demands, generalized ligamentous laxity, underlying deformities, or prior failure may benefit from our recommended reconstruction technique utilizing a hamstring tendon autograft.
- Positive stress test on radiographs should serve as the primary indicator for surgery with 10 degrees or greater talar tilt, 10 mm or greater anterior drawer displacement, or a 5 degrees or 5 mm difference between the affected and contralateral side serving as the baseline for a positive test.
- To ensure successful reconstruction, attention must also be paid to other comorbidities including OCLs, damage peroneal tendons, or improper foot alignment. Appropriate action should be taken to correct all other presenting pathologies.
- When using our reconstruction technique, the ankle must be reduced in maximum posterior translation and eversion when the final screws are secured in the fibular and talar tunnels.
- Augmentation should be considered in revision cases as well as severe primary cases with talar tilt greater than 20 degrees or cases of generalized ligamentous laxity.

T. N. Cabe · S. C. Karnovsky · M. C. Drakos (✉)
Hospital for Special Surgery, Foot and Ankle Service, New York, NY, USA
e-mail: drakosm@hss.edu

Introduction

Ankle sprains are one of the most frequent injuries seen in the lower extremity and occur at a rate of approximately 2 million per year in the United States [1]. Ankle sprains often involve injury to the lateral ankle ligaments [2]. While the majority of people heal from a first sprain with no complications, it has been reported that up to 34% of people will re-sprain their ankle in the 3-year period immediately following their initial sprain. Furthermore, chronic ankle instability has been reported to develop in 20–40% of patients [1, 3]. Chronic instability can be caused by ligaments that are stretched to such a degree that they allow for supra-physiologic range of

M. J. Berkowitz et al. (eds.), *Revision Surgery of the Foot and Ankle*,
https://doi.org/10.1007/978-3-030-29969-9_13

motion as well as by a proprioceptive deficit [1]. Radiographically, chronic instability is commonly defined as over 10 degrees of talar tilt on a stress radiographs, 10 mm of displacement with anterior drawer, or 5 degrees talar tilt and/or 5 mm anterior drawer difference compared to the contralateral side [4].

When chronic instability is present and conservative measures such as physical therapy and bracing have been exhausted, operative treatment is indicated. There are a myriad of operative techniques that exist for repairing ankle instability, including the Chrisman-Snook procedure and the modified Brostrom procedure [4]. Currently, the modified Brostrom is the gold standard, and it has shown overall very positive results [1, 4, 5]. However, despite its overall success, the modified Brostrom as well as other repairs can fail, and a one-size-fits-all approach is probably not optimal.

Failure of an ankle stabilization procedure is indicated by positive stress tests on radiographs as well as a continued feeling of pain of the ankle and/or of "giving out" in patients. Failure can be due to a variety of reasons, including large patients with high demand athletics, generalized ligamentous laxity (Ehlers-Danlos syndrome), an underlying deformity such as a cavovarus foot, or failure of a graft [1, 3, 6–10]. In cases of failure, revision surgery is often indicated. Successful revision operation typically involves an anatomic ligament reconstruction, which can be done using either an allograft or autograft [1]. Different grafts, including semitendinosus auto- and allografts, periosteal flaps, extensor digitorum longus grafts, plantaris grafts, gracilis grafts, and peroneus longus grafts, have all been described as potential options [1–3, 5, 8, 11, 12]. In cases requiring revision, we have recommended using a hamstring autograft. This technique uses three tunnels in the calcaneus, the fibula, and the talus through which either an autograft gracilis, semitendinosus, or both tendons – dependent on size – are woven. The graft is secured in each tunnel using interference screws with the ankle in eversion and posterior translation [13]. In early results, with 33 patients with greater than a 1-year follow-up, we have found significant radiographic and clinical outcome score improvement with this technique.

Case Examples

Case 13.1

History

- A 30-year-old female, presented with an 11-year history of left ankle pain. She reported feeling achiness and dull pains as well as pain with activity at time of initial presentation to the office.
  - Patient reported three bad ankle sprains in the past.
  - Initially treated 10 years ago at an outside facility with a Brostrom-type procedure.
  - She reported improvement after the initial surgery but a continued sense of ankle instability.
  - Physical exam showed 2+ anterior drawer.
  - Radiographs and stress radiographs were taken which demonstrated 14 degrees of varus opening (Fig. 13.1a, b).
  - MRI reviewed which showed no OCL.
  - Attempted conservative treatment which included the use of an ASO lace-up ankle brace as well as physical therapy for 6 months.
- Patient had an additional 3-month physical therapy and felt as though the problem had not gotten better.
- Revision surgery was indicated and included an ankle arthroscopy, lateral ligament reconstruction with hamstring autograft, as well as Brostrom-Gould-type ankle stabilization.

Surgical Plan

Positioning

- Place the patient in a supine position.
- Place a nonsterile tourniquet on the operative thigh.

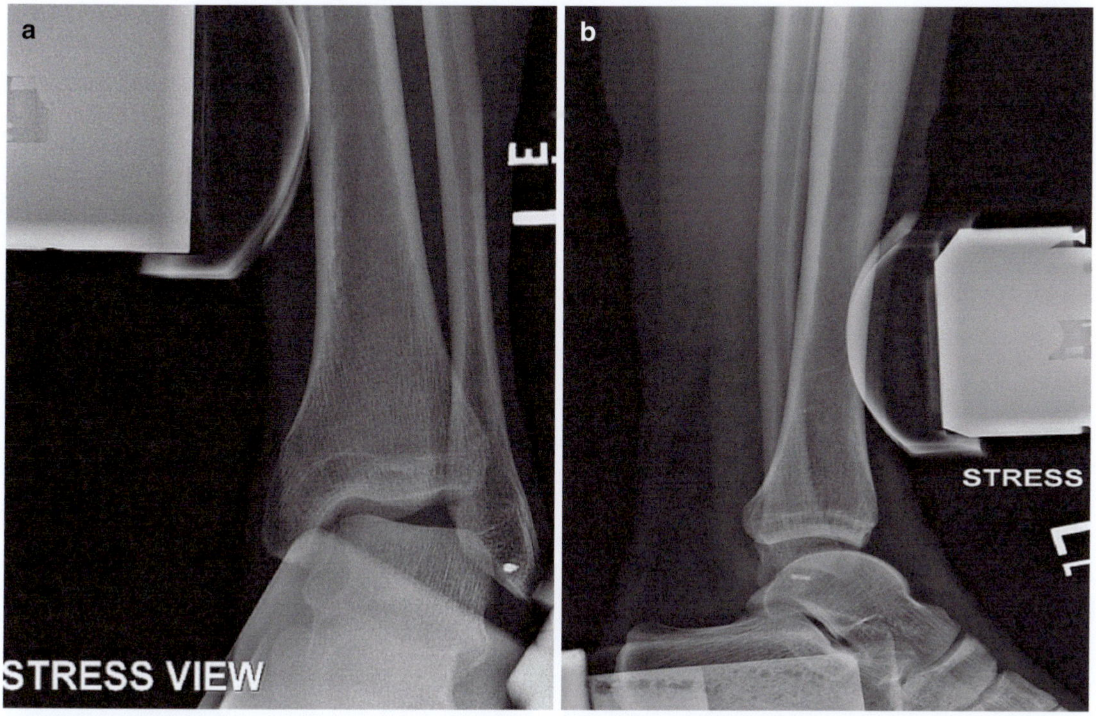

Fig. 13.1 Preoperative anteroposterior (**a**) and lateral (**b**) stress x-rays showing increased talar tilt and anterior drawer, respectively, in **Case 13.1** patient

Ankle Arthroscopy

- The patient was placed in a noninvasive ankle distraction.
- Standard anteromedial and anterolateral ports were established, and a diagnostic arthroscopy was performed.
- A significant impingement lesion was found in both the anteromedial and anterolateral gutters.
  - These lesions were debrided with a 2.9 shaver.
- No full-thickness cartilage defects were found. There were some grade 2 changes which were debrided.

Hamstring Autograft

- A 3 cm incision was made over the medial aspect of the proximal tibia, and dissection was carried out to the level of the sartorial fascia.
- The sartorial fascia was divided in line with its fibers.
- The gracilis was exposed.
- The gracilis was harvested using a Linvatec tendon stripper (ConMed; Utica, NY).
- The muscle was removed from the gracilis, and then it was tubularized using 0 Vicryl suture.
- The graft measured a size 4 mm × 26 cm.

Ankle Reconstruction

- A 5 cm incision was made over the patient's previous incision, and dissection was carried out to the level of the fibula.
- The ATFL, CFL, and capsule were removed off the fibula.
- There were several Ethibond knots and one anchor buried in the bone present which were removed.
- The fibula was then prepared with a curette.
- A separate incision was then made over the calcaneofibular ligament insertion, right behind the peroneal tendons. Dissection was carried out to the level of the calcaneus (Fig. 13.2).
- A 4.5 drill bit was placed at the calcaneus.

- Sutures were then shuttled underneath the peroneal tendons.
- Another drill hole was then placed at the origin of the ATFL (from anterior to posterior across the fibula). This tunnel was size 4.
- A third tunnel was then made at the talus (at the anterior aspect of the lateral process of the talus) (Fig. 13.3a, b).
- Tunnel position was confirmed with fluoroscopy.
- The graft was then placed in the calcaneal tunnel and secured in place using a 4.75 × 15 mm Bio-Tenodesis screw (Fig. 13.4).

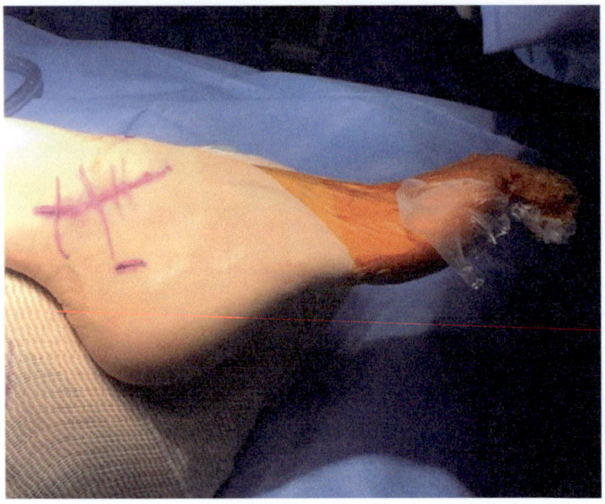

Fig. 13.2 Incision sites are marked at the distal fibula (top mark, approximately 5 cm) and the lateral aspect of the calcaneus below the peroneal tendons (bottom mark, approximately 1 cm)

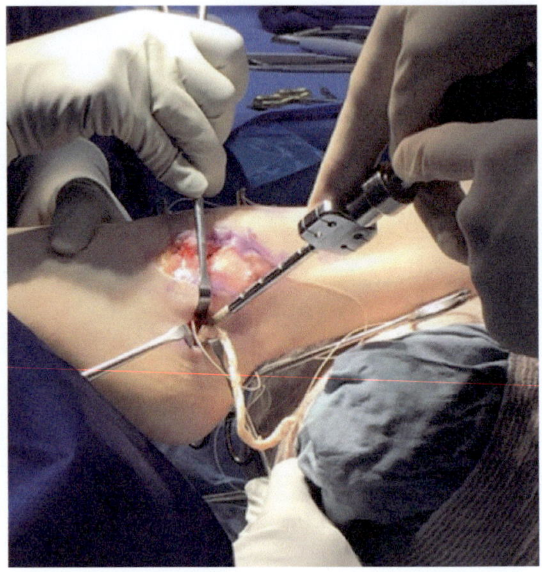

Fig. 13.4 The hamstring autograft is secured in the calcaneal bone tunnel using a Bio-Tenodesis screw

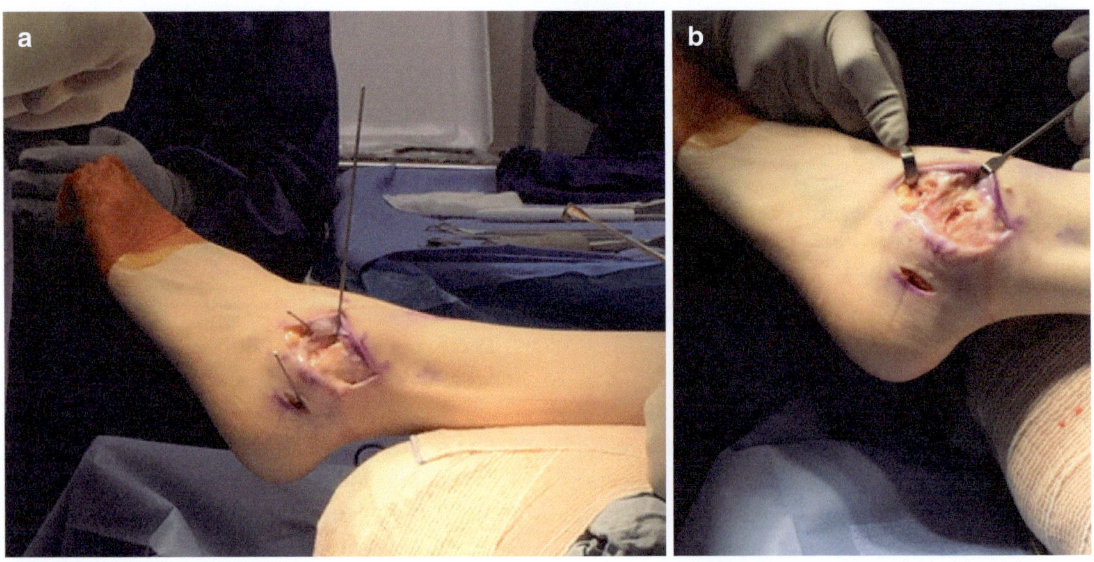

Fig. 13.3 Three bone tunnels are drilled: first in the calcaneus (25 mm deep), then the fibula (completely through the bone), and finally the talus (completely through the bone). Guide wires mark all three locations (**a**), and the three completed tunnels are shown (**b**)

- The graft was shuttled underneath the peroneals and then from posterior to anterior to the fibular tunnel and then underneath the soft tissues through the talar tunnel (Fig. 13.5).
- The ankle was reduced in maximal posterior translation and eversion.
- The graft was then secured in place with a 4 × 10 mm Bio-Tenodesis screw in the talar tunnel and a 4 × 10 mm Bio-Tenodesis screw in the fibular tunnel with the ankle reduced (Fig. 13.6a–c).

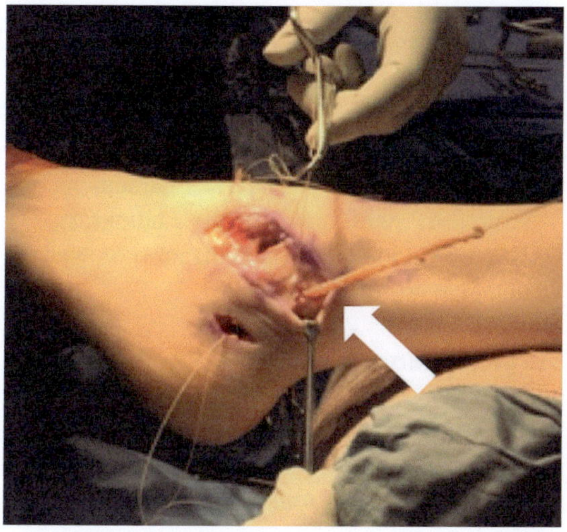

Fig. 13.5 The graft is shuttled under the peroneal tendons, then posteriorly to anteriorly through the fibular tunnel, and finally under the soft tissues and out the medial aspect of the talus through the talar tunnel. The arrow indicated the graft being shuttled under the peroneals

Ankle Stabilization

- Four 2-0 Ethibond sutures were placed in a mattress-type fashion off the periosteal sleeve of the fibula and into the ATFL, CFL, and capsule.
- The ankle was placed into maximum posterior translation as well as eversion, and the sutures were all tied down.
- Three 0 Vicryl sutures were also placed in a mattress-type fashion across the extensor retinaculum, and the ankle was again placed into maximum posterior translation as well as eversion, and the sutures were all tied down.

Closing

- The patient was placed in a non-weight-bearing splint in eversion for 2 weeks.

Postoperative Course

- After the splint was removed, the patient was placed into a cast and was told to remain non-weight-bearing for 4 weeks.
- After 4 weeks in the cast, the patient was placed into a controlled ankle movement (CAM) walker boot and was allowed to progress to partial weight-bearing. She was allowed

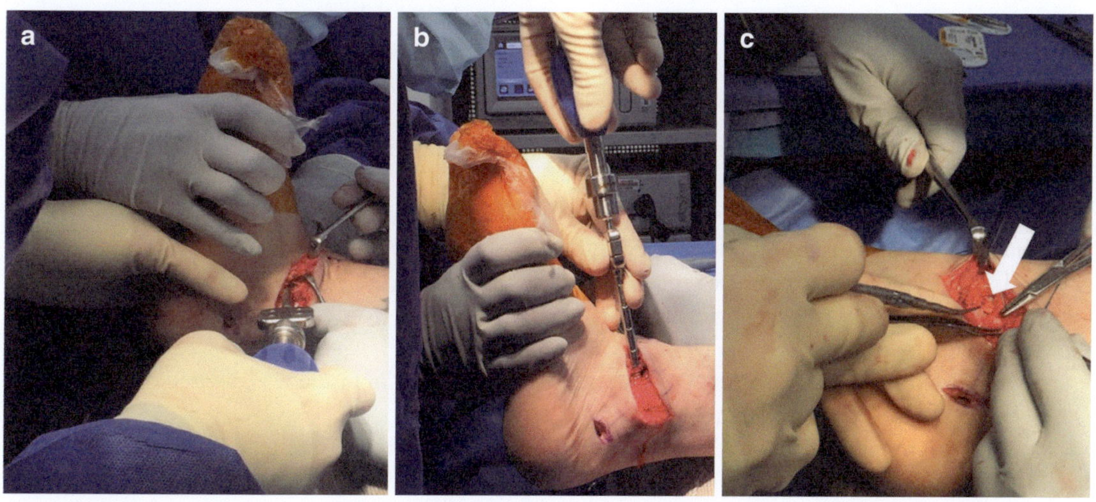

Fig. 13.6 With the ankle reduced in maximal eversion and posterior translation, a Bio-Tenodesis screw is used to secure the graft in the talus (**a**) and the fibula (**b**). The graft is then secured, and the ATFL limb of the graft is pictured (**c**)

to start with 50 pounds and advance 25–50 pounds per week, as guided by her physical therapist.

- At 3 months postoperatively, the patient was instructed to begin wearing sneakers and continue strengthening and stretching in physical therapy. The patient was given an ASO lace-up ankle brace to provide extra support when the ankle still felt symptomatic.
- At 6 months postoperatively, the patient could return to sport (Fig. 13.7).

Implants

- Two 4 × 10 mm Bio-Tenodesis screws
- One 4.75 × 15 mm Bio-Tenodesis interference screw

Pearls and Pitfalls

- Previous stabilization procedure had failed, and the remaining tissue was attenuated.
- It is necessary to evaluate other pathologies including OCLs, peroneal tendons, and foot alignment with this procedure.
- If the patient's tissue was good and poor technique led to the need for revision, a Brostrom-Gould procedure may have been suitable.
- It's unclear why the patient's original surgery failed. We speculate the use of only one anchor could have been a contributing factor.

Case 13.2

History

- A 23-year-old female, presented with a longstanding history of right ankle problems.
  - Patient had multiple ankle sprains (exact number not known) as a child that eventually led to a Chrisman-Snook procedure at an outside facility 10 years prior to presenting to us.
    - This led her to do well for 9 years until she had a very bad sprain falling down stairs 4 months prior to presenting to our office.
  - On physical exam, 1+ anterior drawer noted.
  - Radiographs and stress radiographs were taken. Stress radiographs showed 8 degrees of varus opening (Fig. 13.8a, b).
  - Determination to proceed with conservative treatment which included the use of an ASO lace-up ankle brace as well as physical therapy.
- Patient returned in 2 months and felt as though the problem has not been resolved from conservative treatment.
  - Her MRI was reviewed at this time and showed no tendon remaining from the initial lateral ligament reconstruction. It also showed that she had no OCLs.
- Due to the lack of progression, we advised the patient to undergo a lateral ligament reconstruction with hamstring autograft, a Brostrom-Gould-type stabilization as well as an ankle arthroscopy.

Surgical Plan

Positioning

- Place the patient in a supine position.
- Place a nonsterile tourniquet on the operative thigh.

Ankle Arthroscopy

- The patient was placed in a noninvasive ankle distraction.
- Standard anteromedial and anterolateral ports were established, and a diagnostic arthroscopy was performed.
- A grade 1 change was found in the talar dome and tibial plafond but no full-thickness cartilage lesions.

Hamstring Autograft

- A 3 cm incision was made over the medial aspect of the proximal tibia, and dissection was carried out to the level of the sartorial fascia.
- The sartorial fascia was divided in line with its fibers.
- The gracilis and semitendinosus were exposed. The gracilis was small (only 3.5 mm); therefore the decision was made to use the semitendinosus which was more robust.

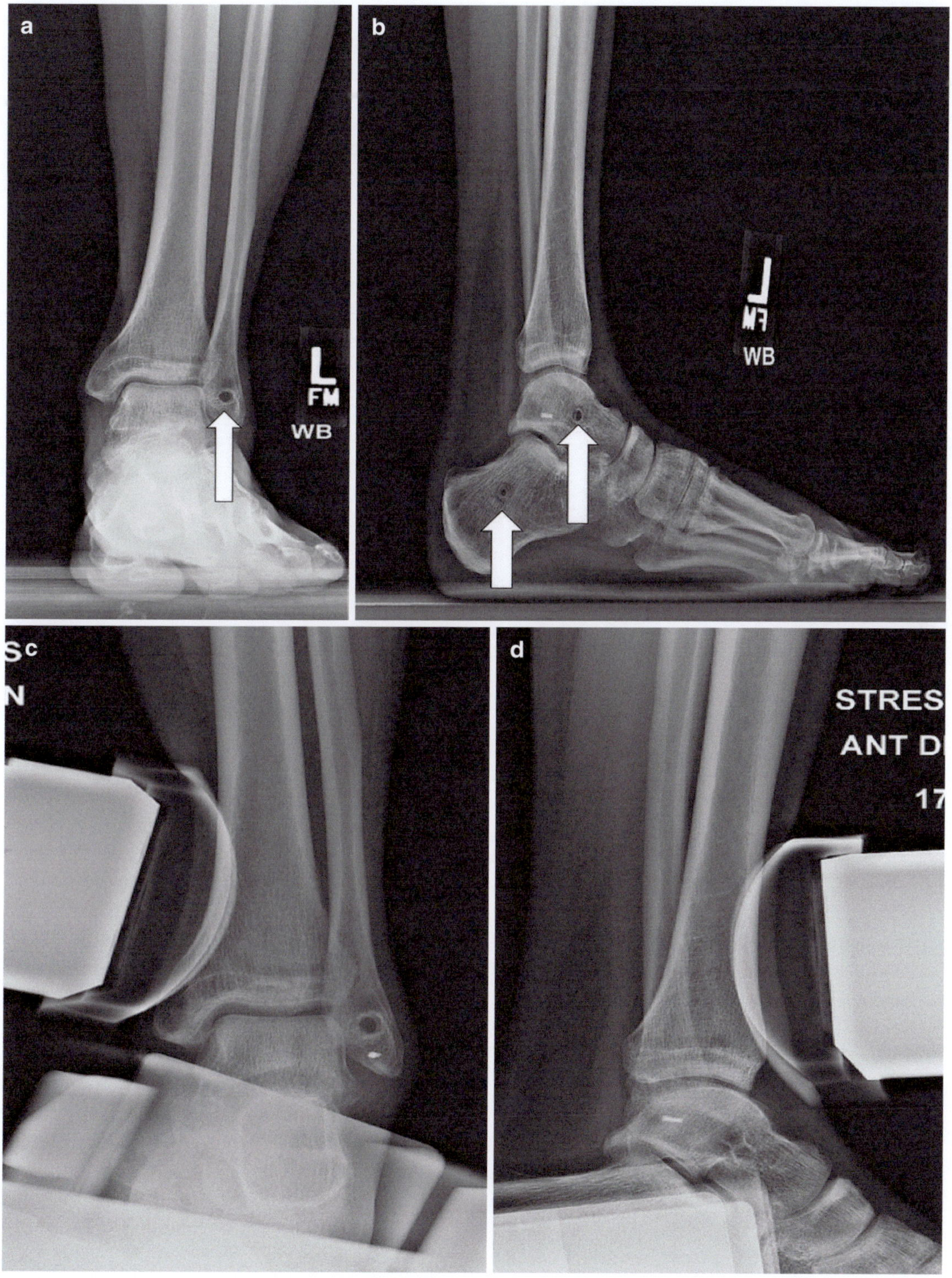

Fig. 13.7 Standard anteroposterior (**a**) and lateral (**b**) postoperative x-rays for **Case 13.1** patient show the location of each of the bone tunnels (arrows). Anteroposterior and lateral postoperative stress test images show a reduced talar tilt (**c**) and anterior drawer (**d**) when compared to preoperative images, indicating a successful repair. Images were taken 8 months postoperatively

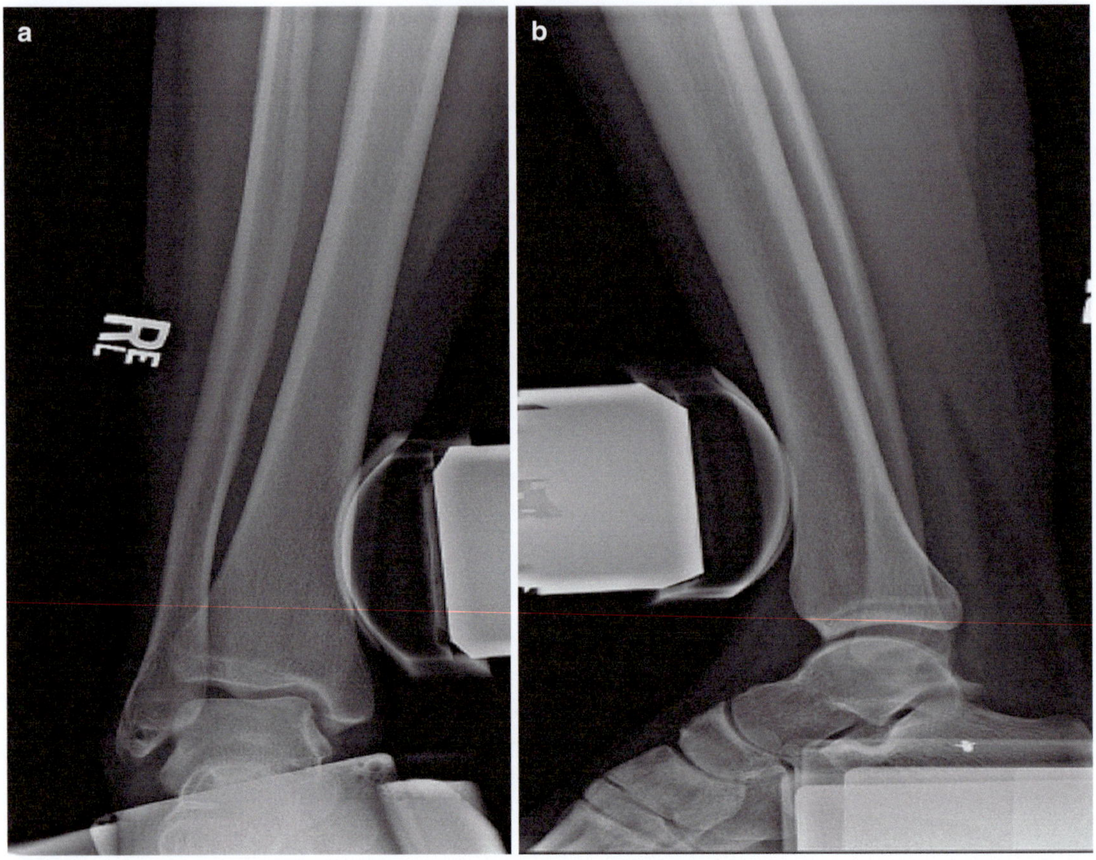

Fig. 13.8 Preoperative anteroposterior (**a**) and lateral (**b**) stress x-rays showing increased talar tilt and anterior drawer, respectively, in **Case 13.2** patient

- The semitendinosus was harvested using a Linvatec tendon stripper (ConMed; Utica, NY).
- Muscle remnants were removed from the semitendinosus using a ruler, and then it was attached to the Graft Master (Smith & Nephew; Andover, MA) and tubularized using 0 Vicryl suture.
- The graft measured a size 4.5 mm.

Ankle Reconstruction

- A 6 cm incision was made over the patient's previous incision, and dissection was carried out to the level of the fibula.
- The ATFL and CFL were removed off the fibula.
- Part of the peroneus brevis was identified.
- There was no tissue within the fibula.
- The distal peroneus tendon was debrided off the subcutaneous tissues.
- The remaining peroneus brevis and the peroneus longus had no focal tears present.
- A separate incision was then made over the calcaneofibular ligament insertion, right behind the peroneal tendons. Dissection was carried out to the level of the calcaneus.
- A 4.5 drill bit was placed at the calcaneus.
- Sutures were then shuttled underneath the peroneal tendons.
- Another drill hole was then placed at the origin of the ATFL (from anterior to posterior across the fibula).
- A third tunnel was then made at the talus (at the anterior aspect of the lateral process of the talus).
- Tunnel position was confirmed with fluoroscopy.
- The graft was then placed in the calcaneal tunnel and secured in place using a 4.75 × 15 mm Bio-Tenodesis screw.

- The graft was shuttled underneath the peroneals and then from posterior to anterior to the fibular tunnel and then underneath the soft tissues through the talar tunnel.
- The ankle was reduced in maximum posterior translation and eversion.
- The graft was then secured in place with a 4 × 10 mm Bio-Tenodesis screw in the talar tunnel and a 4 × 10 mm Bio-Tenodesis screw in the fibular tunnel, while the ankle was reduced.

Ankle Stabilization

- Three 2-0 Ethibond sutures were placed in a mattress-type fashion off the periosteal sleeve of the fibula and into the ATFL, CFL, and capsule.
- The ankle was placed into maximum posterior translation as well as eversion, and the sutures were all tied down.
- Three 3-0 Vicryl sutures were also placed in a mattress-type fashion across the extensor retinaculum, and the ankle was again placed into maximum posterior translation as well as eversion, and the sutures were all tied down.

Closing

- Steri-Strips and a sterile dressing were applied to the wound.
- The patient was placed in eversion in a non-weight-bearing splint for 2 weeks.

Postoperative Course

- After the splint was removed, the patient was placed into a cast and was told to remain non-weight-bearing for 4 weeks
- After 4 weeks in the cast, the patient was placed into a controlled ankle movement (CAM) walker boot and was allowed to progress to partial weight-bearing. She was allowed to start with 50 pounds and advance 25–50 pounds per week, as guided by his physical therapist.
- At 3 months postoperatively, the patient was instructed to begin wearing sneakers and continue strengthening and stretching in physical therapy. The patient was given an ASO lace-up ankle brace to provide extra support when the ankle still felt symptomatic (Fig. 13.9a–d).

Implants

- Two 4 × 10 mm Bio-Tenodesis screws
- One 4.75 × 15 mm Bio-Tenodesis interference screw

Pearls and Pitfalls

- Previous stabilization had failed; Chrisman-Snook is not an ideal procedure, especially in cases of severe chronic ankle instability, frequently leading to subtalar arthrosis and nonanatomic reconstruction.

Case 13.3

History

- A 39-year-old female presented with a long-standing history of right ankle problems.
  - Patient had had over 100 ankle sprains.
  - Patient had a right ankle reconstruction 20 years prior to reporting to us.
  - Patient had Ehlers-Danlos type 3.
  - On physical exam, 2+ anterior drawer was noted.
  - Radiographs and stress radiographs were taken. Stress radiographs showed 12 degrees of varus opening (Fig. 13.10a, b).
  - MRI was reviewed and showed no OCLs.
- Patient was indicated for a lateral ligament reconstruction with hamstring allograft, a Brostrom-Gould-type stabilization as well as an ankle arthroscopy.

Surgical Plan

Positioning

- Place the patient in a supine position.
- Place a nonsterile tourniquet on the operative thigh.

Ankle Arthroscopy

- The patient was placed in a noninvasive ankle distraction.
- Standard anteromedial and anterolateral ports were established, and a diagnostic arthroscopy was performed.
- Significant impingement lesions were found in both the anteromedial and anterolateral gutters.
  - These were debrided with a 2.9 shaver.

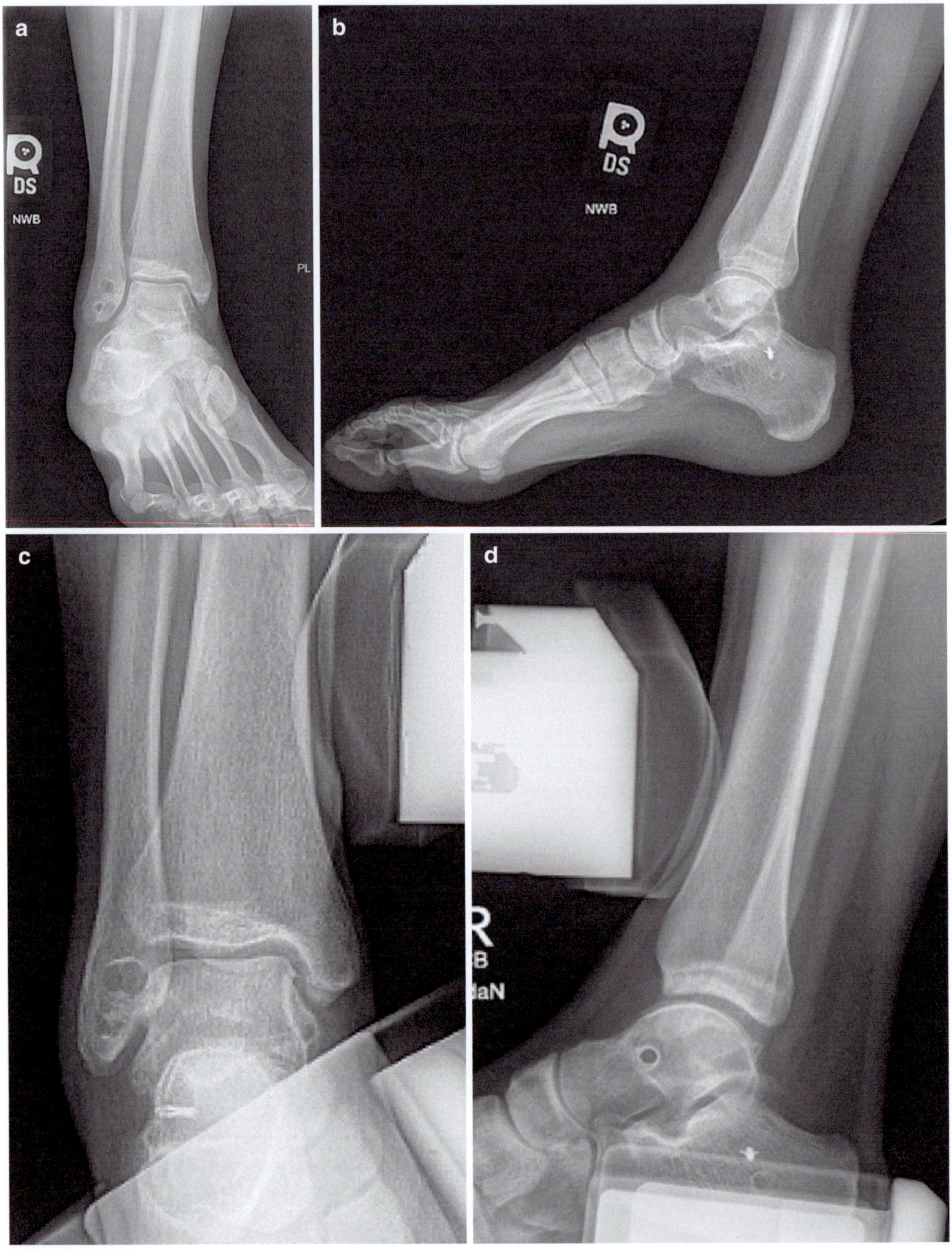

Fig. 13.9 Standard oblique (**a**) and lateral (**b**) 3-months postoperative x-rays for **Case 13.2** patient. Anteroposterior and lateral postoperative stress test images show a reduced talar tilt (**c**) and anterior drawer (**d**) when compared to preoperative images, indicating a successful repair

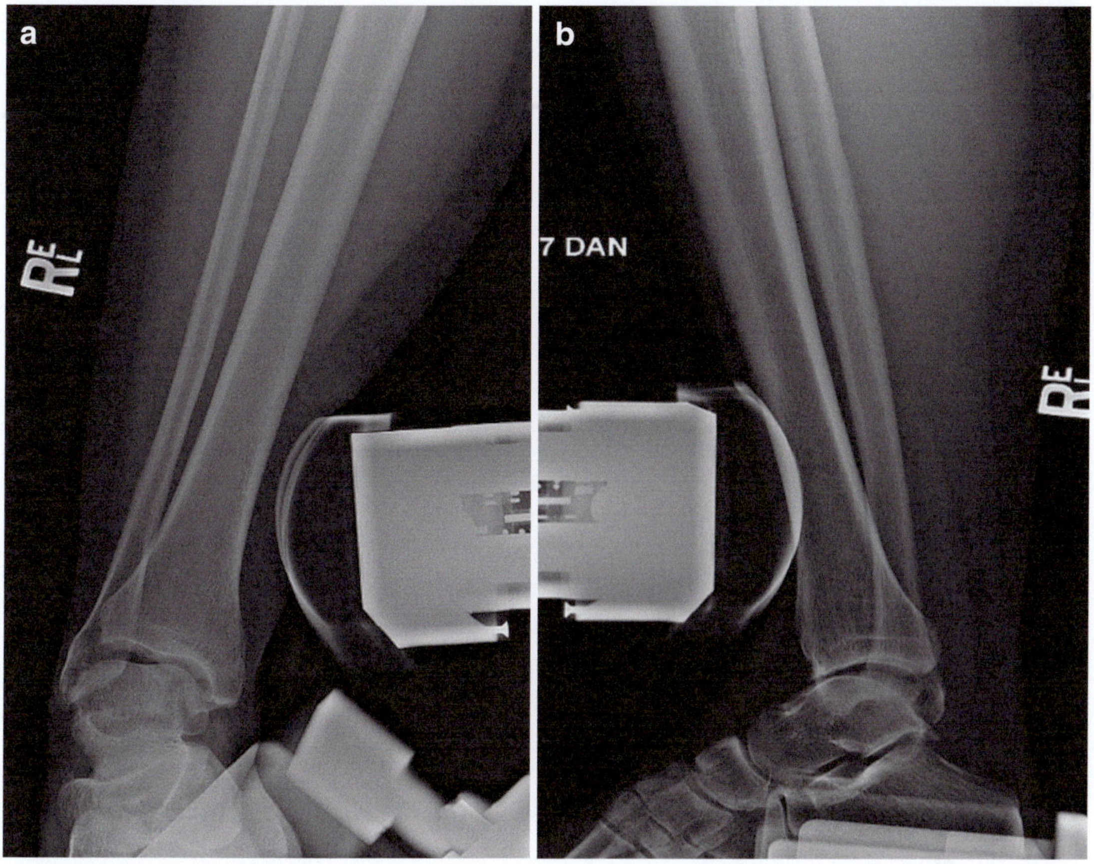

Fig. 13.10 Preoperative anteroposterior (**a**) and lateral (**b**) stress x-rays showing increased talar tilt and anterior drawer, respectively, in **Case 13.3** patient

- A full-thickness (approximately 7 mm) defect was found in the medial talar dome.
- Microfracture holes were placed in this area.
- The patient had an anterior tibial exostosis.
  - This was debrided down with a 4.0 bur.
- Full-thickness cartilage loss was also found over the anterior tibial plafond.
  - This was debrided using a 4.0 bur and filled using BioCartilage + BMAC.
- The patient was taken out of the noninvasive ankle distraction.

Hamstring Allograft

- An allograft was used due to the patient's history of Ehlers-Danlos type 3.
- The allograft was tubularized using 0 Vicryl.
- It measured a size 5 mm × 30 cm.

Ankle Reconstruction

- A 5 cm curvilinear incision was made over the fibula dissection and was carried out to the level of the fibula.
- The ATFL and CFL were removed off the fibula.
- The patient's tissue quality was observed and noted to be patulous without good integrity.
- A separate small incision was made posterior to the fibula to inspect the peroneal tendons, which appeared to be good quality.
- A separate incision was then made over the calcaneofibular ligament insertion, right behind the peroneal tendons. Dissection was carried out to the level of the calcaneus.
- A 5.5 drill bit was placed at the calcaneus.

- Another drill hole was then placed at the origin of the ATFL (from anterior to posterior across the fibula), using a 5 drill bit.
- A third tunnel was then made at the talus (at the anterior aspect of the lateral process of the talus).
- Tunnel position was confirmed with fluoroscopy.
- The graft was then placed in the calcaneal tunnel and secured in place using a 5.5 × 15 mm Bio-Tenodesis screw.
- The graft was shuttled underneath the peroneals and then from posterior to anterior to the fibular tunnel and then underneath the soft tissues through the talar tunnel.
- The ankle was reduced in maximum posterior translation and eversion.
- The graft was then secured in place with a 4.75 × 12 mm Bio-Tenodesis screw in the talar tunnel and a 4.75 × 12 mm Bio-Tenodesis screw in the fibular tunnel with the ankle reduced.

Ankle Stabilization

- Four 2-0 Ethibond sutures were placed in a mattress-type fashion off the periosteal sleeve of the fibula and into the ATFL, CFL, and capsule.
- The ankle was placed into maximum posterior translation as well as eversion, and the sutures were all tied down.
- Three 3-0 Vicryl sutures were also placed in a mattress-type fashion across the extensor retinaculum, and the ankle was again placed into maximum posterior translation as well as eversion, and the sutures were all tied down.

Closing

- Steri-Strips and a sterile dressing were applied to the wound.
- The patient was placed in eversion in a non-weight-bearing splint for 2 weeks.

Postoperative Course

- After the split was removed, the patient was placed into a CAM walker boot and was told to remain non-weight-bearing for 4 weeks
- After 4 weeks in the CAM walker boot, she was allowed to progress to partial weight-bearing. She was allowed to stat with 50 pounds and advance 25–50 pounds per week, as guided by his physical therapist.
- At 3 months postoperatively, the patient was instructed to begin wearing sneakers and continue strengthening and stretching in physical therapy. The patient was given an ASO lace-up ankle brace to provide extra support when the ankle still felt symptomatic.
- At 6 months postoperatively, patient could return to sports (Fig. 13.11a–d).

Implants

- Two 4.75 × 12 mm Bio-Tenodesis screws
- One 5.5 × 15 mm Bio-Tenodesis interference screw

Pearls and Pitfalls

- Previous stabilization not enough with combination of Ehlers-Danlos type 3 syndrome, making use of additional tissue necessary/helpful

Case 13.4

History

- A 41-year-old male presented with a 3-year history of right ankle pain.
  - Patient reported many past ankle sprains (exact number unknown).
  - Patient twisted his ankle and felt a pop the day before presenting to the office.
  - Patient had a right ankle reconstruction 9 years prior to presenting to us that did well for 6 years and had been hurting for the past 3 years.
  - Patient's hindfoot alignment was cavovarus (Fig. 13.12a–c).
  - On physical exam, 2+ anterior drawer noted.
  - Radiographs and stress radiographs were taken. Stress radiographs showed 17 degrees of varus opening (Fig. 13.13a, b).

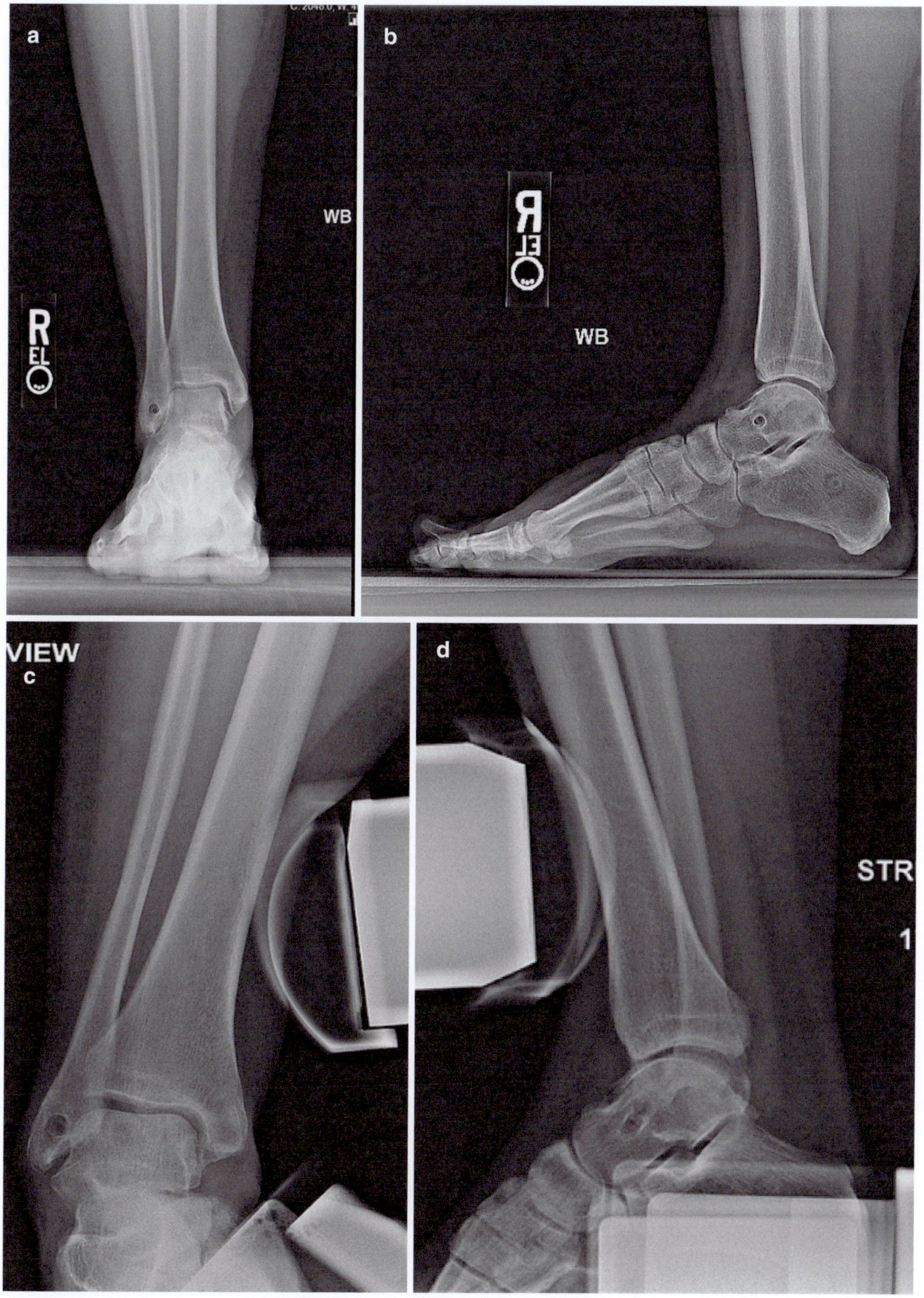

Fig. 13.11 Standard anteroposterior (**a**) and lateral (**b**) 6-months postoperative x-rays for **Case 13.3** patient. Anteroposterior and lateral postoperative stress test images show a reduced talar tilt (**c**) and anterior drawer (**d**) when compared to preoperative images, indicating a successful repair

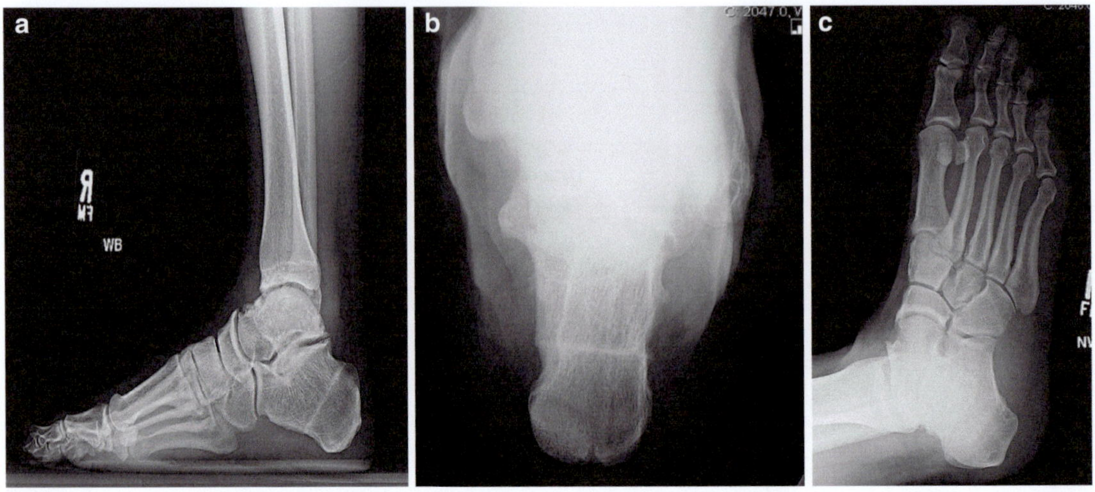

Fig. 13.12 Preoperative x-rays for **Case 13.4** patient showing cavovarus hindfoot alignment (**a**–**c**)

- Patient was indicated for an MRI to further assess the area of interest and, for the interim, was given an ASO lace-up brace to provide extra support.
- Patient returned 3 weeks later to review MRI.
  - MRI showed no OCLs and present peroneal tendons, but peroneal tendinopathy was present.

- Patient was indicated for a lateral ligament reconstruction with hamstring autograft, a lateralizing calcaneal osteotomy, and peroneal tendon reconstruction as well as a Brostrom-Gould-type stabilization and ankle arthroscopy.

Surgical Plan

Positioning

- Place the patient in a supine position.
- Place a nonsterile tourniquet on the operative thigh.

Ankle Arthroscopy

- The patient was placed in a noninvasive ankle distraction.
- Standard anteromedial and anterolateral ports were established, and a diagnostic arthroscopy was performed.
- Significant impingement lesions were found in both the anteromedial and anterolateral gutters.
  - These were debrided with a 2.9 shaver.
- The patient had an 8 mm loose body in the medial gutter which was removed with a grasper.
- The patient had several areas of chondral injury on the talar dome that were all debrided. Of note, all were grade 2 or 3, and none were full-thickness chondral injuries.
- The patient was taken out of the noninvasive ankle distraction.

Hamstring Autograft

- A 3 cm incision was made over the medial aspect of the proximal tibia, and dissection was carried out to the level of the sartorial fascia.
- The sartorial fascia was divided in line with its fibers.
- The gracilis and semitendinosus were exposed.
- The gracilis and semitendinosus were harvested using a Linvatec tendon stripper (ConMed; Utica, NY).
- Muscle remnants were removed from both tendons using a ruler, and then each was attached to the Graft Master (Smith &

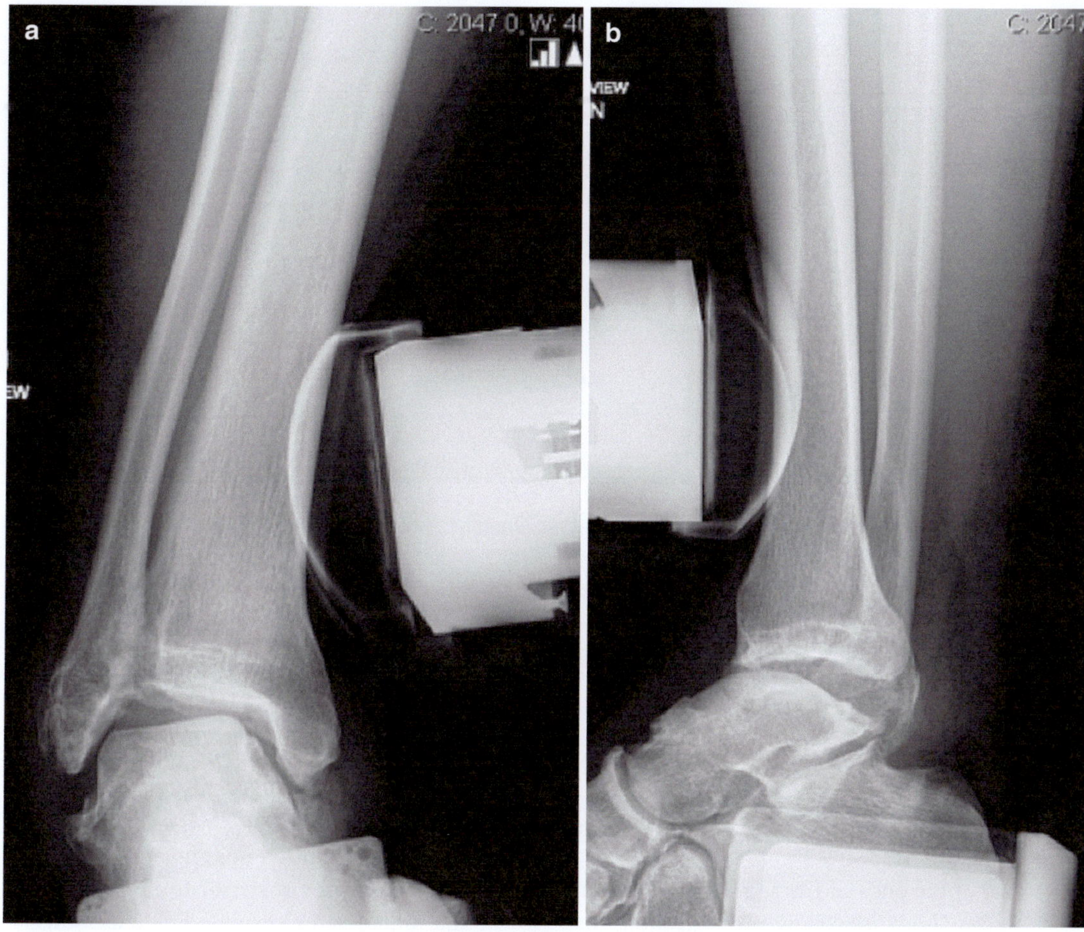

Fig. 13.13 Preoperative anteroposterior (**a**) and lateral (**b**) stress x-rays showing increased talar tilt and anterior drawer, respectively, in **Case 13.4** patient

Nephew; Andover, MA) and tubularized using 0 Vicryl suture.

- The graft measured a size 4.5 mm.

Calcaneal Osteotomy

- A 3 cm incision was made posteriorly on the patient's heel, and dissection was carried down to the level of the calcaneus.
- The lateral aspect of the calcaneus was exposed using a Bovie and a periosteal elevator.
- An oscillating saw was then used to make a posterior calcaneal osteotomy in front of the Achilles, distal to the weight-bearing part of the tibial tuber.
- A curved osteotome was then used to translate the calcaneus 1 cm laterally.
- The osteotome was used to hold the calcaneus in place, and two 6.5 screws were placed percutaneously into the calcaneal tuber across the osteotomy site (Fig. 13.14a–c).

Ankle Reconstruction and Peroneus Brevis Reconstruction

- A 6 cm curvilinear incision was made along the base of the ankle, and dissection was carried out to the level of the fibula.
- The ATFL, CFL, and capsule were removed off the fibula all the way back to the peroneal tendons.
- The patient's peroneus longus was noted to be completely ruptured, and the peroneus brevis was intact but very thin and attenuated with

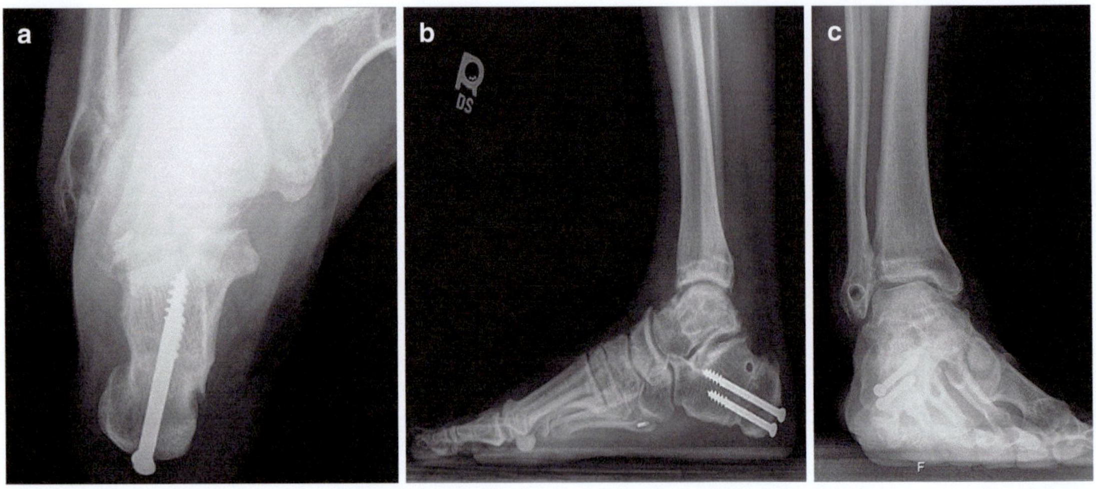

Fig. 13.14 Postoperative x-rays showing corrected hindfoot alignment following calcaneal osteotomy in **Case 13.4**

many fissures and longitudinal tears along the tendon.

- This led to the decision to perform a peroneus brevis reconstruction.
  - An incision was made along the base of the 5th MT, and dissection was carried out to the level of the 5th MT.
  - A drill was used to place a hole in the base of the 5th MT.
  - One of the ends of the semitendinosus was placed in a Krackow-type fashion and secured with a G2 anchor.
  - A kite string maneuver was used to retract the tendon back down to the bone.
  - The tendon was then tunneled in the peroneal tunnel, and a Pulvertaft maneuver was used. The graft was tensioned with the foot in slight neutral and slight eversion.
  - The graft was secured in place using 2-0 Orthocord sutures.
- At this point, the tourniquet was let down.
- A separate incision was then made over the calcaneofibular ligament insertion, right behind the peroneal tendons. Dissection was carried out to the level of the calcaneus.
- A 5.0 drill bit was placed at the calcaneus.
- Another drill hole was then placed at the origin of the ATFL (from anterior to posterior across the fibula), using a 4.5 drill bit.
- A third tunnel was then made at the talus (at the anterior aspect of the lateral process of the talus).
- Tunnel position was confirmed with fluoroscopy.
- The graft was then placed in the calcaneal tunnel and secured in place using a 4.75 × 15 mm Bio-Tenodesis screw.
- The graft was shuttled underneath the peroneals and then from posterior to anterior to the fibular tunnel and then underneath the soft tissues through the talar tunnel.
- The graft was then secured in place with a 4.75 × 15 mm Bio-Tenodesis screw in the talar tunnel and a 4.75 × 15 mm Bio-Tenodesis screw in the fibular tunnel.

Ankle Stabilization

- Four 2-0 Ethibond sutures were placed in a mattress-type fashion off the periosteal sleeve of the fibula and into the ATFL, CFL, and capsule.
- The ankle was placed into maximum posterior translation as well as eversion, and the sutures were all tied down.
- Four 0 Vicryl sutures were also placed in a mattress-type fashion across the extensor retinaculum, and the ankle was again placed into maximum posterior translation as well as eversion, and the sutures were all tied down.

Peroneal Retinaculum Repair

- Three 2-0 Ethibond sutures were used in a pants-over-vest-type fashion so that there was no dislocation of the reconstructed peroneus brevis.

Closing

- Steri-Strips and a sterile dressing were applied to the wound.
- The patient was placed in a non-weight-bearing splint for 2 weeks.

Postoperative Course

- After the splint was removed, the patient was placed into a cast and was told to remain non-weight-bearing for 4 weeks.
- After 4 weeks in the cast, he was allowed to progress to partial weight-bearing in a CAM walker boot. He was allowed to start with 50 pounds and advance 25–50 pounds per week, as guided by his physical therapist.
- At 3 months postoperatively, the patient was instructed to begin wearing sneakers and continue strengthening and stretching in physical therapy. The patient was given an ASO lace-up ankle brace to provide extra support when the ankle still felt symptomatic.

Implants

- Three 4.75 × 15 mm Bio-Tenodesis interference screws
- One G2 Anchor

Pearls and Pitfalls

- Previous stabilization not enough/indicated to fail due to cavovarus foot. Peroneal pathology made problem worse.
- In addition to the stabilization, the cavovarus deformity must be addressed. Possible corrective surgeries include first-ray dorsiflexion osteotomy, flexor lengthening, plantar fascia release, and calcaneal osteotomy. The specific deformity will determine which procedures are necessary.

Summary

Ankle sprains are a very common problem in the United States. While 85% of people with an ankle sprain will recover without operative intervention, it has been reported that 20–40% of patients experience repeated sprains which can eventually lead to chronic ankle instability [1, 3]. The gold standard operation for a patient with symptomatic chronic ankle instability that is not responsive to conservative treatment has been debated over the years. In recent literature, the modified Brostrom has been considered the best option for repair of chronic ankle instability, with success reported in 90% of patients [1, 5, 9]. Despite these high levels of success, there are several reasons that a primary repair, such as a modified Brostrom, can fail. In some patients, failure is due to a more antiquated, nonanatomic procedure, such as a Chrisman-Snook. In others, generalized ligamentous laxity or Ehlers-Danlos syndrome, which leaves patients with lower quality tissue than the average person, can lead to a failed primary repair due to lack of healthy tissue available to provide a sufficient repair. In others, the use of an inappropriate graft, such as a peroneus, can lead to an imperfect, nonanatomic reconstruction and can fail. Furthermore, malalignment of the foot can lead patients to failed ankle stabilization. In patients with a pronounced cavovarus foot and chronic ankle instability, the underlying foot deformity puts the patient at risk of failing treatment unless it is addressed. In a study on the use of augmented repairs, revision surgery was needed in 13 cases following failed primary repairs due to limited (0-2) anchors used during primary reconstruction, a failed Chrisman-Snook procedure, the presence of generalized ligamentous laxity, a case of Ehlers-Danlos disease, and two cases in a cavovarus setting. In difficult cases, we advocate a lateral ligament reconstruction, with either a hamstring autograft or an allograft if the patient's own tissue is not suitable for use, as well as a modified Brostrom and a diagnostic arthroscopy to identify and treat chondral injuries. Care should also be paid to the peroneal tendons and any other concurrent pathology present.

References

1. Shakked R, Sheskier S. Acute and chronic lateral ankle instability diagnosis, management, and new concepts. Bull Hosp Jt Dis (2013). 2017;75(1):71–80.
2. Chrisman OD, Snook GA. Reconstruction of lateral ligament tears of the ankle. An experimental study and clinical evaluation of seven patients treated by a new modification of the Elmslie procedure. J Bone Joint Surg Am. 1969;51:904–12.
3. Jung H-G, Kim T-H, Park J-Y, Bae E-J. Anatomic reconstruction of the anterior talofibular and calcaneofibular ligaments using a semitendinosus tendon allograft and interference screws. Knee Surg Sports Traumatol Arthrosc. 2012;20(8):1432–7.
4. Chrisman OD, Snook GA. Reconstruction of lateral of the ankle ligament tears. J Bone Joint Surg Am. 1969;51-A:904–11.
5. Hennrikus WL, Mapes RC, Lyons PM, Lapoint JM. Outcomes of the Chrisman-Snook and modified-Broström procedures for chronic lateral ankle instability. A prospective, randomized comparison. Am J Sports Med. 1996;24:400–4.
6. Russo A, Giacchè P, Marcantoni E, Arrighi A, Molfetta L. Treatment of chronic lateral ankle instability using the Broström-Gould procedure in athletes: long-term results. Joints. 2016;4:94–7.
7. Huang B, Kim YT, Kim JU, Shin JH, Park YW, Kim HN. Modified Broström procedure for chronic ankle instability with generalized joint hypermobility. Am J Sports Med. 2016;44:1011–6.
8. Ibrahim SA, Hamido F, Al Misfer AK, Ghafar SA, Awad A, Salem HK, et al. Anatomical reconstruction of the lateral ligaments using Gracillis tendon in chronic ankle instability; a new technique. Foot Ankle Surg. 2011;17:239–46.
9. Miller AG, Raikin SM, Ahmad J. Near-anatomic allograft tenodesis of chronic lateral ankle instability. Foot Ankle Int. 2013;34:1501–7.
10. Tourné Y, Mabit C. Lateral ligament reconstruction procedures for the ankle. Orthop Traumatol Surg Res. 2017;103(1S):S171–81.
11. Park CH, Lee W-C. Donor site morbidity after lateral ankle ligament reconstruction using the anterior half of the Peroneus Longus Tendon autograft. Am J Sports Med. 2017;45:922–8.
12. Song B, Li C, Chen N, Chen Z, Zhang Y, Zhou Y, et al. All-arthroscopic anatomical reconstruction of anterior talofibular ligament using semitendinosus autografts. Int Orthop. 2017;41:975–82.
13. Shakked R., DeSandis B, Drakos MC. Lateral ligament reconstruction with hamstring graft for severe and revision cases of ankle instability. E-poster presented at: 2016 AOFAS Annual Meeting; 2016 July 20–23; Toronto, Canada.

Revision Surgery of the Peroneal Tendon

14

Eric Giza, Christopher D. Kreulen,
and Karim Boukhemis

Key Takeaway Points

- It is important to evaluate the initial cause of the symptoms.
- Take into account the structure of the foot (cavus or valgus).
- Repair of the cartilaginous corner is paramount in keeping the peroneal tendons within their groove.
- Do not cause an iatrogenic tenodesis effect by repairing the inferior peroneal retinaculum too tight.
- It is important to check post repair excursion.

Introduction

The peroneus longus tendon originates on the lateral tibial condyle and fibular head and inserts on the plantar aspect of the base of the first cuneiform and first metatarsal. It serves as an ankle and great toe plantar flexor, everter, and helps with longitudinal arch support. The peroneus brevis originates from the lateral fibula and inserts on the base of the fifth metatarsal. The tendons share a common sheath, and the peroneus longus is oriented posterior to the brevis until they cross at the tip of the lateral malleolus. They are split by the peroneal tubercle of the calcaneus just inferior to the tip of the lateral malleolus. The superior peroneal retinaculum (SPR) arises from the lateral malleolus periosteum and inserts on the lateral calcaneus and Achilles tendon [1]. It stabilizes the peroneal tendons in their retromalleolar location. An injury to the SPR can cause peroneal tendon subluxation or dislocation. The peroneal tendons are subject to multiple pathologies including tenosynovitis [2, 3], tears, ruptures, subluxation, dislocation, and painful os peroneum. Determining the cause of continued pain and the pathology behind it can be difficult to determine.

E. Giza · C. D. Kreulen · K. Boukhemis (✉)
University of California at Davis, Department of Orthopaedics, Sacramento, CA, USA

Radiographic Evaluation/Assessment

There are many ways to evaluate peroneal pathology, but first, it is always recommended to obtain standard weight-bearing three-view x-rays of the foot and ankle. This helps to evaluate for any pathologic bony component that may be causing the pain or discomfort. After radiographs are obtained, further imaging can be requested. Historically, tenography has been performed in evaluating the tendons. This is not performed as often today with the advent of MRI. MRI has been the imaging modality of choice in recent

M. J. Berkowitz et al. (eds.), *Revision Surgery of the Foot and Ankle*,
https://doi.org/10.1007/978-3-030-29969-9_14

years. Slowly, dynamic ultrasound has been used more and more to evaluate peroneal tendon pathology [4]. Realistically, a thorough evaluation is accomplished with a combination of MR and ultrasonography together. Of course, despite new technologies and imaging, a full physical exam should clue you in to subluxing peroneal tendons or possibly a painful tenosynovitis. Patients may have a distant history of a severe ankle sprain. Usually, the tendons can be visibly subluxing on exam and/or easily reduced with manipulation. A key maneuver to detect subluxing peroneals or even painful pathology is to ask the patient to dorsiflex and evert the foot and ankle from a plantarflexed, inverted position. Recreation of symptoms can lead you to hone further studies to this area [5]. Another method has been described known as peroneal tunnel compression test for longitudinal peroneus brevis tendon tear [6].

Tears

Peroneal tendon tears can occur from a variety of different etiologies. Acute peroneal tears or dislocations are the result of sudden forced dorsiflexion with a concomitant reflexive contraction of the peroneal muscles [7–9]. Tears can also occur from inversion injuries or recurrent lateral instability. Injuries to the superior peroneal retinaculum can also cause subluxation which leads to mechanical abrasion of the tendons [6, 7, 9–12]. Brevis tears are more likely to occur in the peroneal sulcus. The brevis is under more stress in the region and can have abrasion from the peroneus longus [12–14]. Peroneus longus tears are less common than brevis tears. Both brevis and longus repairs are typically tubularized after debridement if less than 50% of the tendon is involved. If greater than 50% of the tendon is involved, then the tendon is debrided and tenodesed to the peroneus longus or vice versa [12].

Ruptures

Ruptures of the longus or brevis are rare but do occur. Some debate whether the presence of an os peroneum could predispose the peroneus longus to degenerative tearing. Other etiologies have included autoimmune diseases such as rheumatoid arthritis and psoriasis as well as diabetes. This is usually a nontraumatic cause. Treatment with steroid injections can also weaken the tendons and lead to rupture. Multiple treatment modalities have been discussed in the literature including approximation of the tendon ends, suture anchor within the cuboid, and partial tenodesis. Occasionally, a free graft or autograft is necessary to bridge the gap. Rupture in a cross-country skier has been reported in a case report [15]. There have also been reports of simultaneous rupture in bilateral peroneal tendons following steroid injections treated with repair and tenodesis [16]. A professional soccer player also has a rupture after inversion injury with no prior lesions based on previous MRI [17]. Infrequently, a rupture can be preceded by synovitis, seen in a collegiate athlete [18].

Subluxation/Dislocation

Most subluxations/dislocations are caused from a traumatic event. Mostly, these can correspond to an athletic event, most notably alpine skiing, ice skating, and running. The calcaneofibular portion of the SPR lies parallel to the calcaneofibular ligament (CFL), and tears of the CFL could lead to increased strain and instability with the SPR [10, 13]. The mechanism is usually a sudden forceful dorsiflexion and inversion with simultaneous contraction of the peroneals. Most of these injuries are rarely caught acutely, and the patient continues to have symptoms months after the event. The superior peroneal retinaculum is a continuation of the fascia of the lower calf and is the primary restraint to peroneal subluxation/dislocation. An injury to this structure can, and often, lead to peroneal instability. An additional factor that can predispose an individual to recurrent instability is a convex fibular groove or deficient lateral ridge; this is debatable. Immobilization in some form of cast or boot can be offered but only has about 30–50% success [19, 20]. Athletes are commonly repaired surgically with SPR reinforcement [21]. Other techniques have included using the peroneal brevis, tertius, and even a slip of the Achilles. Tendon rerouting techniques have also been described, as well as bone block transfers. Finally, groove-deepening techniques were developed and saw some success [22].

Failure of Repair

Failure of repair may be closely connected with type of repair. Traumatic fracture of the fixation of graft used has been reported, as well as recurrence of pain. Adhesion of the tendons to the fresh bone block was also found [23]. Attenuation of the superior peroneal retinaculum has also been accused of recurrence after repair [24]. A zone of critical hypovascularity has also been suggested for repairs to fail [25]. Other mechanical reasons have been mentioned in the literature including mechanical impingement from the fibular groove, incompetence of the peroneal retinaculum, presence of a sharp posterior fibular ridge, dynamic compression between the peroneus longus and brevis, and finally the presence of a peroneus quartus muscle.

Septic Tenosynovitis

Schade et al. [26] report a case of septic peroneal tenosynovitis following lateral ankle reconstruction using allograft. The patient developed a postoperative infection, and eventually, the peroneal tendons desiccated. They were then excised from the musculotendinous junction to the base of the fifth metatarsal, and silicon rods were placed temporarily along with an external fixator. After the patient received the appropriate antibiotics, he had autograft tensor fascia lata rolled and used to reconstruct to the peroneal tendons. He also had Achilles tendon autograft to reconstruct the super peroneal retinaculum. The patient eventually returned full muscle strength and no objective ankle instability.

Fibular Groove Deepening/ Subluxation

The peroneal tendons do not have much support with a convex or flat "sulcus." Eleven percent of specimens had a flat "sulcus," and 7% were convex [27]. This can be deepened using a more minimally invasive technique described by Anderson. They reported good outcomes on 20 patients without quantifying their results [22, 28]. Kollias reported on 12 ankles in 11 patients that underwent fibular groove deepening. At mean of 6-year follow-up, 11 ankles were pain-free, 10 had full ROM, 10 returned to previous sport, and no recurrent subluxation [29].

Tendon Transfer

Wapner et al. performed a retrospective analysis on seven patients who underwent two-stage peroneal revision surgery. The seven patients had undergone at least two previous surgeries. The patients all had lateral ankle pain. They underwent debridement and placement of a 6 mm hunter rod. Three months later, they underwent FHL transfer and hunter rod removal. The reconstructed tendons were attached to the brevis distally. At 8.5 years, 7/8(1/8 WCpt) were doing well, did not use a brace, and returned to work. Only the workers' comp patient failed to return to work and used a brace [30].

Seybold et al. compared the FHL and FDL tendons for transfer. They found that the FHL tendon is larger, 5.1 mm compared to 4.5 mm, has less bulk in the retromalleolar groove, is longer, and would not cause tibial nerve compression. They recommend the FHL as the tendon transfer of choice for peroneal reconstruction [31].

Allograft

Rapley et al. used acellular dermal matrix allograft on 11 patients [32]. Two had prior surgery for debridement and instability repair, four had previous tenodesis, and all had either longitudinal tearing or completer rupture. Seven of the repairs had a gap jump, and in four of the repairs, the matrix was used to augment which allowed for earlier rehabilitation. Ten of the eleven patients had complete resolution of their symptoms, and 11/11 returned to previous level of sport. AOFAS mean was 93.5 (75–100). The rehab allowed active motion after week 1 and discontinuance of external immobilization after week 3. Pellegrini et al. have recently described a primary allograft technique. Reconstruction of the peroneal tendons using semitendinosus allograft has recently expanded the treatment armamentarium of peroneal tendon pathology and should be considered when addressing this problem [33].

Mook et al. used peroneal tendon or semitendinosus allograft for reconstructing brevis tears in 14 patients. Average length of segment was 10.8 cm with no difference in outcome based on graft length. SF-12, VAS, and LEFS scores all improved. Benefits include single-stage and no donor site morbidity and availability of allograft [34].

Autograft

Pellegrini et al. [35] wrote a case report on the reversal of peroneal tenodesis and reconstruction using TFL autograft. The patient had lateral ankle pain after multiple surgeries for clubfoot. She had tenodesis of the brevis to longus. The tendon was reconstructed using TFL autograft and Pulvertaft weave. She also had the fibular groove deepened using Anderson's technique [29]. Seventeen months after surgery, the patient had a significant reduction in pain and resumed normal activities [35].

Surgical Planning

First, it is important to obtain quality weight-bearing images of the foot and ankle. This helps to rule out any abnormal bony architecture or anatomy. Commonly with recurrent injury to the peroneals, there is an anatomic variant or a previously missed pathology such as a rim fracture of the distal fibula. A rim fracture was found to occur 15–50% of all cases of peroneal subluxation [36]. If these x-rays are found to be normal, it is recommended to obtain an MRI to evaluate the soft tissues. This will help determine if there is any lateral ankle instability, peroneus quartus, or need for SPR augmentation that needs to be addressed at the same time. Finally, it is important to determine if the patient suffers from any collagen disorders (Marfan, Ehlers-Danlos) that could change treatment.

Cases

Case 14.1

History

A 47-year-old female with history of stroke during childbirth. Previous surgery with calcifications within the longus. Distant history of stroke and previous surgery for foot drop. Tibiotalarcalcaneal nail, with peroneal debridement with fibular osteotomy. Able to actively evert/invert. Initially, tear was debrided successfully. Three years later, developed osteophyte and pain over lateral aspect with subsequent abrasion/tear because of this. Subsequent discussions regarding next operative plan involved the longus to brevis transfer. The patient agreed to move forward given the fact she had continued pain laterally with no relief after conservative measures and previous surgeries.

Reasons for Failure

- Continued abrasion from osteophyte

Surgical Plan

- Reevaluate tendon quality with possible debridement vs allograft vs tenodesis.

Approach

Previous incision for peroneal approach was performed, and significant scarring was encountered. The peroneal longus was determined to have additional tearing of >60%.

It has significant scarring and lacked a substantial amount of excursion. The prominent osteophyte was excised which was clearly causing fraying/tearing to the tendon. After proximal and distal adhesions were removed and adequate excursion of the brevis was noted, the proximal and distal ends of the longus were tenodesed to the brevis. This was then wrapped in an amniotic allograft membrane to prevent further scarring and promote gliding.

Implants

- 2-0 fiber wire
- Amniotic allograft membrane

Pearls and Pitfalls

- Clear communication with physical therapy as to not overly stress repair to early.
- Important to address the overall deformity, such as a varus hindfoot, in conjunction with soft tissue procedures.
- Recreation of the cartilaginous corner is paramount in preventing subluxation after repair of any kind.
- Prevent stenosis from tight closure of cartilaginous corner or inferior peroneal retinaculum at the peroneal tubercle (Figs. 14.1, 14.2, 14.3, and 14.4).

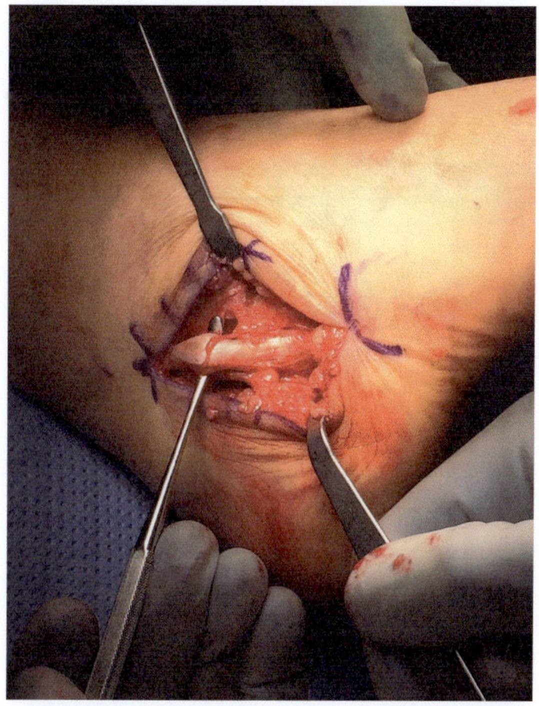

Fig. 14.1 Initial approach and evaluation of peroneal tendons (peroneal longus exposed)

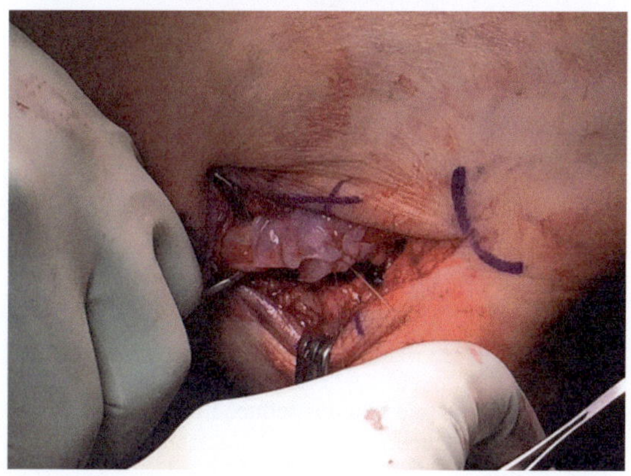

Fig. 14.2 After tenodesis of longus to brevis, the tendons are wrapped in amniotic membrane to prevent adhesions

Case 14.2

History

A 46-year-old male, very active, who sustained an initial rolling injury to his ankle. Continued to have right lateral ankle pain with no relief despite conservative measures. Found to have a cavus deformity with lateral posterior malleolus pain. Imaging revealed partial tear of the longus. After long discussion with the patient, he did not want a calcaneus osteotomy; instead, he just wanted attempted repair/debridement of the tissues. The patient underwent minimal surgery with debridement of the longus. During physical therapy within 6 weeks of his operation, the patient ruptures his peroneal longus.

Reasons for Failure

- Aggressive physical therapy

Surgical Plan

- Will evaluate tendon for ability to primarily tenodese to brevis or if requires allograft patch to obtain adequate tenodesis to brevis. Include

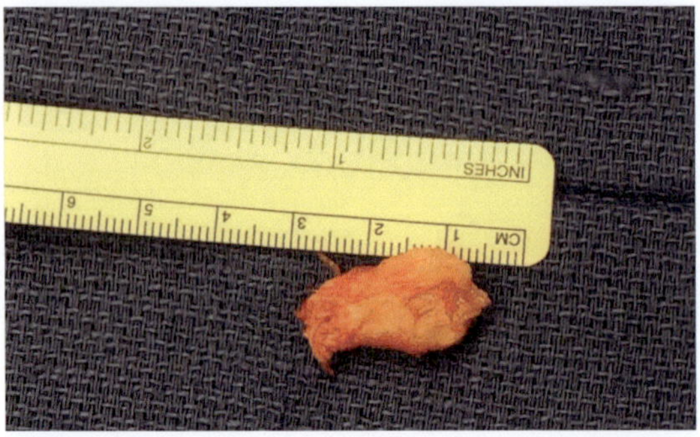

Fig. 14.3 Large osteophyte after excision

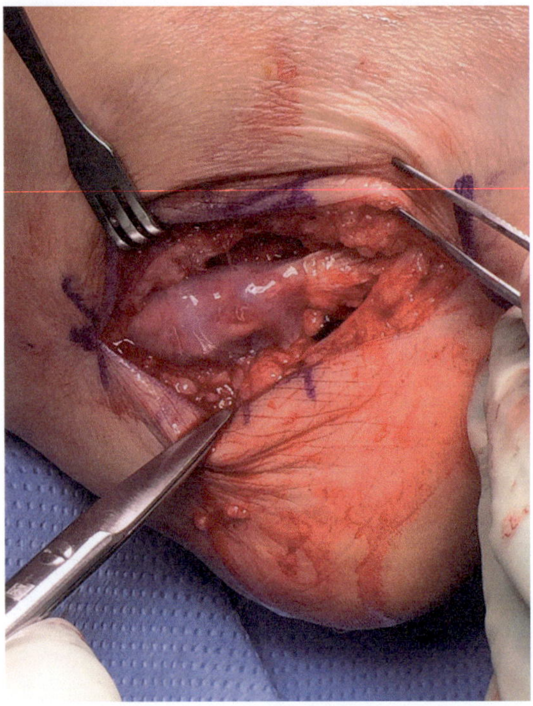

Fig. 14.4 Tenodesed tendons reduced posterior to fibula with adequate excursion

calcaneus osteotomy to prevent further stressing the repair.

Approach

The calcaneus osteotomy was performed first. This incision was cheated slightly posterior to allow a large enough skin bridge between the peroneal incision. After the osteotomy, the lateralization was fixated with two cannulated, headless screws. Previous incision over peroneals was opened with the patient in the lateral position. The longus rupture was immediately visualized, and given the extent of fraying and poor tissue, an allograft patch was selected to improve the tenodesis. The tenodesis was performed proximally and distally to the peroneal brevis. Excursion was tested after this was performed and determined to be appropriate.

Implants

- Arthrex headless cannulated screws

Allograft

- Fiber wire

Pearls and Pitfalls

- Clear communication with physical therapy as to not overly stress repair to early.
- Important to address the overall deformity, such as a varus hindfoot, in conjunction with soft tissue procedures.
- Recreation of the cartilaginous corner is paramount in preventing subluxation after repair of any kind.
- Prevent stenosis from tight closure of cartilaginous corner or inferior peroneal retinaculum at the peroneal tubercle (Figs. 14.5, 14.6, 14.7, 14.8, 14.9, 14.10, and 14.11).

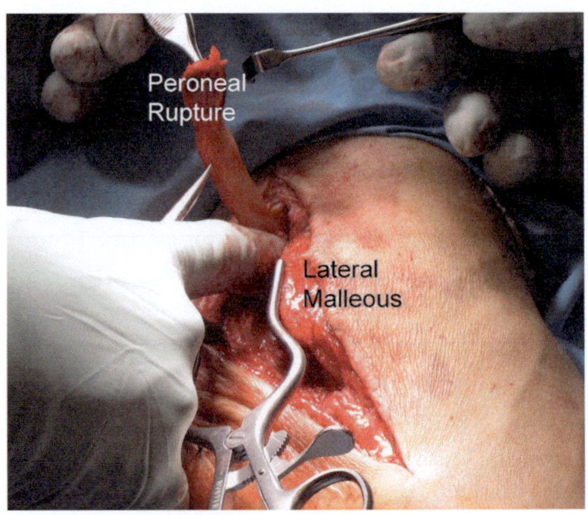

Fig. 14.5 Initial dissection and peroneal rupture easily visualized

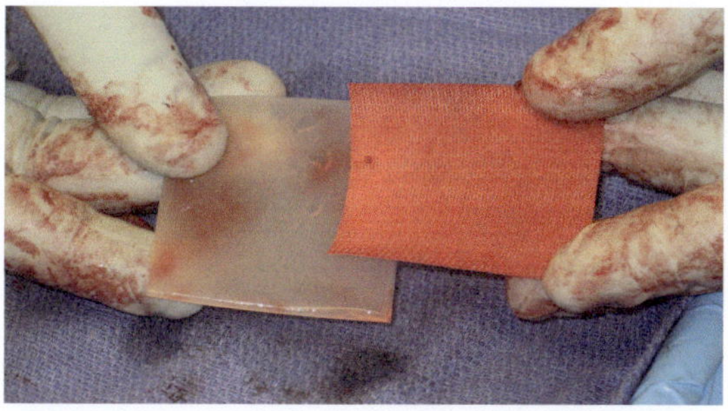

Figs. 14.6 Allograft patch construction 1

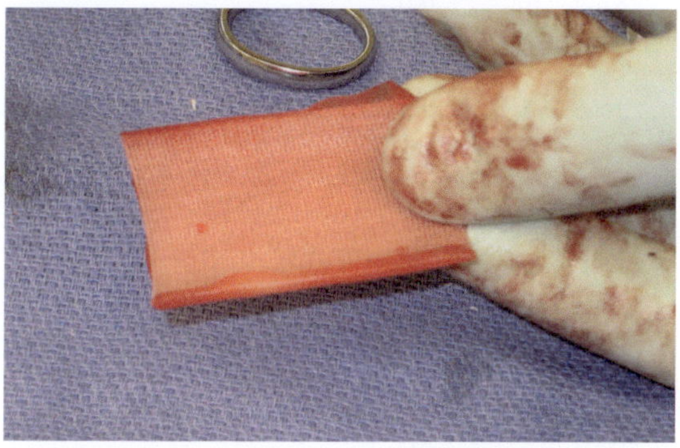

Figs. 14.7 Allograft patch construction 2

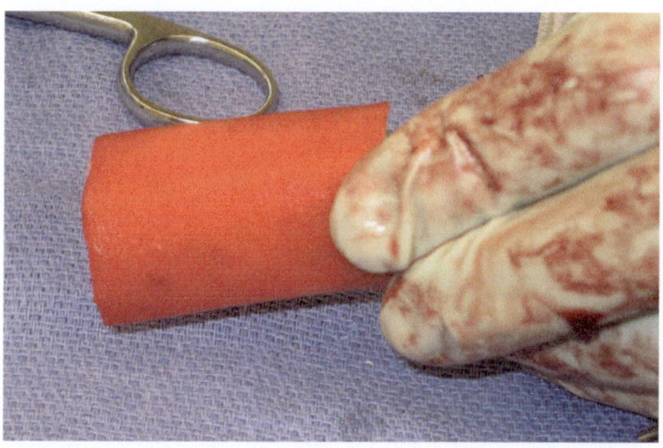

Figs. 14.8 Allograft patch construction 3

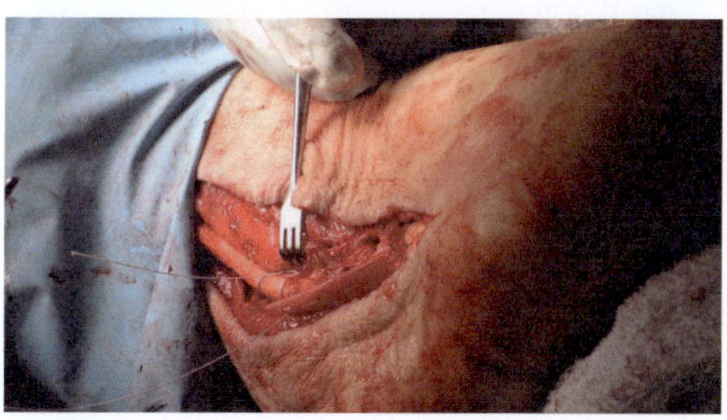

Fig. 14.9 Allograft patch placement around peroneals

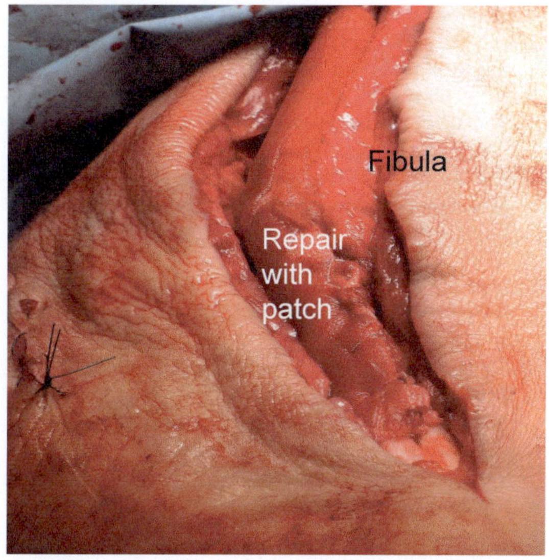

Fig. 14.10 Completed peroneal tenodesis with allograft reinforcement

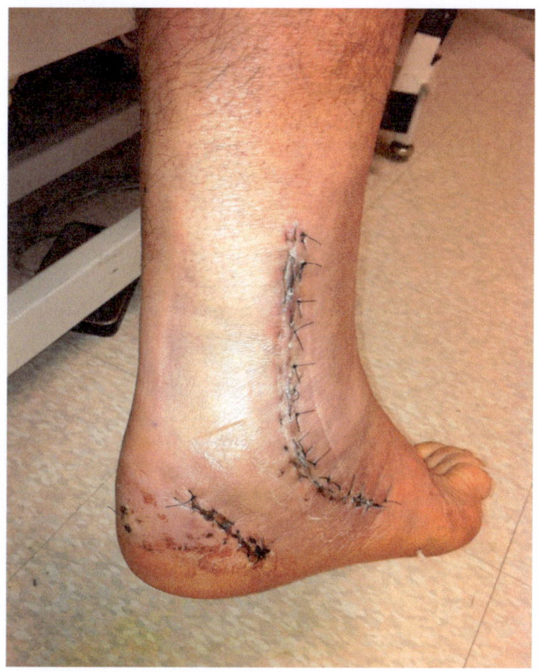

Fig. 14.11 Two-week follow-up with routine healing

References

1. Davis WH, Sobel M, Deland J, Bohne WH, Patel MB. The superior peroneal retinaculum: an anatomic study. Foot Ankle Int. 1994;15(5):271–5.

2. Hildebrand O. Tendovaginitis chronica deformans und Luxation der Peronealsehnen. Langenbeck's Arch Surg. 1907;86(5):526–31.
3. Hackenbroch M. Eine seltene Lokalisation der stenosierenden Tendovaginitis (an der Sehnenscheide bei Peroneen). Münch Med Wschr. 1927;74:932–5.
4. Khoury NJ, el-Khoury GY, Saltzman CL, Kathol MH. Peroneus longus and brevis tendon tears: MR imaging evaluation. Radiology. 1996;200:833–41.
5. Hammerschlag WA, Goldner JL. Chronic peroneal tendon subluxation produced by an anomalous peroneus brevis: case report and literature review. Foot Ankle. 1989;10:45–7.
6. Sobel M, Geppert MJ, Olson EJ, Bohne WH, Arnoczky SP. The dynamics of peroneus brevis tendon splits: a proposed mechanism, technique of diagnosis, and classification of injury. Foot Ankle. 1992;13(7):413–22.
7. Clarke HD, Kitaoka HB, Ehman RL. Peroneal tendon injuries. Foot Ankle Int. 1998;19(5):280–8.
8. Arrowsmith SR, Fleming LL, Allman FL. Traumatic dislocations of the peroneal tendons. Am J Sports Med. 1983;11(3):142–6.
9. Munk RL, Davis PH. Longitudinal rupture of the peroneus brevis tendon. J Trauma Acute Care Surg. 1976;16(10):803–6.
10. Geppert MJ, Sobel M, Bohne WH. Lateral ankle instability as a cause of superior peroneal retinacular laxity: an anatomic and biomechanical study of cadaveric feet. Foot Ankle. 1993;14(6):330–4.
11. DiGiovanni BF, Fraga CJ, Cohen BE, Shereff MJ. Associated injuries found in chronic lateral ankle instability. Foot Ankle Int. 2000;21(10):809–15.
12. Squires N, Myerson MS, Gamba C. Surgical treatment of peroneal tendon tears. Foot Ankle Clin. 2007;12(4):675–95.
13. Redfern D, Myerson M. The management of concomitant tears of the peroneus longus and brevis tendons. Foot Ankle Int. 2004;25(10):695–707.
14. Sobel M, Bohne WH, Levy ME. Longitudinal attrition of the peroneus brevis tendon in the fibular groove: an anatomic study. Foot Ankle. 1990;11(3):124–8.
15. Konradsen L, Sommer H. Ankle instability caused by peroneal tendon rupture: a case report. Acta Orthop Scand. 1989;60(6):723–4.
16. Madsen BL, Noer HH. Simultaneous rupture of both peroneal tendons after corticosteroid injection: operative treatment. Injury. 1999;30(4):299–300.
17. Verheyen CC, Bras J, van Dijk CN. Rupture of both peroneal tendons in a professional athlete. Am J Sports Med. 2000;28(6):897–900.
18. Wind WM, Rohrbacher BJ. Peroneus longus and brevis rupture in a collegiate athlete. Foot Ankle Int. 2001;22(2):140–3.
19. Escalas F, Figueras JM, Merino JA. Dislocation of the peroneal tendons. Long-term results of surgical treatment. J Bone Joint Surg Am. 1980;62:451–3.
20. McLennan JG. Treatment of acute and chronic luxations of the peroneal tendons. Am J Sports Med. 1980;8:432–6.
21. Alm A, Lamke LO, Liljedahl SO. Surgical treatment of dislocation of the peroneal tendons. Injury. 1975;7:14–9.
22. Shawen SB, Anderson RB. Indirect groove deepening in the management of chronic peroneal tendon dislocation. Tech Foot Ankle Surg. 2004;3:118–25.
23. Beck E. Operative treatment of recurrent dislocation of the peroneal tendons. Arch Orthop Trauma Surg. 1981;98:247–50.
24. Maffulli N, Ferran NA, Oliva F, Testa V. Recurrent subluxation of the peroneal tendons. Am J Sports Med. 2006;34(6):986–92.
25. Sobel M, Geppert MJ, Hannafin JA, et al. Microvascular anatomy of the peroneal tendons. Foot Ankle. 1992;13:469–72.
26. Schade VL, Harsha W, Rodman C, Roukis TS. Peroneal tendon reconstruction and coverage for treatment of septic peroneal tenosynovitis: a devastating complication of lateral ankle ligament reconstruction with a tendon allograft. J Foot Ankle Surg. 2016;55(2):406–13.
27. Edwards ME. The relations of the peroneal tendons to the fibula, calcaneus, and cuboideum. Am J Anat. 1928;42(1):213–53.
28. Mendicino RW, Orsini RC, Whitman SE, Catanzariti AR. Fibular groove deepening for recurrent peroneal subluxation. J Foot Ankle Surg. 2001;40(4):252–63.
29. Kollias SL, Ferkel RD. Fibular grooving for recurrent peroneal tendon subluxation. Am J Sports Med. 1997;25(3):329–35.
30. Wapner KL, Taras JS, Lin SS, Chao W. Staged reconstruction for chronic rupture of both peroneal tendons using Hunter rod and flexor hallucis longus tendon transfer: a long-term followup study. Foot Ankle Int. 2006;27(8):591–7.
31. Seybold JD, Campbell JT, Jeng CL, Myerson MS. Anatomic comparison of lateral transfer of the long flexors for concomitant peroneal tears. Foot Ankle Int. 2013;34(12):1718–23.
32. Rapley JH, Crates J, Barber A. Mid-substance peroneal tendon defects augmented with an acellular dermal matrix allograft. Foot Ankle Int. 2010;31(2):136–40.
33. Pellegrini MJ, Adams SB, Parekh SC. Allograft reconstruction of peroneus longus and brevis tendons tears arising from a single muscular belly. Case report and surgical technique. Foot Ankle Surg. 2015;21(1):e12–5.
34. Mook WR, Parekh SG, Nunley JA. Allograft reconstruction of peroneal tendons: operative technique and clinical outcomes. Foot Ankle Int. 2013;34(9):1212–20.
35. Pellegrini MJ, Adams SB, Parekh SG. Reversal of peroneal tenodesis with allograft reconstruction of the peroneus brevis and longus: case report and surgical technique. Foot Ankle Spec. 2014;7(4):327–31.
36. Church CC. Radiographic diagnosis of acute peroneal tendon dislocation. AJR Am J Roentgenol. 1977;129:1065–8.

Revision Achilles Tendon Reconstruction

15

Roshan T. Melvani and Stuart D. Miller

Key Takeaway Points

- Most acute tendon repairs involve damaged and somewhat degenerated tissues from an acute-on-chronic injury; some of these will fail with large gaps of sufficient tendon.
- The turndown flaps work well but require extensive dissection and have risk for significant scar formation.
- Dual semitendinosus allograft reconstruction offers preservation of the proximal muscle tendon unit and strength.
- The need for flexor hallucis longus tendon transfer with preservation of the gastrocsoleus motor unit has yet to be determined.

Introduction

The importance of a functioning Achilles tendon for normal gait underlies the need for adequate reconstruction in the event of problems with repair or initial surgical manipulation. Since many Achilles tendon ruptures are acute on chronic (these tendons often have pathologic evidence of chronic changes and microtears despite being previously asymptomatic), the repaired tendon might have less than optimal strength. Thus, revision Achilles tendon reconstruction often requires excision of a large segment of tendon.

Large segmental Achilles tendon defects present a difficult problem to treating surgeons. Multiple procedures including fascial turndowns [1, 2], local autograft tendon transfers [3, 4], allograft reconstruction [5], and synthetic grafts [2, 6, 7] have been utilized to reconstruct these defects with varying degrees of success. The use of a semitendinosus autograft reconstruction has been described [4, 8, 9, 10, 11, 12] and has demonstrated good results [11]. However, autograft harvesting is limited because it yields only one graft. Additionally, it requires a second surgical site incision and often causes significant postoperative knee pain [13]. Allografts have demonstrated equivalent utility in orthopedic tendon repair to autograft, and their ready availability has led to widespread use [8]. The benefits of a long turndown procedure versus allograft reconstruction have yet to be well-studied.

The utility of a flexor hallucis longus (FHL) tendon transfer to the calcaneus continues to be investigated. The musculotendinous transfer does help greatly when no gastrocnemius motor function remains (i.e., old long-standing Achilles

R. T. Melvani (✉) · S. D. Miller
MedStar Union Memorial Hospital, Department of Orthopaedic Surgery, Baltimore, MD, USA

M. J. Berkowitz et al. (eds.), *Revision Surgery of the Foot and Ankle*,
https://doi.org/10.1007/978-3-030-29969-9_15

failure with scarring and contraction of the gastrocsoleus complex) [14, 15]. The need for FHL transfer in addition to a functioning Achilles tendon reconstruction continues to be debated; these authors prefer to reserve the FHL for a later salvage attempt if needed.

Causes for Failure

A common element of problems after Achilles reconstruction is adhesion of the tendon to adjacent tissues and lack of motion. This should be lessened with aggressive postoperative range of motion exercises, even starting 1 week after surgery. Many surgeons like a nonbinding barrier sheet such as TenoGlide or AmnioFix around the reconstructed tendon.

Weakness of the reconstructed tendon often occurs with an overly long construct. The tendon should be adjusted to be slightly tight in some plantar flexion at the time of closure, and some stretching should be anticipated. One of the causes of dissatisfaction after primary Achilles rupture repair is leaving the repaired tendon too long, which results in a gait abnormality. A moderately tensioned Achilles usually stretches out to a satisfactory length after rehabilitation, but a poorly tensioned Achilles does not contract. Treatment for a poorly tensioned Achilles tendon usually requires another operative procedure for shortening.

Catastrophic failure of the reconstruction can be very intimidating. Aggressive reinforcement with sutures and intraoperative stretch testing can help avoid this dismal event. Patient education toward appropriate cessation of weight-bearing for 6 weeks can improve compliance. The authors and their partners do not use a cast, but rather a splint for the first week, followed by a walker boot whenever up for the next 5 weeks. At 6 weeks, a gradual weight-bearing protocol begins, accompanied by physical therapy guidance.

Infection remains a looming threat in this region of challenged vascularity. Caution with soft tissue handling has been significant, and in similar respect to total ankle arthroplasty tissues, care with gentle retraction and limited use of mechanical retractors seems to improve the damage. Staged debridements are rarely needed and threaten to lose a viable gastrocsoleus muscle unit to scar tissue and retraction if prolonged immobilization occurs.

Pain after Achilles tendon repair has been reported, and the posterior branch of the sural nerve can be at risk. Nerve involvement can be diagnosed with local anesthetic injection; a persistent neuroma may require surgical removal.

Evaluation and Assessment

The evaluation of the frustrated patient with a failed Achilles tendon repair can present many pitfalls. The most common mode of failure is catastrophic overload, but issues such as possible infection should be evaluated via standard means of inflammatory markers and imaging. A severe infection will require thorough debridement and great care before implanting any nonviable tissue which may be easily infected or colonized. Often, a period of antibiotic treatment will be indicated, along with normalized inflammatory markers after an antibiotic holiday, before a salvage procedure can be attempted. Such a delay might lead to contraction and scarring of the proximal gastrocnemius and soleus muscles and then lose the option for reconstruction other than flexor hallucis longus transfer.

The skin and soft tissues will be stressed, and adequate circulation should be assured; any lack of palpable pulses probably merits vascular studies. Some patients may have a local area of skin damage which might merit plastic surgery evaluation preoperatively—preferable to the emergent consult after a postoperative wound dehiscence. In cases of known tissue coverage issues, preoperative planning with plastic surgeons may determine the necessity of a free flap or vascularized local tissue transfer. Other factors in wound healing, such as the diabetes control, should be assessed, and many surgeons delay the procedure until optimized (such as hemoglobin A_1C being below 8). Nicotine and tobacco products certainly add morbidity to these procedures, and cessations should be strongly encouraged during preoperative counseling; other medical assistance may be necessary in achieving this goal.

The need for a period of non-weight-bearing can be quite onerous, especially when compounded in a revision situation; preoperative physical therapy evaluation may be beneficial. A rolling knee walker may improve mobility, but these devices are often poorly tolerated in patients who have undergone an ipsilateral total knee arthroplasty. Learning to negotiate stairs while preserving or maintaining non-weight-bearing restrictions can be difficult, and pre-procedure rehabilitation can be very instrumental.

An important issue in revision surgery centers around the etiology of repair failure. Most Achilles tendon ruptures are acute on chronic injuries; perhaps the repaired tendon was poor-quality tissue unable to sustain loading. The surgeon should be prepared to do an extensive resection of tendon and be prepared for a large defect repair. The benefits of a long turndown flap versus an allograft rebuilding have not been resolved: both procedures offer good results. Performing a revision procedure in an outpatient surgicenter where limited allograft selection is available may limit surgical options.

Surgical Planning

The key element of this procedure centers on length of repair and quality of the remaining muscle tissue. Most patients preserve the gastrocsoleus motor function and will do well with either a turndown or allograft procedure. Patients with long-standing tendon dysfunction may have a nonfunctioning gastrocsoleus and will need augmentation with an FHL transfer. A small (2–3 centimeter) defect can be repaired directly and some gastrocnemius length recovered through a small Strayer type lengthening. Key decision-making often occurs intraoperatively, and the surgeon must be prepared for a variety of options.

The patient is usually positioned prone. While many procedures for revision Achilles can be performed from a supine position, the operative exposure and difficulty of determining proper tension and length seems to be more challenging.

Case Examples

Case 15.1 Turndown Procedure

History

This is a 39-year-old woman presented with persistent pain and drainage over 6 years after an acute Achilles tendon repair augmented with a xenograft patch. This unfortunate woman had a palpable fluid subcutaneous bulge on exam (Fig. 15.1a) with significant pain.

Reasons for Failure

The popularity of these grafts was reversed with episodes of immunologic reaction and drainage, probably related to graft preparation.

Surgical Plan

Her MRI (Fig. 15.1b, c) revealed a large cystic-appearing mass in the region of the repair site that extended into the subcutaneous skin.

Approach

With removal of the graft material and damaged tendon, a large 10 cm gap was measured (Fig. 15.1d, e). With a negative Gram stain taken intraoperatively and lack of systemic reaction consistent with infection, a decision was made to perform immediate reconstruction using a turndown flap. Multiple intraoperative cultures were taken as precaution.

Implants

A 10x2 cm free flap of gastrocnemius-soleus complex was advanced into the distal Achilles stump. The extensive incision needed to prepare and harvest the turndown can be intimidating. Tension should be adjusted to moderate tension just less than neutral at the ankle (Fig. 15.1f). She had an easy and uneventful recovery.

Pearls and Pitfalls

These extensive dissections threaten to scar quickly. Range of motion begins as soon as the skin seems to be healing, usually at 7–10 days postoperatively. Weight-bearing can start much later at 6 weeks.

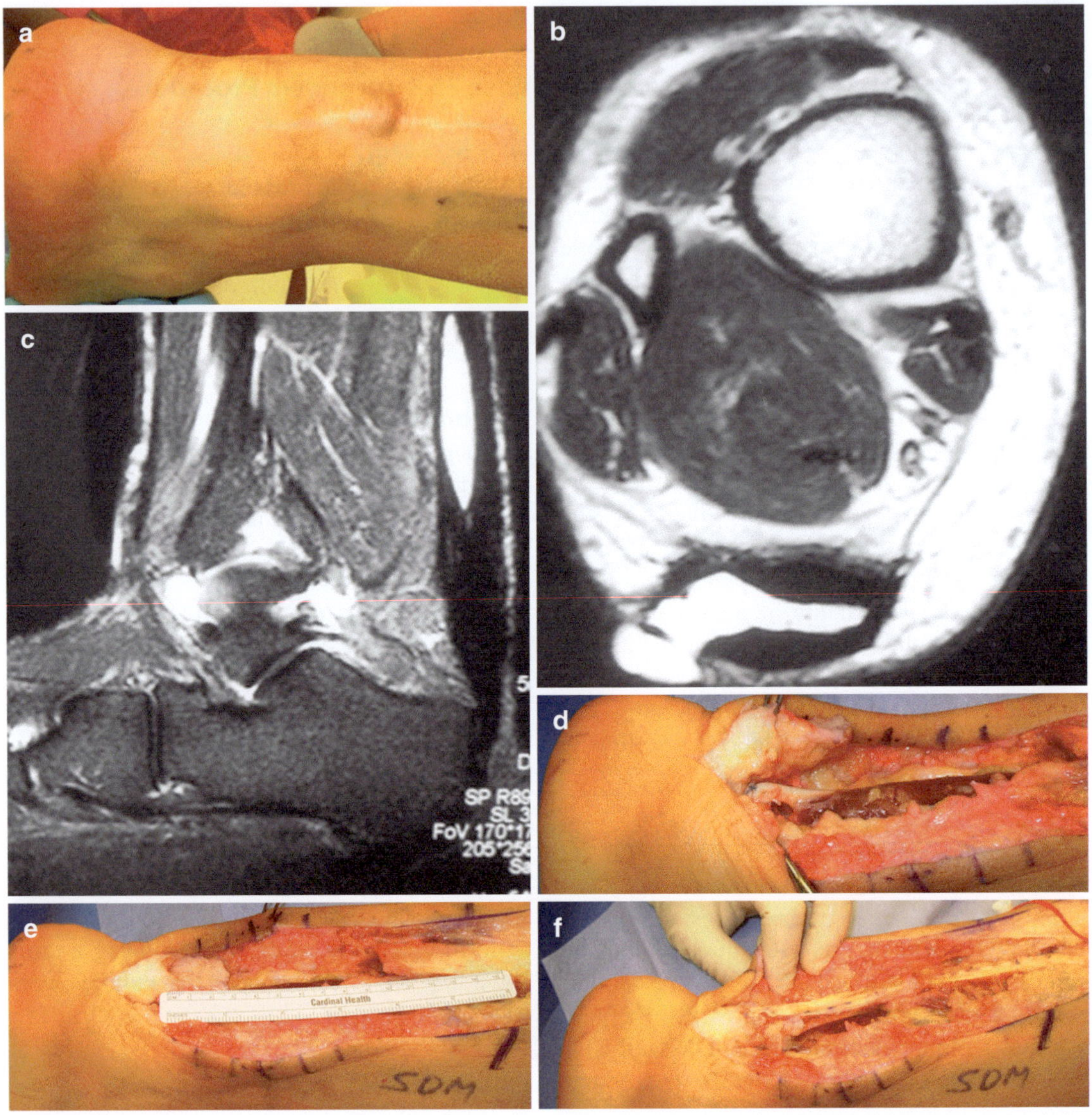

Fig. 15.1 (**a**) Ballotable cyst seen on physical exam. (**b**, **c**) Axial and sagittal MRI cuts showing cyst formation and tendon defect (two separate figs in files and chapter). (**d**) Intraoperative tendon defect. (**e**) Intraoperative measurement of approx. 10 mm defect. (**f**) Intraoperative FHL transfer into calcaneus

Case 15.2 V-Y Lengthening

History

This primary care physician had primary repair of an acute Achilles tendon rupture. Repair was done with a simple loop rather than Krakow style multiple loop stitch, and he presented with an infected draining sinus tract (Fig. 15.2a).

Reasons for Failure

Repair had been done with a simple loop rather than Krakow style multiple loop stitch. The construct was not very strong, and the repair had pulled apart (Fig. 15.2b).

Surgical Plan

The difficulty of decision-making to stage reconstruction versus immediate reconstruc-

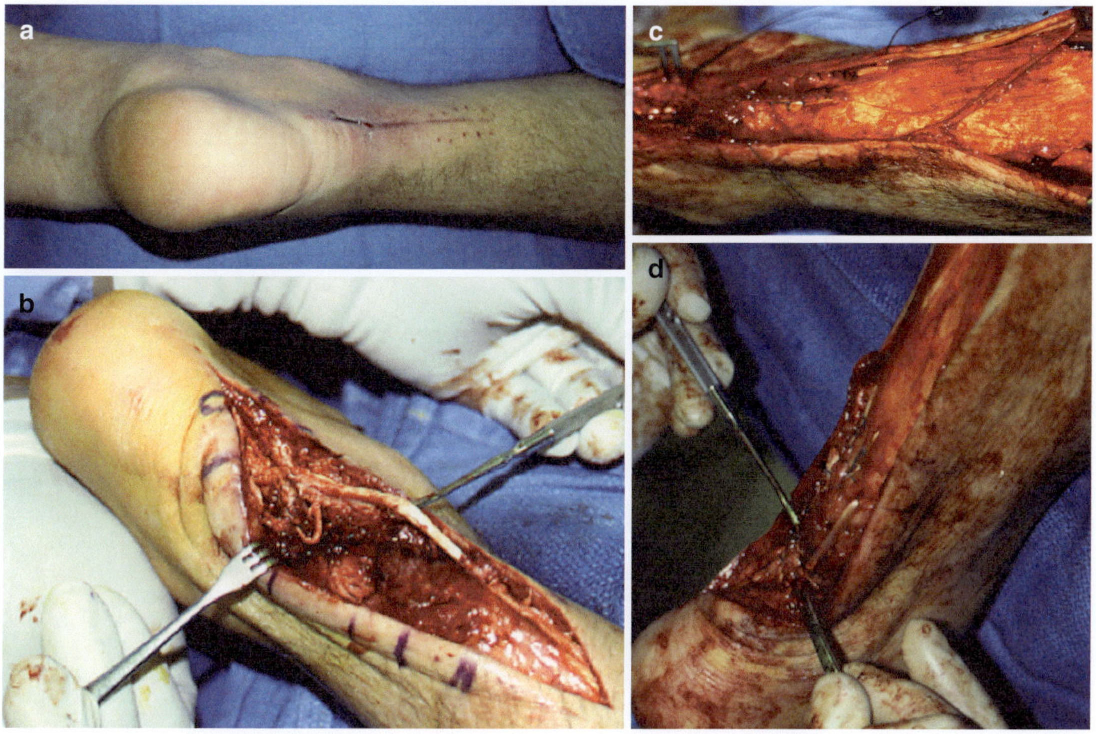

Fig. 15.2 (**a**) Preoperative infected draining sinus tract. (**b**) Intraoperative tendon defect. (**c**) Intraoperative V-Y lengthening. (**d**) Intraoperative completion with plantaris weave

tion should not be underestimated. Performing immediate repair risks further infection of the new repair. On the other hand, delaying repair would cause retraction of the gastrocsoleus muscle tendon construct and may cause enough scarring to prevent its later use in repair.

Approach

The relatively benign bacteriology (methicillin-sensitive *Staphylococcus aureus*) combined with the patient's excellent health led to a mutual decision to immediately reconstruct the tendon with a two-in-one pattern [16] (Fig. 15.2c, d).

Implants

His tendon was repaired with nonabsorbable suture (Ethibond, Ethicon, LLC, Somerville, NJ). The patient did well and returned to normal activities by 8 weeks. Even at a year, he noted some weakness which finally resolved by 18 months.

Pearls and Pitfalls

Repair of early failures can be challenging. This case went well despite worries of infection; more recently, the authors have advocated local antibiotics in the surgical site (Stimulan beads with vancomycin and gentamicin, Biocomposites Inc., Wilmington, NC). Recovery from these cases can be prolonged.

Case 15.3 Semitendinosus Allograft Reconstruction

History

This 35-year-old female had multiple prior Achilles tendon reconstructions for insertional Achilles tendinosis (Fig. 15.3a) and presented after many failed attempts (Fig. 15.3b).

Reasons for Failure

Multiple surgical procedures produce more and more scar tissue formation. Coupled with overly

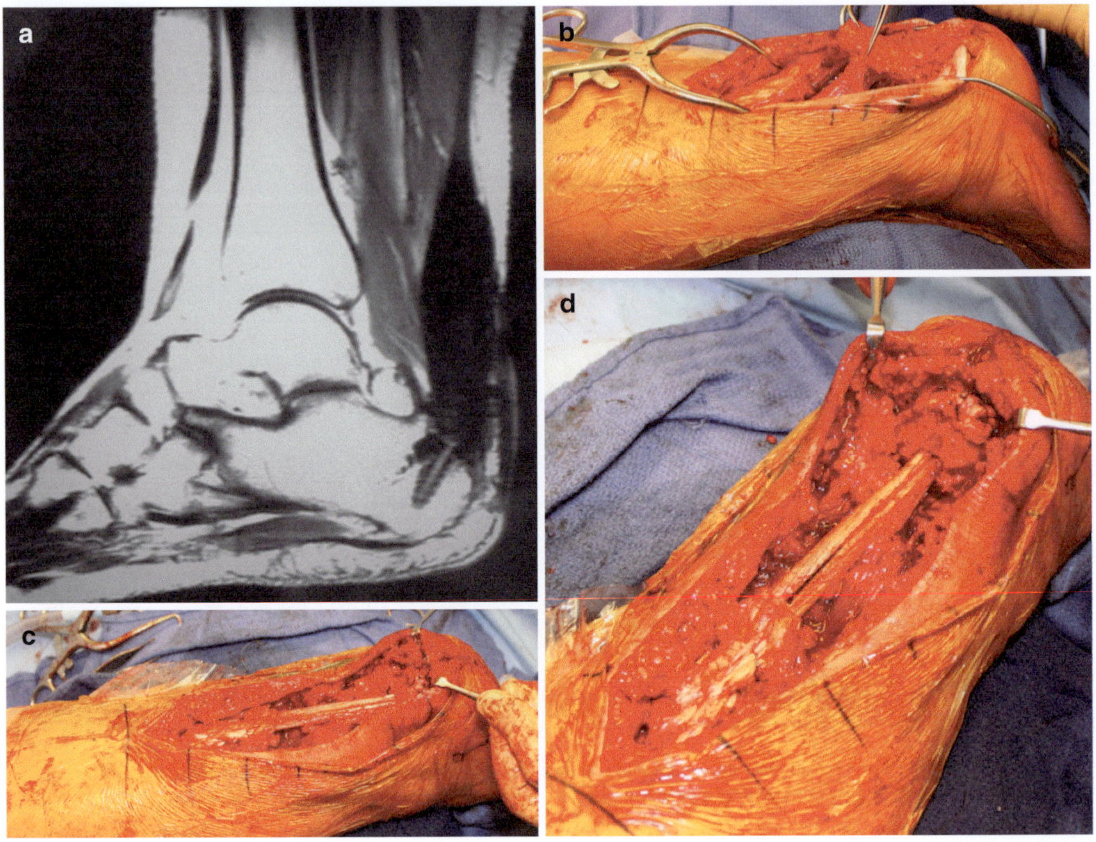

Fig. 15.3 (**a**) Preoperative sagittal MRI cut of tendon defect. (**b**) Intraoperative tendon defect with significant scar. (**c**) Intraoperative completion. (**d**) Intraoperative completion (cephalad view)

cautious rehabilitation with limited motion after surgery, the Achilles tendon can often scar down and become dysfunctional.

Surgical Plan

A plan to remove the damaged tissue and assess the quality of the proximal muscle tendon motor unit was envisioned. Decisions to add the FHL graft augmentation depended upon mobility and strength of the remaining tissues after debridement.

Approach

Via an extensile 12 centimeter posteriorly based incision, a large 10 centimeter defect was encountered along with her prior FHL transfer (Fig. 15.3c).

Implants

Two semitendinosus allografts were fashioned and tubularized using running locking Krakow stitches with Ethibond shuttled through drill holes in the calcaneus and suture upon themselves while the proximal portion was anchored using Pulvertaft weaves into the gastrocsoleus complex (Fig. 15.3d). FHL muscle belly and proximal tendon stump were reattached using allograft with Pulvertaft weave into proximal myotendinous junction. The foot was appropriately tensioned in approximately 10 degrees of plantar flexion.

Postoperatively, the patient was placed in a resting splint in near neutral. She began physical therapy at 6 weeks and was transitioned out of CAM boot at 3 months. She is now over 2 years out from surgery and doing well.

Pearls and Pitfalls

Early motion after this procedure is essential to prevent the common formation of scar tissue in the reconstructed Achilles tendon. Decisions as to securing the tendon to the bone and then Pulvertaft weaving into the tendon (as was done here) or to Pulvertaft weave first are uncertain. With limited assistance, the authors have found it a bit easier to Pulvertaft first since securing the weave under tension can be challenging.

Case 15.4 Turndown Flap and FHL Transfer

History

This 56-year-old female had a previous debridement for Achilles tendonitis and reinsertion of her tendon using suture anchors. Her symptoms persisted, and her imaging showed a significant amount of heterotopic ossification (Fig. 15.4a) within her tendon along with degenerative changes (Fig. 15.4b).

Reasons for Failure

The prior surgery resulted in severe scar formation without adequate power and function.

Surgical Plan

The dysfunctional tendon is needed to be removed, and the proximal muscle tendon unit should still be functional for motor power. A turndown procedure was chosen at the time.

Approach

A 10 centimeter posteriorly based incision was made with exploration of the Achilles tendon showing significant degeneration with intrasubstance calcification. After the tendon was lifted off the distal insertion and found to be significantly thickened and of poor quality, 6 cm of the tendon was resected.

Implants

A turndown procedure was performed with the middle third of the proximal tendon incised to obtain approximately 8 centimeters of length and attached with Ethibond suture (Fig. 15.4c). The FHL distal end of the FHL tendon was harvested for transfer. An extensive ostectomy was needed given the significant amount of heterotopic bone and Haglund's deformity. The harvested turndown and FHL were attached into the calcaneus via bone tunnels (Fig. 15.4d, e) and tensioned to maintain approximately 15 degrees of plantar flexion with appropriate passive dorsiflexion to neutral. She was splinted in 20 degrees of plantar flexion. She has not had any major issues postoperatively.

Pearls and Pitfalls

The turndown procedure utilizes a long extensile incision. Care must be taken to protect the sural nerve and its variable branches. Early motion remains a mainstay of rehabilitation to prevent scar tissue binding postoperatively.

Case 15.5 Semitendinosus Allograft Reconstruction and FHL Transfer

History

This case involves a 30-year-old male who sustained a primary Achilles tendon rupture after a work-related heavy lifting incident and went onto to have multiple reconstructive procedures. He presented with significant pain and dysfunction.

Reasons for Failure

MRI demonstrated extensive signal changes in the tendon. The prior surgical procedures had left his tendon scarred and dysfunctional.

Surgical Plan

The scarred tissue needed to be removed, and a healthy bed established. If no contractility of the proximal muscle tendon unit was found, then an FHL transfer would have to suffice.

Approach

A 10 centimeter posterior incision was made, and upon exploration, there was significant intrasubstance degeneration of the tendon. Approximately 6 centimeters of tendon had to be resected until the native appearance of the tendon appeared healthy.

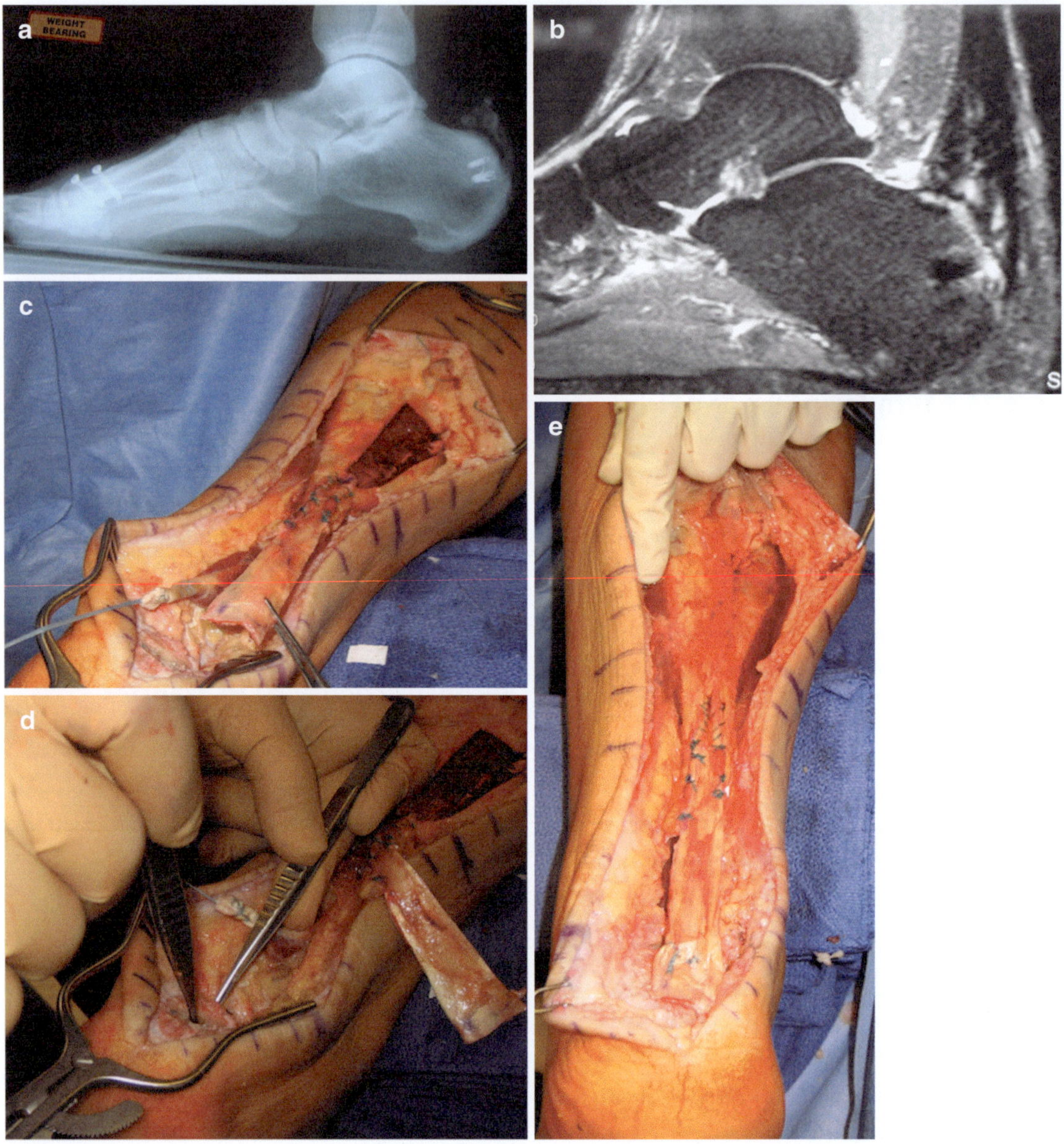

Fig. 15.4 (**a**) Preoperative lateral ankle XR. (**b**) Preoperative sagittal MRI cut of tendon defect. (**c**) Intraoperative turndown. (**d**) Intraoperative turndown with calcaneal bone tunnels. (**e**) Intraoperative completion

Implants

An allograft reconstruction was performed with semitendinosus allograft fashioned with Pulvertaft weaves proximally (Fig. 15.5a, b) and Krakow stitches distally attached via drill holes in the calcaneus and sutured upon themselves with Ethibond (Fig. 15.5c). Tension was appropriately set in 15 degrees of plantar flexion. An FHL transfer was performed for augmentation. Collagen matrix was placed around the tendon reconstruction site so as to avoid postoperative adhesions given the significant amount of scarring encountered during the approach (Fig. 15.5d, e). He is doing well 2 years out and notes significant improvement of his symptomatology.

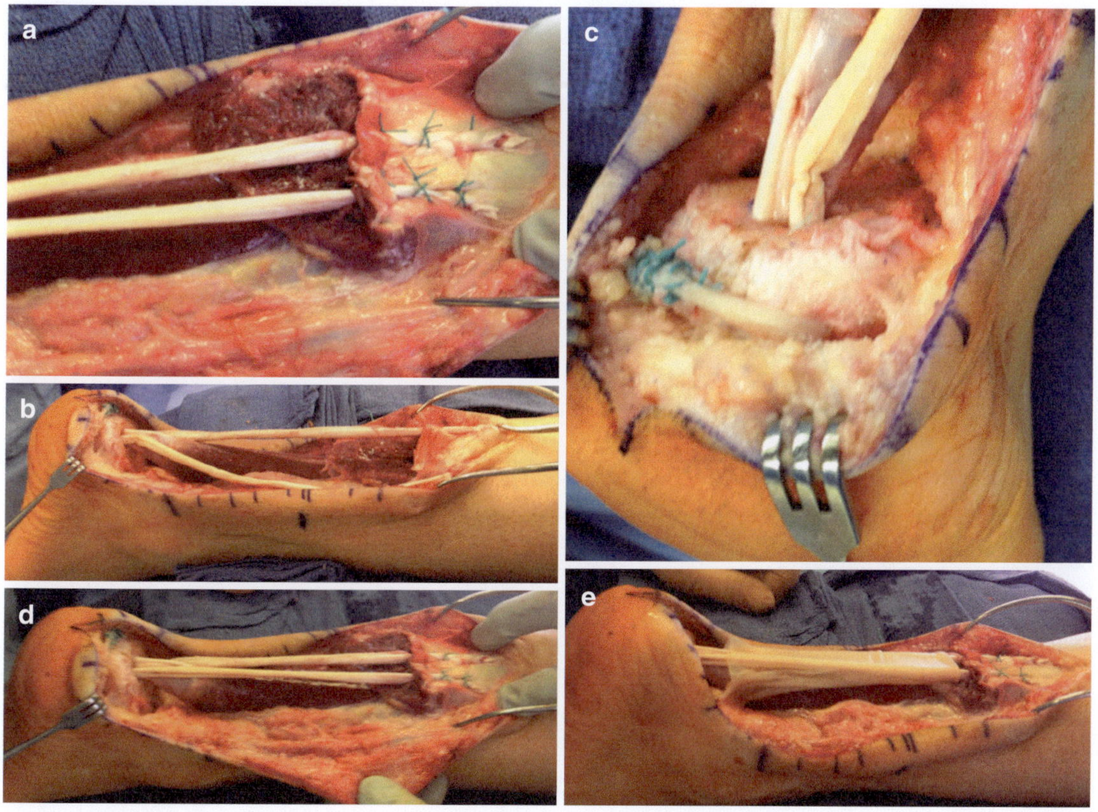

Fig. 15.5 (a) Proximal Pulvertaft weave. (b) Intraoperative tensioning of first semitendonosis graft with foot in plantar flexion. (c) Distal fixation in calcaneal bone tunnels. (d) Intraoperative completion. (e) Intraoperative completion with collagen matrix application

Pearls and Pitfalls

When extensive scar formation of an Achilles tendon reconstruction prevents adequate recovery, the entire repaired tissue might require removal and replacement with allograft.

Case 15.6 Semitendinosus Allograft Reconstruction

History

This patient is a 34-year-old female who had a history of posterior tibial tendon dysfunction and underwent a flexor digitorum longus transfer in the past. She presented with symptoms of persistent Achilles tendonitis approximately 9 months after undergoing a debridement with tendon reattachment and sural nerve resection. She had undergone postoperative physical therapy and rehabilitation with several months of postoperative symptom relief.

Reasons for Failure

Her imaging on presentation showed significant degenerative changes of the tendon (Fig. 15.6a).

Surgical Plan

With her previous history of tendon transfer, we did not feel a flexor hallucis longus tendon transfer would be optimal.

Approach

There was extensive scar tissue appreciated during the dissection, and upon exploration, the Achilles tendon was found to be thickened and degenerated about its midsubstance (Fig. 15.6b). As the insertion was further debrided, suture anchors were encountered and removed.

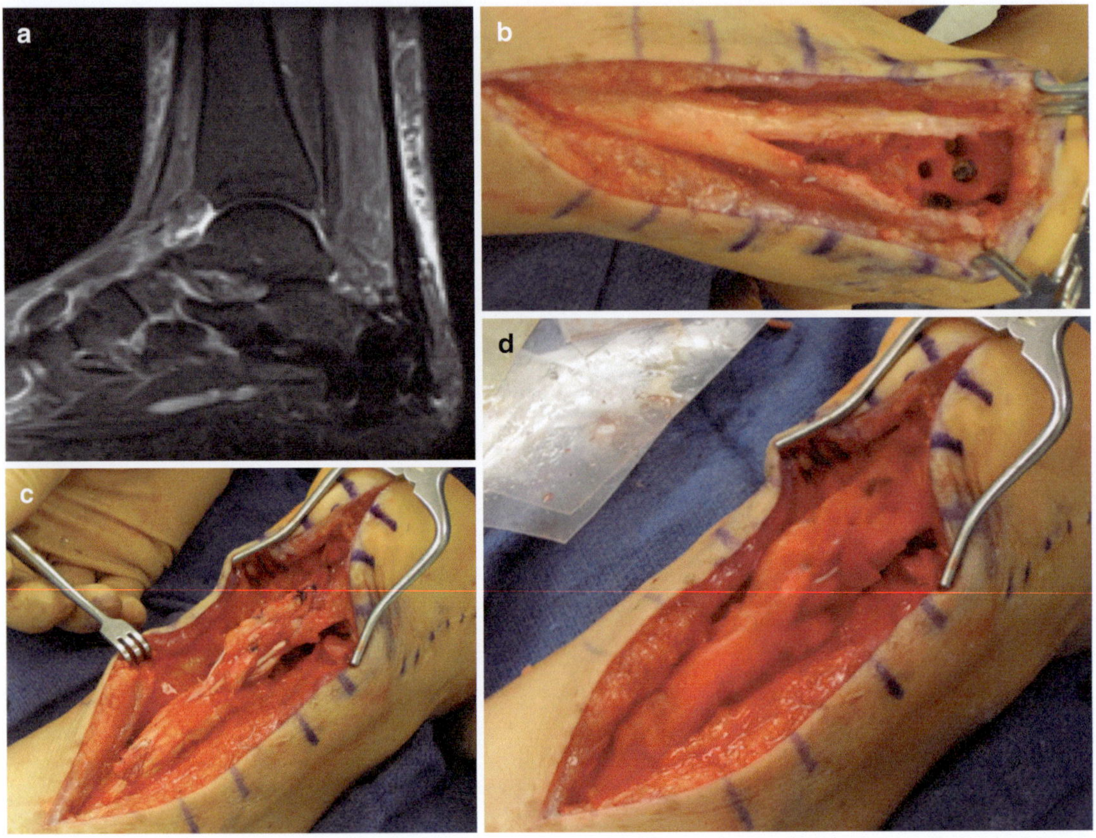

Fig. 15.6 (**a**) Preoperative sagittal MRI cut of tendon defect. (**b**) Intraoperative tendon defect. (**c**) Intraoperative completion. (**d**) Intraoperative completion with collagen matrix application

Implants

A semitendinosus allograft was placed into the calcaneus using a tenodesis screw. Approximately 20% of the distal tendon was remaining after debridement, and the graft was then attached via Pulvertaft weaves into the proximal segment and sutured with the appropriate tension in 15 degrees of plantar flexion (Fig. 15.6c). A collagen matrix was then wrapped around the tendon to avoid scarring as seen during the exposure (Fig. 15.6d). She is now 5 years postop and has minimal pain about her Achilles tendon site.

Pearls and Pitfalls

An allograft may present a fine alternative to FHL transfer in complicated patients. Collagen wrapping might be helpful to prevent postoperative scarring of the tendon.

Summary

Large segmental Achilles tendon defects cause significant impairment of gait. They also present a difficult problem to treating surgeons. From a scientific standpoint, no evidence-based recommendations exist for treatment of these injuries. Present studies evaluating reconstructive techniques are limited by sample size, retrospective methods, and lack of objective long-term follow-up. Achilles tendon turndown procedures and semitendinosus allograft reconstruction are good options for large segmental defects and can be augmented with an FHL transfer. A large intraoperative dissection is required, and preoperative preparation is essential for success.

References

1. Bosworth DM. Repair of defects in the tendo Achillis. J Bone Joint Surg Am. 1956;38:111–4.
2. Giza E, Frizzell L, Farac R, Williams J, Kim S. Augmented tendon Achilles repair using a tissue reinforcement scaffold: a biomechanical study. Foot Ankle Int. 2011;32(5):S545–9.
3. Mann RA, Holmes GBJ, Seale KS, Collins DN. Chronic rupture of the Achilles tendon: a new technique of repair. J Bone Joint Surg Am. 1991;73(2):214–9.
4. Wapner KL, Pavlock GS, Hecht PJ, Naselli F, Walther R. Repair of chronic Achilles tendon rupture with flexor hallucis longus tendon transfer. Foot Ankle. 1993;14:443–9.
5. McCoy BW, Haddad SL. The strength of achilles tendon repair: a comparison of three suture techniques in human cadaver tendons. Foot Ankle Int. 2010;31(8):701–5.
6. Fideler BM, Vangsness CT Jr, Lu B, Orlando C, Moore T. Gamma irradiation: effects on biomechanical properties of human bone-patellar tendon-bone allografts. Am J Sports Med. 1995;23(5):643–6.
7. Nellas ZJ, Loder BG, Wertheimer SJ. Reconstruction of an Achilles tendon defect utilizing an Achilles tendon allograft. J Foot Ankle Surg. 1996;35(2):144–8.
8. Dumbre Patil SS, Dumbre Patil VS, Basa VR, Dombale AB. Semitendinosus tendon autograft for reconstruction of large defects in chronic Achilles tendon ruptures. Foot Ankle Int. 2014;35(7):699–705.
9. Guclu B, Basat HC, Yildirim T, Bozduman O, Us AK. Long-term results of chronic Achilles tendon ruptures repaired with V-Y tendon plasty and fascia turndown. Foot Ankle Int. 2016;37(7):737–42.
10. Hsu NN, Tan EW, Miller SD. Dual semitendinosus allograft reconstruction of large defects in chronic Achilles tendinopathy. Tech Foot Ankle Surg. 2016;15(4):202–9.
11. Maffulli N, Del BA, Spiezia F, et al. Less-invasive semitendinosus tendon graft augmentation for the reconstruction of chronic tears of the Achilles tendon. Am J Sports Med. 2013;41(4):865–71.
12. Maffulli N, Longo UG, Gougoulias N, Denaro V. Ipsilateral free semitendinosus tendon graft transfer for reconstruction of chronic tears of the Achilles tendon. BMC Musculoskelet Disord. 2008;9:100.
13. Ardern CL, Webster KE. Knee flexor strength recovery following hamstring tendon harvest for anterior cruciate ligament reconstruction: a systematic review. Orthop Rev (Pavia). 2009;1(2):e12.
14. Ozaki J, Fujiki J, Sugimoto K, Tamai S, Masuhara K. Reconstruction of neglected Achilles tendon rupture with Marlex mesh. Clin Orthop. 1989;(238):204–8.
15. Sebastian H, Datta B, Maffulli N, Neil M, Walsh WR. Mechanical properties of reconstructed Achilles tendon with transfer of peroneus brevis or flexor hallucis longus tendon. J Foot Ankle Surg. 2007;46(6):424–8.
16. Beskin JL, Sanders RA, Hunter SC, Hughston JC. Surgical repair of Achilles tendon ruptures. Am J Sports Med. 1987;15(1):1–8.

Part IV

Arthritis and Reconstruction

Revision of the Failed Flatfoot Reconstruction

16

Todd A. Irwin

Key Takeaway Points

- Thorough history and physical examination, including knowledge of the previous operation(s) by review of operative notes, is important to understand what aspect of the failed flatfoot is causing symptoms.
- Radiographic evaluation must include the ankle in order to evaluate for resultant or causative tibiotalar deformity or instability.
- Determining overall alignment is an important first step that will aid the direction of surgical planning.
- Previous reconstructions that are well aligned may have resultant degenerative changes or nonunion as reasons for failure.
- Residual deformity may be present in the ankle/hindfoot and/or the midfoot/forefoot that has to be addressed.
- Combining bone work (realignment osteotomies or arthrodesis) with soft tissue reconstructions (tendon transfers, ligament reconstructions) may be needed to achieve a good result.

Introduction

The adult acquired flatfoot deformity (AAFD) is a complex clinical scenario with multiple presentations and treatment options. These treatments have evolved significantly over the previous 20–30 years [1–6]. Originally described as primarily due to posterior tibial tendon (PTT) dysfunction, it is now understood that this deformity develops secondary to failure of both static and dynamic structures [7–10]. In addition to insufficiency of the posterior tibial tendon, there is progressive stress/strain on the deltoid-spring ligament complex, hindfoot valgus due to stress/strain on the subtalar joint, abduction through the transverse tarsal joints, and medial column instability through multiple joints (Table 16.1). Contracture of the gastrocnemius-soleus complex and the Achilles tendon also plays an important role in the deformity, though it is debated whether the resultant force accentuates the problem or is a primary cause [11].

Surgical correction of the AAFD has similarly evolved. The first step in surgical planning involves defining whether the deformity is flexible or rigid.

T. A. Irwin (✉)
OrthoCarolina Foot and Ankle Institute, Carolinas Medical Center, Charlotte, NC, USA
e-mail: todd.irwin@orthocarolina.com

M. J. Berkowitz et al. (eds.), *Revision Surgery of the Foot and Ankle*,
https://doi.org/10.1007/978-3-030-29969-9_16

Table 16.1 Overview of physiologic components of the adult acquired flatfoot deformity

Posterior tibial tendon insufficiency and degeneration
Stress/strain on the deltoid-spring ligament complex
Stress/strain on the subtalar joint and transverse tarsal joint capsules resulting in progressive hindfoot valgus and abduction through the transverse tarsal joints
Plantar collapse of the talar head with associated external rotation of the subtalar joint and dorsomedial peritalar subluxation
Shortening of the gastrocnemius-soleus complex and/or Achilles tendon accentuating the hindfoot valgus force
Possible medial column collapse through naviculocuneiform and/or tarsometatarsal joint
Relative unopposed pull of the peroneus brevis with possible contracture
Compensatory forefoot supination deformity in order to achieve plantigrade foot

In the flexible clinical setting, original attempts at addressing the posterior tibial tendon dysfunction with tendon transfers in isolation failed [8, 9]. Adding osteotomies to the hindfoot and midfoot has improved functional outcomes and the durability of the reconstruction [2, 3, 5, 6, 12–15]. Arthrodesis of isolated joints has also been utilized in the flexible flatfoot in combination with other procedures to achieve a more robust reconstruction or in the setting of arthritis [16–18]. In the rigid flatfoot, triple arthrodesis has been utilized for many decades with success [19, 20]. Recent modifications to this surgical strategy include only fusing certain joints, most commonly the subtalar and talonavicular (TN) joints, and leaving the calcaneocuboid (CC) joint in its native position as long as there are no significant degenerative changes [21–23]. Significant clinical challenges arise when the progressive flatfoot deformity, either flexible or rigid, creates valgus instability at the ankle joint [24, 25]. This problem can be seen both at initial presentation and late after an initial attempt at surgical correction.

Causes of Failure

The complex nature of flatfoot reconstruction results in potential complications of each procedure in isolation, which may ultimately lead to failure of the reconstruction. While complications may be seen radiographically, addressing these complications is only necessary if the patient is symptomatic. The most common complication after flatfoot reconstruction is likely undercorrection, which can occur if all components of the deformity are not recognized or certain components are not fully corrected [26]. A common site of unrecognized deformity is along the medial column where instability and resultant sag can occur in any of the joints, in particular the naviculocuneiform (NC) joint [14, 16, 27]. Overcorrection is another potential complication, though less common [28]. This frequently results in symptoms similar to a cavovarus foot such as lateral column overload pain or increased pressure underneath the first ray. Nonunion and malunion are other potential causes of failure any time osteotomies or arthrodesis procedures are undertaken as part of the flatfoot reconstruction. Symptomatic nonunion may need to be addressed at the specific site alone if the overall alignment is well maintained, such as with lateral column lengthening nonunion. Alternatively, malunion may result in undercorrection or overcorrection, which may need to be addressed with revision osteotomies or arthrodesis. Determining the appropriate procedure for salvage of the failed flatfoot reconstruction can be difficult, and diligent clinical and radiographic evaluation must be undertaken.

Patient Evaluation

Evaluation of the failed flatfoot reconstruction begins with understanding what was done during the index procedure. A thorough history and physical examination are paramount to understanding the patient's complaints. This includes obtaining the patient's preoperative radiographs and operative report if done elsewhere. Physical examination must include observation of the patient standing from the front and the back, as well as close inspection of the location of prior incisions. Any history of infection or wound healing difficulty may have pertinent implications for revision surgery. The location of the patient's pain must be elucidated and then determined if this pain is secondary to overall deformity or issues with the bone such as nonunion. Radiographic evaluation includes standing anteroposterior (AP), lateral, and oblique foot radiographs, with comparison to the contralateral side. Standing bilateral AP and mortise ankle radiographs also need to be evaluated to determine if tibiotalar incongruity or supramalleolar deformity is present, either as a compensatory deformity or possibly as a cause of the failure. Hindfoot alignment views can provide important information regarding the relationship of the hindfoot and point of contact of the calcaneus to the long alignment of the tibia [29]. Long-leg alignment views may also be utilized if more proximal deformity such as genu varum or varus proximal tibias is suspected. Advanced imaging such as computed tomography (CT) can help evaluate for nonunion of prior arthrodesis. Weight-bearing CT scans are increasing in popularity and can help to further evaluate hindfoot alignment or specific areas of bone impingement that non-weight-bearing studies may otherwise miss [30].

Surgical Planning

As noted above, the first step in surgical planning is determining the cause of failure and what specifically is causing the patient's symptoms, which will then lead to an individualized plan. During the assessment, the surgeon should be evaluating whether joint sparing procedures or arthrodesis will be required. Determining overall alignment is critical and should be addressed first. When alignment is acceptable, evaluating for arthritic change in unfused joints versus nonunion of fused joints or osteotomies should be undertaken next. When residual deformity is present, determining if the deformity is localized to the forefoot, the midfoot, or the hindfoot (including the ankle) or a combination is extremely important. Depending on the site of deformity and what was done prior, decisions can then be made regarding corrective osteotomy versus realignment arthrodesis. The contribution of soft tissue structures should also not be overlooked. Residual Achilles and/or gastrocnemius contractures need to be recognized and treated. Similarly, an overlooked deltoid-spring ligament complex insufficiency needs to be addressed. As with any revision procedure, planning the incisions required relative to prior incisions, including length of time since the index operation, may affect surgical approaches. Evaluating location of previously placed hardware, which specific system was used (as outlined in the operative reports or medical records), whether it needs to be removed, and whether the hardware is intact or broken are other important factors to consider. Finally, bone graft is often required in revision situations. With deformity correction, structural graft (autograft versus allograft) may be required. Alternatively, in the setting of nonunion or arthrodesis, bone grafting +/− biologic augmentation is often utilized, and several options are available. Importantly, if autograft is used, the location of prior autograft harvest must be determined and the plan modified if necessary. A proposed algorithm is provided in Fig. 16.1.

Cases

Case 16.1

History

- A 68-year-old female with a midfoot injury about 19 years prior to presentation that developed into a progressive flatfoot deformity.
- Two years prior to presentation, she had surgical intervention at an outside institution, including a posterior tibial tendon debridement and advancement with a suture anchor into the navicular, as well as first tarsometatarsal (TMT) arthrodesis.
- She presented with complaints of difficulty with ambulation and lateral hindfoot pain.
- Physical examination revealed significant and asymmetric pes planovalgus deformity, tenderness along the sinus tarsi and posterior tibial tendon, 0/5 strength to the posterior tibial tendon, Achilles tightness, and residual forefoot supination with correction of the hindfoot valgus.
- Foot radiographs revealed severe pes planus, talonavicular uncoverage with increased AP talo-first metatarsal angle compared to the

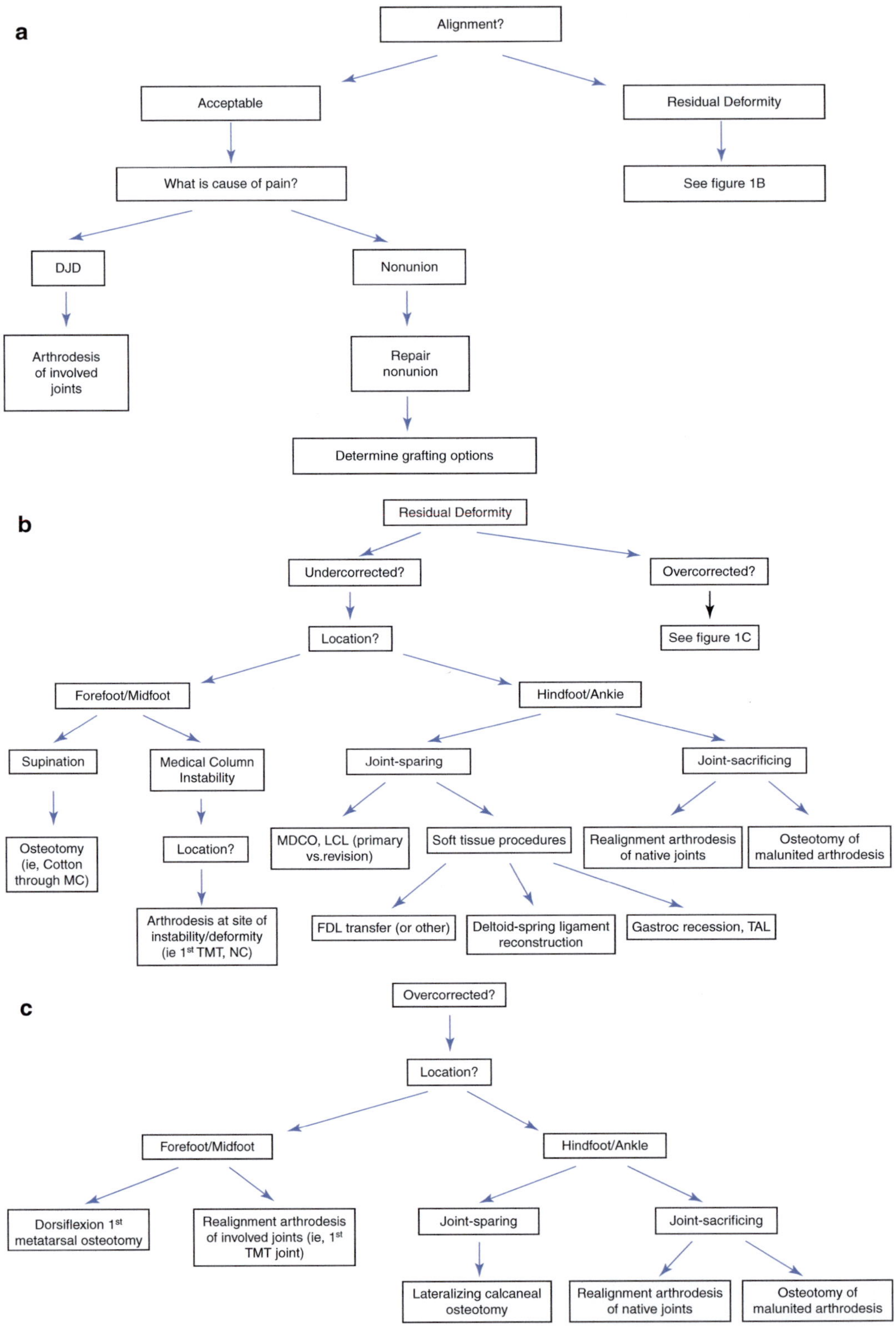

Fig. 16.1 (**a**) Proposed algorithm for revision of the failed flatfoot reconstruction. A DJD, degenerative joint disease; (**b**) residual deformity undercorrected. MC, medial cuneiform; TMT, tarsometatarsal; NC, naviculocuneiform; MDCO, medial displacement calcaneal osteotomy; LCL, lateral column lengthening; FDL, flexor digitorum longus; TAL, tendo-Achilles lengthening; (**c**) residual deformity overcorrection. TMT, tarsometatarsal

opposite side, small accessory navicular, suture anchor in the navicular, and a well-fused first TMT joint (Fig. 16.2a, b).

Potential Reasons for Failure

- Inadequate medial soft tissue stabilization utilizing likely diseased posterior tibial tendon advancement in isolation
- Failure to address the hindfoot valgus deformity
- Incomplete deformity correction of the medial column, leaving the foot with residual supination

Surgical Plan and Approach

- Flexor digitorum longus (FDL) transfer into navicular for dynamic inversion due to diseased PTT
- Medial displacement calcaneal osteotomy (MDCO) to correct hindfoot valgus:
  - Posterior tuberosity segment was translated medially and inferiorly to increase calcaneal pitch (Fig. 16.2c, d).
  - Lateral column lengthening (LCL) to address transverse tarsal joint abduction:
    - Tricortical allograft wedge
- Plantarflexion medial cuneiform osteotomy (Cotton) to address residual forefoot supination:
  - Tricortical allograft wedge
- Percutaneous triple hemisection tendo-Achilles lengthening to address Achilles contracture
- Final radiographs 1.5 year postoperative (Fig. 16.2e, f)

Implants

- 6.5 mm partially threaded cannulated screw for fixation of the MDCO
- 3.5 mm cortical screw for fixation of the LCL
- 2.4 mm cortical screw for fixation of the Cotton osteotomy

Case 16.2

History

- A 48-year-old male with a history of progressive left flatfoot deformity, initially treated with realignment subtalar arthrodesis, flexor digitorum longus (FDL) tendon transfer to the navicular, opening wedge medial cuneiform (Cotton) osteotomy, and gastrocnemius recession.
- Complained of pain, swelling, and recurrent deformity 5 months after the index procedure.
- Standing foot radiographs demonstrated significant instability at the talonavicular joint with sagittal plane collapse and foot abduction (Fig. 16.3a, b).
- Standing ankle radiographs demonstrated valgus instability with deltoid ligament incompetence at the ankle that was not present preoperatively (Fig. 16.3c).
- CT scan demonstrated subtalar joint arthrodesis nonunion (Fig. 16.3d).

Potential Reasons for Failure

- Unrecognized deltoid-spring ligament instability
- Medial column ligamentous instability that may have been more appropriately treated with arthrodesis of the first tarsometatarsal (TMT) joint or naviculocuneiform (NC) joint, as opposed to an opening wedge medial cuneiform (Cotton) osteotomy

Surgical Plan and Approach

- Revision subtalar joint arthrodesis with iliac crest bone graft and biologic augmentation to address the subtalar joint nonunion:
  - Utilizing same sinus tarsi incision:
    - Iliac crest bone graft lateral to anterior superior iliac spine (ASIS)
    - Mesenchymal stem cell bone matrix (biologic allograft)
- Talonavicular joint arthrodesis to address the abduction deformity and medial column instability:
  - Dorsal approach just lateral to tibialis anterior
- This approach was essentially conversion to a modified triple arthrodesis, though the calcaneocuboid joint was not included in the arthrodesis (Fig. 16.3e–g):
  - Screw was placed from navicular into the anterior process for added construct rigidity (Fig. 16.3f).
- Deltoid ligament reconstruction with allograft to address the valgus instability of the ankle

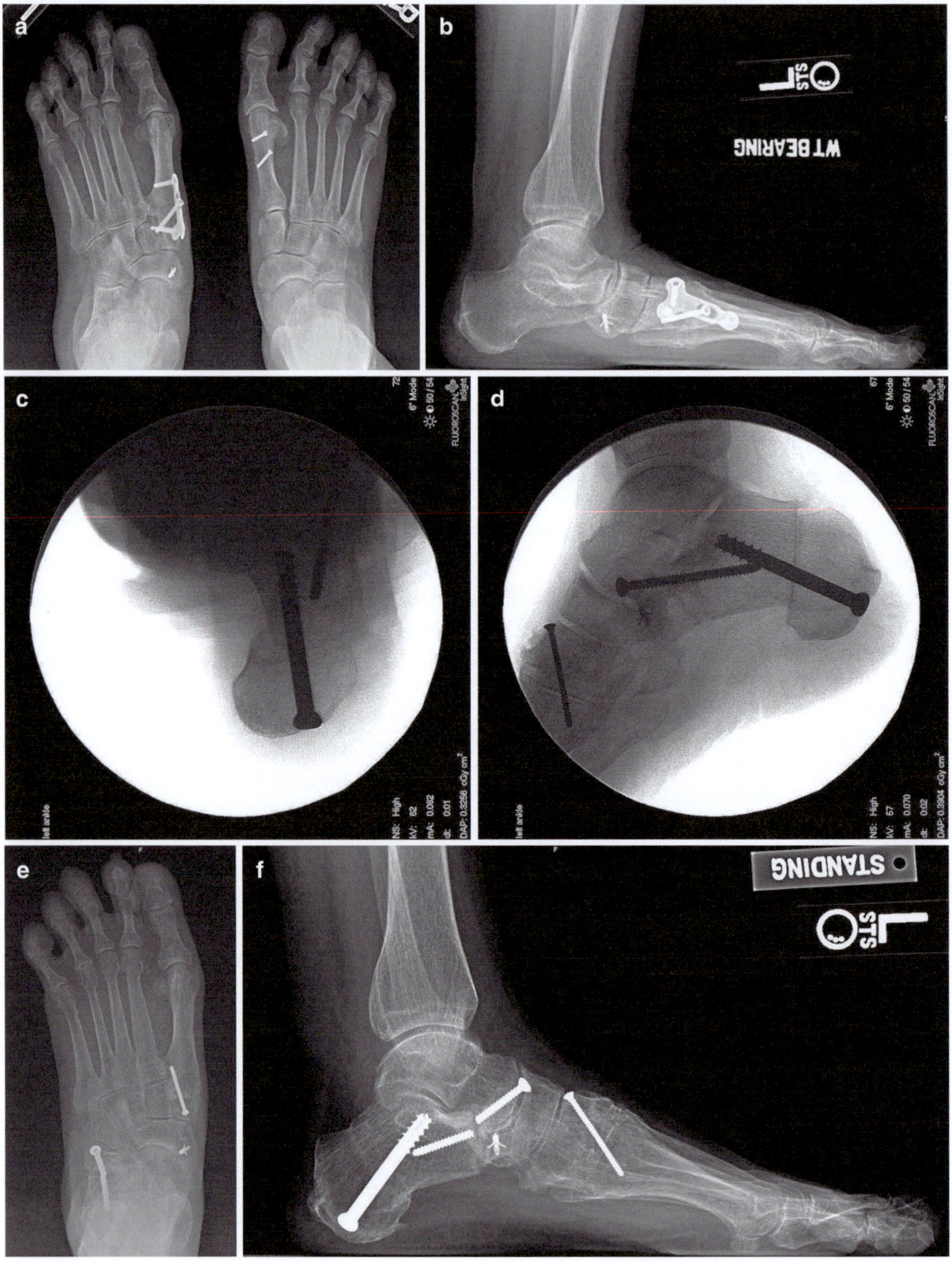

Fig. 16.2 Preoperative AP and lateral foot radiographs (**a**, **b**). Intraoperative axial and lateral heel view (**c**, **d**). 1.5-year postoperative AP and lateral foot radiographs (**e**, **f**). Note the improved talonavicular coverage and presence of stable pseudarthrosis with broken screw through LCL that was asymptomatic

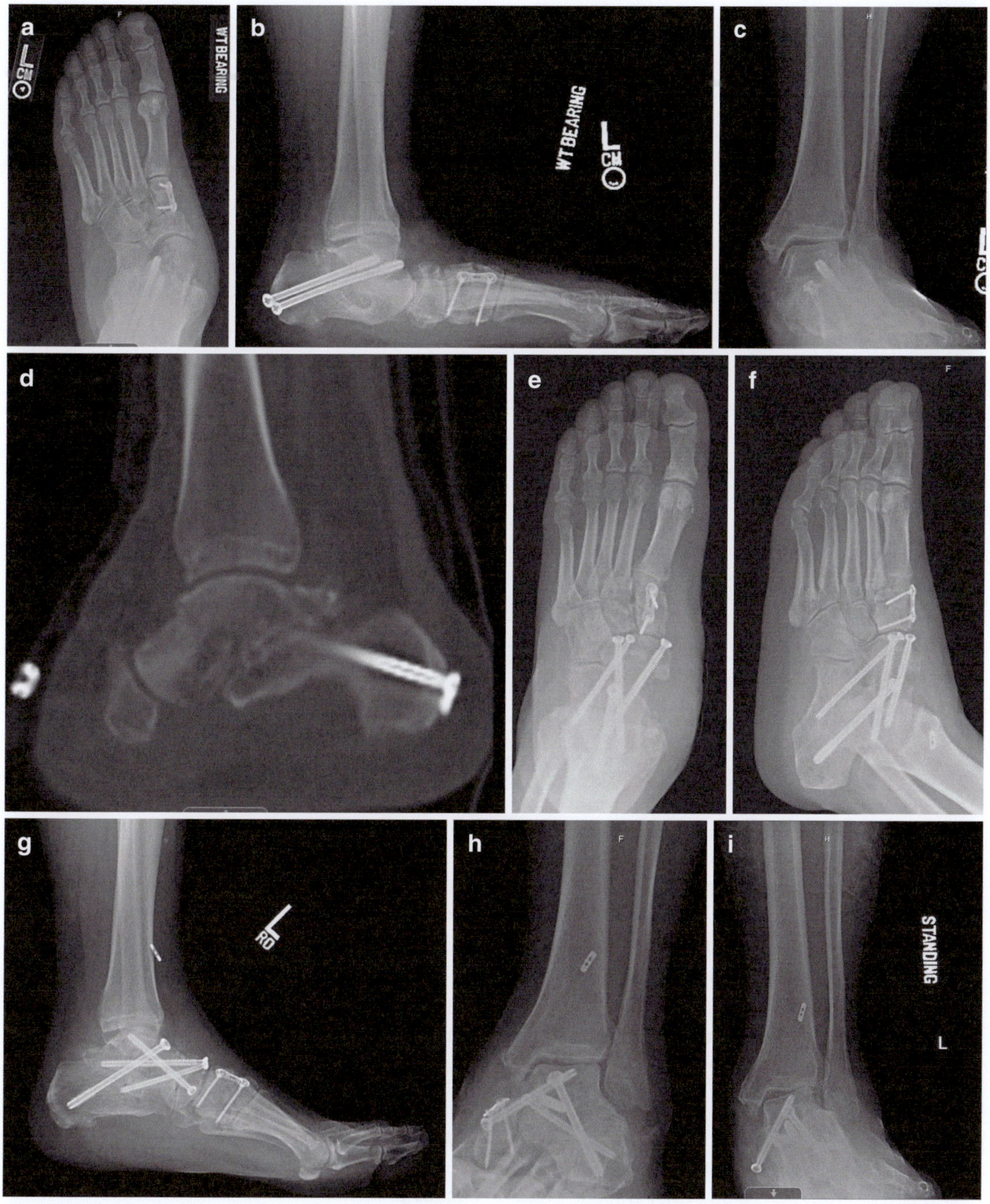

Fig. 16.3 Preoperative AP and lateral foot radiographs and mortise ankle radiograph (**a**–**c**). Preoperative sagittal CT scan slice demonstrating nonunion through subtalar joint (**d**). Two-week postoperative non-weight-bearing AP, oblique and lateral foot radiographs, and mortise ankle radiograph (**e**–**h**). Five-month postoperative standing mortise ankle and AP and lateral foot radiographs demonstrating improved foot alignment but significant residual valgus talar tilt (**i**–**k**). Three-month postoperative mortise and lateral ankle radiograph after conversion to ankle fusion

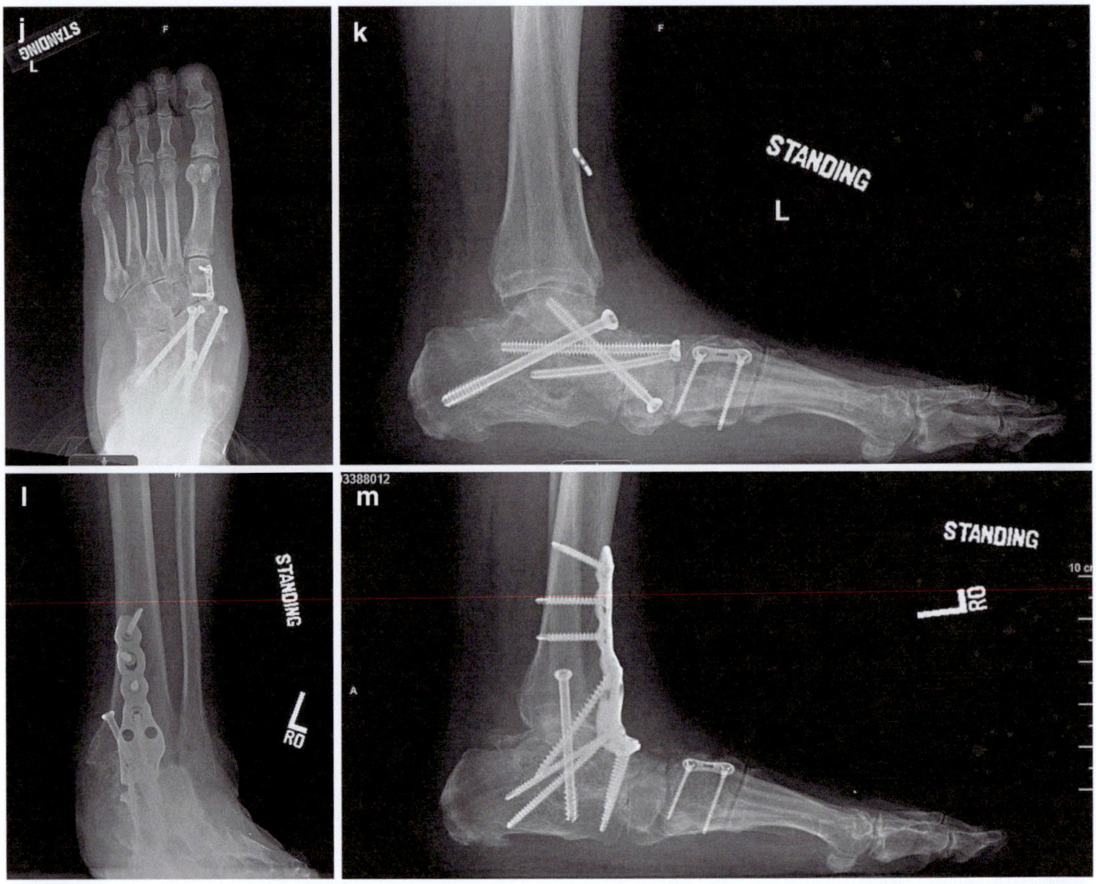

Fig. 16.3 (continued)

and deltoid ligament incompetence (Fig. 16.3h):
  - Through extensile medial incision from the previous incision for the FDL transfer
  - Semitendinosus allograft docked into the medial malleolus, talar body, and sustentaculum of the calcaneus

Implants

- Subtalar and talonavicular arthrodesis:
- 7.0 and 5.5 mm partial and fully threaded cannulated titanium screws.
- The fully threaded screws across the talonavicular joint are placed in lag fashion.
- The screw from the navicular to the anterior process of the calcaneus is a set screw, without lag technique.
- Deltoid ligament allograft reconstruction:
- Suture button device securing the folded over semitendinosus allograft into a reamed hole in the medial malleolus with button on the anterolateral tibia.
- Allograft limbs in the talus and sustentaculum secured with interference screws. Suture buttons on the far side of each bone can also be considered.

Case 16.3

History

- Same patient as in **Case 16.1**.
- At 5 months post-op, patient was clinically improved but had moderate residual hindfoot valgus.
- Standing ankle radiographs demonstrated progressive ankle valgus instability and failure of the deltoid ligament reconstruction (Fig. 16.3i).

- Foot radiographs revealed a well-aligned and well-fused modified triple arthrodesis (Fig. 16.3j, k).

Potential Reasons for Failure

- Inadequate allograft tissue, with possible stretch or creep
- Failure of the implants:
  - Poor fixation in the docking sites
  - Poor bone quality secondary to extended period of immobilization and non-weight-bearing during the initial postoperative period

Surgical Plan and Approach

- Options included conversion to ankle arthrodesis versus staged total ankle arthroplasty:
  - Ankle arthrodesis would result in a pantalar arthrodesis and expected significant functional limitations but would leave open the possibility of conversion to later total ankle arthroplasty at a more appropriate age.
  - Total ankle arthroplasty would likely require a staged revision deltoid ligament reconstruction, followed by total ankle arthroplasty with likely need for multiple revisions in future due to the patient's relatively young age.
- Patient opted to proceed with ankle arthrodesis (Fig. 16.3l, m):
  - Anterior ankle approach

Implants

- Anterior ankle fusion plate
- 6.7 mm partially threaded cancellous screw across medial aspect of ankle joint to help reduce the valgus instability
- Recombinant human platelet-derived growth factor in b-tricalcium phosphate granules for biologic augmentation

Case 16.4

History

- A 54-year-old male with history of right flatfoot reconstruction involving FDL transfer, medial displacement calcaneal osteotomy, lateral column lengthening with tricortical allograft, and gastrocnemius recession that was complicated by lateral column lengthening nonunion.
- Correction of the lateral column lengthening nonunion was addressed with insertion of a trabecular metal wedge prior to presentation.
- Patient presented with continued lateral column pain and swelling.
- Foot radiographs demonstrated well-maintained arch alignment with possible collapse of the anterior process of the calcaneus distal to the metal wedge. Broken hardware was noted from the previous nonunion (Fig. 16.4a–c).
- CT scan revealed a thin, fractured anterior process distal to the metal wedge, with degenerative changes present in the calcaneocuboid joint (Fig. 16.4d, e):
  - There was some evidence of bony incorporation into the metal wedge.
- Selective steroid injection into the calcaneocuboid joint provided symptomatic relief.

Potential Reasons for Failure

- Insufficient anterior process remaining after bone prep and revision grafting:
  - Based on the location of the metal wedge, as well as placement of the broken screw distally, it is likely the initial osteotomy through the anterior process was too distal.
- Poor biology associated with trabecular metal wedge:
  - It is unclear what bone graft and/or biologics was used during the initial revision procedure, though there was some evidence of bone incorporation.

Surgical Plan and Approach

- Calcaneocuboid joint bone block arthrodesis through lateral approach:
  - Based on the thin shelf of anterior process with fracture into the CC joint and the presence of a metal wedge, it was felt the entire anterior process involving the metal wedge required resection (Fig. 16.4f, g).

- Structural autograft utilizing vascularized medial femoral condyle (MFC) with anastomosis to the dorsalis pedis artery (performed by a hand surgeon colleague) (Fig. 16.4h, i):
  - Based on the size and depth of the void after resection, the vascularized (MFC) graft was placed medial in the joint, with a tricortical iliac crest allograft placed laterally for structural support.
- Final radiographs and CT scan at 1 year postoperative (Fig. 16.4j–m).

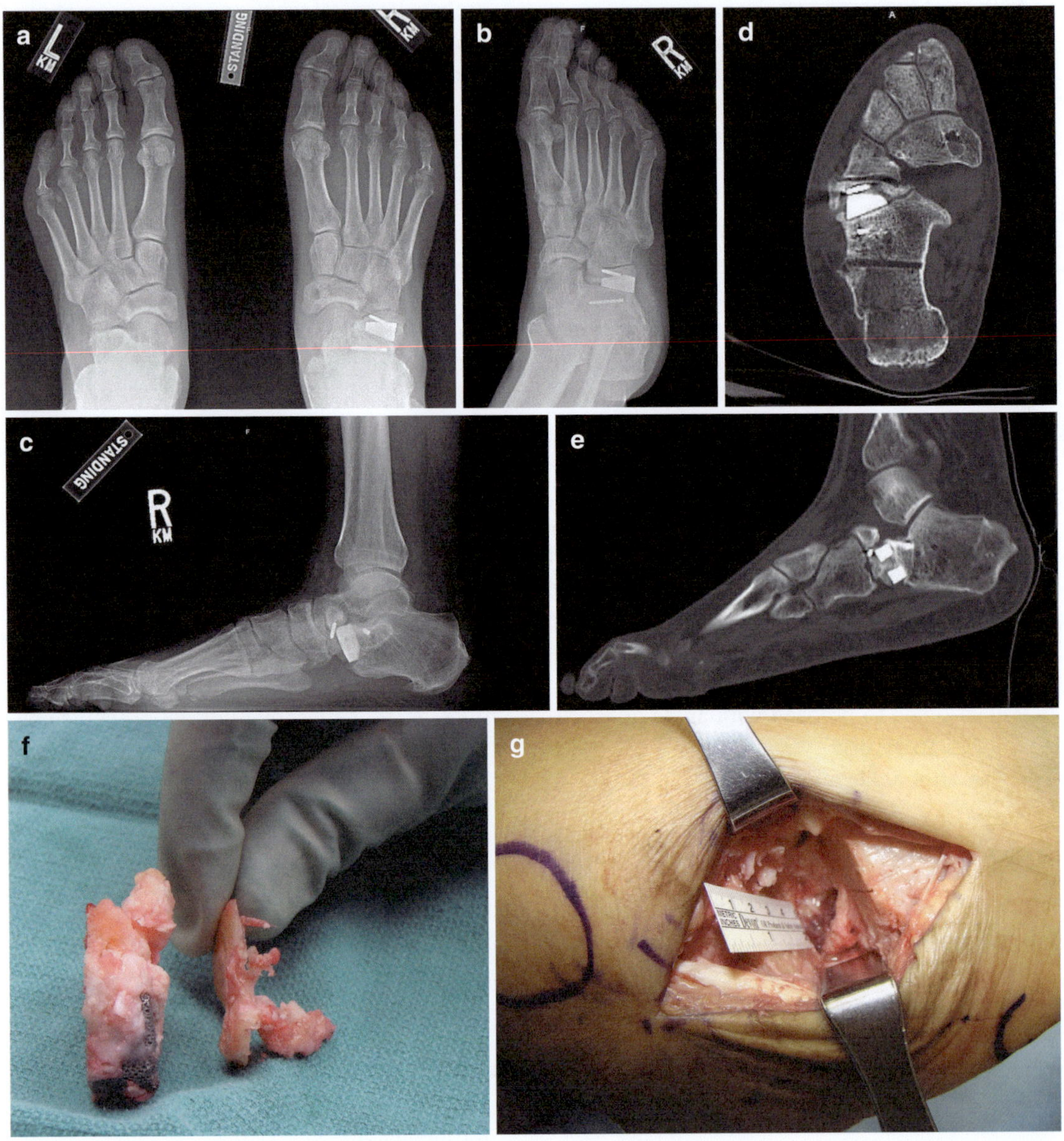

Fig. 16.4 Preoperative AP and oblique and lateral foot radiographs (**a**–**c**). Preoperative axial and sagittal CT scan reconstructions (**d**, **e**). Note the thin distal shelf of anterior process, with fracture into the calcaneocuboid joint and some bone incorporation into the metal wedge. Clinical picture of resected anterior process, articular surface of the cuboid, and the resultant void in the lateral column (**f**, **g**). Example of vascularized pedicle graft from the medial femoral condyle, both prior to and after implantation (**h**, **i**). One-year postoperative AP, oblique and lateral foot radiographs, and sagittal CT scan reconstruction (**j**–**m**)

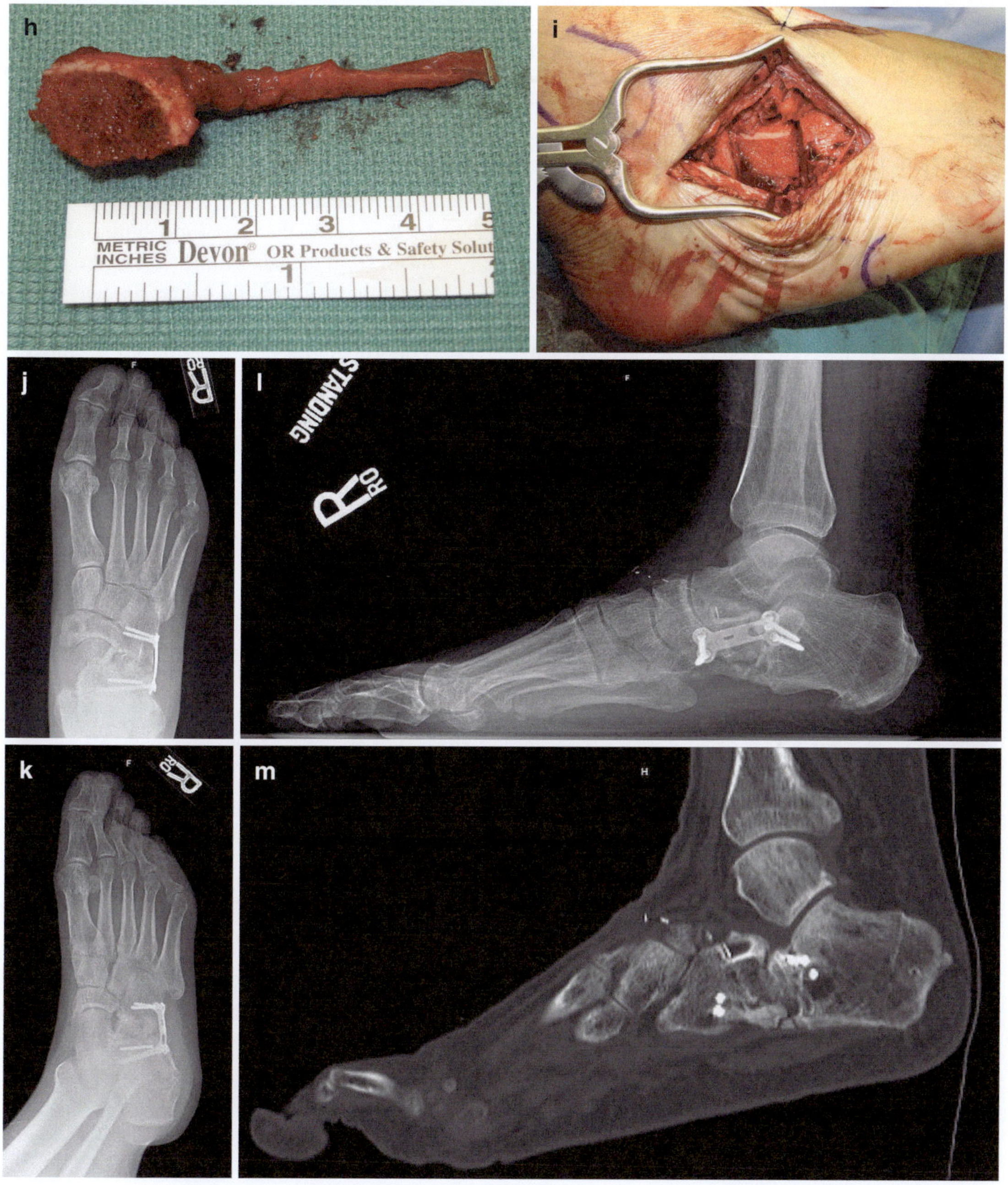

Fig. 16.4 (continued)

Implants

- Locking titanium H-plate along the lateral column

Case 16.5 (Courtesy of Carroll P. Jones, MD)

History

- Different patient than in **Case 16.2** but similar history.
- Most recent revision included removal of trabecular metal wedge and placement of tricortical iliac crest allograft that went on to nonunion (Fig. 16.5a, b).
- Patient complaining of isolated lateral column pain with well-maintained alignment both clinically and radiographically.

Surgical Plan and Approach

- Distal anterior process was intact and therefore kept in place to avoid large bone void (Fig. 16.5c).
- Structural autograft into void in anterior process, combined with calcaneocuboid and subtalar arthrodesis:
  - In this case, the structural autograft was taken from the superior aspect of the posterior tuberosity of the calcaneus and backfilled with tricortical allograft (Fig. 16.5d).
  - Tricortical iliac crest autograft would be another option.
  - Recombinant human platelet-derived growth factor in B-tricalcium phosphate granules was added for biologic graft.
- Final radiographs and CT scan at 1 year postoperative (Fig. 16.5e–g).

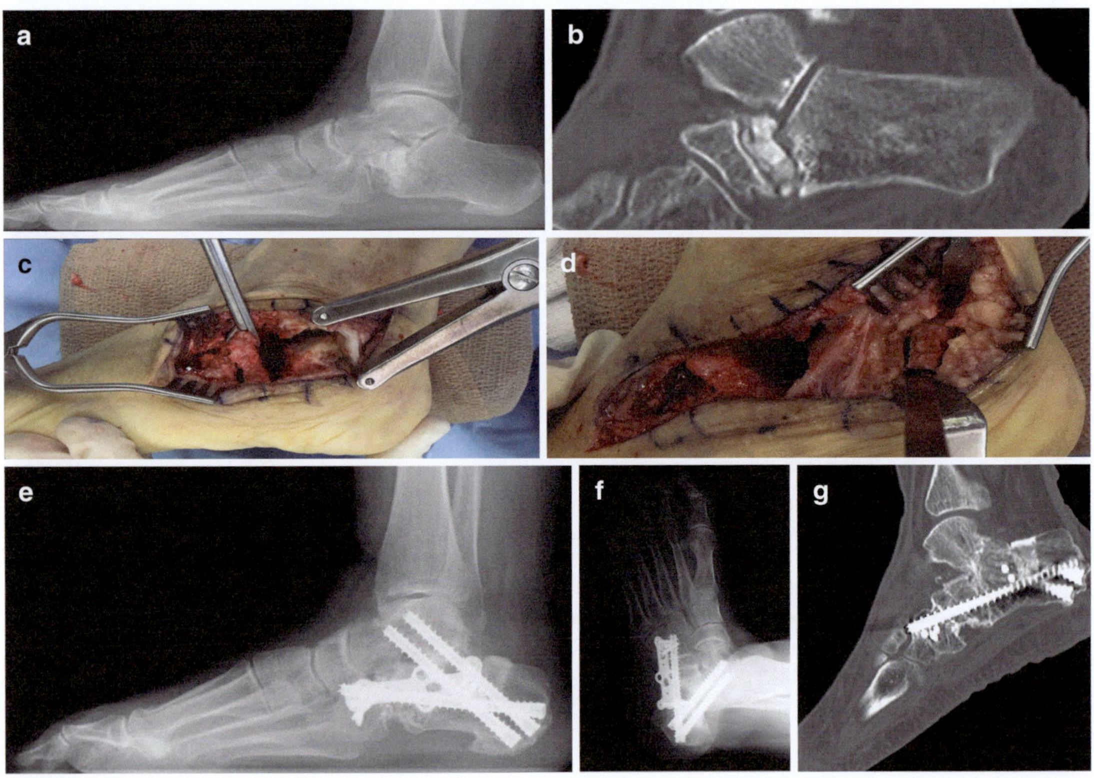

Fig. 16.5 Preoperative lateral foot radiograph and sagittal CT scan reconstruction (**a**, **b**). Clinical picture of intact anterior process (held by pituitary rongeur), with defect after graft removed (**c**). Clinical picture of structural autograft being harvested from posterior calcaneus tuberosity (between the Hohmann retractors, **d**). Six-month postoperative lateral and oblique foot radiographs and sagittal CT scan reconstruction (**e**–**g** (Courtesy of Carroll P. Jones, MD)

Implants

- Locking plate along lateral column
- Partially threaded titanium variable pitch cannulated screws across subtalar joint and lateral column

Case 16.6

History

- A 45-year-old male with history of talocalcaneal coalition and significant associated flatfoot deformity treated with triple arthrodesis about 2 years prior to presentation.
- He presented with complaints of persistent deformity and primarily lateral hindfoot pain.
- Physical examination revealed severe rigid pes planovalgus deformity, well-healed incisions, tenderness to palpation in the sinus tarsi and subfibular region, and gastrocnemius tightness per the Silfverskiold exam (Fig. 16.6a, b).
- Radiographs revealed a well-fused triple arthrodesis with staple fixation across the talonavicular and CC joint and screw fixation across the subtalar joint. There is significant residual pes planovalgus radiographic alignment with an apex plantar lateral talo-first metatarsal angle and increased AP talo-first metatarsal alignment indicating significant residual forefoot abduction (Fig. 16.6c, d).

Potential Reasons for Failure

- Inadequate deformity correction when performing the triple arthrodesis resulting in an undercorrected hindfoot fusion:
  - In situ fusion likely performed instead of addressing the hindfoot valgus and talocalcaneal alignment through the subtalar joint and the forefoot abduction and supination through the transverse tarsal joints.

Surgical Plan and Approach

- Biplanar closing wedge midtarsal osteotomy at site of prior talonavicular arthrodesis (Fig. 16.6e, f).
- Biplanar opening wedge midtarsal osteotomy at site of prior CC arthrodesis, utilizing removed autograft bone from the medial side:
  - Another option would have been a medial-based biplanar closing wedge osteotomy across the entire transverse tarsal fusion [31].
- Medial displacement calcaneal osteotomy to address residual hindfoot valgus.
- Peroneus brevis and longus tendon Z-lengthening to remove deforming force and lateral soft tissue contracture.
- Gastrocnemius recession to address equinus contracture.
- Consideration could also be made for further medial column arthrodesis through either the NC or TMT joints.
- Radiographs at 6 months postoperative and clinical pictures at 3 months postoperative (Fig. 16.6g–j).

Implants

- 5.5 mm partially threaded cannulated titanium screws across the talonavicular closing wedge osteotomy
- Titanium H-plate for fixation of the CC opening wedge osteotomy
- 7.0 mm partially threaded cannulated titanium screw across the MDCO

Case 16.7

- A 23-year-old male with a history of remote injury leading to multiple prior surgeries, including a medial displacement calcaneal osteotomy, lateral column lengthening, and FDL transfer secondary to apparent posterior tibial tendon insufficiency. He also had multiple peroneal tendon procedures ultimately resulting in FHL transfer.
- He presented with complaints of primarily lateral ankle instability, apprehension of instability, mild ankle pain, and mild lateral column foot pain.
- Physical examination revealed asymmetric cavovarus hindfoot and midfoot alignment and 1+ laxity to the lateral ankle ligaments. Coleman block test resulted in improvement from varus hindfoot to neutral hindfoot position (Fig. 16.7a, b).

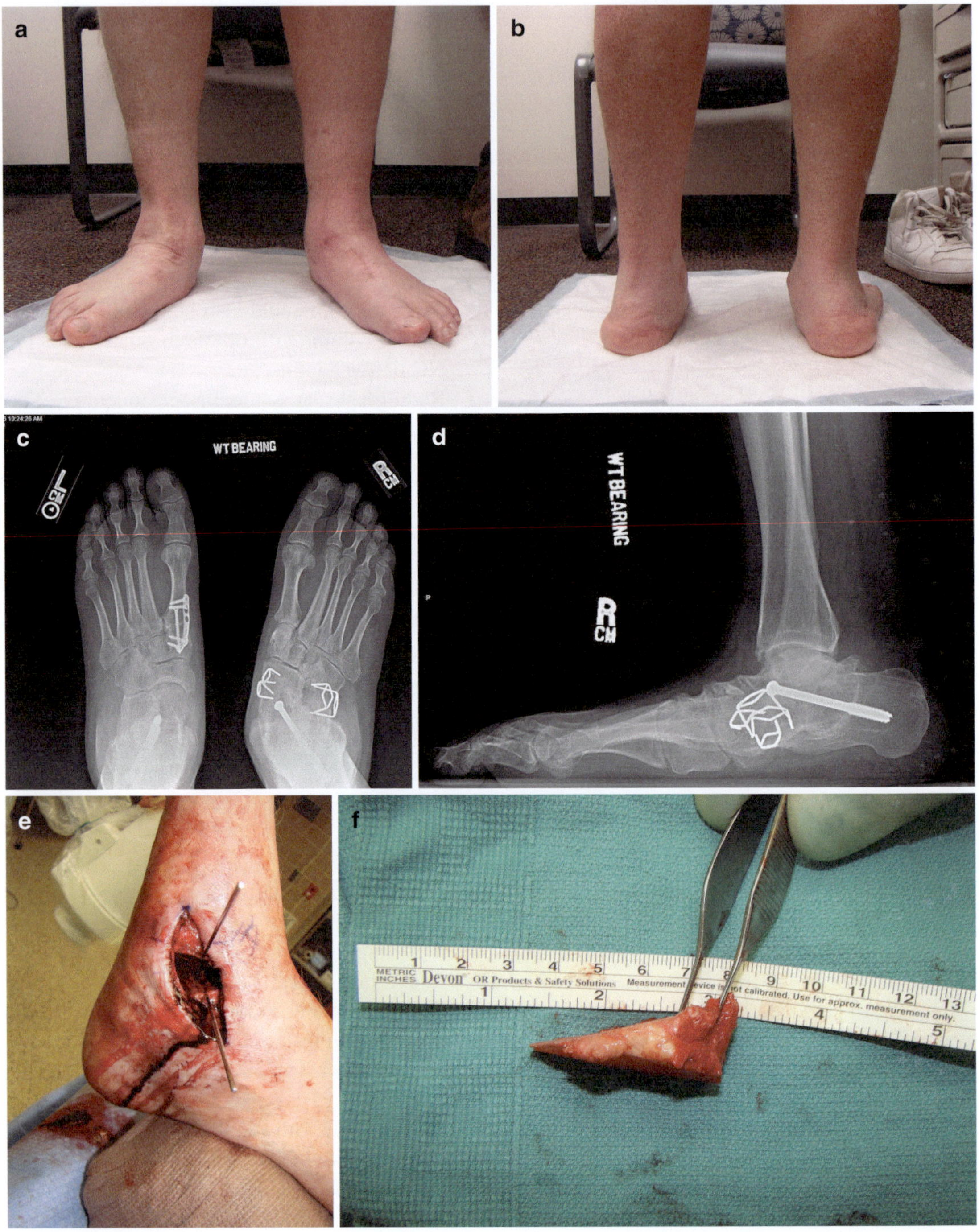

Fig. 16.6 Preoperative standing clinical pictures (**a**, **b**). Preoperative AP and lateral foot radiograph (**c**, **d**). Clinical picture of medial- and plantar-based wedge removed from prior site of talonavicular fusion (**e**, **f**). Six-month postoperative AP and lateral foot radiographs (**g**, **h**). Three-month postoperative clinical pictures (**i**, **j**)

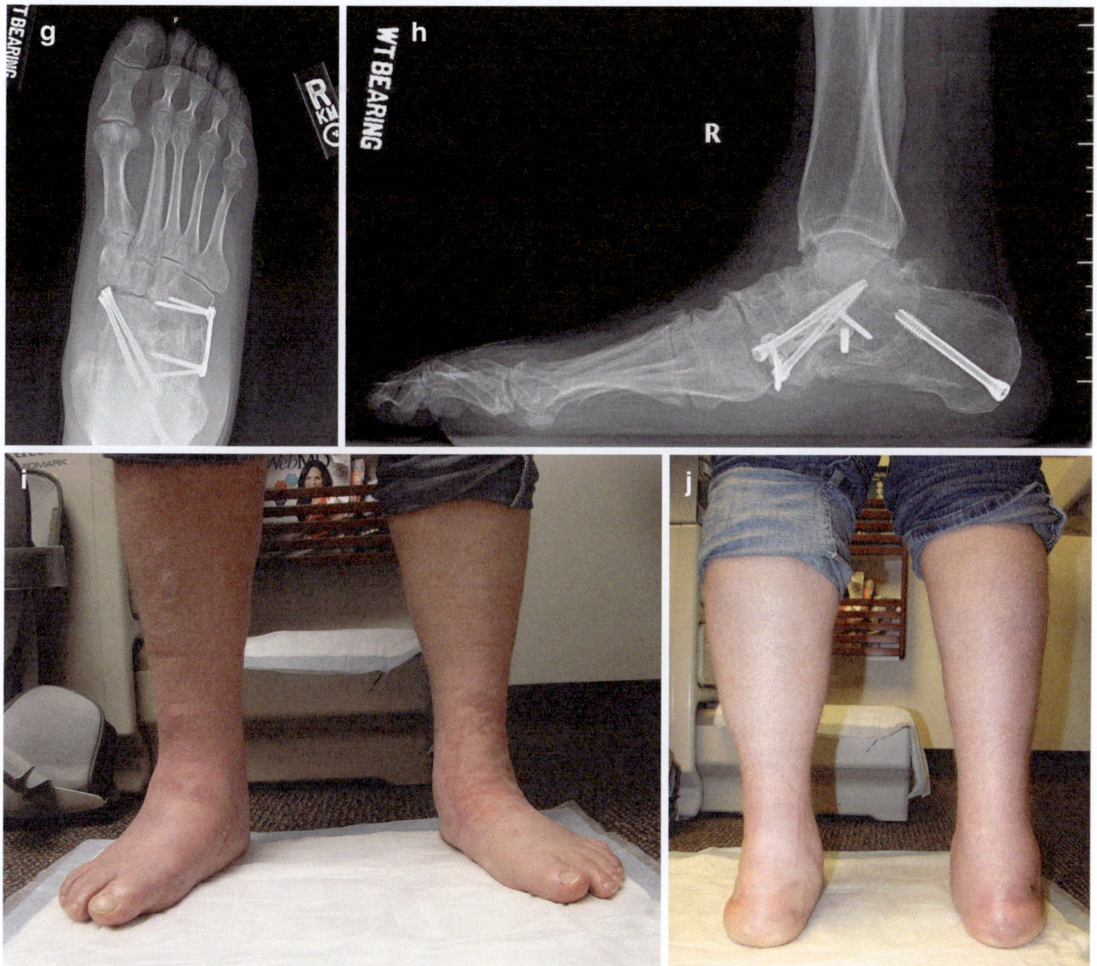

Fig. 16.6 (continued)

- Radiographs revealed cavus foot deformity, asymmetric talonavicular coverage, and moderate hindfoot varus (Fig. 16.7c–e).

Potential Reasons for Failure

- Overcorrection of a mild flatfoot through multiple osteotomies:
  - Possibly excessive medial displacement of the MDCO
  - Possibly excessive lengthening of the lateral column through the LCL
  - A combination of both of the above leading to overcorrection
- Eversion and external rotation weakness secondary to insufficient peroneals, leading to ankle instability that is exacerbated by his hindfoot alignment.

Surgical Plan and Approach

- Revision calcaneal osteotomy through lateral approach:
  - Lateral closing wedge osteotomy (Dwyer) to address the hindfoot varus.
  - Posterior tuberosity segment was also slightly translated laterally (avoiding excessive shift due to concerns of tibial nerve compression) and superiorly to decrease the calcaneal pitch (Fig. 16.7f, g).
- Dorsiflexion first metatarsal osteotomy through dorsal approach to address the cavus alignment by elevating the first ray (Fig. 16.7f, h)
- Modified Brostrom-Gould lateral ligament reconstruction through lateral approach:

- Suture tape device was used for augmentation.
- Clinical pictures at 7 months postoperative (Fig. 16.7i, j)

Implants

- 4.5 mm partially threaded headless cannulated titanium screws x2 for fixation of the calcaneal osteotomy
- 2.0 mm plate and screws for fixation of the dorsiflexion first metatarsal osteotomy
- Suture tape device with anchors in the fibula and talus, combined with pants-over-vest suture repair, for stabilization of the lateral ankle ligament reconstruction

Pearls and Pitfalls

- Inadequate correction of the medial column is a common cause of failure of initial flatfoot reconstruction:
  - Medial column osteotomy or realignment arthrodesis is often required in revision cases.
- Triple arthrodesis malunion often results in residual midfoot abduction, supination, and hindfoot valgus:
  - Realignment osteotomy through the involved joints, often with biplanar wedge removal, may be required.
- Recognize tilt in the tibiotalar joint or deformity in the supramalleolar tibia as potential causes of failure.
- In the setting of ligamentous laxity, low threshold for arthrodesis of involved joints may improve outcomes and durability of the reconstruction.
- Revision of a lateral column lengthening through the anterior process of the calcaneus may have difficult healing potential:
  - Care should be undertaken to preserve the anterior process as much as possible. Diligent use of bone graft and/or biologics may be required.
- Overcorrected flatfoot correction through either joint-sparing or joint-sacrificing procedures results in a clinical scenario similar to a cavovarus foot and can be treated with similar surgical techniques.

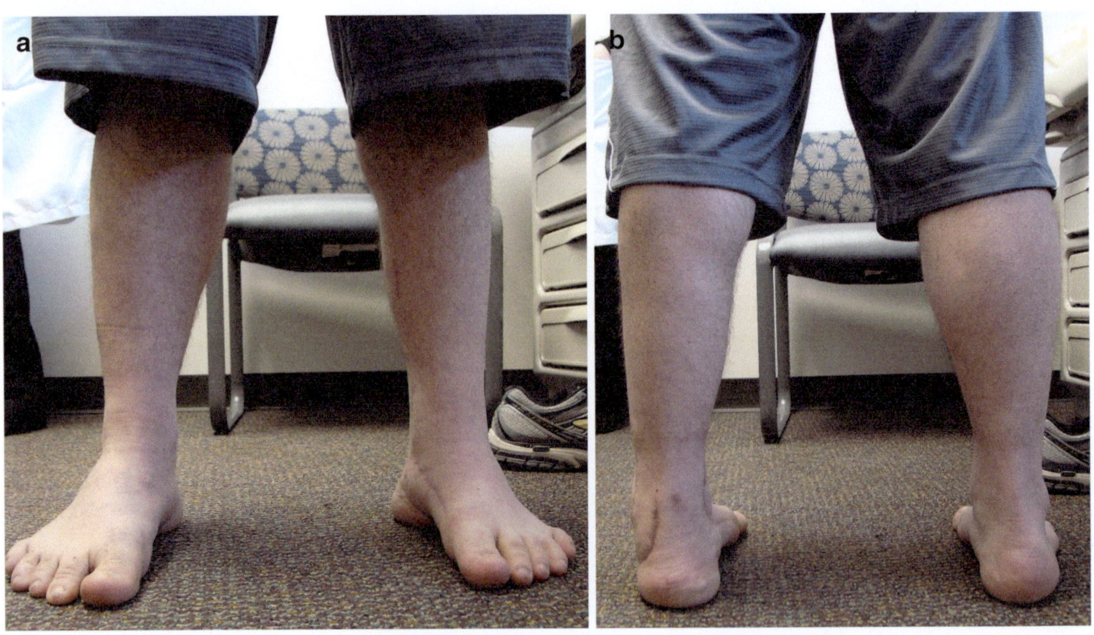

Fig. 16.7 Preoperative anterior and posterior clinical pictures (**a**, **b**). Preoperative AP and lateral and axial foot radiographs (**c**–**e**). Four-month postoperative AP and lateral and axial foot radiographs (**f**–**h**). Seven-month postoperative clinical pictures

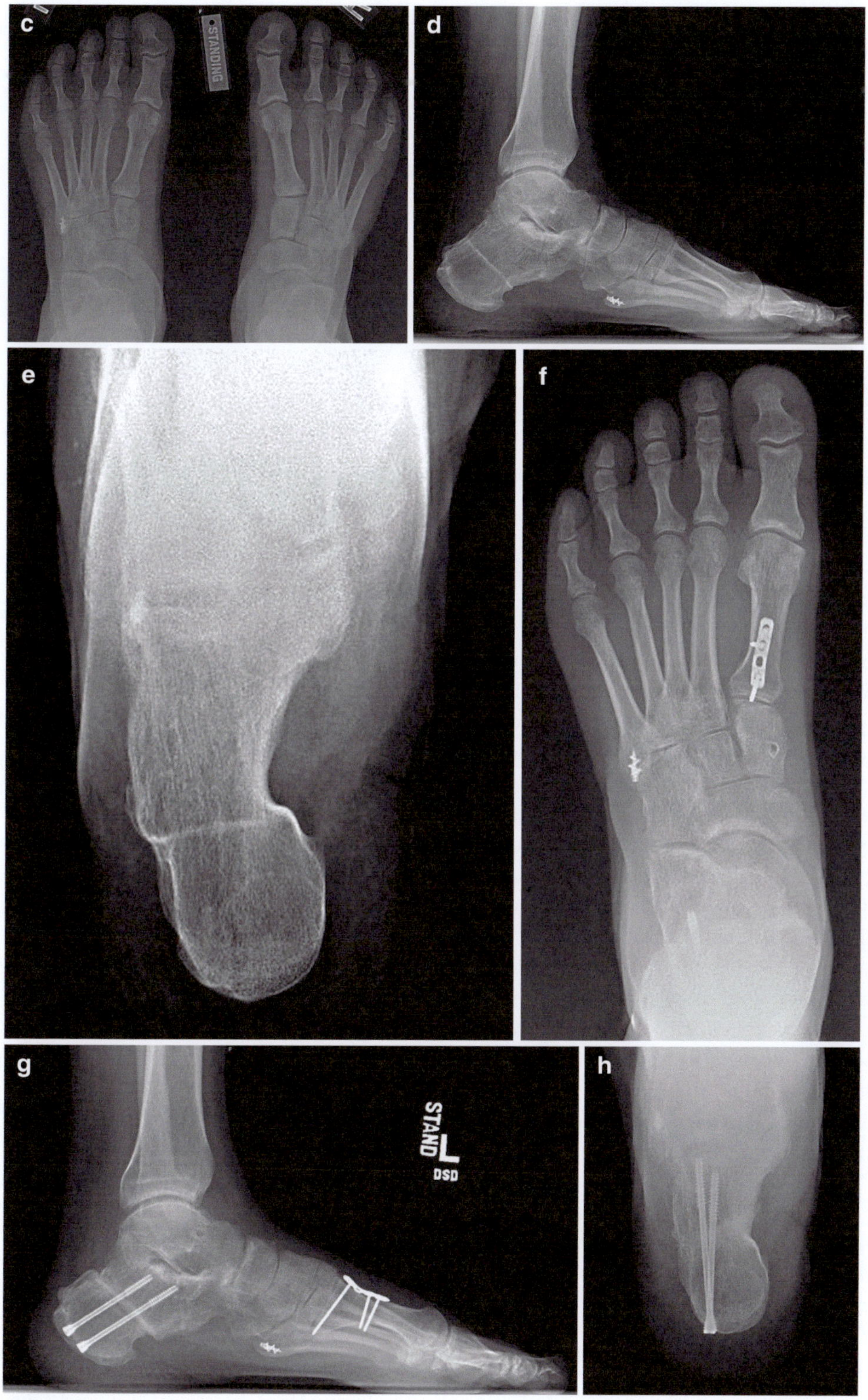

Fig. 16.7 (continued)

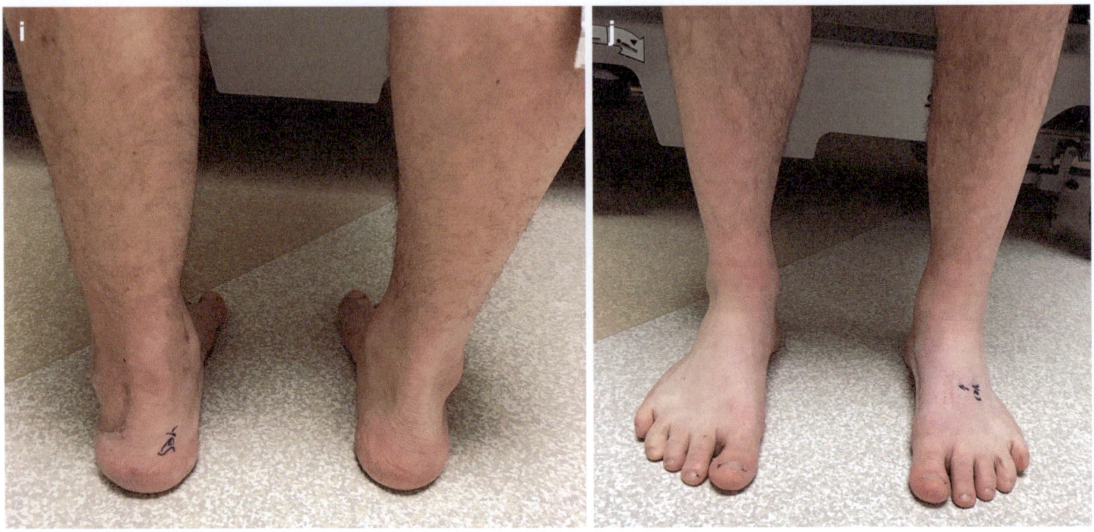

Fig. 16.7 (continued)

Summary

Revision of the failed flatfoot reconstruction is a challenging clinical problem. Diligent evaluation of the patient is required to determine the location and cause of symptoms. Residual deformity and its location are important to determine and are often an important contributor to the patient's symptoms. If there is no residual deformity, symptoms are likely secondary to complications at the specific site of prior procedures. Surgical correction of the failed flatfoot reconstruction is often required. A combination of osteotomies, arthrodesis, and soft tissue procedures such as tendon transfers or tendon lengthenings may be required for adequate correction. Preoperative planning is paramount to achieving a good clinical outcome that results in a durable, functional, plantigrade foot and ankle.

References

1. Sangeorzan BJ, Mosca V, Hansen ST Jr. Effect of calcaneal lengthening on relationships among the hindfoot, midfoot, and forefoot. Foot Ankle. 1993;14:136–41.
2. Toolan BC, Sangeorzan BJ, Hansen ST Jr. Complex reconstruction for the treatment of dorsolateral peritalar subluxation of the foot. Early results after distraction arthrodesis of the calcaneocuboid joint in conjunction with stabilization of, and transfer of the flexor digitorum longus tendon to, the midfoot to treat acquired pes planovalgus in adults. J Bone Joint Surg. 1999;81-A:1545–60.
3. Moseir-Laclair S, Pomeroy G, Manoli A II. Intermediate follow-up on the double osteotomy and tendon transfer procedure for stage II posterior tibial tendon insufficiency. Foot Ankle Int. 2001;22(4):283–91.
4. Hadfield MH, Snyder JW, Liacouras PC, Owen JR, Wayne JS, Adelaar RS. Effects of medializing calcaneal osteotomy on Achilles tendon lengthening and plantar foot pressures. Foot Ankle Int. 2003;24:523–9.
5. Myerson MS, Badekas A, Schon LC. Treatment of stage II posterior tibial tendon deficiency with flexor digitorum longus tendon transfer and calcaneal osteotomy. Foot Ankle Int. 2004;25(7):445–50.
6. Vora AM, Tien TR, Parks BG, Schon LC. Correction of moderate and severe acquired flexible flatfoot with medializing calcaneal osteotomy and flexor digitorum longus transfer. J Bone Joint Surg Am. 2006;88(8):1726–34.
7. Johnson KA, Strom DE. Tibialis posterior tendon dysfunction. Clin Orthop Relat Res. 1989;239:196–206.
8. Mann RA, Thompson FM. Rupture of the posterior tibial tendon causing flatfoot. J Bone Joint Surg Am. 1985;67-A:556–61.
9. Funk DA, Cass JR, Johnson KA. Acquired adult flat foot secondary to posterior tibial-tendon pathology. J Bone Joint Surg Am. 1986;68-A:95–102.
10. Myerson MS. Adult acquired flatfoot deformity: treatment of dysfunction of the posterior tibial tendon. Instr Course Lect. 1997;46:393–405.

11. DiGiovanni CW, Langer P. The role of isolated gastrocnemius and combined achilles contractures in the flatfoot. Foot Ankle Clin. 2007;12:363–79.
12. Kou JX, Balasubramaniam M, Kippe M, et al. Functional results of posterior tibial tendon reconstruction, calcaneal osteotomy, and gastrocnemius recession. Foot Ankle Int. 2012;33(7):602–11.
13. Guyton GF, Jeng C, Krieger LE, et al. Flexor digitorum longus transfer and medial displacement calcaneal osteotomy for posterior tibial tendon dysfunction: a middle-term clinical follow-up. Foot Ankle Int. 2001;22(8):627–32.
14. Aiyer A, Dall GF, Shub J, et al. Radiographic correction following reconstruction of adult acquired flat foot deformity using the cotton medial cuneiform osteotomy. Foot Ankle Int. 2016;37(5):508–13.
15. Silva MG, Tan SH, Chong HC, et al. Results of operative correction of grade IIB tibialis posterior tendon dysfunction. Foot Ankle Int. 2015;36(2):165–71.
16. Ajis A, Geary N. Surgical technique, fusion rates, and planovalgus foot deformity correction with naviculocuneiform fusion. Foot Ankle Int. 2014;35(3):232–7.
17. Johnson JE, Cohen BE, DiGiovanni BF, et al. Subtalar arthrodesis with flexor digitorum longus transfer and spring ligament repair for treatment of posterior tibial tendon insufficiency. Foot Ankle Int. 2000;21(9):722–9.
18. Stephens HM, Walling AK, Solmen JD, et al. Subtalar repositional arthrodesis for adult acquired flatfoot. Clin Orthop Relat Res. 1999;365:69–73.
19. Sangeorzan BJ, Smith D, Veith R, Hansen ST. Triple arthrodesis using internal fixation in treatment of adult foot disorders. Clin Orthop Relat Res. 1993;294:299–307.
20. Ahmad J, Pedowitz D. Management of the rigid arthritic flatfoot in adults: triple arthrodesis. Foot Ankle Clin. 2012;17(2):309–22.
21. Knupp M, Schuh R, Stufkens SA, et al. Subtalar and talonavicular arthrodesis through a single medial approach for the correction of severe planovalgus deformity. J Bone Joint Surg Br. 2009;91:612–5.
22. Sammarco VJ, Magur EG, Sammarco GJ, et al. Arthrodesis of the subtalar and talonavicular joints for correction of symptomatic hindfoot malalignment. Foot Ankle Int. 2006;27(9):661–6.
23. Schuh R, Salzberger F, Wanivenhaus AH, et al. Kinematic changes in patients with double arthrodesis of the hindfoot for realignment of planovalgus deformity. J Orthop Res. 2013;31(4):517–24.
24. Davis WH. Is this my ankle or my foot? Foot Ankle Clin. 2017;22:587–95.
25. Miniaci-Coxhead SL, Weisenthal B, Ketz JP, Flemister AS. Incidence and radiographic predictors of valgus tibiotalar tilt after hindfoot fusion. Foot Ankle Int. 2017;38:519–25.
26. Hunt KJ, Farmer RP. The undercorrected flatfoot reconstruction. Foot Ankle Clin. 2017;22:613–24.
27. Kadakia AR, Kelikian AS, Barbosa M, Patel MS. Did failure occur because of medial column instability that was not recognized, or did it develop after surgery? Foot Ankle Clin. 2017;22:545–62.
28. Irwin TA. Overcorrected flatfoot reconstruction. Foot Ankle Clin. 2017;22:597–611.
29. Saltzman CL, el-Khoury GY. The hindfoot alignment view. Foot Ankle Int. 1995;16(9):572–6.
30. Yoshioka N, Ikoma K, Kido M, et al. Weight-bearing three-dimensional computed tomography analysis of the forefoot in patients with flatfoot deformity. J Orthop Sci. 2016;21(2):154–8.
31. Haddad SL, Myerson MS, Pell RF, Schon LS. Clinical and radiographic outcome of revision surgery for failed triple arthrodesis. Foot Ankle Int. 1997;18:489–99.

Revision of the Cavovarus Foot

17

Arthur Manoli II

Key Takeaway Points

- Usually from malposition after the initial fixation or reconstructive surgery.
- This type of cavovarus is usually stiff with the hindfoot in varus and the forefoot pronated.
- It can be from unrecognized initial postural traits and/or from inadequate soft tissue releases at time of initial surgery.
- Most cases are revision fusions coupled with soft tissue releases.
- In most situations, a medial release is necessary and the Achilles or gastrocnemius muscle needs to be lengthened.

Introduction

Many of the pathological problems of the foot may require a patient to have a hindfoot fusion (arthrodesis). This is usually a subtalar, triple, tibiotalocalcaneal, or talonavicular fusion. It is not uncommon for the foot to be malaligned after these procedures. The foot may be fused in excessive heel valgus (flatfoot) or excessive varus (cavus). This review will focus on the later, the cavovarus deformity.

Brief Review of the Problem and Literature

When the foot is fused in cavus with the heel in varus, the patient usually also has a pronated forefoot. They may also have a bean-shaped foot with an externally rotated talus [1].

Revision subtalar and triple osteotomies have become more commonplace since the techniques have been described to do them through the area of the deformity [2, 3] and alternative techniques using nearby osteotomies have also been described [4]. We prefer to do the revision osteotomies at the area of original fusions, as it corrects the deformity at the original site, and it doesn't produce compensatory deformities.

We have also noticed the need for pairing the osteotomies with a medial release of the subtalar and talonavicular joint. A medial release was originally emphasized to do by Daniels' group when a severe varus ankle received an arthroplasty [5]. It is also critical to use when revising cavovarus feet [6].

A. Manoli II (✉)
Wayne State University, Detroit, MI, USA

Department of Orthopaedic Surgery, Michigan State University, East Lansing, MI, USA

Department of Orthopaedic Surgery, Michigan International Foot and Ankle Center, St. Joseph Mercy Hospital—Oakland, Pontiac, MI, USA

M. J. Berkowitz et al. (eds.), *Revision Surgery of the Foot and Ankle*,
https://doi.org/10.1007/978-3-030-29969-9_17

Causes of Failure

The causes of failure of the original procedure are many. A common cause of failure is failing to recognize a preexisting cavovarus foot preoperatively. Approximately one-quarter of the population has a mild, subtle cavovarus foot [7, 8]. This can be familial and has been difficult to identify in the past. With increasing recognition of the existence of a peek-a-boo heel in these patients, it has been easier to identify the subtle cavus foot. In acute trauma, one can always stand the patient and observe the other, if uninjured, foot, for these characteristics. If the patient has a normal cavus on the other side, there's a good chance that they'll have it in the involved side. The patient could have been functioning satisfactorily with normal joints, but when the foot is stiffened, they may not be able to function, as the stiffened foot cannot change and adapt.

In patients who have had prior hindfoot procedures, it is important to recognize the shape of the opposite contralateral foot. This gives one an idea of what the patients' "normal" is and if one needs to restore it to the normal shape or add some correction to the native cavovarus situation. Bilateral standing radiographs and a CT scan to include both feet are essential, if possible, for comparison and decision-making.

Recently, there has been interest in trying to relate preexisting skeletal deformity to traumatic injuries in orthopedics. Wong and Clare have found 57.6% of high-energy talar fractures had a cavovarus foot on the contralateral side [9]. Also in the foot, Gallagher et al. found an anatomic predisposition to ligamentous Lisfranc injury with different metatarsal lengthens [10]. Kang and Park even found a predisposing effect of elbow alignment on the elbow fracture type in children [11].

Other causes of failure are failure to perform an adequate soft tissue release prior to fusing the subtalar or triple complex. Generally, in the cavovarus foot, the posterior tibial tendon and, occasionally, subtalar and talonavicular joint capsules are contracted and should be released. Even in a cavovarus foot, there may be a talocalcaneal or calcaneonavicular tarsal coalition present. We resect these if they exist [12].

The most common surgery that is done for revision of a cavovarus foot is a revision subtalar fusion or a revision triple arthrodesis. Occasionally, it is necessary to add an ankle fusion to fully correct and stabilize the foot [2]. Soft tissue releases are usually necessary.

Evaluation and Assessment

Accurate evaluation is essential to plan the corrective procedures. The patient should be evaluated in a standing position first, with their shoes and socks removed. When viewed from the front, the patients usually have a peek-a-boo heel visible on the medial side of the foot, suggesting a varus heel [8] (Fig. 17.1a). This is confirmed by viewing the patient from the rear, looking for heel varus or a medial inserting Achilles tendon. A Coleman block test is then performed in all patients that exhibit heel varus.

The classic Coleman block test is performed by having the patient stand on a piece of wood or a book, hanging the first and second toes off of the medial aspect of the block, and seeing if the heel corrects out of varus to a more normal slight valgus position [13]. In most normal patients, the heel corrects into a normal slight valgus position. In these patients, there usually has been a stiffening due to a fusion of the subtalar joint, so one does not expect much correction of the heel varus. A small bit of correction may be possible because of the ankle rotating and tipping into slight valgus.

In cases with prior fusion surgery, there will be a stiff foot in cavovarus, with a pronated forefoot and a plantarflexed first ray. The posterior tibial tendon will be contracted and tight, and the flexor digitorum longus and the flexor hallucis longus tendon may also be contracted giving claw toes.

Generally, these patients will also have a tight gastrocnemius muscle or a tight Achilles tendon. Almost always, they have contracture of the posterior tibial tendon and occasionally the medial hindfoot joint capsules of the talonavicular and subtalar joints. In most cases, the original operating surgeon failed to identify the contracted medial tissues resulting in undercorrection of a

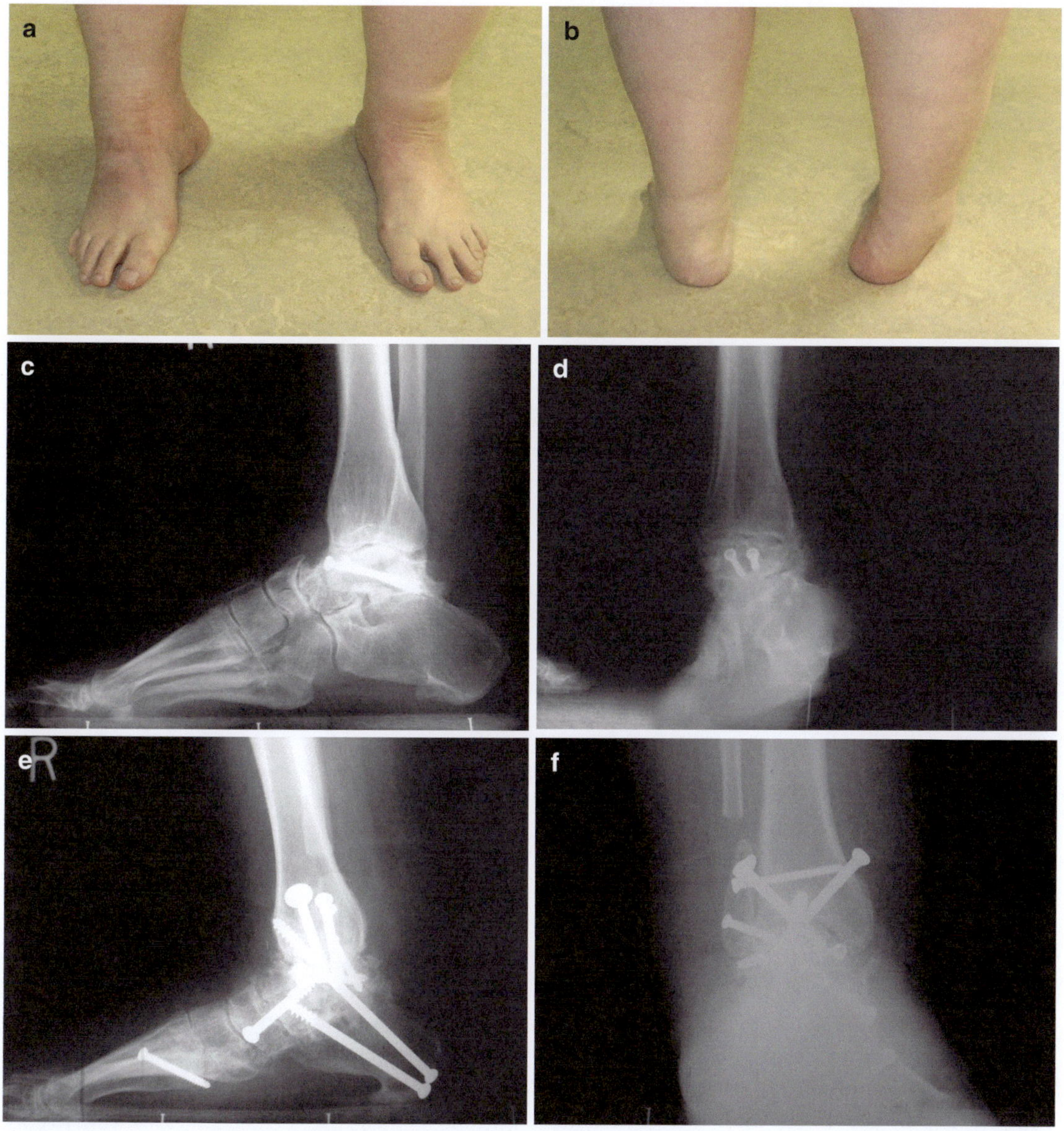

Fig. 17.1 (**a**) Photo of **Case 17.1**, after the initial fixation of a talar fracture. The right foot had surgery and is in more cavovarus than the normal left foot. Note that the peek-a-boo heel is more visible on the right than the left. (**b**) When the patient in **Case 17.1** is viewed from the rear, the heel varus is very obvious. (**c**) Lateral radiograph illustrates a healed talar fracture with posttraumatic arthritis of the ankle and subtalar joints. There is irregularity of the talar dome. (**d**) Preoperative anteroposterior radiograph of the ankle. There is irregularity of the talar dome due to posttraumatic arthritis and spotty avascular necrosis. The varus heel is even seen. (**e**) Lateral view of the final construct. The implants used were the 6.5 mm solid screws across the major joints (ankle, subtalar, and talonavicular) and a single 4.0 mm solid screw for the dorsiflexion osteotomy of the first metatarsal. (**f**) Anteroposterior view of the final construct. (**g**) A lateral approach is used to perform a transfibular ankle fusion. It is curved distally in the distal portion, so a subtalar fusion could be added through a single incision. (**h**) A medial approach was used for a posterior tibial tendon tenotomy, a release of the talonavicular and subtalar joints, a talonavicular fusion, and a first metatarsal dorsiflexion osteotomy. The anteromedial incision was used by the initial surgeon. (**i**) Final postoperative views of both feet. The cavovarus deformity on the right has been corrected. (**j**) Rear view of both feet. There is less heel varus on the right, compared to the normal left side. The percutaneous "stab" incisions to lengthen the Achilles tendon can be seen on the right side

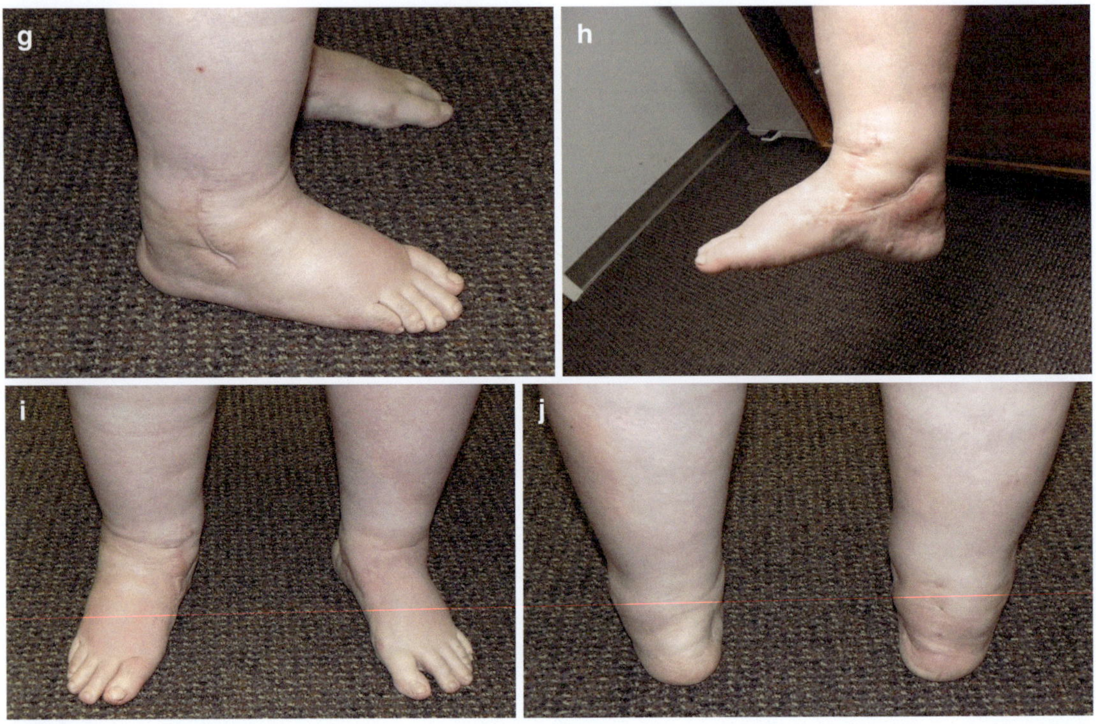

Fig. 17.1 (continued)

cavovarus foot. It is especially important to identify these contracted tissues in order to obtain a correction at the time of revision.

The triceps surae is evaluated with the Silfverskiöld test, and the amount of equinus of the foot is noted. Ideally, the foot should be passively corrected to neutral or a few degrees of dorsiflexion with the knee straight and the patient in a sitting position [14]. If it does not approach neutral and the dorsiflexion improves with flexing of the knee, then the gastrocnemius muscle is tight. If there is no improvement of dorsiflexion with the knee flexed, then the entire Achilles tendon complex is tight. Either the gastrocnemius muscle is loosened or the entire Achilles must be loosened in order to obtain correction.

Standing radiographs of the feet and ankles with oblique views of the foot should be obtained.

A CT scan of both feet and ankles is also essential for the pre-op plan.

Surgical Planning

Most patients that need revision surgery of the cavovarus need one or more of these: a revision subtalar fusion, a revision triple arthrodesis, an ankle fusion, a medial release, and a Holt-type triple cut of the Achilles tendon or a gastrocnemius muscle slide procedure. These can be used in various combinations or alone if necessary. Oftentimes, a dorsiflexion osteotomy of the first, second, and third metatarsals may be necessary, as well, to correct a pronated forefoot which is made worse as the hindfoot is corrected out of varus [15].

Revision Subtalar Fusion

A revision subtalar fusion is indicated in those cases which have previously been fused with the heel in varus. Generally, there is a lateral scar, and this can be used to approach the fusion mass. The peroneal muscles and their overlying sural nerve should be identified and lifted off of the calcaneus and protected. The extensor digitorum brevis muscle is removed from its origin on the anterior process of the calcaneus. The sinus tarsi is identified and cleaned of the local fat. The previous subtalar fusion site is visible in most cases. Unless the fusion is ancient, the edges of the previous fusion can usually be identified, and a small osteotome can be used to outline the previous joints, and additional osteotomes are used to deepen the osteotomy through the fusion mass as one approaches the medial surface (Fig. 17.4e). Care should be taken not to cut through the medial cortex; rather, we prefer to get close to the medial cortex and then use a large lamina spreader to spread and break through the cortex (Fig. 17.2g). Curettes can remove additional bone carefully in the medial aspect. If the osteotomy resembles the previous position and shape of the subtalar joint, external rotation of the foot through the calcaneus allows it to straighten the foot, and a physiologic valgus is produced. If the foot does not rotate through the osteotomy, an additional medial incision is made, and the posterior tibial tendon is sectioned, and if necessary, the subtalar and talonavicular joint capsules can be released to allow the rotation.

As the osteotomy is done through cancellous bone, it heals rapidly, and minimal screw fixation can be placed across it to hold the position. Usually, the valgus that is produced in the hind-

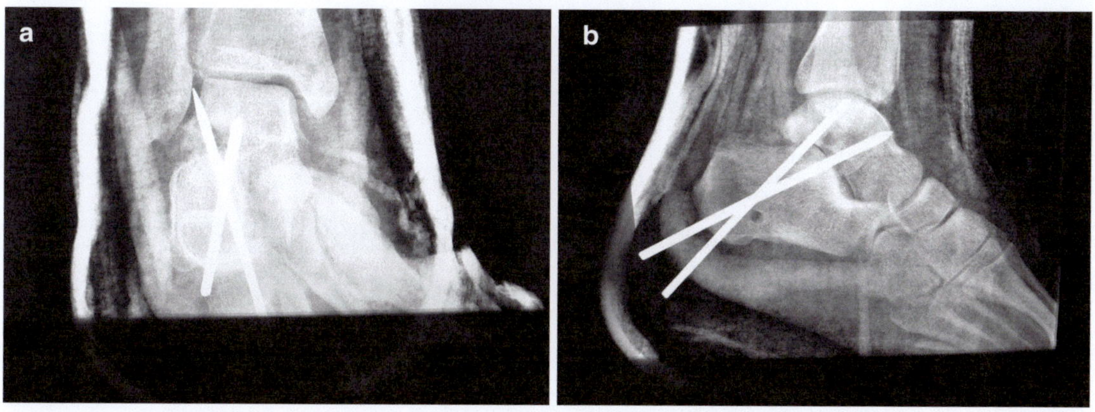

Fig. 17.2 (**a**) Anteroposterior radiograph after subtalar dislocation was reduced and pinned. The calcaneus fracture through the primary fracture line not repaired. (**b**) Lateral radiograph after subtalar dislocation was reduced and pinned. (**c**) Photograph of the feet after the initial triple arthrodesis. There is a significant peek-a-boo heel on the right side. (**d**) Lateral photograph of the right foot. Note the high arch. Although the first ray appears elevated, when the hindfoot is corrected, the first ray will be more plantarflexed. Here, we were demonstrating to the patient that it may be necessary to elevate it. Ultimately, it was not necessary to elevate it. (**e**) Standing radiographs of both of the feet after the first triple arthrodesis. In the anteroposterior view, one can see that the right foot is supinated compared to the normal left foot. (**f**) Lateral radiograph after the initial triple arthrodesis. Note the supination and elevation of the first ray. (**g**) Technique of revision triple arthrodesis. Through a lateral incision, the previous subtalar and talonavicular joint areas are identified. A small osteotome is used to outline the lateral and dorsal areas where the joints were previously. The joints are gradually cut apart. Eventually, a lamina spreader is inserted, and the joints can be pried apart and loosened (above). In a cavovarus deformity, the distal foot is rotated laterally through these joints. When this is done, the heel everts through the subtalar joint. The calcaneocuboid joint does not usually need to be recut in this procedure, but if it is fused in a poor position, it may need to be osteotomized, also. (**h**) Medial release. Here, the posterior tibial tendon is identified, and 1–2 cm is resected. If more correction is needed, the talonavicular and subtalar joints may need to be opened. (**i**) Lateral radiograph after the osteotomies are performed and fixed. As the osteotomies are through cancellous bone areas, minimal fixation is all that is necessary. Note that the first ray was plantarflexed when the hindfoot was placed in the correct position. (**j**) Anteroposterior radiograph after the revision triple arthrodesis. (**k**) Axial view of the heel after the corrective osteotomies. There is still some mild medial positioning of the calcaneal tuberosity, as the initial calcaneal fracture displacement was not addressed. (**l**) Photograph of the feet after the corrective osteotomies. Compare to Figure (**c**). (**m**) Photograph of the feet after the corrective osteotomies. The right Achilles tendon was lengthened with a four-cut technique

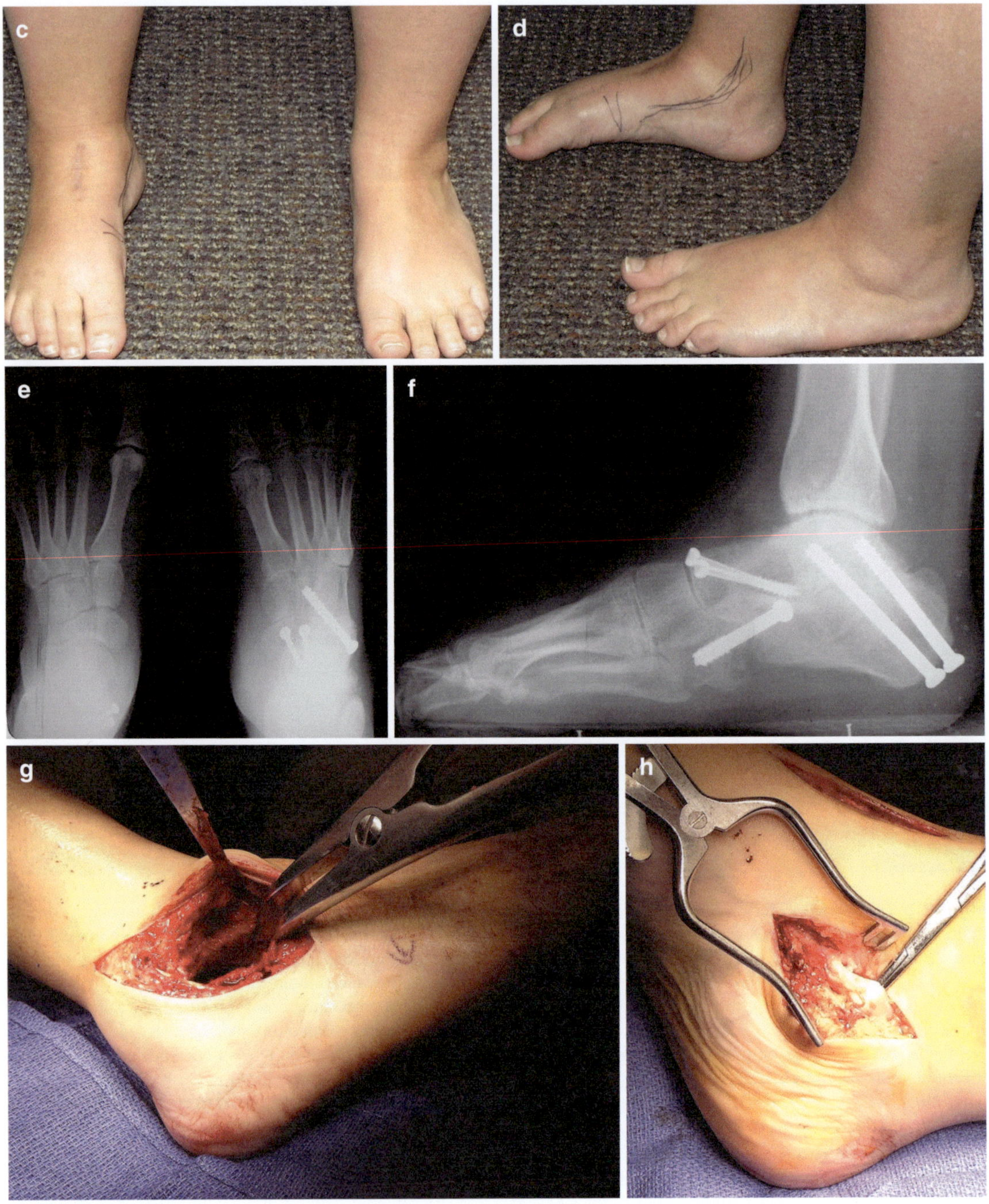

Fig. 17.2 (continued)

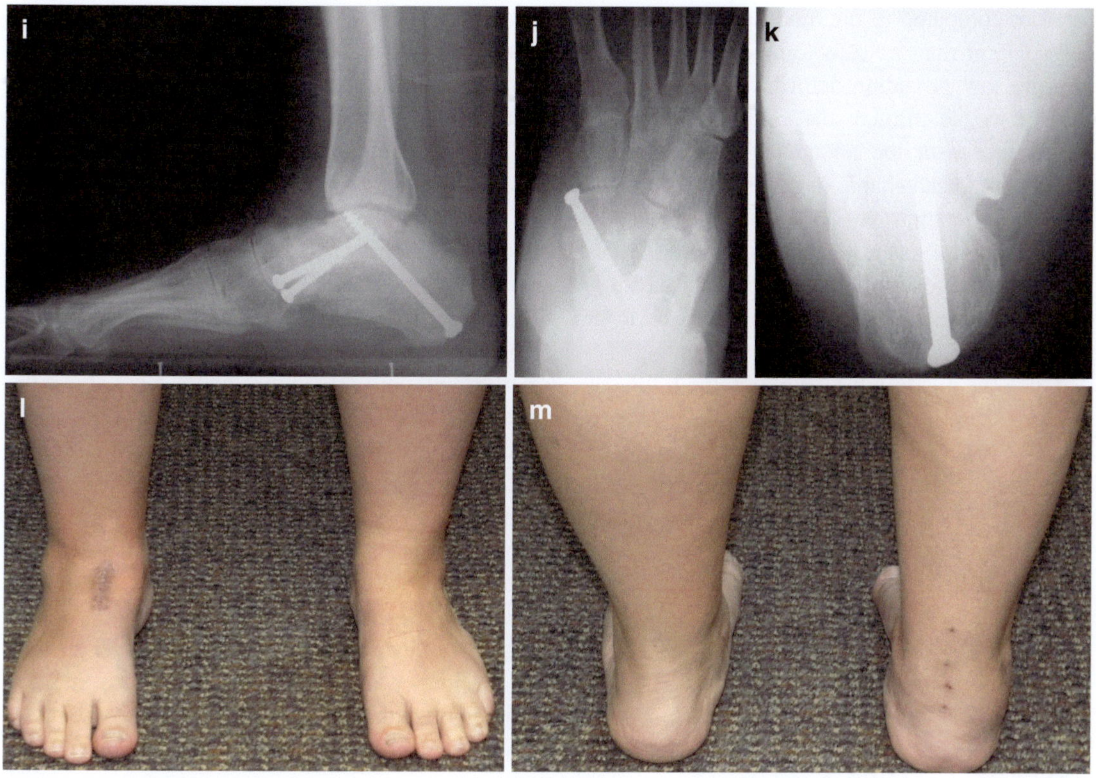

Fig. 17.2 (continued)

foot is sufficient. If it is insufficient, one can take off the bone from the talar or calcaneal surface laterally to provide a little more heel valgus [3].

When this procedures is performed, obtaining heel valgus will also rotate the forefoot and pronate the medial first metatarsal and further plantarflex it (and occasionally the second and third also) necessitating a dorsiflexion osteotomy as described below [15].

Revision Triple Arthrodesis

A revision triple arthrodesis is indicated for a previous triple arthrodesis which has been fused in varus [2, 3]. The approach is similar to that of a revision subtalar fusion; however, the talonavicular joint area is also exposed. One can extend the distal portion of the subtalar osteotomy incision from the lateral side, or one could make an additional medial incision over the fused talonavicular joint and expose the area from the medial side. In some instances, one may choose to do both. A slightly curved osteotomy thru the talonavicular joint is performed with osteotomes. One should free this up until it moves easily. This allows the foot to rotate laterally through the talonavicular and subtalar joints.

A medial release is usually required to obtain enough rotation to abduct the foot and allow the heel to face more laterally. Routinely, the posterior tibial tendon is sectioned, and a large portion of it is removed, so it doesn't hook up again. If the subtalar and talonavicular joints don't move well, the medial incision can be deepened and expanded, so these joints can have capsulotomies. Most of the rotation can be obtained through the talonavicular and subtalar joints. As the foot is rotated laterally, the heel moves into a valgus position, because of the shape of the subtalar joint. If the heel does not move into enough valgus, additional bone can be removed from either the talar or the calcaneal side of the subtalar joint, as described by Stephens [3].

On rare occasions, there may be a persistence to be a rotational or bean-shaped deformity of the forefoot compared to the hindfoot. The calcaneocuboid joint may be osteotomized and rotated to improve any pronation deformity, or a V-shaped, closing wedge through the calcaneocuboid joint can couple with the talonavicular osteotomy to improve the bean shape. If this is done, care must be taken to not improve *all* of the metatarsus adductus or the bean shape. If all of the bean shape is taken out, the foot will face too lateral, because of the external rotation that is seen in the ankle in a cavus foot [1, 16, 17].

Once the position has been obtained, the osteotomies can be fixed with large lag screws. Because the osteotomies are done through cancellous bone, they all heal rapidly. If the screws are placed at an angle to the surface of the bone, the screw-hole sites are prepared as described by Manoli and Hansen [18].

Ankle Fusion

An ankle fusion may be necessary to correct ankle arthritis which has developed in a previously fused cavovarus foot. Usually, a standard transfibular ankle fusion is performed by osteotomizing the fibula, denuding the surfaces of the joint of their cartilage surfaces through the lateral approach, and drilling small 2.0 mm drill holes through the subchondral bone to encourage blood supply to the joint surfaces [19]. The ankle is positioned at neutral or a couple of degrees of dorsiflexion and pushed posteriorly in the mortise to diminish the anterior lever arm of the foot. A heel cord lengthening is almost always required to obtain the desired position. Any coronal plane tipping is corrected, and if needed, long pieces of the inner fibula can be used to shim the joint into place. Additional pieces of the inner fibula are used to fill any voids in the joint. Large lag screws are placed in three planes to fix the construct [20, 21] (Figs. 17.1d–f and 17.5c–e).

Achilles Lengthening

In many cases, an Achilles tendon lengthening is necessary to provide the proper positioning of the hindfoot. Generally, the technique of Hatt and Lamphier is very satisfactory [22]. With the percutaneous technique, a number 15 scalpel blade is used in the midline posteriorly approximately 1–2 cm proximal to the insertion of the Achilles on the calcaneus. The scalpel is placed into the middle of the tendon turned medially, and a medial hemisection is carefully performed. The scalpel is rotated through approximately a 90° arc, and with direct palpation, the medial one-half of the tendon's inside border is cut. A similar vertical stab incision is then performed more proximally, about 5 cm above the first incision. This hemisection is also done there medially. Next, a third percutaneous incision is made between the other two, in the middle of the tendon, and is directed laterally. Then, the foot is stretched to neutral. The incomplete incisions separate below the skin providing length to the Achilles as the fibers slide apart [23]. On rare occasions a fourth stab incision or an open Z-plasty lenghening of the tendon and posterior capsulotomy may be needed if the deformity is severe.

Gastrocnemius Slide Procedure

If, after using the Silfverskiöld test, the Achilles complex is only tight in the superficial portion, a gastrocnemius slide procedure can be performed [14]. There are numerous ways to perform this, which include a Strayer, Vulpius, piecrust, and others [24, 25, 26]. In recent years, we have gone to the Bauman procedure [27]. It is easy and reliable. The interval between the gastrocnemius and soleus muscles is found through a small medial incision between the two muscles, just proximal to the distal portion of the gastrocnemius insertion. Deep retractors are used to identify the anterior surface of the gastrocnemius tendon, and it is incised transversely. Dorsiflexion of the foot allows the edges of cut tendon to separate.

First (or Second, Third) Metatarsal Dorsiflexion Osteotomy

If the hindfoot is corrected from a varus to a valgus position, most of the time in the cavovarus foot, a preexisting plantarflexed first ray will develop more plantarflexion [15]. After the hindfoot is fixed in the appropriate position, one should check and see if the first, or occasionally second and third, metatarsal heads are excessive by plantarflexed. If that is the case, it is important to perform dorsiflexion osteotomy of at least the first ray. If the hindfoot is fused, obviously, the fused joints will not move, but, any open joint will tend to tip into varus if this is not done. Then, the patient will continue to walk on the lateral border of the foot. It is important to remember this forefoot-hindfoot relationship, as any change in one will affect the other.

For example, if one performs a triple arthrodesis and there is a plantarflexed first ray, the *ankle* joint will tend to tip into varus, and the patient will continue to walk on the lateral border of the foot.

The dorsiflexion osteotomy is done through a small incision just distal to the first tarsometatarsal joint. It is a closing wedge, V-shaped osteotomy. A single screw can hold it well. The osteotomy heals quickly as it is through cancellous bone. We usually use a 4.0 mm fully threaded screw, placed with a lag screw technique (Fig. 17.4i, j). As the screw is coming in at an angle to the cortex of the bone, the pilot hole technique of Manoli and Hansen is used [18]. Leeuwesteijn et al. have found in eighty first metatarsal osteotomies in CMT (some severe) that usually, all that is needed is an osteotomy of the first metatarsal [28]. But, we have noted that occasionally the second and third metatarsal heads may be prominent in the sole after the first is osteotomized. These bones can be repaired with a couple of small dorsiflexion procedures at the base of the bones. These can be fixed with K-wires (Fig. 17.3d, e).

Case Examples

Case 17.1

Case History

A 45-year-old-female, a seat-belted driver, had a right talar neck fracture 2 years previously in a motor vehicle accident (MVA). The patient underwent open reduction and internal fixation (ORIF) of the fracture. When the patient stood on it, postoperatively, it was noticed that there was a varus positioning of the foot (Fig. 17.1a, b).

Reason for Failure

The operating surgeon tried to repair the foot to be close to anatomically correct. The contralateral foot was also a varus foot, though of a lesser degree. The patient also developed some avascular necrosis of talar body and degenerative arthritis of the ankle and subtalar joint. (Fig. 17.1c, d).

Surgical Plan

The plan was to convert the arthritic hindfoot to an ankle, subtalar, and talonavicular joint release and fusion; excision of the posterior tibial tendon, with an Achilles lengthening; and a dorsiflexion osteotomy of first metatarsal (Fig. 17.1e, f).

Approach

Lateral transfibular ankle fusion and sinus tarsi approach for subtalar fusion (Fig. 17.1g). Medial approaches were used for a posterior tibial tendon excision, talonavicular and subtalar joint release, talonavicular fusion, and first metatarsal dorsiflexion osteotomy (Fig. 17.1h). A percutaneous triple-cut approach lengthened the Achilles tendon.

Implants

6.5 mm solid screws were used across the major joints (ankle, subtalar, talonavicular joints); a 4.0 mm solid screw was used to fix the dorsiflexion osteotomy of first metatarsal (Fig. 17.1e, f).

Pearls and Pitfalls

Medial release of joint capsules and tenotomy of posterior tibial tendon were necessary to obtain correction of the foot. External rotation of the foot through the subtalar joint osteotomy after release of the medial tissues corrected the internal rotation and inversion of the hindfoot (Fig. 17.1i, j).

Case 17.2

Case History

A 22-year-old-female was in a MVA 3 years previously. She sustained a right calcaneus fracture with a concurrent subtalar fracture dislocation. The injury was initially reduced and pinned (Fig. 17.2a, b). Subsequently, a triple arthrodesis was performed for a painful varus deformity (Fig. 17.2c, d).

Reason for Failure

The initial triple arthrodesis was done without full correction of the deformity. No heel cord lengtheing or medial release were performed at the time (Fig. 17.2e, f).

Surgical Plan

Removal of hardware, revision triple arthrodesis, medial soft tissue release, Achilles lengthening, and dorsiflexion osteotomy of first metatarsal were performed.

Approach

Lateral approach for revision triple arthrodesis, medial approach for medial release, posterior tibial tendon tenotomy, and dorsal approach for first metatarsal dorsiflexion osteotomy (Fig. 17.2g, h).

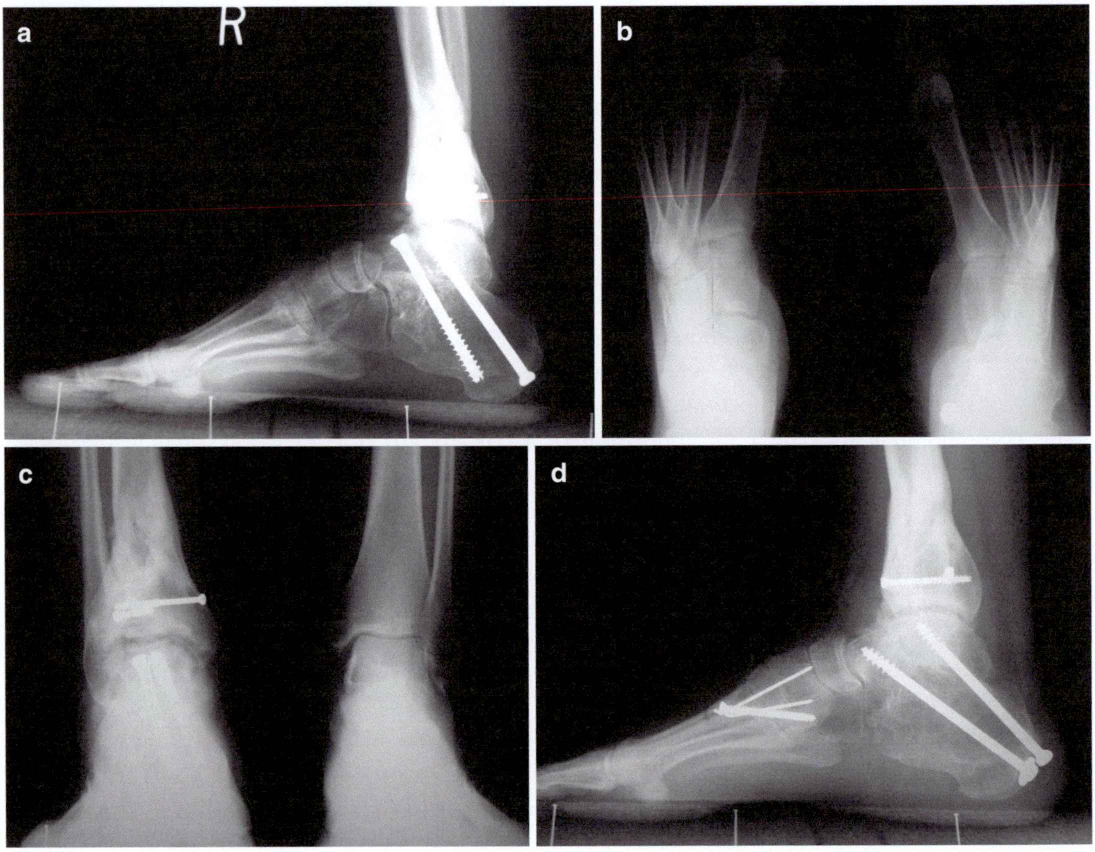

Fig. 17.3 (**a**) This tibial pilon and calcaneal fracture combination underwent an initial open reduction and internal fixation. It subsequently underwent calcaneal hardware removal and a subtalar fusion. Note the very high arch seen on the lateral view. (**b**) Anteroposterior view of both feet. Note the excessive supination of the right foot, compared to the left foot, which also has mild supination. (**c**) Anteroposterior view of both ankles. The patient had a fracture of the distal tibia which underwent open reduction/internal fixation. There is a very mild varus tip of the right ankle. (**d**) Standing radiograph of the right foot after revision of the subtalar fusion, a medial release, and a dorsiflexion osteotomy of the first, second, and third metatarsal. (**e**) Standing anteroposterior radiograph of both feet postoperatively. The supination deformity of the right foot seen in Figure 3b has been corrected. (**f**) Photograph of both feet postoperatively showing very mild peek-a-boo heels. On the right side, more heel can be seen due to the mild varus deformity seen in the ankle in Figure (**c**). (**g**) Photograph of both feet postoperatively. The heel varus is slightly more on the right side due to the mild varus in the ankle seen in Figure (**c**). (**h**) Medial view of the right foot, showing the medial release incision

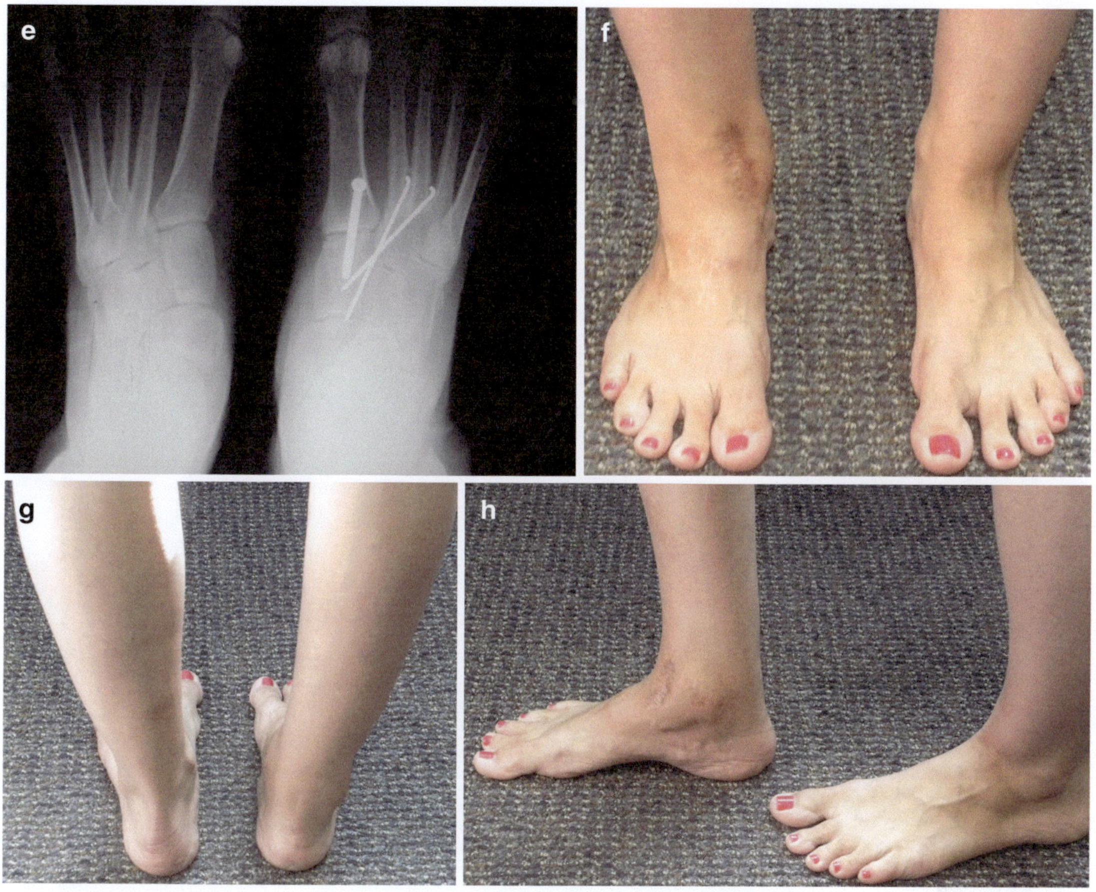

Fig. 17.3 (continued)

Implants

6.5 mm solid screws and 4.0 mm solid screw (Fig. 17.2i–k).

Pearls and Pitfalls

The deformity was never reduced. A revision triple arthrodesis was performed through the previous subtalar and talonavicular joints. At revision, the Achilles was lengthened with a percutaneous four-cut approach, and the posterior tibial tendon was excised (Fig. 17.2l, m).

Case 17.3

Case History

A 29-year-old female was riding on the back of a motorcycle when it crashed. She sustained a right tibial pilon fracture and a right calcaneal fracture. Both injuries underwent open reduction and internal fixation. Later, a subtalar fusion was performed (Fig. 17.3a–c).

Reason for Failure

The patient had a mild cavus foot on the contralateral, uninvolved, and uninjured side. The operating surgeon performed a subtalar fusion using large screws; however, no medial release was performed, and the resulting fusion was in varus. The patient was walking, painfully, on the lateral side of her foot.

Surgical Plan

The plan was to perform a revision subtalar arthrodesis with a medial release and sectioning of the posterior tibial tendon after the fusion

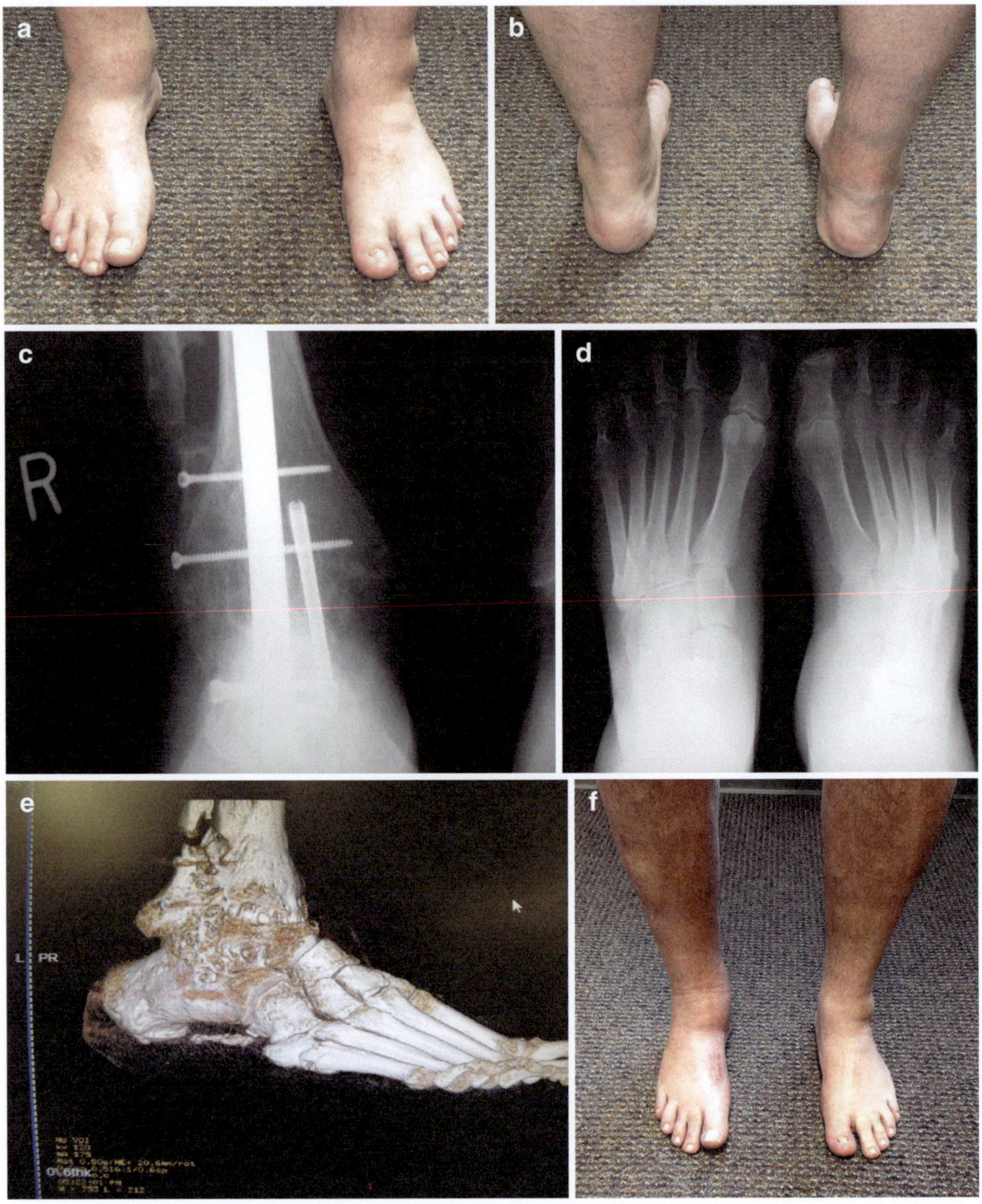

Fig. 17.4 (**a**) Photograph of both feet after the initial subtalar fusion on the right. There is a peek-a-boo heel bilaterally, worse in the operated-on right side than his normal left side. The right foot is "bean-shaped." (**b**) Excessive heel varus on the right compared to the left. (**c**) Anteroposterior radiograph of the tibial-talar-calcaneal (TTC) fusion on the right. (**d**) Anteroposterior radiograph of both feet. There is more supination and metatarsus adductus on the right, compared to the left. Note the stress fracture of the right fifth metatarsal from walking on the lateral border of the foot. (**e**) Three-dimensional reconstruction of the CT scan of the right foot. There has been a subtalar fusion. Note that, although it has been 2 years since the fusion, the "scar" of the subtalar joint can still be seen. The talus and the calcaneus are somewhat "stacked," with the calcaneus internally rotated, and sitting under the head of the talus, more than usually. This is a non-weight-bearing view, so the calcaneocuboid and talonavicular joints are also internally rotated, contributing to the bean-shaped foot. The healing stress fracture of the fifth metatarsal is seen. (**f**) Photograph after the revision subtalar fusion. The peek-a-boo heel is much improved, and it is about equal to the uninvolved left side. (**g**) Rearview of the patient after the revision subtalar fusion on the right. There is slightly more heel valgus, compared to the uninvolved left side. (**h**) Medial view of the right foot, showing the incision for the medial release and the dorsal incision for the dorsiflexion osteotomy of the first metatarsal. (**i**) Lateral radiograph after the revision procedure. (**j**) Anteroposterior view of the right foot after the revision procedure. Healing fifth metatarsal fracture healed uneventfully

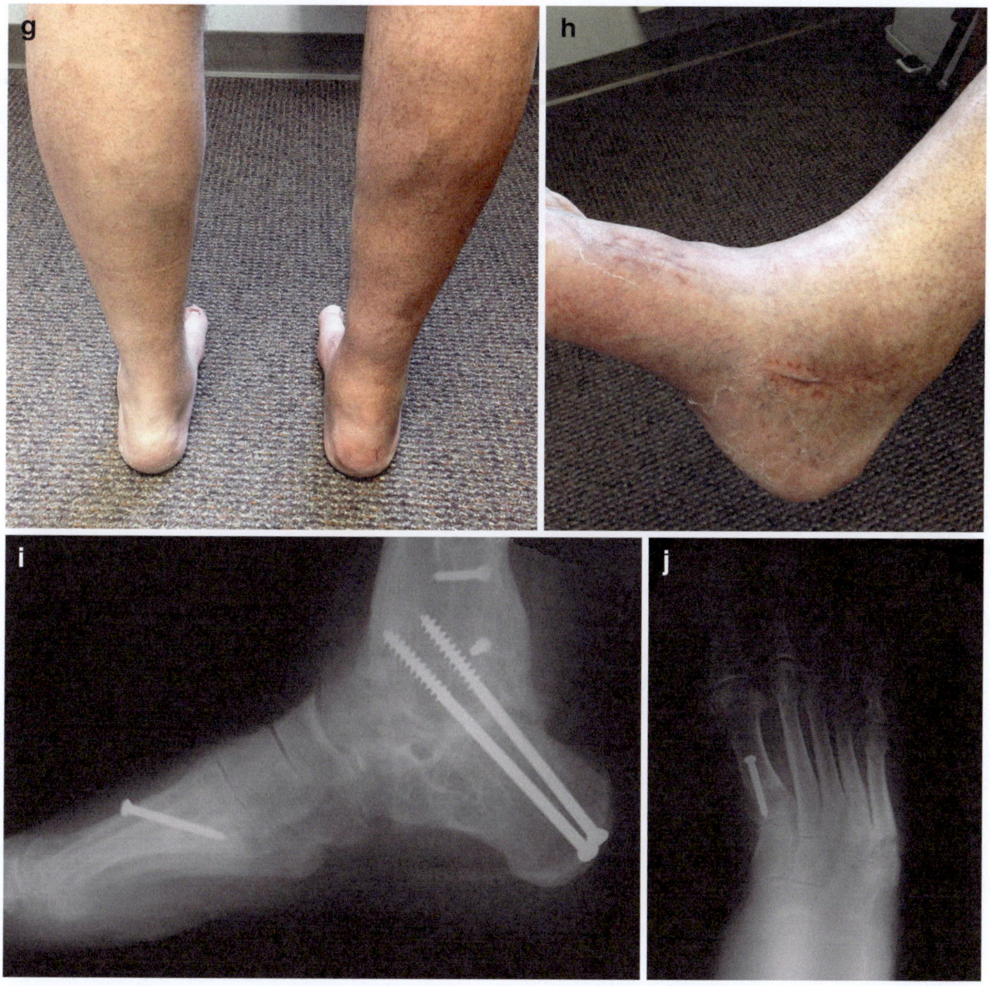

Fig. 17.4 (continued)

hardware was removed. This was done through a lateral incision for the bone work and a medial incision for the soft tissue release. No Achilles tendon lengthening was necessary. A dorsiflexion osteotomy of the first, second, and third metatarsal was also performed for excessive residual forefoot pronation (Fig. 17.3d, e).

Approach

A lateral approach to the subtalar joint area was performed. The joint had been fused previously; however, a remnant of where the joint was previously could be detected. A small osteotome was used there to outline the previous edges of the joint. Osteotomes were advanced through the previous joint areas, re-creating them.

The medial release was done with sectioning of the posterior tibial tendon. The foot could be repositioned by rotating through the unfused talonavicular joint. As this was done, the hindfoot was placed into a normal position, and the bones were fixed with screws (Fig. 17.3f–h).

Implants

Two 6.5 mm leg screws were used across the osteotomy site. Also, a 4.0 mm screw and 0.62 in pins were used to fix the osteotomies of the first thru third metatarsal osteotomies.

Pearls and Pitfalls

It is important to observe the contralateral, uninvolved foot to see what its posture is. If it has a cavus foot posture, one must consider performing a medial release, with at least sectioning of the posterior tibial tendon on the injured side to ensure that the foot is not fixed in excessive hindfoot varus. Occasionally, an Achilles lengthening may be necessary in addition to the medial release, although it was not necessary in this case. A dorsiflexion osteotomy of the first thru third metatarsals was necessary; as when the calcaneus is externally rotated and everted, the medial forefoot is moved more plantarward. If this is not done, the patient will get tipping of the *ankle* above the fusion when they begin to walk (Fig. 17.3d–f).

Case 17.4

Case History

A 47-year-old male was involved in an MVA approximately 2 years previously. He underwent a tibial-talar-calcaneal (TTC) nailing for severe talus and calcaneal fractures. He found that he was walking on the lateral border of his foot postoperatively. This was painful, and with the stiff hindfoot, it was very difficult to walk on unlevel ground (Fig. 17.4a, b).

Reason for Failure

The uninjured left side had a peek-a-boo heel, indicating that it was likely that the injured side started out a subtle cavus foot, also. It was noticed that the involved foot had more heel varus and a bean-shaped foot.

Surgical Plan

The plan was to remove the originally placed hardware and perform a revision subtalar fusion with a medial release to reposition the hindfoot (Fig. 17.4c, d).

Approach

Through a lateral approach above the peroneal tendons, the original subtalar joint edges could be identified (Fig. 17.4e). A small osteotome was used to break through the cortex of the original joint. This was expanded deeper into the body of the fused bones between the talus and the calcaneus. Once one is approximately 3/4 of the way through the bone, a large lamina spreader can be used to gently open the revision osteotomy, and it can be completed using curettes (Fig. 17.2g). A medial release can be done through separate medial incision. Here, the posterior tibial tendon was resected. The subtalar joint was repositioned by externally rotating the calcaneus through the osteotomy until heel valgus was obtained; the subtalar osteotomy was then fixed with two screws.

Implants

Because the osteotomy is primarily through cancellous bone, it tends to heal rapidly. Here, two 6.5 mm lag screws were used across subtalar osteotomy to hold it until it was healed.

Pearls and Pitfalls

Unless the fusion is many years old, generally, one can identify the edges of the previous fusion. A small osteotome is used to begin the osteotomy using these edges as a guide (Fig. 17.4e). A pitfall is not releasing the posterior tibial tendon and occasionally the medial subtalar and talonavicular joint. If one does not release it, it is difficult to get the surfaces of the osteotomy to move and to externally rotate to the proper position.

Final Photographs (Fig. 17.4f–j)

Case 17.5

Case History

A 39-year-old male had a right triple arthrodesis performed as a teenager for a clubfoot. Immediately after surgery, the patient noticed that his ankle was in mild equinus. Over time, the foot drifted into varus and collapsed. The collapse progressed until the man could not put any weight on extremity (Fig. 17.5a–c).

Reason for Failure

Patients who have a varus deformity, especially with ankle equinus, can increase the deformity over time [29]. It is believed that a mechanically

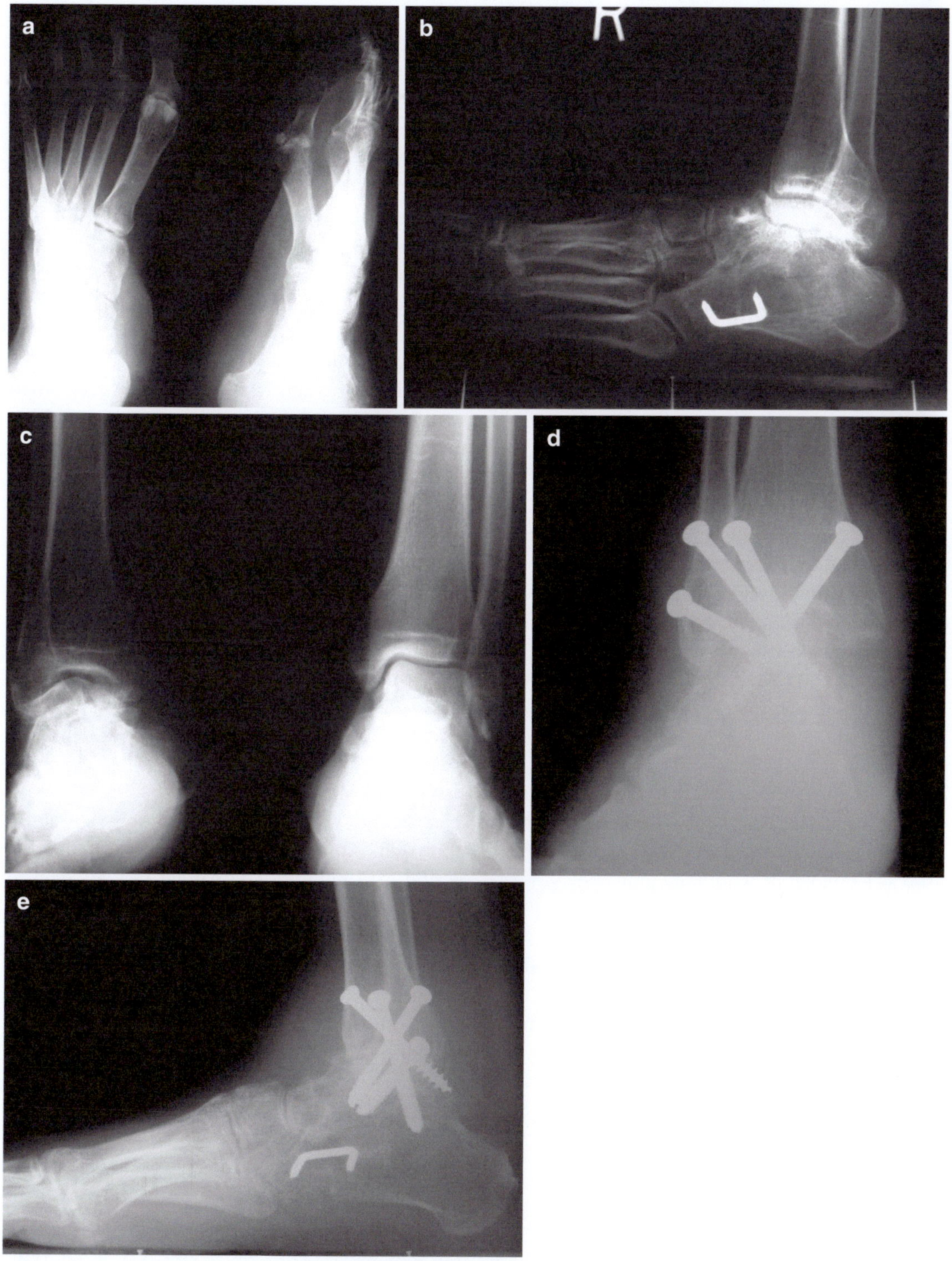

Fig. 17.5 (**a**) Anteroposterior, standing radiograph of both feet. There is severe supination of the right foot. (**b**) Lateral standing view of the right foot and ankle. There is severe supination of the right foot. Although there is an appearance of avascular necrosis of the talus, it is just an artifact from the extreme positioning. (**c**) Anteroposterior standing view of the right ankle. There is severe tipping of the dome of the talus in the ankle mortise. The cortex of the dome of the ankle is what is giving the appearance of avascular necrosis of the talus. (**d**) Anteroposterior standing view of the right ankle after the transfibular ankle fusion and medial release. (**e**) Standing lateral view of the right foot and ankle after the ankle fusion and medial release

advantaged peroneus longus muscle overpowers its antagonist muscle, the anterior tibial muscle. With time, this pulls the foot into more equinus, and in this case, the equinus progressed so much that his lateral ankle ligaments became dysfunctional and the foot collapsed into a direct medial position. He could no longer stand on this severely dysfunctional extremity.

Surgical Plan
The triple arthrodesis was actually in a satisfactory position; however, his ankle joint completely fell into a varus position. It was elected to fuse his ankle in a straight position after resecting the posterior tibial tendon.

Approach
A transfibular ankle fusion was performed by osteotomizing the fibula proximal to the joint, removing the articular cartilage of the ankle with curettes, perforating the subchondral bone with small 2.0 mm drill holes, and fixing the ankle in a satisfactory position. The Achilles tendon was tight, and it was released with a triple-cut percutaneous technique (Fig. 17.5d, e).

Implants
Four 6.5 mm stainless steel leg screws were used to fuse the ankle. The inner portion of the fibula was removed, and the cancellous bone of it was used as a bone graft within the joint.

Pearls and Pitfalls
Patients who have hindfoot reconstructive fusions that have some residual equinus deformity can gradually have progression of the equinus component due to overpull of the long peroneal tendon. Eventually, this can cause adjacent joints to fail.

Case 17.6

Case History
A 59-year-old-female, who was involved in a head-on MVA, sustained a talus and a medial malleolar fracture. She underwent open reduction and internal fixation of both fractures with small screws. Eventually, both fractures were displaced (Fig. 17.6a, b). A reoperation was performed and an infection and avascular necrosis of the talar body developed (Fig. 17.6c, d). The hardware and talar body were removed, and antibiotic beads were placed (Fig. 17.6e, f).

After 3 months, the foot was still in varus (Fig. 17.6e–h). The beads were removed, and a modified Blair fusion with a medial release was performed [30]. At 3 years postoperatively, the foot remained plantigrade, and patient was pain-free and had a jog of total "talocalcaneal" motion.

Reason for Failure (1)
The initial fractures were fixed with very small screws which failed. The talar fixation was from the lateral side. Perhaps a plate and larger screws from the medial side would have fared better in the talus.

Surgical Plan (1)
After the initial fracture fixation with small screws, a reoperation using larger, 4.0 mm, screws.

Reason for Failure (2)
This operation failed by developing a deep wound infection and avascular necrosis of the talar body.

Surgical Plan (2)
The body was removed through a lateral approach. Antibiotic beads were inserted for a period of 3 months. The patient was allowed to walk on the beads.

Surgical Plan (3)
The plan following the beads was to remove them and perform a modified Blair fusion with a medial release, if possible.

Approach
A modified Blair fusion was performed through a transfibular and anterior approach. The fibula was sectioned, and a portion was removed to move it proximally, so the tip would not strike the calcaneus. The beads and any other talar body debris were removed. Usually, when performing a modified Blair fusion, we used a large 6.5 mm screw from the back of the tibia through the front cortex of the tibia and place it into the

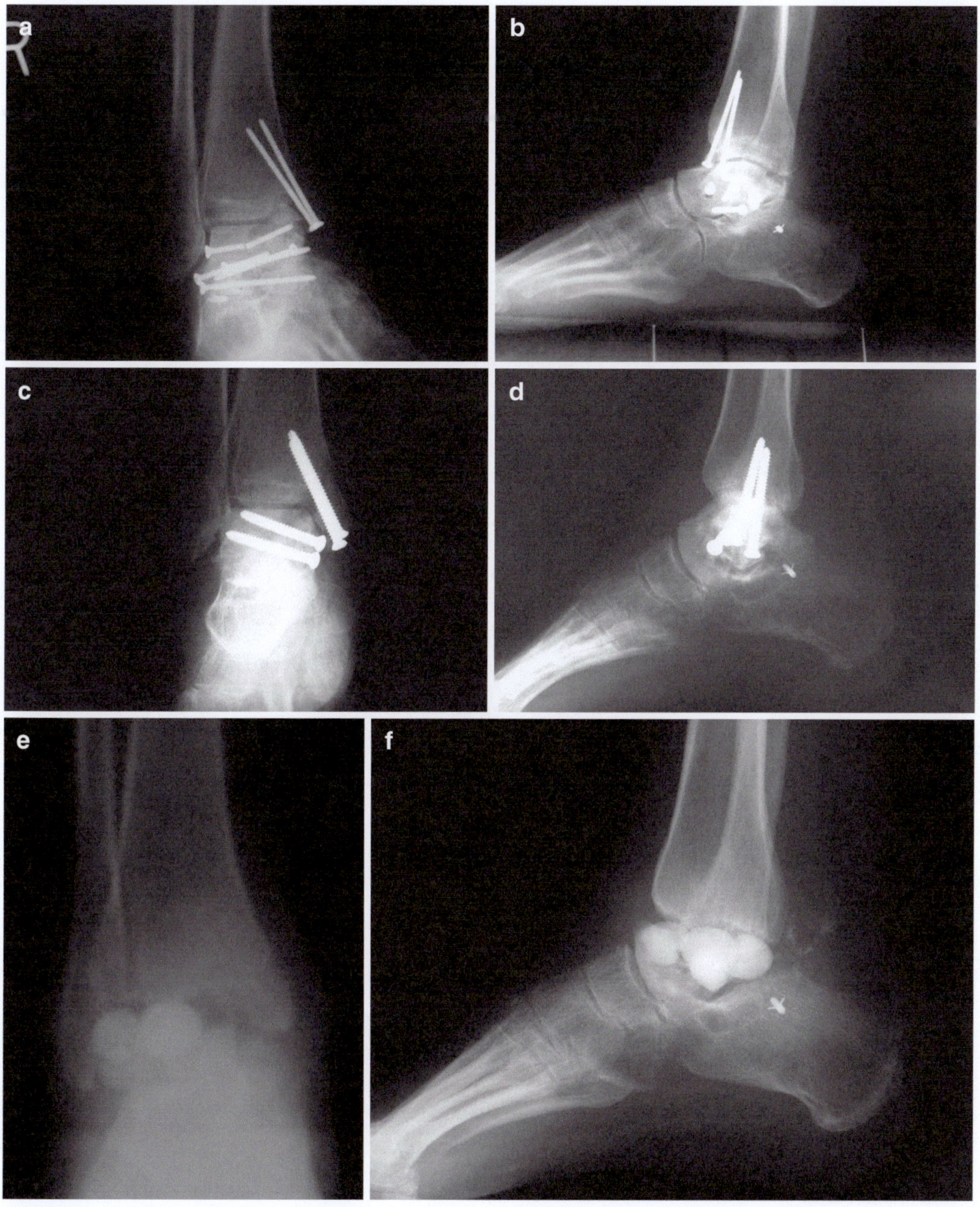

Fig. 17.6 (**a**) Anteroposterior standing view of the right ankle 6 months after initial fixation of the talus and medial malleolar fracture. (**b**) Lateral standing foot and ankle radiograph after the initial fixation. (**c**) Anteroposterior standing view of the right ankle after fracture revision operation. (**d**) Lateral standing foot and ankle radiograph after fracture revision operation. (**e**) Anteroposterior radiograph of ankle after infection and avascular necrosis developed. The talar body was removed, and antibiotic beads were placed. (**f**) Lateral radiograph of ankle after infection and avascular necrosis developed. The talar body was removed, and antibiotic beads were placed. (**g**) Photograph of the feet with the antibiotic beads in place. There is varus of the right heel. (**h**) Rearview photo of both heels illustrating the heel varus on the right. (**i**) Standing anteroposterior radiograph of the ankle after a modified Blair fusion with a medial release. (**j**) Standing lateral radiograph of the ankle after a modified Blair fusion with a medial release. There is a painless jog of talocalcaneal motion. (**k**) Anteroposterior photo of the feet/ankles after a modified Blair fusion with a medial release. The peek-a-boo heel has been corrected on the right. (**l**) Posterior photo of the feet/ankles after a modified Blair fusion with a medial release. The heel varus has been corrected

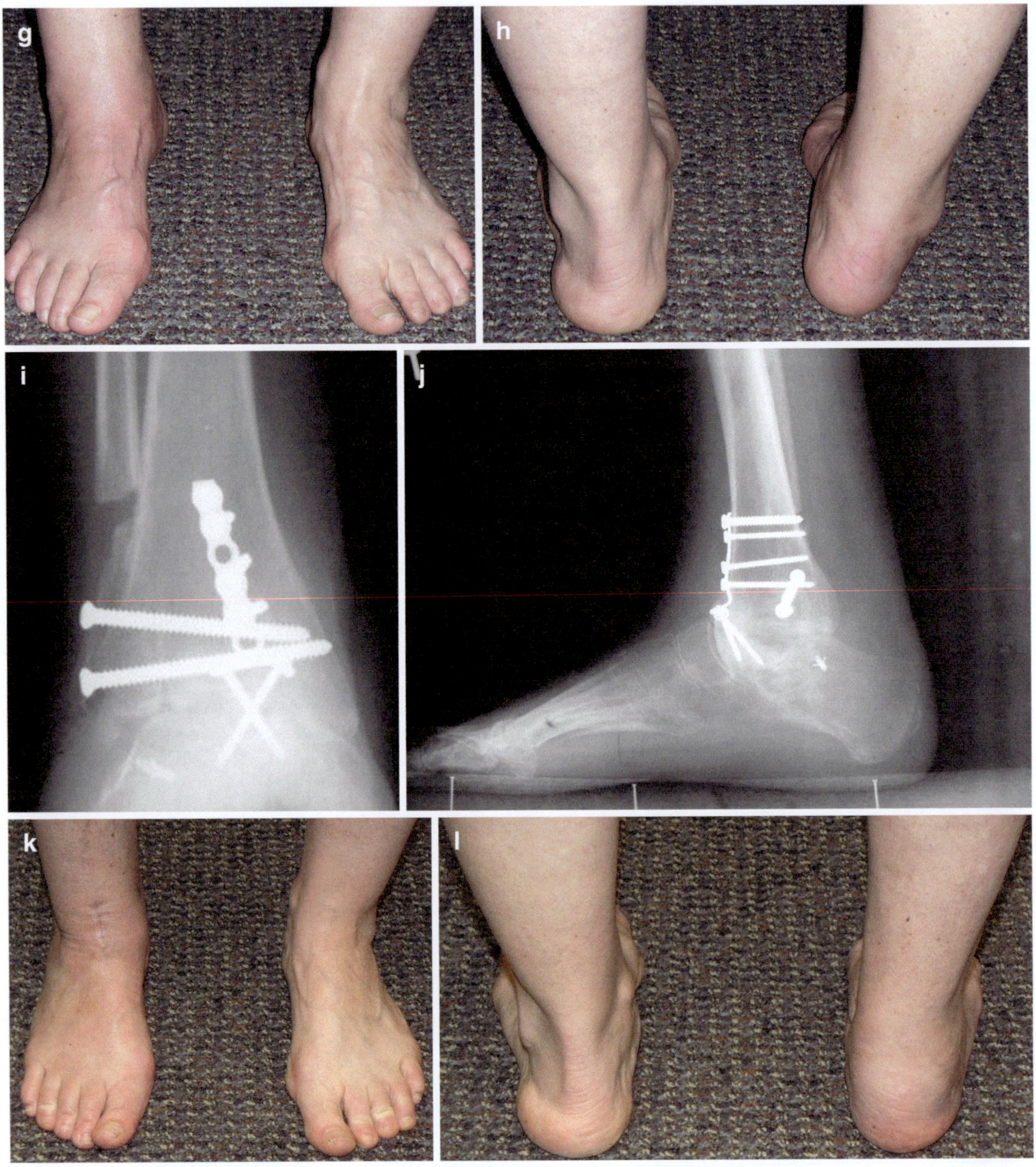

Fig. 17.6 (continued)

head and neck fragment. Here, the head and neck fragment was so small that we decided to use an alternative fixation of a plate and screws (Fig. 17.6i, j).

Implants

A small T-type plate was bent and placed on the front of the tibia and the dorsum of the talus and fixed in place with 2.7 mm screws. This construct was chosen because of the small size of the residual talar head. The bone from the inner fibula was taken and used between the head and neck and the tibia as a bone graft to help ensure healing of the talar fragment to the front of the tibia.

Pearls and Pitfalls

The modified Blair fusion is useful in cases of talar body avascular necrosis, particularly with an infection within the body. The body is removed, and the head and neck of the remaining talus are fixed to the front of the tibia (Fig. 17.6k, l). In most cases, there is motion in the talonavicular joint and the "pseudarthrosis" of the "talocalcaneal" articulation. The alternative operation would be a large allographic block or femoral head allograft to replace the entire talar body. These large grafts may be difficult to heal by revascularization in the relatively avascular bed that remains. Infection complicates the use of all allographs.

Summary

A hindfoot fusion procedure may cause patients to have further problems if there is malalignment, particularly cavovarus. A careful analysis of the deformity will provide the surgeon with the details of what group of procedures will provide a total and long-lasting correction. A plantigrade, stable, painless foot is the ultimate goal.

References

1. Lloyd-Roberts GC, Swann M, Catterall A. Medial rotation osteotomy for severe residual deformity in clubfoot. A preliminary report on a new method of treatment. J Bone Joint Surg Br. 1974;56(1):37–43.
2. Pomeroy G, Manoli A. Techniques of revision talocalcaneal arthrodeses. Tech Orthop. 1996;11(4):347–54.
3. Stephens M, Saleh J. Calcaneal dome osteotomy: a new procedure for revising triple arthrodesis. Foot Ankle Int. 1994;15(7):368–71.
4. Joseph TN, Myerson MS. Correction of multiplanar hindfoot deformity with osteotomy, arthrodesis, and internal fixation. Instr Course Lect. 2005;54:269–76.
5. Trajkovski T, Pinsker E, Cadden A, Daniels T. Outcomes of ankle arthroplasty with preoperative coronal-plane varus deformity of 10° or greater. J Bone Joint Surg Am. 2013;95(15):1382–8.
6. Manoli A, Graham B. Clinical and new aspects of the subtle cavus foot. a review of an additional twelve year experience. FussSprungg. 2018, (in press) https://doi.org/10.1016/j.fuspru.2017.11.006.
7. Apostle KL, Sangeorzan BJ. Anatomy of the varus foot and ankle. Foot Ankle Clin. 2012;17(1):1–11.
8. Manoli A 2nd, Graham B. The subtle cavus foot, "the underpronator". Foot Ankle Int. 2005;26(3):256–63.
9. Wong C, Clare M. Pes cavus in talar neck fractures: an anatomic predisposition? Presented at the annual meeting of the American Academy of Orthopaedic Surgeons, Las Vegas. Mar 24, 2015. Paper 133, p. 82.
10. Gallagher SM, Rodriguez NA, Andersen CR, Granberry WM, Panchbhavi VK. Anatomic predisposition to ligamentous Lisfranc injury: a matched case-control study. J Bone Joint Surg Am. 2013;95(22):2043–7.
11. Kang S, Park SS. Predisposing effect of elbow alignment on the elbow fracture type in children. J Orthop Trauma. 2015;29(8):e253–8.
12. Lisella JM, Bellapianta JM, Manoli A. Tarsal coalition resection with pes planovalgus hindfoot reconstruction. J Surg Orthop Adv. 2011;20(2):102–5.
13. Coleman SS, Chesnut WJ. A simple test for hindfoot flexibility in the cavovarus foot. Clin Orthop. 2008;123:60–2.
14. Singh D. Nils Silfverskiöld (1888-1957) and gastrocnemius contracture. Foot Ankle Surg. 2013;19(2):135–8. Epub 2013 Jan 16
15. Fortin PT, Guettler JH, Manoli A. Idiopathic cavovarus foot and lateral ankle instability: recognition and treatment implications relating to ankle arthritis. Foot Ankle Int. 2002;23(11):1031–7.
16. Berkowitz MJ, Kim DH. Fibular position in relation to ankle stability. Foot Ankle Int. 2004;25(5):318–21.
17. Peden, S, Tanner J, Manoli A. The posterior fibula of the cavus foot deformity. J Surg Orthop Adv. 2018;27(4):255–60.
18. Manoli A, Hansen ST Jr. Screw hole preparation in foot surgery. Foot Ankle. 1990;11(2):105–6.
19. Manoli A, Beals TC, Hansen ST Jr. Technical factors in hindfoot arthrodesis. Instr Course Lect. 1997;46:347–56.
20. Monroe MT, Beals TC, Manoli A. Clinical outcome of arthrodesis of the ankle using rigid internal fixation with cancellous screws. Foot Ankle Int. 1999;20(4):227–31.
21. Holt ES, Hansen ST, Mayo KA, Sangeorzan BJ. Ankle arthrodesis using internal screw fixation. Clin Orthop Relat Res. 1991;268:21–8.
22. Hatt RN, Lamphier T. Triple hemisection: a simplified procedure for lengthening the Achilles Tendon. N Engl J Med. 1947;236(5):166–9.
23. Salamon ML, Pinney SJ, Van Bergeyk A, Hazelwood S. Surgical anatomy and accuracy of percutaneous achilles tendon lengthening. Foot Ankle Int. 2006;27(6):411–3.
24. Pinney SJ, Sangeorzan BJ, Hansen ST Jr. Surgical anatomy of the gastrocnemius recession (Strayer procedure). Foot Ankle Int. 2004;25(4):247–50.
25. Yoshimoto M, Kura H, Matsuyama T, Sasaki T, Yamashita T, Ishii S. Heel cord advancement combined with Vulpius' lengthening of the gastrocnemius. Clin Orthop Relat Res. 2005;434:213–6.
26. Manoli A. The gastrocnemius slide procedure using the piecrust technique article in techniques in foot & ankle. Surgery. 2009;8(1):30–3.

27. Herzenberg JE, Lamm BM, Corwin C, Sekel J. Isolated recession of the gastrocnemius muscle: the Baumann procedure. Foot Ankle Int. 2007;28(11): 1154–9.
28. Leeuwesteijn AE, de Visser E, Louwerens JW. Flexible cavovarus feet in Charcot-Marie-tooth disease treated with first ray proximal dorsiflexion osteotomy combined with soft tissue surgery: a short-term to mid-term outcome study. Foot Ankle Surg. 2010;16(3):142–7.
29. Beals TC, Manoli A. Late varus instability with equinus deformity. Foot Ankle Surg. 1990;4(2):77–81.
30. Van Bergeyk A, Stotler W, Beals T, Manoli A. Functional outcome after Modified Blair arthrodesis for talar osteonecrosis. Foot Anlle Int. 2003;24(10): 765–70.

18 Revision of Malunion and Nonunion After Hindfoot Arthrodesis

Justin Roberts, John D. Maskill, John G. Anderson, and Donald R. Bohay

Key Takeaway Points

- Revision hindfoot arthrodesis is challenging and requires an intimate understanding of the anatomy and biomechanics of the hindfoot, midfoot, and forefoot and the normal relationship and interaction between them.
- A wide variety of pathology and deformity can be treated with hindfoot arthrodesis. It is critical to understand the underlying pathology that led to the index procedure, as this will likely be the key to the cause of failure and the plan for a successful revision.
- The goal of revision should be to obtain a well-balanced, plantigrade foot with a solid fusion. Many surgical reconstruction options are available. Surgical planning must be individualized based on the underlying pathology and the type and degree of deformity present.
- Successful management of hindfoot nonunions requires medical optimization of the patient; meticulous debridement of the pseudoarthrosis down to healthy, bleeding bone; a rigid internal fixation construct for mechanical stability; and biologic augmentation with bone graft or substitute.
- The goal of hindfoot malunion reconstruction is to achieve a plantigrade foot. This often involves complex osteotomies with bone blocks and/or wedges, as well as osteotomies or arthrodeses through the midfoot and forefoot to achieve a balanced foot.
- Literature is scarce to guide treatment in these difficult scenarios. Success can be achieved through precise surgical planning and surgical technique while respecting the basic principles of deformity correction, bone healing, and internal fixation.

J. Roberts
The Orthopaedic Clinic Association, Phoenix, AZ, USA

J. D. Maskill · J. G. Anderson (✉) · D. R. Bohay
Orthopaedic Associates of Michigan, Grand Rapids, MI, USA
e-mail: john.anderson@oamichigan.com

Introduction

Hindfoot arthrodesis is a time-honored procedure for deformity correction that has been well documented and accepted in the orthopedic literature for almost 100 years [1, 2]. Originally used for the treatment of clubfeet and paralytic deformities

M. J. Berkowitz et al. (eds.), *Revision Surgery of the Foot and Ankle*,
https://doi.org/10.1007/978-3-030-29969-9_18

caused by polio, the methods and indications have vastly expanded over the years. Current indications include a wide range of pathologic conditions including post-traumatic arthritis and deformity, inflammatory arthropathies, neurologic disorders, congenital abnormalities, and adult acquired flatfoot deformity (AAFD).

While hindfoot arthrodesis remains a powerful tool for deformity correction that generally produces satisfactory results, it is technically demanding, and complications are not uncommon. The most common cited complication after hindfoot arthrodesis is nonunion. Rates vary in the literature, but isolated subtalar arthrodesis has nonunion rates as high as 20% [3–7]. Contemporary series for triple arthrodesis have nonunion rates up to 23% [6, 8–13]. Isolated calcaneocuboid arthrodesis has nonunion rates that can approach 30% [14]. In general, nonunion rates have decreased over the years with advances in internal fixation. However, with the advent of computed tomography (CT) as the preferred method to evaluate bony consolidation, nonunion rates may be underestimated in the literature.

Although nonunion rates have decreased with modern internal fixation techniques and biologic augmentation, malunion in an overcorrected or undercorrected position continues to be a significant challenge [15]. In their early review of 80 triple arthrodeses, Angus and Cowell noted residual deformity in 62% of feet postoperatively [8]. Wilson et al. showed that 14 of 300 feet undergoing triple arthrodesis had poor positioning, necessitating additional procedures to achieve correction [11]. Manoli's review of triple arthrodesis results found a malunion rate of 6%, with 2 varus and 2 valgus malunions out of 63 procedures [16].

Haddad et al. reviewed the causes for failure of 29 patients undergoing revision triple arthrodesis and found that the failed index arthrodesis produced multiplanar deformity necessitating systematic correction [17]. The most common deformity was equinovarus with or without rocker bottom deformity (10 feet), followed by hindfoot varus (8 feet), hindfoot valgus (5 feet), and rocker bottom deformity alone (2 feet) [17]. Successful revision was able to be achieved in 87%. Hindfoot arthrodesis remains a technically demanding procedure with less than ideal outcomes. Complications can be minimized at the time of index procedure with careful preoperative planning, meticulous surgical technique, critical intraoperative assessment of the correction clinically and radiographically, and rigid internal fixation.

Patient Evaluation

The evaluation of a patient with pain and/or deformity following hindfoot arthrodesis begins with a thorough history. Understanding the reason for the index procedure is extremely important and may provide insight to the reason for failure. A pertinent medical history should be taken, focusing on factors that may predispose to complications, such as smoking status, diabetes, neuropathy, peripheral vascular disease, and nutritional status. These issues must be optimized prior to proceeding with surgical reconstruction.

Physical exam begins with a critical evaluation of patient alignment, not only of the hindfoot but proximally and distally as well. Standing evaluation may reveal any gross deformity of the hindfoot in varus or valgus. The entire lower extremity should be examined especially for angular and torsional deformity. It is not uncommon for foot deformity to be compensatory for more proximal abnormalities in the lower extremity. The presence of excessive tibia vara or femoral anteversion requires compensatory pronation of the foot and ankle in order for the foot to contact the ground in a plantigrade position [18]. Cavovarus deformities are often associated with external tibial torsion. Reconstruction and realignment of the foot without addressing the torsional deformity may cause marked external rotation of the foot in relation to the tibia. The patient should be counseled accordingly, and a rotational tibial osteotomy may be necessary to prevent this occurrence [19].

It is critical to understand the relationship of the hindfoot to the midfoot and forefoot. Hindfoot deformity correction and arthrodesis may unmask a primary or compensatory deformity of the forefoot, which may be the cause of the patient's primary complaints after surgery. The forefoot should be assessed for residual plantarflexion (pronation) or dorsiflexion (supination) of the first ray in both the sitting and standing position. Insufficiency of the first metatarsal segment should be evaluated by checking for first cuneiform-metatarsal joint hypermobility or instability. Residual forefoot deformity often has to be addressed at the time of hindfoot revision to help ensure a satisfactory result.

Gastrocnemius tightness is critical to assess via Silfverskiold testing. If no attempt at a triceps surae lengthening procedure was performed at the index procedure, or if intervention was attempted but the patient still lacks adequate ankle dorsiflexion, great consideration must be given to a lengthening procedure at the time of revision. This will allow for optimal restoration of the anatomy of the hindfoot while reducing midfoot and forefoot pressures [20]. Furthermore, it addresses an underlying problem that was likely a main driver of the initial deformity in the first place.

Careful neurovascular examination is also an essential part of the evaluation. Muscle motor testing is performed to examine for weakness or overactivity that may drive deformity. The skin, capillary refill, and pulses are assessed for evidence of vascular deficiency. Finally, all previous surgical scars are noted, as these will often dictate placement of incisions at time of revision.

Imaging begins with standard weight-bearing foot and ankle series. The arthrodesis sites are inspected for bony consolidation. The adequacy of internal fixation type and technique should be heavily scrutinized. Adjacent joints of the midfoot and ankle are evaluated for degenerative changes.

Standard foot and ankle radiographic parameters are used to assess for residual deformity and malunion. Special attention should be given to talocalcaneal and talo-first metatarsal angles on both anteroposterior (AP) and lateral radiographs, as well as talonavicular coverage.

In the revision scenario, CT is an invaluable resource for preoperative planning. CT scanning is more powerful for identifying bony consolidation at arthrodesis sites when compared to standard radiographs [21]. Weight-bearing CT scan, when available, is also an excellent method to assess three-dimensional alignment, with higher reliability than standard radiographs [22] and non-weight-bearing CT [23].

Surgical Techniques

Once a thorough clinical and radiographic evaluation has been completed, cause for failure is identified, and a surgical plan is designed and implemented. The goal of revision surgery is to achieve a well-balanced, plantigrade foot with restoration of the normal relationships of the hindfoot to the midfoot and forefoot. Reconstruction necessitates an individualized approach based on the type and degree of deformity, patient activity, and expectations. Given the wide variety of underlying pathology in this patient population, there is no one "cookbook" approach to surgical reconstruction. General principles and considerations to achieve success in these challenging scenarios will be discussed further in the coming sections.

Nonunion

Nonunion is generally defined as failure of osseous bridging at the arthrodesis site after 6 months. Recent research has only just begun to evolve this definition and its consequences on patient outcome. While it is clear that CT is the modality of choice for assessing nonunion [21], defining and quantifying the amount osseous bridging at the nonunion site still needs exploration. Glazebrook et al. have shown that patient outcomes increase if there is 25–50% of osseous bridging seen on CT scan, versus those with 0–25% of bridging. Recently, it has also been confirmed that failure to achieve arthrodesis leads to a decrease in patient-reported outcomes compared to those patients who achieve a solid fusion [24]. Based on this limited evidence, an algorithm for managing patients with suspected nonunion can be fashioned (Fig. 18.1).

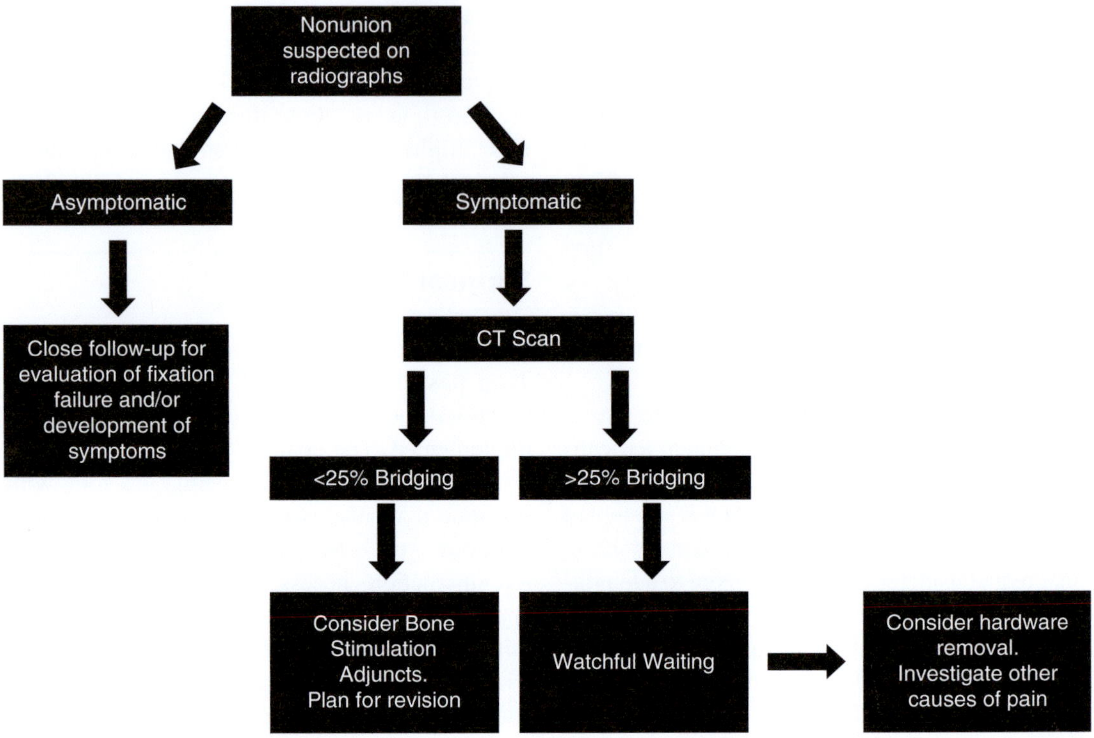

Fig. 18.1 Algorithm for management of hindfoot nonunions

If the patient has a symptomatic nonunion necessitating revision and the foot is well aligned, the decision-making becomes relatively straightforward as the only goal is to achieve a solid fusion to reduce pain and instability from pseudoarthrosis. Basic principles of bony healing must be considered to decipher the cause of the nonunion. Failure of bone healing can be broken down into insufficient biologic healing potential, inadequate fixation and mechanical stability, infection, or a combination of these factors. It should be emphasized again that an attempt should be made to optimize the patient's health status with regard to risk factors for nonunion prior to proceeding with surgery.

The site of nonunion is taken down and then meticulously debrided of all fibrous tissue. A combination of curettes, rongeurs, and osteotomes is used to manually scrape the nonunion site down to healthy, bleeding bone. Manual removal of all tissue is preferred over using a saw or burr, in order to preserve as much bony anatomy as possible and to prevent heat necrosis. As the joint surfaces are debrided, the bone stock must be critically evaluated. Achieving healthy opposing bony surfaces may create large voids and gaps that should be filled with grafting material. In the case of severe bone loss, structural allograft may be necessary, so the joint can maintain appropriate length and not lead to deformity through shortening of the medial or lateral columns.

Once the articular surfaces have been denuded of all remaining non-osseous tissue, the arthrodesis is prepared by drilling multiple holes through the subchondral bone using a small drill or K-wire. In nearly every revision scenario, biologic augmentation is used to increase odds of union. Proximal tibia autograft is an excellent choice for bone graft in the revision scenario; however, a variety of bone graft substitutes are available for use. Bone graft or substitute is then packed into the arthrodesis site, and the joint is reduced into the desired position and held with provisional fixation. It is critical to ensure that the joint surfaces are opposed with no gaps.

Rigid internal fixation is mandatory. Compression screws are used across the joint surfaces if possible. Positional screws should be used if compression will lead to relative shortening across the joint and lead to deformity. Screw tracts can be reused by utilizing larger-diameter screws than were used at the primary arthrodesis. This can be especially helpful for revision of the subtalar joint. At the surgeon's discretion, additional stability can be obtained through neutralization plating. A variety of anatomic non-locking and locked plates are available, which can be particularly helpful for the talonavicular and calcaneocuboid joints. If there is any question about the quality of fixation, more hardware should be added to the construct to improve stability (Figs. 18.2 and 18.3). Postoperative protocol includes strict non-weight-bearing and immobilization in a boot or cast at the surgeon's discretion. Weight-bearing status may be progressed once there is evidence of healing on radiographs, usually between 8 and 12 weeks. The surgeon should error on the side of longer weight-bearing status if severe bone loss required significant structural grafting.

Infection should always be on the differential as the cause of a suspected nonunion. If the clinical suspicion is low or equivocal for infection at the time of revision, cultures should be sent from the pseudoarthrosis material, and revision can proceed as planned. If the intaoperative cultures return positive results unexpectedly, infectious disease should be consulted for targeted intravenous antibiotics to suppress the infection until a stable fusion can be obtained. Once bony consolidation has been confirmed postoperatively, fixation may be removed in order to eradicate any potential nidus for deep infection.

If the clinical picture is obviously consistent with an infection preoperatively (erythema, draining purulence, etc.), thorough debridement and removal of hardware are warranted. Antibiotic-laden bone cement can be used at the time of debridement to elute high-dose local antimicrobial therapy, as well as to relatively maintain the normal lengths and relationships of the hindfoot joints. Cultures should be taken at the time of surgery, and infectious disease should be consulted for targeted intravenous antibiotic management. Once the infection has been cleared, removal of the antibiotic cement and revision arthrodesis can be performed, usually 3–6 months after initial debridement.

Malunion

Surgical planning in the malunion scenario is much more complicated. It deserves mention that prevention of a malunion through good surgical planning and technique is the best way of handling this situation. The general principles for alignment during primary hindfoot arthrodesis will be discussed briefly. At the time of index procedure, the surgeon must have a good understanding of the underlying pathology causing arthritis and deformity. This allows appropriate planning for additional maneuvers or procedures to fully address the deformity and balance the foot. Deformity should be approached systematically from proximal to distal with the goal of achieving a foot that is balanced and plantigrade. Correction begins with restoration of hindfoot alignment with placement of the calcaneal tuberosity in neutral to slight valgus position beneath the long axis of the tibia. Proper reduction of the talus on the calcaneus is critical to restore their normal relationship. The talar head should rest in line with the medial border of the anterior process of the calcaneus. Too wide of a talocalcaneal angle on the AP and lateral views allows for plantarflexion and medial deviation of the talus, leading to dorsal-lateral peritalar subluxation. The opposite is true with hindfoot parallelism, in which the talus is not divergent with the calcaneus on the AP view and is too horizontal on the lateral view, leading to plantar-medial peritalar subluxation.

Attention is then drawn to reduction of the navicular on the talus to provide adequate talonavicular coverage. Finally, the axis of the talus should point in line with the first metatarsal axis on both the AP and lateral views (Fig. 18.4). Attention to these basic principles in both the primary and revision setting will lead to optimal patient outcomes. Unfortunately, especially in

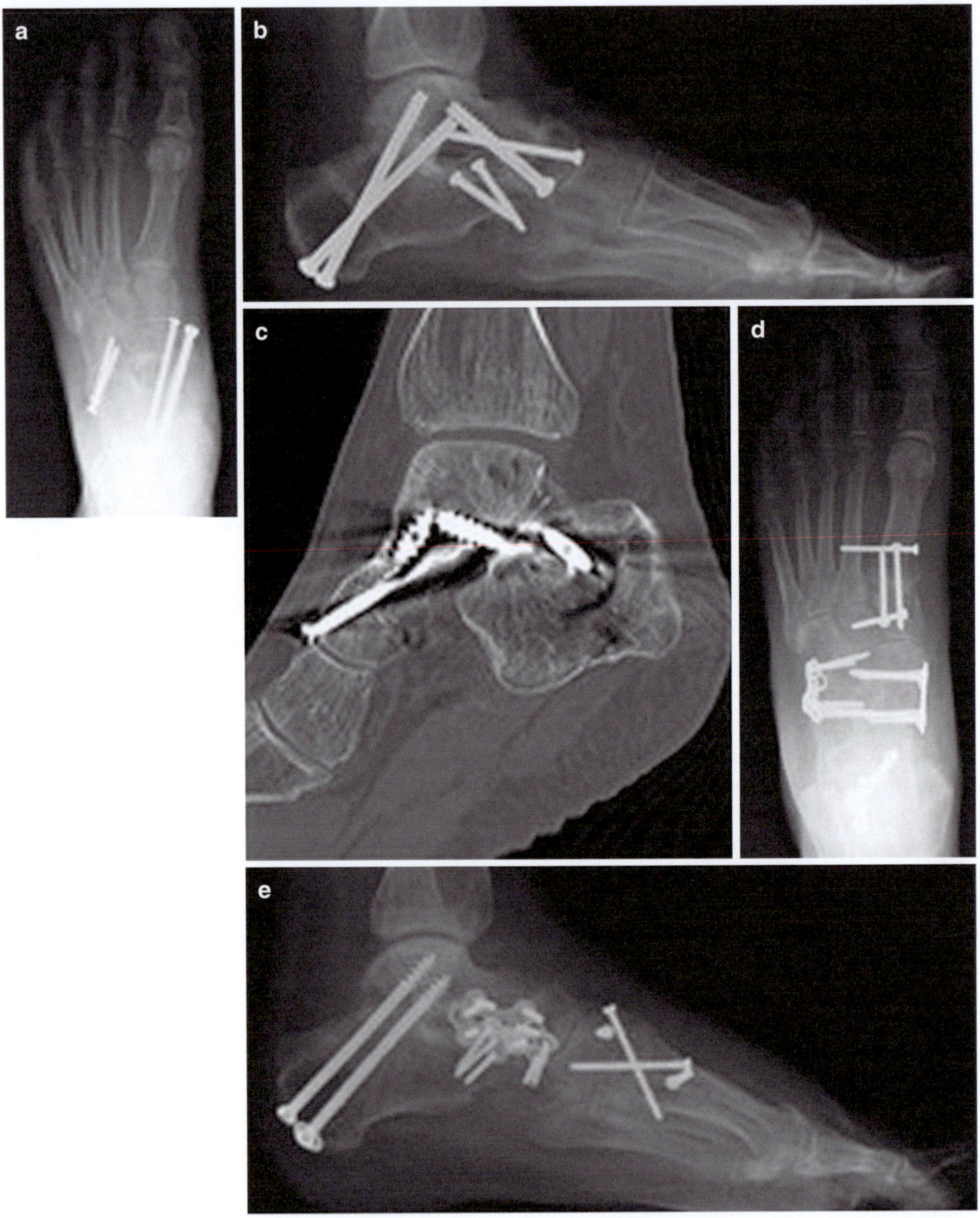

Fig. 18.2 (**a**, **b**) Radiographs of a 44-year-old male who underwent triple arthrodesis and developed a symptomatic nonunion. (**c**) CT scan showing lack of osseous bridging at the subtalar and talonavicular joints. Calcaneocuboid joint was also involved. (**d**, **e**) Radiographs following revision of all three joints with proximal tibial autograft. Modified Lapidus procedure was used to correct residual hindfoot varus due to instability of the medial column

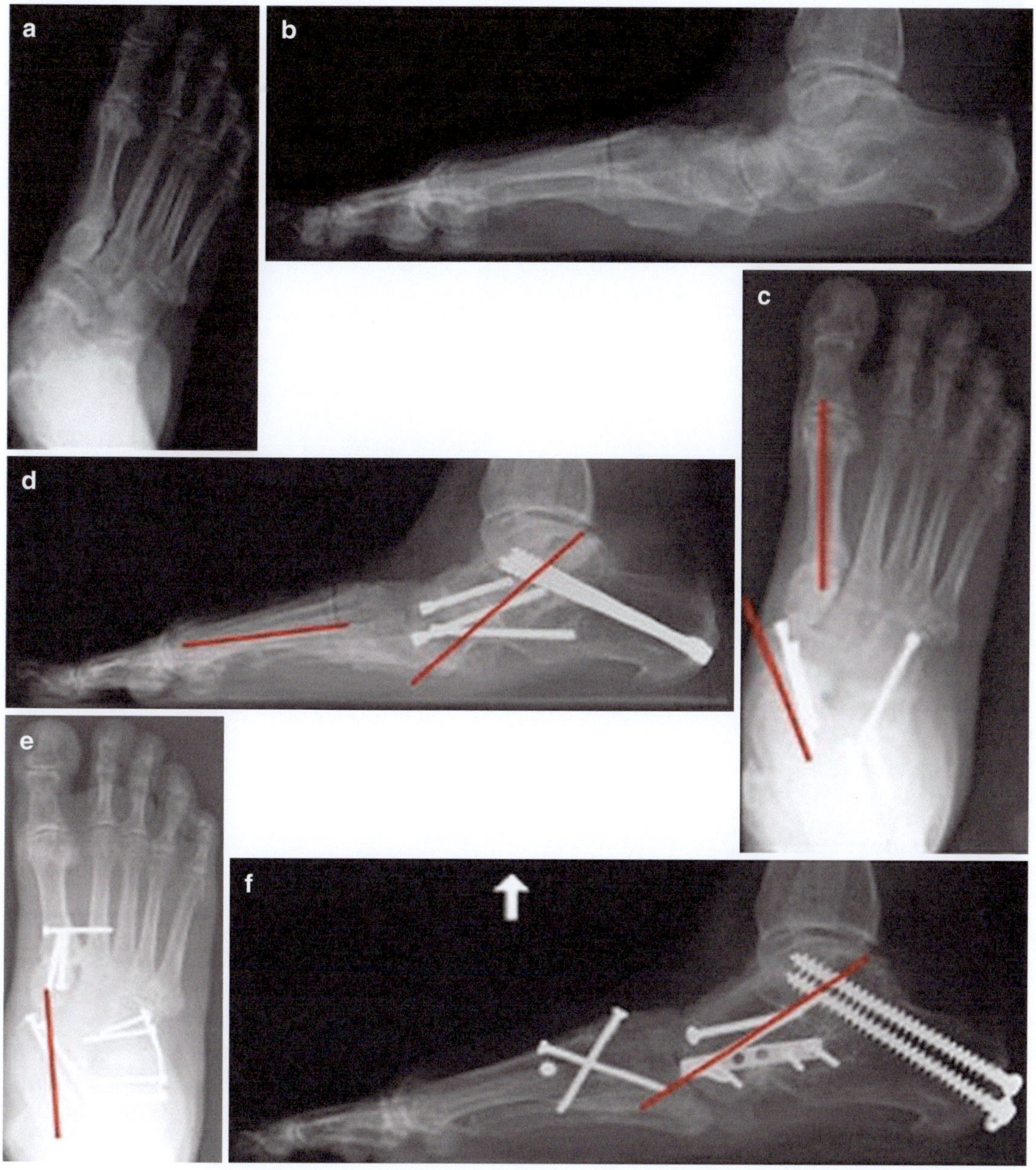

Fig. 18.3 (**a**, **b**) Patient was evaluated for rigid flat foot deformity. (**c**, **d**) He was treated by an outside surgeon with a triple arthrodesis. Note that he was nearly fused in situ with very little correction. He developed painful nonunions and was unhappy with the continued deformity of his foot. (**e**, **f**) He underwent revision triple arthrodesis. Note the improvement in talonavicular coverage and talo-first metatarsal angles. There is some residual plantarflexion deformity of the talus on the lateral view. Residual forefoot varus was treated with a first metatarsal-cuneiform arthrodesis and a first to second metatarsal arthrodesis to restore forefoot balance

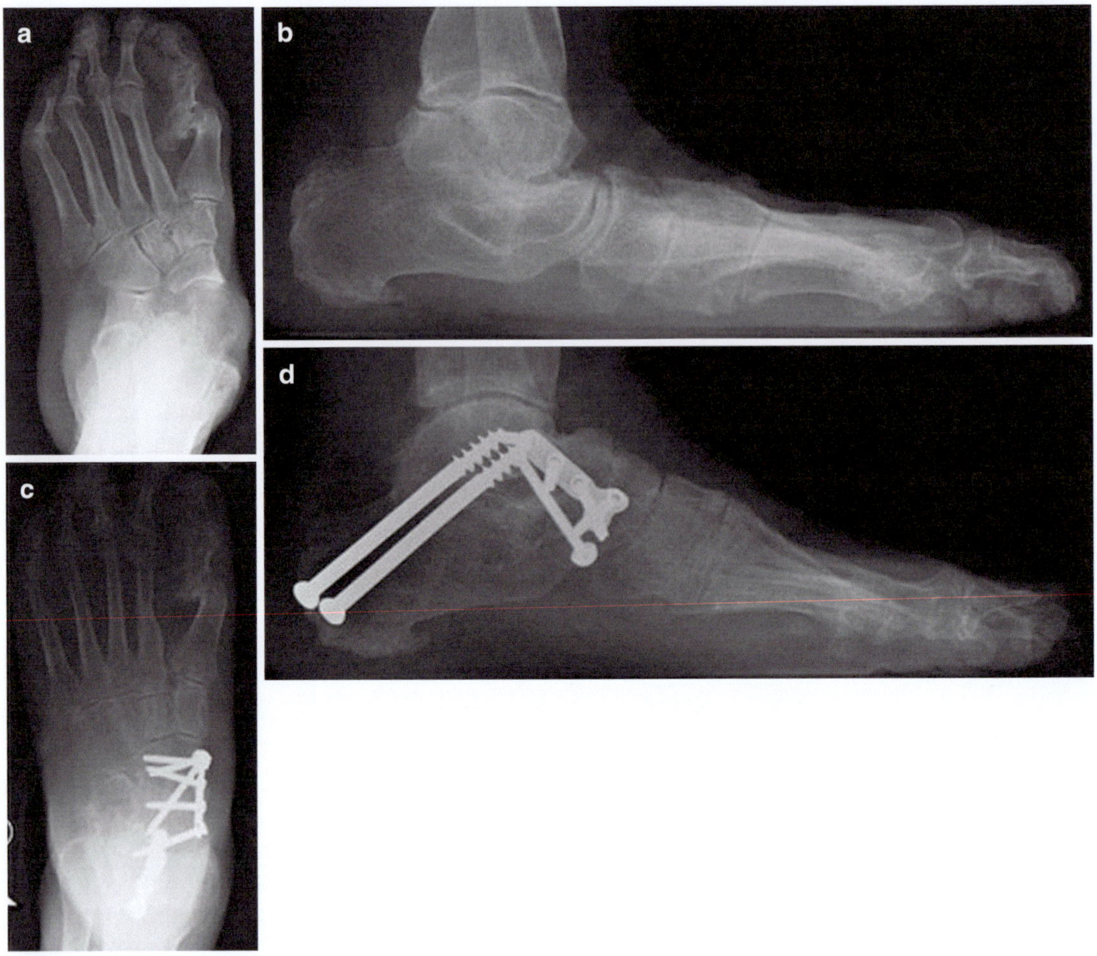

Fig. 18.4 Proper hindfoot double arthrodesis technique (**a**, **b**). A patient with severe rigid flatfoot deformity. (**b**, **c**) Status post triple arthrodesis. Note the significant improvement in talocalcaneal angles, talar coverage, talo-first metatarsal angles, and calcaneal pitch

revision scenarios, the path to achieving the normal relationships above is not always straightforward, and multiple options are available based on the type and magnitude of deformity.

Hindfoot Varus/Valgus

The first step in correction of a hindfoot deformity is to address equinus based on results of Silfverskiold testing. Most commonly, the gastrocnemius is the source of the equinus and can be reliably improved with a gastrocnemius recession. If equinus does not improve with the knee flexed, tendoachilles lengthening is performed, usually through a percutaneous hemisection technique. If the equinus is not addressed, it is often impossible to correct and unwind the deformity in the hindfoot.

The primary deformity in the hindfoot can be simplified into varus and valgus. Again, critical analysis of the etiology for the index procedure allows the surgeon to understand the underlying deformity to develop a precise surgical reconstruction plan for correction. Primary rigid hindfoot varus deformity may be generalized into neurologic, post-traumatic, congenital, and idiopathic [25]. Neurologic causes include hereditary motor and sensory neuropathies (MNSN), cerebral injury from stroke or traumatic brain injury, and anterior horn spinal cell disease or spinal cord lesion. Calcaneus and talus fracture malunion are common causes of post-traumatic hindfoot varus. Congenital deformities include tarsal coalition, residual clubfoot, and intrinsic abnormal morphology in the architecture of the calcaneus and subtalar joint [26]. As discussed previously, hindfoot varus can be compensatory for external tibial torsion. Varus hindfoot malunion can cause lateral border overload with painful callosities or even stress fractures, peroneal tendon damage, lateral ankle instability, and varus tibiotalar arthritis.

The simplest way to address varus malunion is to perform an osteotomy through the tuberosity of the calcaneus. This can be a lateral translational osteotomy, laterally based closing wedge osteotomy, or a combination of the two. In severe deformity, trying to correct the varus deformity through a tuberosity osteotomy alone may not provide the needed correction. An osteotomy through the talocalcaneal fusion mass can also be performed, as described by Haddad et al. [17]. This is a laterally based closing wedge osteotomy that is performed at the level of the subtalar joint and is a powerful tool and our preferred method for hindfoot varus correction. Furthermore, other operative considerations may have to be considered based on the underlying anatomy. This is not uncommon in post-traumatic reconstruction, especially where the sequelae of trauma to the calcaneus or talus lead to hindfoot arthrodesis "in situ" without restoring the normal anatomy at the time of index open reduction and internal fixation (ORIF) or subsequent first arthrodesis. Hindfoot varus due to medial collapse malunion of the talar neck, for example, may require medial column lengthening procedure in addition to a valgus-producing hindfoot osteotomy to restore balance to the foot (Fig. 18.5).

In the case of calcaneal malunion sequelae, correcting hindfoot varus without addressing the lateral wall blowout would lead to continued subfibular pain and impingement, and a lateral wall exostectomy must be performed. If ankle range of motion (ROM) and impingement are an issue due to loss of calcaneal height, this may also need to be addressed with bone block or structural allograft. In the case of neuromuscular deformity, various soft tissue procedures, such as peroneus longus to brevis transfer and tibialis posterior tenotomy or transfer, may be needed to remove the driving forces of the initial deformity. These additional considerations add to the complexity and technical demands of the case, but have the best chance of restoring optimal patient outcomes.

The most common cause of a rigid hindfoot valgus deformity necessitating hindfoot arthrodesis is adult acquired flatfoot deformity (AAFD). Other causes of hindfoot valgus deformity include tarsal coalition, inflammatory arthropathies, cerebral palsy, and traumatic injuries to the talus, calcaneus, Chopart, and midfoot joints. The most common scenario for revision of hindfoot valgus nonunion is the undercorrection of a rigid adult acquired flatfoot deformity. Residual hindfoot valgus may cause laterally based pain from subfibular impingement or fibular stress fracture. Furthermore, with the hindfoot laterally positioned under the weight-bearing axis, deltoid ligament strain and attenuation can occur leading to rapid deterioration of the tibiotalar joint. The simplest method to correct this deformity is to perform a medial displacement osteotomy through the tuberosity of the calcaneus. However, this is usually not adequate depending on the underlying deformity. The subtalar fusion can be osteotomized, and hindfoot position can be restored through lateral opening or medial closing wedge. Medial translation through the osteotomy may have to be performed as well. In some instances, the subtalar joint has intrinsic lateral translation (Fig. 18.6). Failure to translate the osteotomy medially predisposes the patient to continued subfibular pain and impingement.

Forefoot Abduction/Adduction

Forefoot abduction/adduction deformities can be corrected through the power of the Chopart joint, with the goal being to balance the medial and lateral columns of the foot. Relative shortening of the lateral column compared to medial column will lead to forefoot abduction, as is commonly

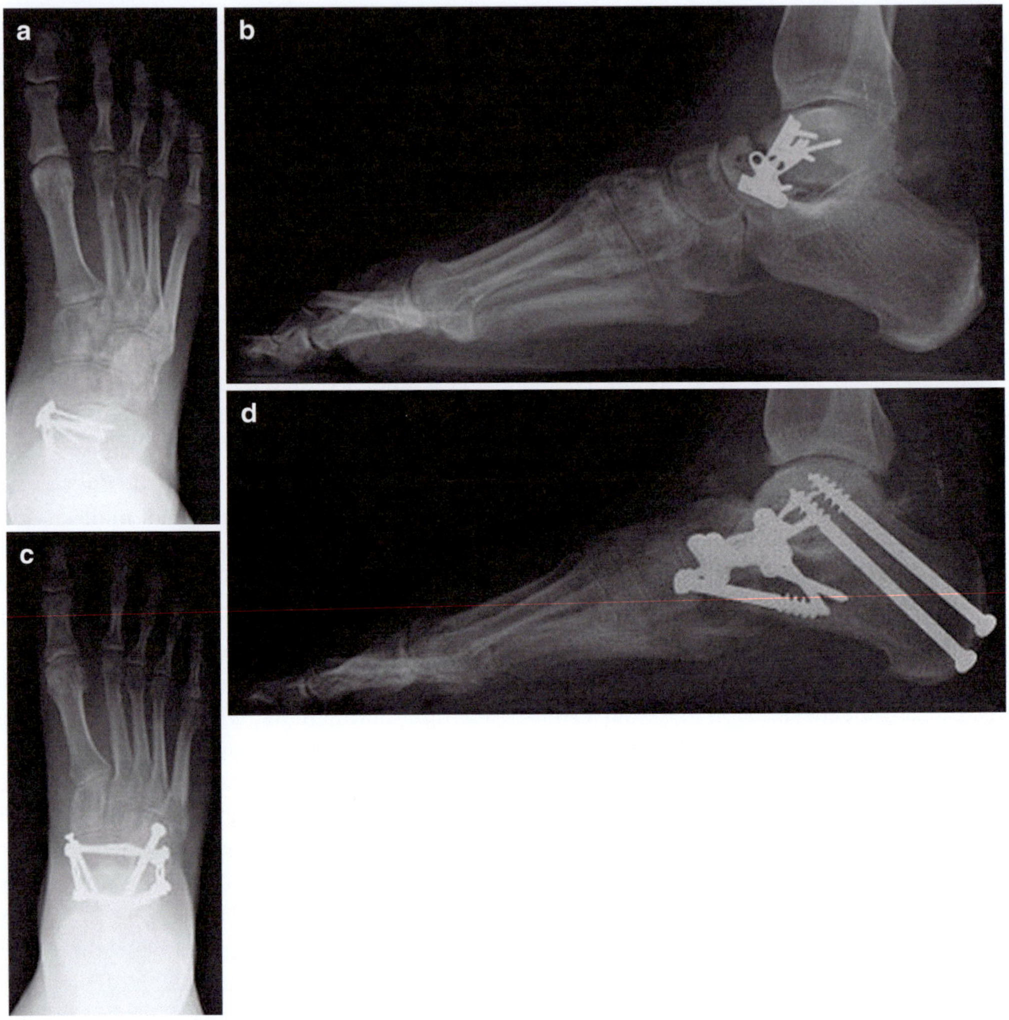

Fig. 18.5 (**a**, **b**) Patient was evaluated following a talar neck fracture malunion with collapse into varus. (**c**, **d**) Reconstruction was performed with triple arthrodesis, utilizing a bone block through the talar malunion to restore medial column length

seen in adult acquired flatfoot. Shortening of the medial column, such as with talar neck fracture malunion, will lead to forefoot adduction (Fig. 18.4). In the case of a malunited Chopart fusion, abduction of the forefoot can be corrected by medial closing wedge osteotomy through the fusion mass, while an adduction deformity can be corrected with a laterally based closing wedge osteotomy [17]. Rotation can also be used through this same osteotomy to help correct residual forefoot supination/pronation [17].

If the Chopart joint has yet to be fused, arthrodesis of the talonavicular joint, with or without the calcaneocuboid joint, will lead to adequate correction with attention to re-establishing talonavicular coverage and talo-first metatarsal angles (Fig. 18.7).

Midfoot

When revising the hindfoot malunion, careful attention must be given to the midfoot's contribution to the patient's pain and deformity. Adult acquired flat foot deformity, for example, is not infrequently accompanied by arthritic changes in

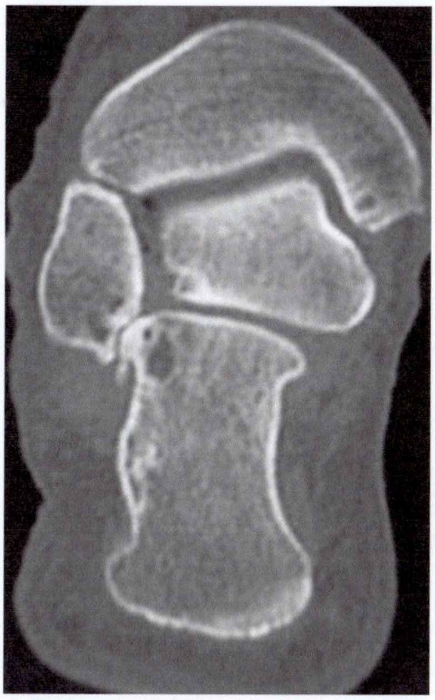

Fig. 18.6 CT scan showing intrinsic lateral translation of the patient's native subtalar joint

the midfoot as the dorsal aspects of the joints collapse in compression and the plantar midfoot gaps under tension. This may lead to sag through the TMT joints or naviculo-cuneiform joints, which can be addressed by including the affected joints in the arthrodesis.

Forefoot Pronation/Supination

Correction of hindfoot deformity through revision arthrodesis will often unmask a forefoot deformity that, left untreated, will lead to unsatisfactory results. Care must be taken with any hindfoot arthrodesis procedure to evaluate and correct forefoot deformity to achieve proper foot balance. After correction of hindfoot valgus, there is often elevation of the first ray (supination) that must be addressed. If there has been a previous Chopart fusion, an internal derotational osteotomy can be performed through the Chopart joint [17]; however, it may be easier and more preferable to address the deformity through the midfoot. This can be achieved through a dorsal opening wedge osteotomy of the medial cuneiform (Cotton osteotomy). Another reliable method to bring down the first ray is first tarsometatarsal arthrodesis. The first metatarsal can be translated plantarly on the medial cuneiform to stabilize the first metatarsal segment in a plantarflexed position. This is especially helpful in adult acquired flat foot, where medial column insufficiency through the first TMT joint is often one of the underlying deformities.

After correction of a hindfoot varus deformity, residual pronation of the forefoot often must be addressed. A dorsiflexion osteotomy of the first metatarsal can be performed to bring the first metatarsal segment up. A dorsiflexion arthrodesis of the first TMT joint is another powerful tool to stabilize the medial column. Addressing the forefoot deformity at the midfoot or forefoot level allows much more precise fine-tuning of the deformity that is much more difficult to achieve more proximally through Chopart joint.

Finally, the surgeon needs to realistically judge the amount of surgical trauma and operative time necessary to achieve complete correction. In complex revision scenarios, attempting to reconstruct and balance the entire foot may be too much to do in one sitting. A staged correction may be prudent in an attempt to decrease wound and infectious complications.

Results

There is scant evidence to guide treatment for revision hindfoot arthrodesis, with only a few case series in the literature. Stephens and Saleh were of the first to describe a technique for revising triple arthrodesis [27]. In this series, a crescenteric calcaneal dome osteotomy was used to provide multiplanar correction in five patients, one with hindfoot valgus due to pes planus and four with equinovarus due to clubfoot or polio. Although very limited numbers, they reported 100% satisfaction with no complications.

Haddad et al. presented the results of 28 patients who underwent revision for failed triple arthrodesis [17]. A systematic approach was used to correct deformity from proximal to distal. Hindfoot valgus was corrected with a medial dis-

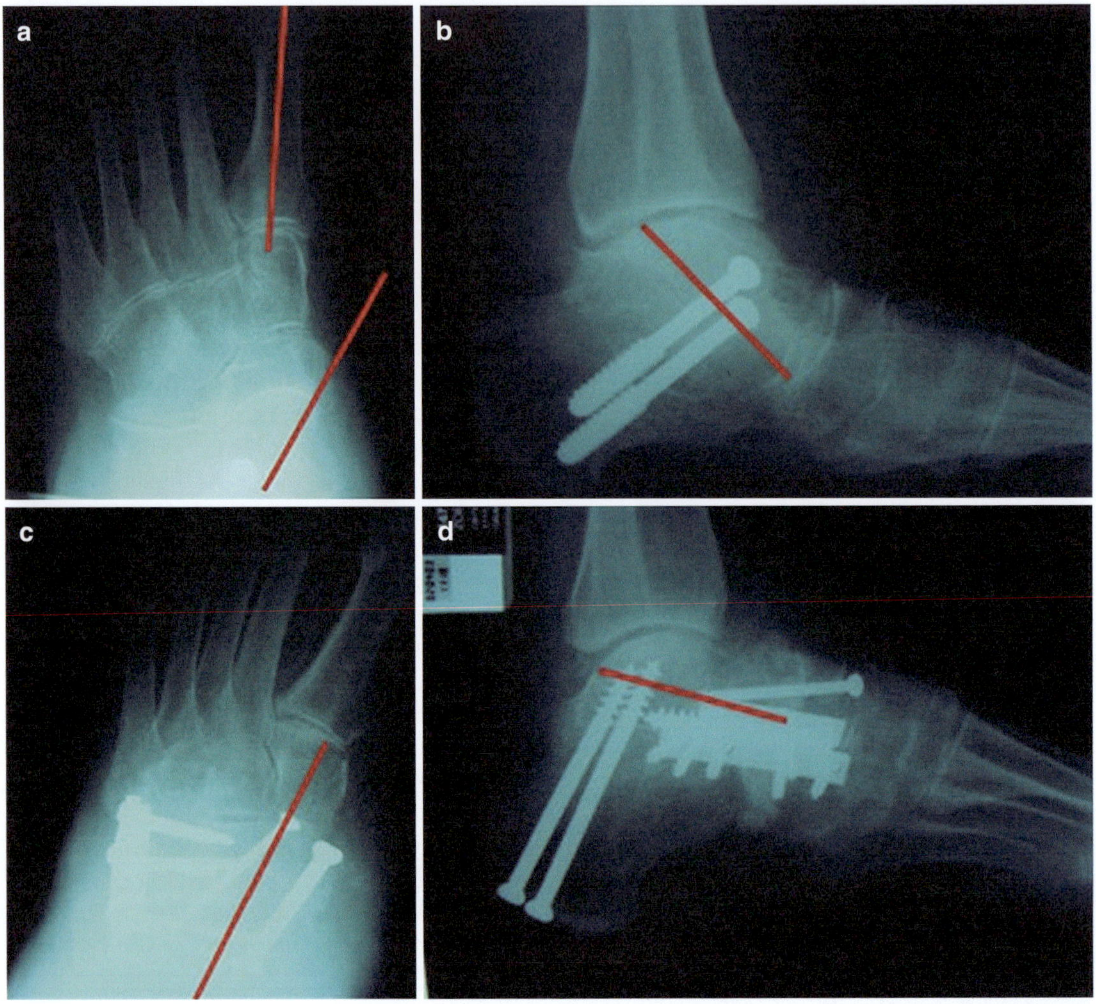

Fig. 18.7 (**a**, **b**) Patient was seen for evaluation of continued pain and deformity following in situ fusion of the subtalar joint for adult acquired flat foot. Note the dorsal-lateral peritalar subluxation allowing for significant forefoot abduction. (**c**, **d**) Correction necessitated revising the subtalar fusion and adding Chopart joint fusion with grafting of the lateral column to significantly improve forefoot abduction

placement calcaneal osteotomy, while hindfoot varus was addressed with either a lateral closing wedge osteotomy through the subtalar joint or a lateral closing and translational osteotomy through the calcaneal tuberosity. Forefoot supination/pronation deformities were corrected with transverse osteotomy through the transverse tarsal fusion mass and derotation to bring the forefoot plantigrade. Medial or lateral closing wedge osteotomies through the fusion mass were also used to treat forefoot abduction or adduction, respectively. Finally, rocker bottom deformity was revised with plantar closing wedge osteotomy. Following reconstructions, the American Orthopaedic Foot & Ankle Society (AOFAS) hindfoot scores improved on average from 31 to 59, with average satisfaction rated as 7.8 out of 10, and all patients saying that would have the operation again. They reported four (14%) major complications: one patient requiring debridement and three weeks of IV antibiotics for deep infection and symptomatic malunion in three patients necessitating repeat osteotomies.

Another analysis of 21 patients with rheumatoid arthritis and a failed triple arthrodesis showed that 12 of the failures (57%) were due to a misjudgment in surgical technique [28]. They reported an 86% fusion rate with complications including two valgus malunions, one distal fibular stress fracture, and two superficial infections.

Finally, Toolan presented the results of five patients treated with a biplanar osteotomy through the midfoot to correct rocker bottom deformity after failed triple arthrodesis. One hundred percent satisfaction was obtained with an average increase in AOFAS hindfoot score from 33 to 70 and statistically significant improvement in all radiographic indices measured [29].

There are multiple surgical options when undertaking revision hindfoot arthrodesis. Surgeons should proceed with caution when attempting to correct multiplanar deformity through single osteotomies. More often than not, multiple osteotomies at different locations will be needed to achieve a plantigrade foot.

Summary

Correction of nonunion and malunion of the hindfoot is challenging. Prior to embarking on surgical revision, the surgeon needs to identify the underlying pathologic process and critically evaluate the deformity clinically and radiographically. Good results can be expected if restoration of normal relationships between the hindfoot, midfoot, and forefoot can be obtained to achieve a balanced foot. Complications can be minimized with meticulous surgical technique and rigid internal fixation. The literature is sparse to guide operative intervention. More research is needed to elucidate outcomes for these complex revision scenarios.

References

1. Ryerson E. Arthrodesis operations on the feet. J Bone Joint Surg. 1923;5:453–71.
2. Hoke M. An operation for stabilizing paralytic feet. J Bone Joint Surg. 1921;3(10):494–507.
3. Mann RA, Beaman DN, Horton GA. Isolated subtalar arthrodesis. Foot Ankle Int. 1998;19(8):511–9.
4. Haskell A, Pfeiff C, Mann R. Subtalar joint arthrodesis using a single lag screw. Foot Ankle Int. 2004;25(11):774–7.
5. Scranton PE. Comparison of open isolated subtalar arthrodesis with autogenous bone graft versus outpatient arthroscopic subtalar arthrodesis using injectable bone morphogenic protein-enhanced graft. Foot Ankle Int. 1999;20(3):162–5.
6. Flemister AS, Infante AF, Sanders RW, Walling AK. Subtalar arthrodesis for complications of intra-articular calcaneal fractures. Foot Ankle Int. 2000;21(5):392–9.
7. Easley ME, Trnka HJ, Schon LC, Myerson MS. Isolated subtalar arthrodesis. J Bone Joint Surg Am. 2000;82(5):613–24.
8. Angus PD, Cowell HR. Triple arthrodesis. A critical long-term review. J Bone Joint Surg Br. 1986;68(2):260–5.
9. Graves SC, Mann RA, Graves KO. Triple arthrodesis in older adults. Results after long-term follow-up. J Bone Joint Surg Am. 1993;75(3):355–62.
10. Pell RF, Myerson MS, Schon LC. Clinical outcome after primary triple arthrodesis. J Bone Joint Surg Am. 2000;82(1):47–57.
11. Wilson FC, Fay GF, Lamotte P, Williams JC. Triple arthrodesis. A study of the factors affecting fusion after three hundred and one procedures. J Bone Joint Surg Am. 1965;47:340–8.
12. Sangeorzan BJ, Smith D, Veith R, Hansen ST. Triple arthrodesis using internal fixation in treatment of adult foot disorders. Clin Orthop. 1993;294:299–307.
13. Smith RW, Shen W, Dewitt S, Reischl SF. Triple arthrodesis in adults with non-paralytic disease. A minimum ten-year follow-up study. J Bone Joint Surg Am. 2004;86–A(12):2707–13.
14. Toolan BC, Sangeorzan BJ, Hansen ST. Complex reconstruction for the treatment of dorsolateral peritalar subluxation of the foot. Early results after distraction arthrodesis of the calcaneocuboid joint in conjunction with stabilization of, and transfer of the flexor digitorum longus tendon to, the midfoot to treat acquired pes planovalgus in adults. J Bone Joint Surg Am. 1999;81(11):1545–60.
15. Seybold JD. Management of the malunited triple arthrodesis. Foot Ankle Clin. 2017;22(3):625–36.
16. Bednarz PA, Monroe MT, Manoli A. Triple arthrodesis in adults using rigid internal fixation: an assessment of outcome. Foot Ankle Int. 1999;20(6):356–63.
17. Haddad SL, Myerson MS, Pell RF, Schon LC. Clinical and radiographic outcome of revision surgery for failed triple arthrodesis. Foot Ankle Int. 1997 Aug;18(8):489–99.
18. Hansen ST. Functional reconstruction of the foot and ankle. Philadelphia/London: Lippincott Williams & Wilkins; 2000.
19. Hansen ST. The cavovarus/supinated foot deformity and external tibial torsion: the role of the posterior tibial tendon. Foot Ankle Clin. 2008;13(2):325–328, viii.
20. Armstrong DG, Stacpoole-Shea S, Nguyen H, Harkless LB. Lengthening of the Achilles tendon in diabetic patients who are at high risk for ulceration of the foot. J Bone Joint Surg Am. 1999;81(4):535–8.

21. Coughlin MJ, Grimes JS, Traughber PD, Jones CP. Comparison of radiographs and CT scans in the prospective evaluation of the fusion of hindfoot arthrodesis. Foot Ankle Int. 2006;27(10):780–7.
22. de Cesar Netto C, Schon LC, Thawait GK, da Fonseca LF, Chinanuvathana A, Zbijewski WB, et al. Flexible adult acquired flatfoot deformity: comparison between weight-bearing and non-weight-bearing measurements using cone-beam computed tomography. J Bone Joint Surg Am. 2017;99(18):e98.
23. Hirschmann A, Pfirrmann CWA, Klammer G, Espinosa N, Buck FM. Upright cone CT of the hindfoot: comparison of the non-weight-bearing with the upright weight-bearing position. Eur Radiol. 2014;24(3):553–8.
24. Krause F, Younger ASE, Baumhauer JF, Daniels TR, Glazebrook M, Evangelista PT, et al. Clinical outcomes of nonunions of hindfoot and ankle fusions. J Bone Joint Surg Am. 2016;98(23):2006–16.
25. Younger ASE, Hansen ST. Adult cavovarus foot. J Am Acad Orthop Surg. 2005;13(5):302–15.
26. Deben SE, Pomeroy GC. Subtle cavus foot: diagnosis and management. J Am Acad Orthop Surg. 2014;22(8):512–20.
27. Stephens M, Saleh J. Calcaneal dome osteotomy: a new procedure for revising triple arthrodesis. Foot Ankle Int. 1994;15(7):368–71.
28. Mäenpää H, Lehto MU, Belt EA. What went wrong in triple arthrodesis? An analysis of failures in 21 patients. Clin Orthop. 2001;7(391):218–23.
29. Toolan BC. Revision of failed triple arthrodesis with an opening-closing wedge osteotomy of the midfoot. Foot Ankle Int. 2004;25(7):456–61.

Revision of Nonunion and Malunion: Ankle Arthrodesis

19

Paul T. Fortin and Douglas N. Beaman

Key Takeaway Points

- Determination of cause of failure is paramount to assure successful revision.
- Infection, bone loss, and neuropathy pose significant challenge.
- Staged reconstruction often necessary.
- Familiarity with multiple surgical techniques such as circular fixation necessary.
- Amputation rather than limb salvage indicated in some cases.

Introduction

The statistical likelihood of successful revision ankle arthrodesis is much lower than with primary arthrodesis; therefore, a thorough understanding of the factors leading to failure is critical [1–5]. Infection, nonunion, malunion, and adjacent joint arthritis are the most common reasons for revision. Because of the significant reconstructive challenges with failed ankle fusion in many patients, revision arthrodesis should be considered an alternative to amputation. Anderson reported a 15% amputation rate in patients treated for nonunion with compression screw fixation. Easley reported that 11% of patients in their series of revision ankle fusion treated primarily with external fixation required amputation [3]. Careful preoperative planning and expertise with multiple reconstructive techniques are necessary to assure successful revision.

P. T. Fortin (✉)
Oakland University William Beaumont, School of Medicine, Royal Oak, MI, USA
e-mail: pfortin@miorthosurgeons.com

D. N. Beaman
Mid Columbia Medical Center, Department of Orthopaedic Surgery, The Dalles, OR, USA

Nonunion

Nonunion is the most common perioperative complication of ankle arthrodesis, and when it occurs, patients have predictably poorer outcomes [6, 7]. The diagnosis of nonunion is not always obvious and is often not accurately predicted by surgeon assessment with plain radiographs and is underestimated compared to blinded CT assessment of union [7]. The extent of osseous bridging seen on CT correlates with clinical outcomes, and asymptomatic nonunions are rare [6]. The rate of nonunion is highly variable and reported to occur in 0–40% of cases [5, 8, 9]. Cobb reported 70% nonunion rate in patients who were actively smoking at the time of surgery [10]. In addition to tobacco use, numerous risk factors for nonunion

M. J. Berkowitz et al. (eds.), *Revision Surgery of the Foot and Ankle*,
https://doi.org/10.1007/978-3-030-29969-9_19

have been cited including neuropathy, inadequate fixation, previous subtalar fusion, history of open fracture, preoperative varus alignment, age, osteonecrosis, noncompliance, obesity, and unemployment [7, 9, 11].

Chalayon reviewed the results of 215 uncomplicated open ankle fusions. Patients with neuropathy, segmental bone loss, simultaneous subtalar fusion, or infection were excluded. The overall nonunion rate was 9% with 19% of patients requiring further surgery due to complications. Nonunion was three times more likely to occur in patients who had previously undergone subtalar fusion and two times more likely in patients with preoperative varus alignment. Identification of patients at risk for nonunion is important and potentially allows for the identification of modifiable factors that might result in improved fusion rates. A nonunion risk assessment model for foot and ankle fusion procedures has been developed and validated [12]. Preliminary studies suggest that it is a reliable and useful tool to stratify risk and improve patient outcome. Examples of modifiable risk factors include obesity, smoking, glucose control, and surgical site stability. The importance of surgical variables such as surgical approach, type of implant, and use of bone graft is debated. A number of newer-generation ankle fusion implants/devices are well suited for revision cases particularly where there is bone loss and a need for greater stability. Several studies have questioned the morbidity of autogenous bone grafting and have shown equivalency with alternatives such as allograft, stem cell, and growth factor products [13, 14].

Malunion

The incidence of malunion after ankle fusion is not well defined and is likely underreported. It often occurs in conjunction with other factors leading to revision surgery such as nonunion and adjacent joint arthritis and therefore is not independently reported in most series. In earlier series using more limited fixation methods, malunion and malposition occurred in as many as 25% of patients [15]. In a more recent series of patients treated with circular fixation for complicated revision of failed ankle fusions, malunion was the reason for revision surgery in over half of the patients [5]. Correction of deformity to restore a plantigrade foot is paramount to achieving a successful revision and is often the most challenging aspect of salvage arthrodesis. Equinus and varus are the most common positions of malunion and result in abnormal force transmission thru the foot and knee. Positioning the foot in equinus, for instance, leads to recurvatum and medial collateral laxity at the knee [16]. The magnitude of deformity and the status of soft tissue dictate the method of correction (gradual vs. acute) as well as the operative approach to avoid compromised soft tissue planes. In cases of mild to moderate deformity from malunion with adequate soft tissues, corrective osteotomy with internal fixation is indicated. More severe multi-planar deformities particularly those with compromised soft tissues are best treated with gradual correction utilizing with small-wire fixation. Paley reported [5] on 21 patients who underwent revision of a failed ankle fusion with circular fixation. Eighteen patients had a limb length discrepancy greater than 2 cm, 11 patients had malunion at the site of the fusion, and 7 patients had a simultaneous infection. Union was achieved in all patients. All but two patients had less than 5 degrees of residual deformity, and two patients had residual limb length discrepancies greater than 1.5 cm. Residual infection was present in only one patient. The authors suggest that despite a high complication rate, circular external fixation addresses the issues of deformity, limb length discrepancy, bone loss, and infection, and it is a worthwhile limb-sparing procedure in these challenging patients.

Causes for Failure

A thorough evaluation of the reasons for failure is necessary to assure successful revision. Causes of failure can largely be grouped into host factors, technical issues, and idiopathic cause.

Some of the common host factors associated with failure include noncompliance, neuropathy, insufficient or avascular bone, smoking, obesity, poor soft tissues, and nutritional deficiency. Technical factors are numerous and undoubtedly underreported. They include inadequate fixation, insufficient bone grafting, malposition, unrecognized foot deformity, unrecognized tibial axis deformity, and inadequate preoperative risk assessment. Identification of modifiable risk factors is paramount. The rate of foot and ankle infections after elective surgery has been reported to be greater than 5% and is higher than that reported in other parts of the body [17]. In a retrospective cohort series evaluating the effect of diabetes on ankle and hindfoot fusion, the postoperative infection rate was 17 times higher in patients with diabetes [18]. Diabetic patients with HbA1c > 7% had an infection rate five times higher than diabetic patients with well-controlled diabetes, and noninfectious complications were twice as likely in patients with diabetes as in those without. Tobacco use and peripheral neuropathy were also identified as independent risk factors of infectious and noninfectious complications. Revision ankle arthrodesis, itself, is a significant risk factor for nonunion, with a 20% nonunion rate, a 38% reoperation rate, and an 11% amputation rate [3]. Adjacent joint arthritis has been proposed by some to also represent a complication of ankle arthrodesis. This often results in revision surgery such as fusion of the symptomatic adjacent joints or conversion total ankle arthroplasty. Subtalar fusion rate has been shown to be only 61% if done in patients that have previously undergone ankle arthrodesis [19].

Evaluation

When evaluating a patient for revision ankle arthrodesis, questions that must be answered are the following:

- Is there infection or other metabolic causes of failure?
- Does the patient have neuropathy?
- Is there significant bone loss?
- Will soft tissue tolerate another extensile surgical procedure?
- What is the patient's willingness/capability of compliance?

In some cases of nonunion, infection is ongoing and very apparent. Subclinical infection must be considered; however, in all cases of nonunion, baseline labs including C-reactive protein and CBC should be obtained. In addition to evaluation for infection, other metabolic causes of nonunion should be investigated. This includes a comprehensive metabolic panel, vitamin D levels, and thyroid function studies. The risk of nonunion from the use of nonsteroidal anti-inflammatories and immunosuppressive drugs is controversial [20]. Any elevation in inflammatory markers warrants further investigation. Triple-phase bone/indium scans can help establish the diagnosis and location of infection when clinical and laboratory findings are equivocal. Dual imaging with technetium-99 and indium-111 also helps differentiate neuropathic osteoarthropathy from infection [21]. Staged reconstruction with bone biopsy and definitive operative debridement is indicated when the presence of infection has been established. In addition to bone and soft tissue culture, the explants should be cultured. The sensitivity of conventional cultures has been shown to be poor with a false-negative rate of 35%. This is particularly common in patients that have previously received antimicrobial agents [22]. Unrecognized or subclinical neuropathy is often subtle and can significantly compromise any further surgical endeavors no matter how robust the fixation. Evaluation should include a good clinical examination including 5.07 monofilament testing, fasting blood glucose, and HbA1c. Formal neurologic evaluation should be considered in high-risk patients. This includes cases of extensive bone loss and unexplained loss of fixation when the clinical evaluation for neuropathy is equivocal.

Vascularity must be assessed, and in patients without strongly palpable pedal pulses, noninvasive arterial Doppler studies should be obtained. Absolute toe pressures less than 50–60 mmHg warrant formal vascular surgical evaluation. Soft tissue assessment includes a historical inquiry of any wound healing issues or infection with prior surgery and documentation of surgical scars, skin grafts and/or flaps, or any areas of impending skin ulceration. A thorough deformity analysis must be performed of the foot and entire limb. Particularly in cases of malunion, consequential or compensatory deformity of the foot can occur in conjunction with the ankle deformity. An example of this includes cases of compensatory varus of the hindfoot associated with valgus malunion of the ankle and distal tibia. Neglecting the position of the hindfoot can result in a non-plantigrade foot when the ankle deformity is corrected. Similarly, the medial column/first ray commonly compensates for hindfoot deformity with plantar flexion or forefoot valgus in cases of hindfoot varus and dorsiflexion or forefoot varus in cases of hindfoot valgus. Range of motion of the subtalar and transverse tarsal joint complex is important. A mobile subtalar joint compensates for coronal plane deformity of the tibia. Likewise, immobility of the subtalar joint can accentuate any coronal plane tibial axis deformity. Knee and tibial axis alignment should be assessed clinically and radiographically. In cavovarus feet, the tibiotalar joint can seemingly be positioned appropriately, but the foot often remains unbalanced, and patients often experience ongoing foot pain and ambulatory impairment. Forefoot and midfoot cavus in these patients result in a "functional equinus" with forefoot overload which is often more pronounced beneath the first metatarsal head as a result of its plantar-flexed position or what is referred to as forefoot valgus (Fig. 19.1a–c). In addition to standing x-rays of the foot and ankle, hindfoot alignment views and standing long-leg alignment views should be obtained especially in cases of malunion. CT is invaluable to determine the extent of bone loss and adequacy for future fixation and to look for any other sources of the patient's symptoms such as adjacent joint arthritis, screw penetration, or lateral gutter arthritis/impingement not adequately addressed by tibiotalar fusion (Fig. 19.2a, b). Patient compliance with weight-bearing instruction and tobacco use is impossible to accurately determine, but it is very important to gauge when considering further surgery. Anticipated noncompliance may preclude another surgical

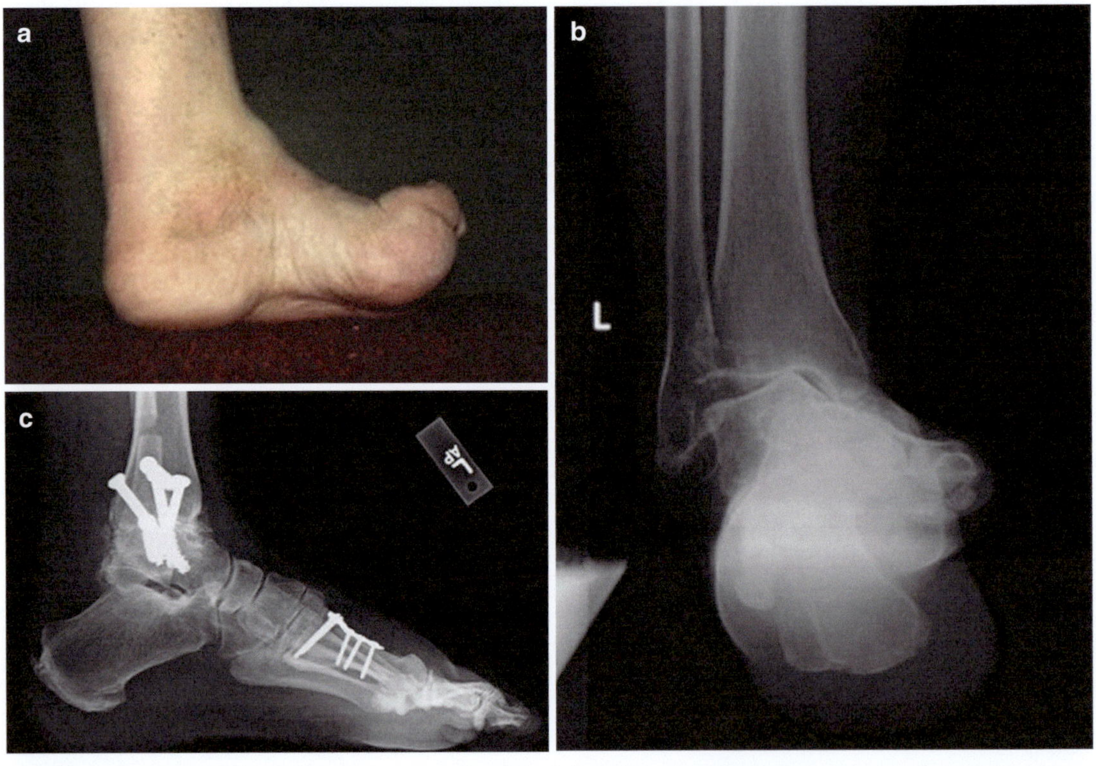

Fig. 19.1 (**a–c**) Foot alignment must be thoroughly evaluated when planning for ankle arthrodesis. In patients with cavovarus, failure to address a plantar-flexed first ray will lead to an unbalanced foot when tibiotalar joint varus is corrected. Dorsiflexion osteotomy of the first ray is necessary in this situation

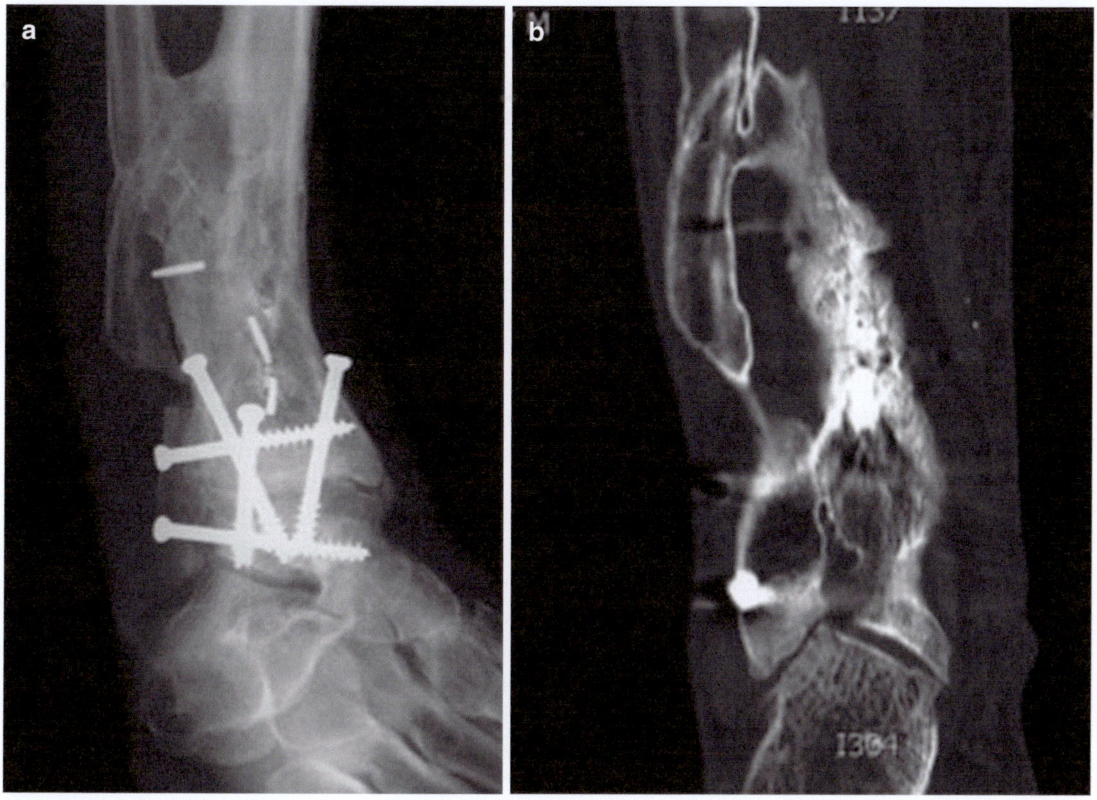

Fig. 19.2 (**a**, **b**) Subfibular impingement can be a source of ongoing ankle pain following otherwise successful ankle arthrodesis that requires revision surgery

endeavor that is destined to fail, or it may alter the method of surgical intervention. In complicated cases of bone loss, infection, poor soft tissue, and deformity, a pointed discussion should be had with the patient regarding their willingness and capability of undergoing a limb salvage procedure with a prolonged recovery versus amputation. In a recent risk assessment for amputation in patients undergoing tibiotalocalcaneal (TTC) fusion, the odds of major amputation were six times higher in patients undergoing revision arthrodesis. Other significant risk factors for amputation were a previous ulceration and neuropathic arthropathy [23].

Surgical Planning

From a very basic standpoint, a differentiation between complicated and uncomplicated cases should be made. An uncomplicated case is one with normal inflammatory markers, no significant bone loss, no neuropathy, or no metabolic bone disease in a compliant patient. These cases are often failures because of inadequate joint preparation or poor fixation and are relatively easy to salvage with rigid internal fixation and bone grafting. This can be accomplished with compression screws or plating [3, 8, 24]. More commonly, however, revision cases are complicated and require careful surgical planning and familiarity with a wide range of reconstructive options. When infection is suspected, staged reconstruction with hardware removal, debridement, bone biopsy, and possible antibiotic spacer is indicated. In addition to bone cultures, cultures of the explants should also be considered. In musculoskeletal infection, microbes are often in a sessile state with a slow metabolic rate that makes it difficult to get useful culture information and makes antibiotics less effective [25]. Sonication is a technique that has been reported to be useful in disrupting biofilm and releasing sessile microorganisms that may otherwise go unrecognized on routine culture [22]. This technique has been used in prosthetic joint infection and may prove to have utility in confirming infection in cases using other forms of internal fixation. Spanning external fixation is sometimes necessary when there is gross instability from bone loss or open wounds that require access for wound management. Anticipated noncompliance with weight-bearing restrictions is also an indication for external fixation. A spanning small-wire fixator will allow these patients to weight-bear and not compromise the stability of the fusion. The pattern and extent of bone loss often dictate the method of fixation and needs for bone grafting. Bone loss in the talus is particularly challenging and necessitates creative methods of fixation. If plate fixation is planned, it must allow for multidirectional screw trajectories that make use of the bone that has structural integrity. Some implants have more points of fixation in the talus and are better than others in this regard, and preoperative imaging should be studied closely to determine the optimal means of fixation. The choice of autogenous graft versus the multitude of commercially available bone graft substitutes is debated [13, 26]. The importance of adequate grafting, no matter the type, however, is not contested and has been substantiated [27, 28]. In a recent study, 81% of joints with adequate graft fill were successfully fused at 24 weeks versus only 21% of joints without adequate graft fill. Large segmental defects will often require structural grafting or bone-lengthening techniques for skeletal restoration. Prior surgical incisions and the soft tissue status need to be considered when planning the surgical approach. Especially in patients with a history of trauma, the anterior soft tissue is sometimes tenuous and not suited for another extensile approach or bulky anterior implants. Posterior and lateral approaches should be considered in those circumstances. The posterior approach typically allows for adequate coverage of implants and is invaluable in many of these cases. Percutaneous osteotomy techniques can be helpful when correcting malunion in the setting of compromised soft tissue. Acute correction of deformity can result in soft tissue and/or neurovascular compromise, and unless bone decompression and shortening are planned, consideration should be given to gradual correction with external fixation [5]. Acute correction of varus deformity can be associated with traction injury of the tibial nerve, and decompression of the tibial and plantar nerves should be considered. Wedge and dome osteotomy in the supramalleolar area allow for acute correction of mild to moderate deformity. In most cases of malunited ankle fusion, the deformity's center of rotation of angulation (CORA) is at the level of the ankle joint, and the osteotomy is above this level to allow for fixation. This can lead to translation of the mechanical axis that may have to be addressed (Fig. 19.3a–d). Especially in developmental and traumatic cases, limb length discrepancies sometimes coexist with ankle arthritis and, if significant, may need to be addressed. Equinus malunion will often mask a significant limb length discrepancy because the plantar-flexed posture of the foot effectively lengthens the extremity, and when this is corrected, the extremity is effectively shortened. In cases of extreme bone loss, uncontrolled infection, and neuropathy in patients unwilling or incapable of prolonged recovery, amputation is often the best option.

Cases

Case 19.1

History

- A 64-year-old nondiabetic and non-neuropathic.
- Persistent ankle pain 10 months following ankle fusion for large osteochondral lesion that failed microfracture debridement (Fig. 19.4a).
- Radiographs show apparent union – CT demonstrates nonunion (Fig. 19.4b–d).
- Inflammatory marker studies normal.

Reason for Failure

- Lack of adequate grafting of medial tibial defect

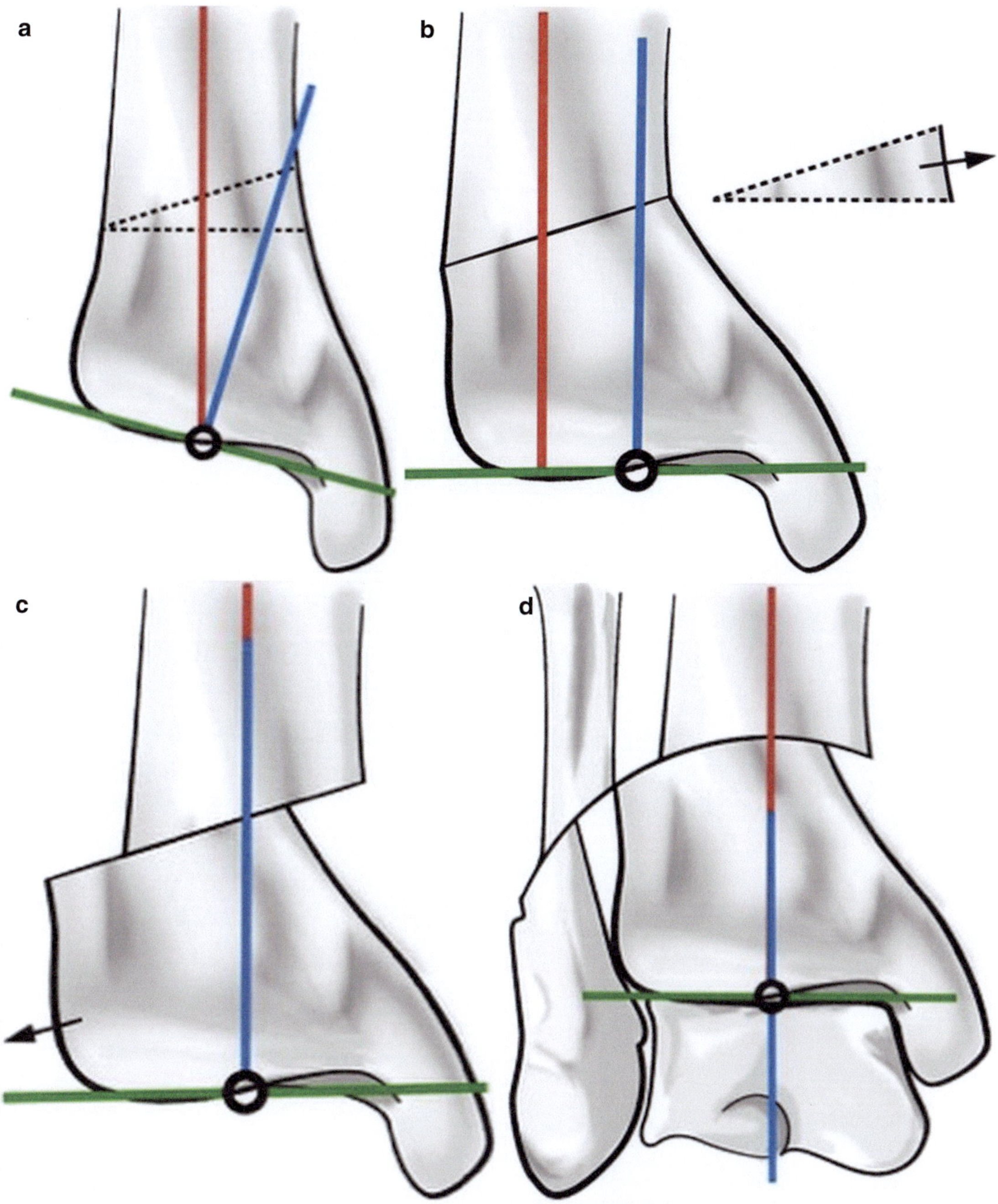

Fig. 19.3 In malunited ankle fusion, the center of rotation of angulation (CORA) is usually located at the level of the ankle joint (**a**). Acute correction is often performed thru a wedge osteotomy at a site remote from the CORA resulting in translation of the mechanical axis of the tibia requiring compensatory translation to restore normal mechanical axis alignment (**b**, **c**). With a dome osteotomy, rotation along the radius of curvature of the osteotomy results in compensatory translation (**d**)

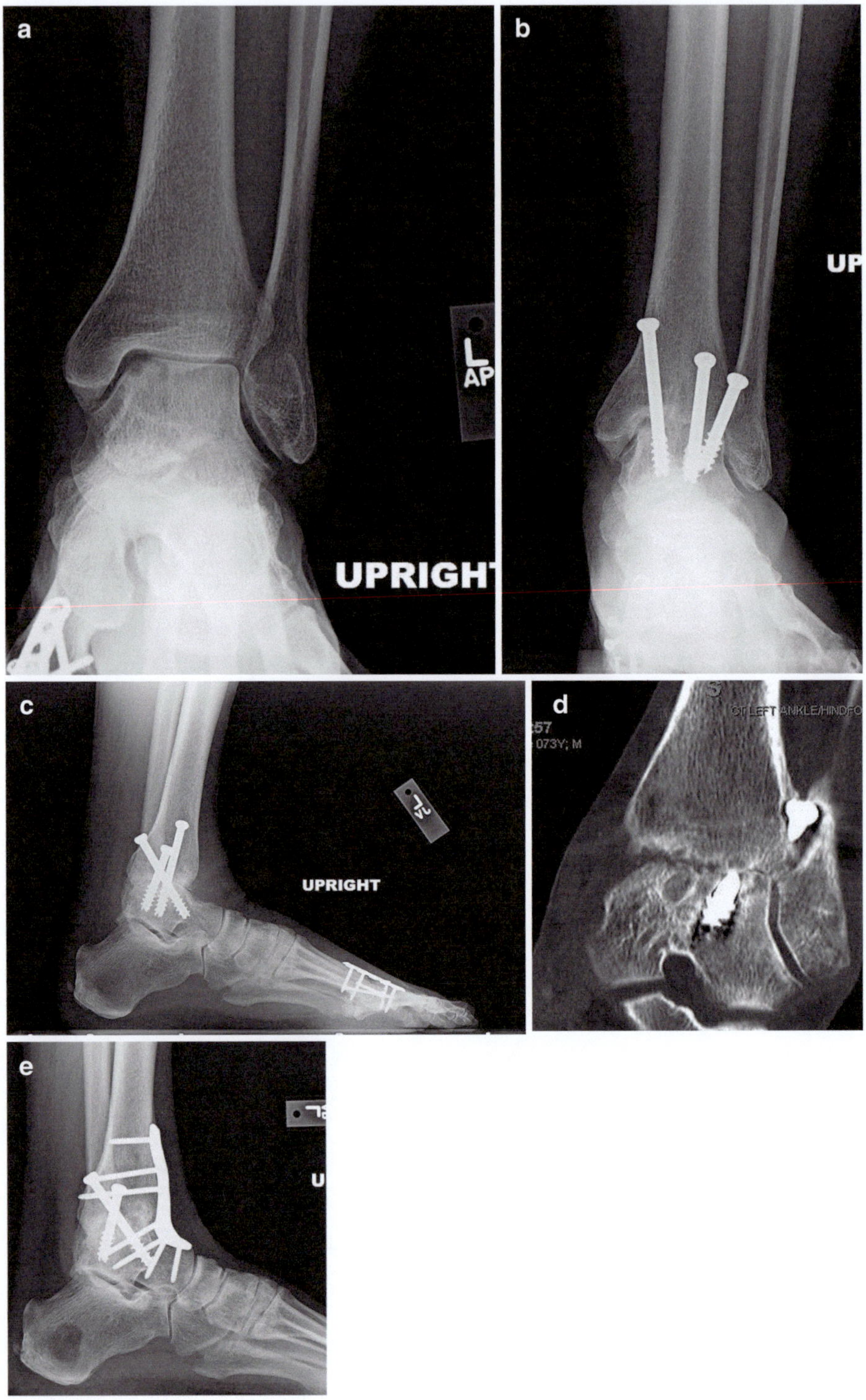

Fig. 19.4 Large osteochondral defect of the medial dome of the talus in a 67-year-old patient that had refractory pain following two previous debridement/microfracture procedures (**a**). Radiographs and CT scan 9 months following ankle arthrodesis using compression screws showing nonunion with persistent medial tibiotalar defect from inadequate bone grafting (**b**–**d**). Revision arthrodesis with bone grafting and anterior plate fixation that has multidirectional screw trajectories (**e**)

Surgical Plan
- Curettage of all interposed fibrous tissue
- Autogenous bone graft from calcaneus
- Augmented fixation with anterior plate
- Multidirectional screw capability in the talus

Approach
- Anterior approach thru previous incision

Implants
- Anterior ankle fusion plate with multidirectional screw option (Fig. 19.4e)

Pearls and Pitfalls
- Multiple-site intraoperative cultures of the bone and explant.
- CT scan in conditions of apparent union that remain painful useful to determine adequacy of healing.
- Bone grafting should be considered in cases of bone loss/defects.

Case 19.2

History
- A 56-year-old with two prior attempts at ankle fusion
- The fibula harvested for bone graft at most recent attempted fusion
- Lateral wound healing issues associated with prolonged drainage
- Valgus collapse with progressive lateral tibial bone loss (Fig. 19.5a, b)

Reasons for Failure
- Inadequate fixation.
- Poor joint preparation.
- Fibular resection along with inadequate fixation resulted in progressive valgus collapse.

Surgical Plan
- Because of history of prolonged drainage, poor soft tissues, and multiple prior surgery, multi-planar external fixation was chosen.

Approach
- Combined medial and lateral approach
- Guide pin placed orthogonal to tibial axis and used as a cutting guide (Fig. 19.5c, d)
- Planar cuts of the tibia and talus minimizing amount of bone resection and correcting valgus malunion

Implants
- Multi-planar external fixation with talar drop wire for compression across fusion site (Fig.19.5e–g)

Pearls and Pitfalls
- Fibular resection destabilizes the ankle and compromises salvage/revision options.
- Multi-planar external fixation useful in situation of poor soft tissue and/or presumed infection.

Case 19.3

History
- A 55-year-old with history of open injury with traumatic loss of medial malleolus
- Progressive talar tilt and bone loss (Fig. 19.6a–c)
- Ankle arthrodesis with dual plating and autogenous bone grafting
- Successful arthrodesis but patient complained of lateral forefoot pain and knee pain secondary to varus alignment (Fig. 19.6d, e)
- Good soft tissue status
- No history of incisional healing issues or infection

Reason for Failure
- Improper intraoperative positioning with varus malunion

Surgical Plan
- Multiple drill-hole dome osteotomy
- Low-energy osteotomy that minimizes change in mechanical axis (Fig. 19.6f–i)
- Broad surface area for healing

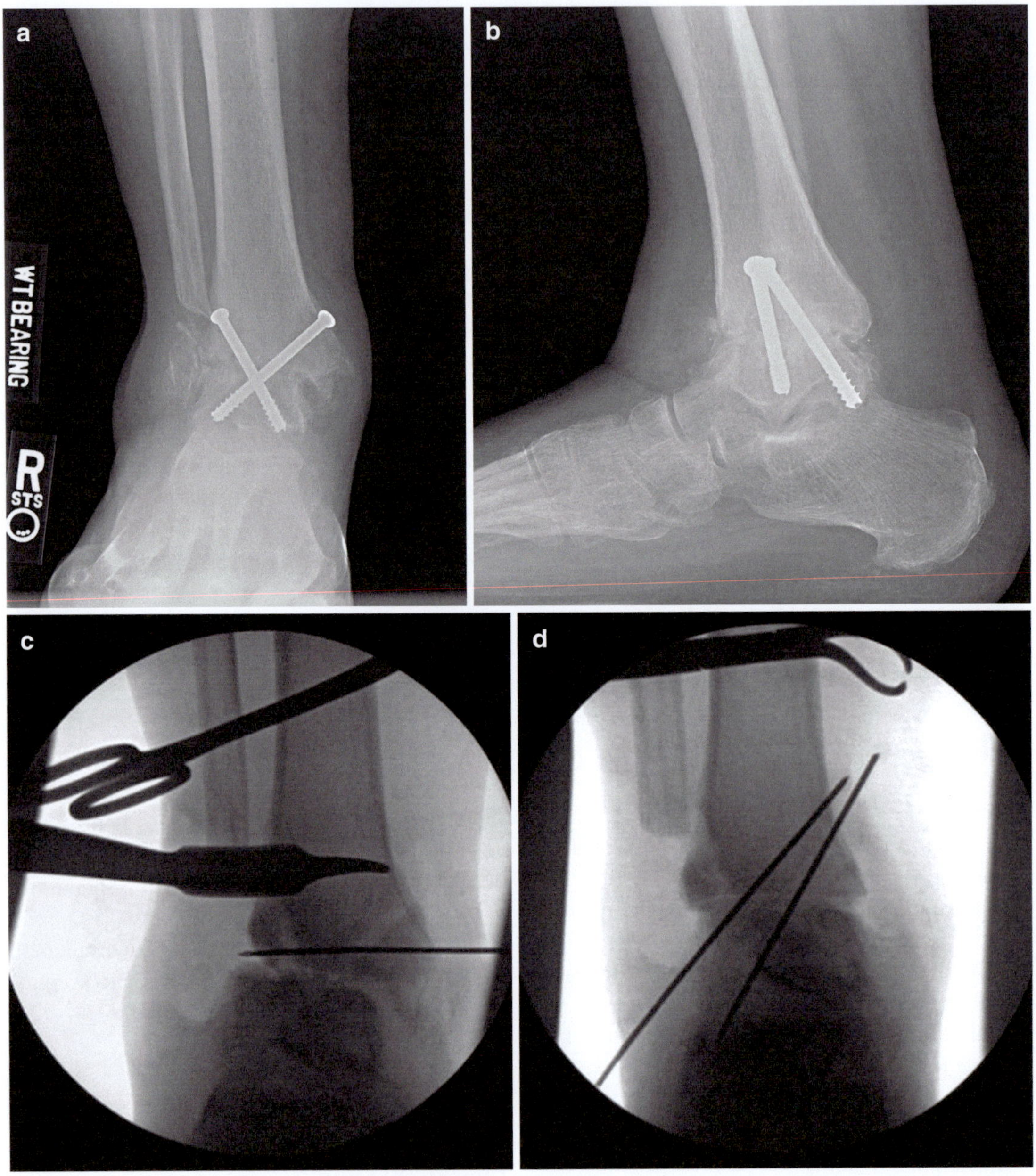

Fig. 19.5 Nonunion after two attempts at ankle fusion with compression screw fixation. The patient had a history of delayed healing with prolonged drainage from the lateral incision with poor lateral soft tissues. Most of the fibula had been harvested and used as bone graft for the second attempt at fusion. Valgus collapse and nonunion ensued (**a**, **b**). Because of concerns for indolent infection and poor soft tissues, external fixation was chosen. Thru combined medial and lateral approaches, planar cuts were made in the tibia and talus correcting valgus malunion (**c**, **d**). Multi-planar external fixation with a talar drop wire for compression thru the fusion site (**e**, **f**). Postoperative CT scan 4 months following surgery demonstrating healing across the fusion (**g**)

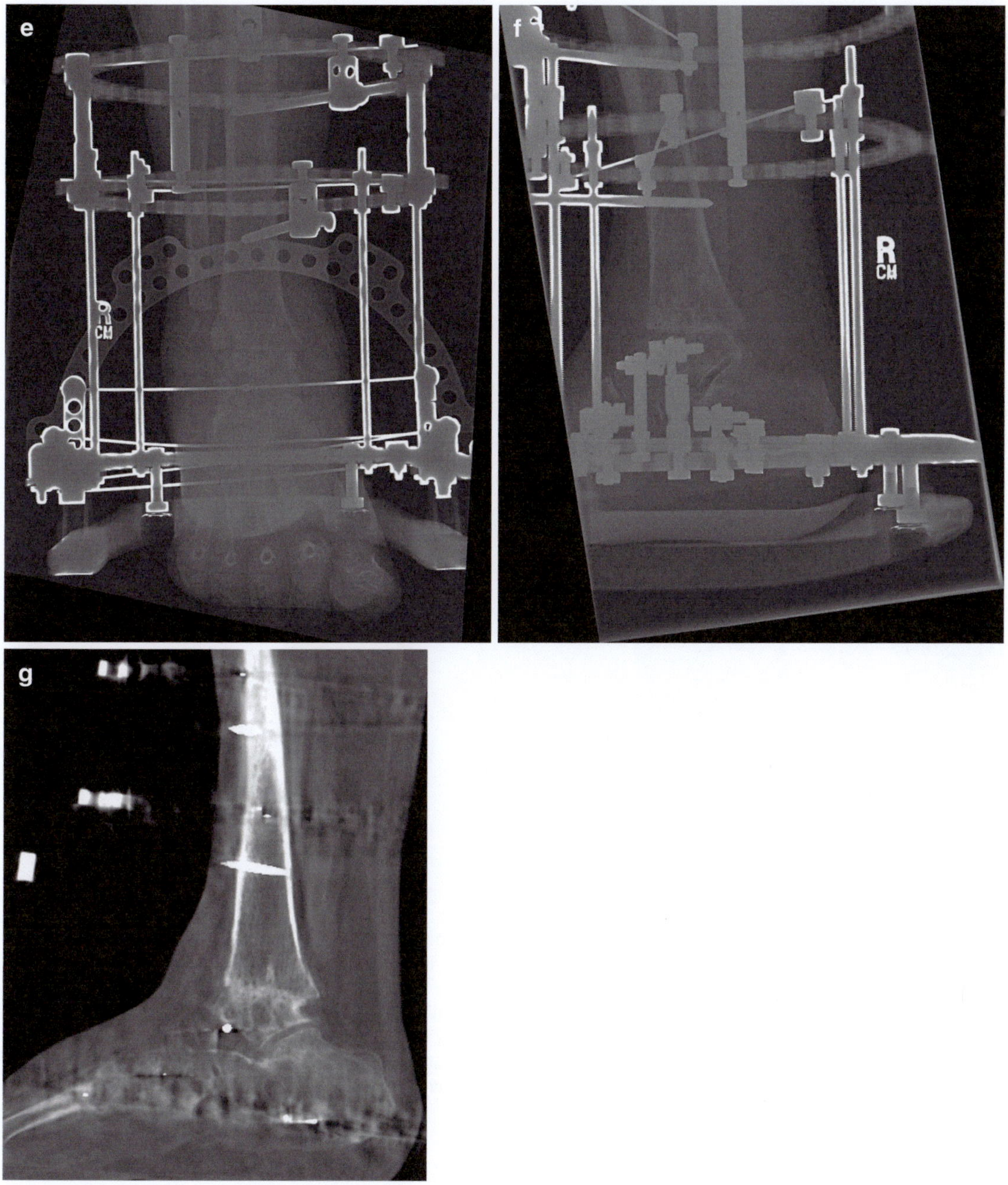

Fig. 19.5 (continued)

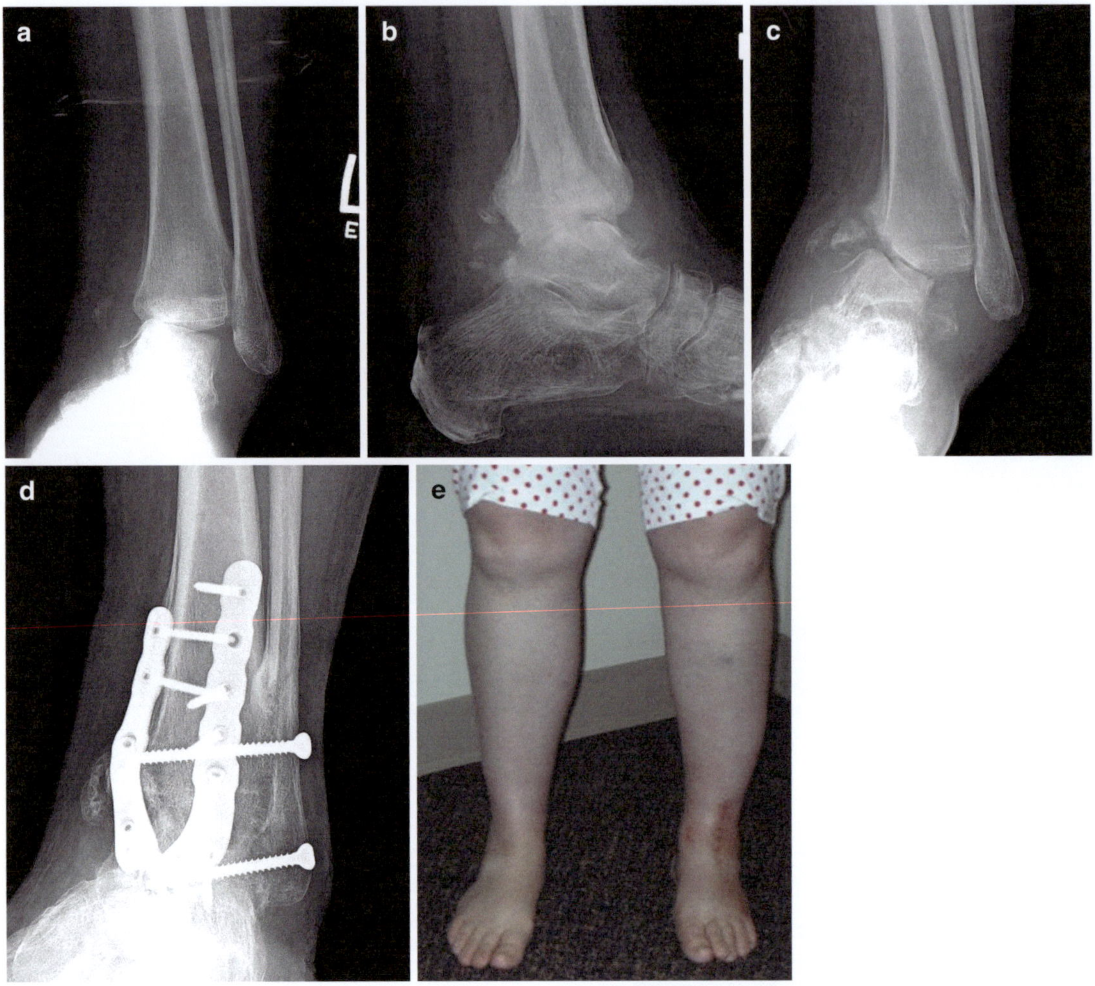

Fig. 19.6 A 56-year-old with a history of open ankle fracture traumatic loss of the medial malleolus resulting in progressive varus collapse and medial tibial bone loss. Patient also had history of maturity-onset diabetes and peripheral neuropathy (**a–c**). Ankle arthrodesis performed using dual plating and bone grafting which resulted in consolidation across the arthrodesis (**d**). Incomplete correction of the varus deformity coupled with genu varum resulted in malunion with painful weight-bearing on the lateral border of the foot (**e**). Correction of varus malunion with a dome osteotomy using multiple drill-hole guide and thin osteotome. This is a low-energy technique that results in a broad surface area in metaphyseal bone that facilitates healing. Osteotomy stabilized with anterolateral plate (**f–i**)

- Guides available to assist as a template for drilling
- "Connect the dots" with thin osteotome

Approach

- Anterior approach thru previous incision

Implants

- Anterolateral distal tibial locking plate

Pearls and Pitfalls

- Not suitable for large-magnitude deformity because of soft tissue and/or neurovascular compromise.
- Negligible shortening or mechanical axis deviation.
- Broad surface area with dome osteotomy facilitates healing.
- Limited utility for multi-planar deformities.

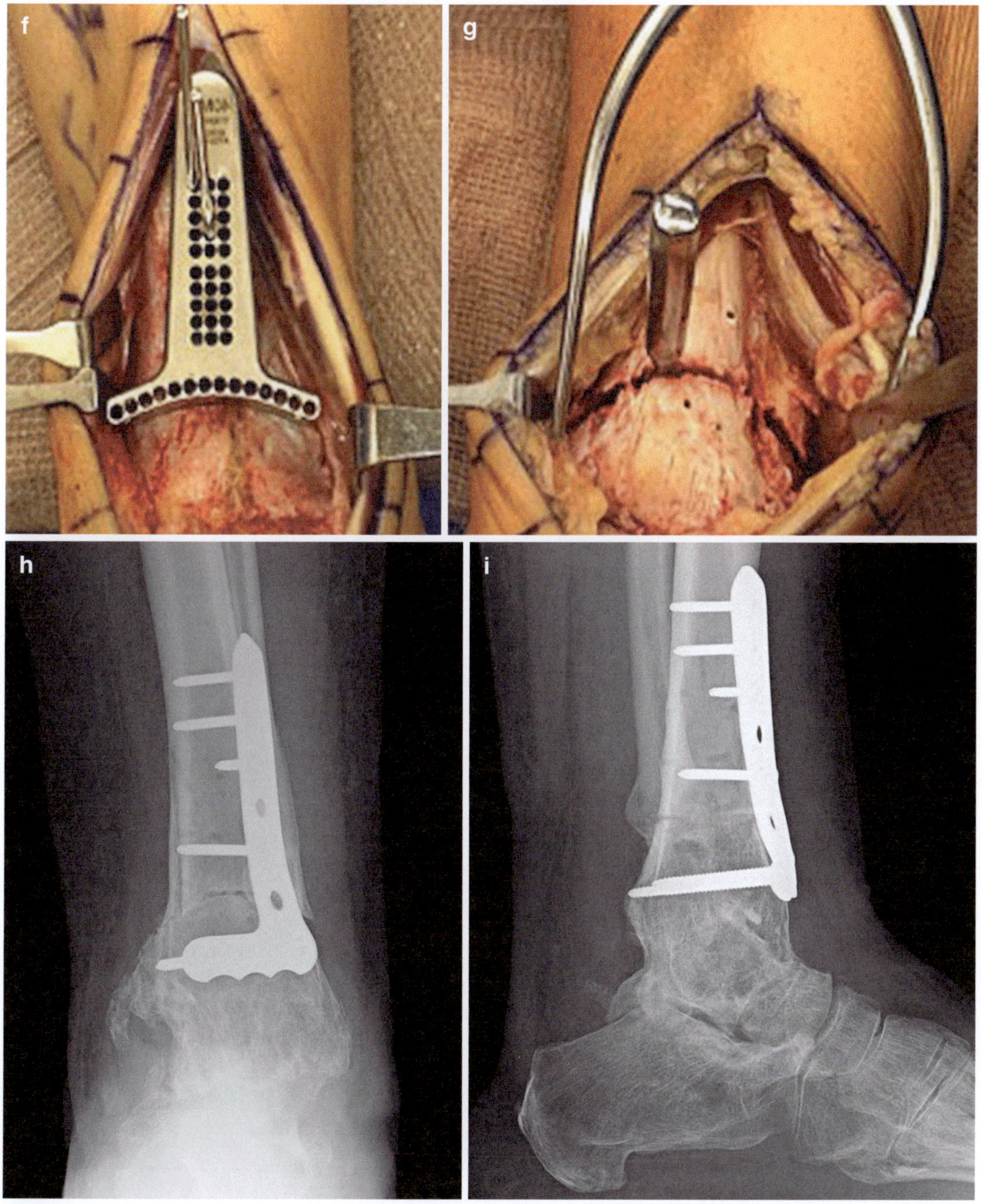

Fig. 19.6 (continued)

Case 19.4

History

- A 64-year-old sustained multiple lower-extremity injuries resulting in ankle and hindfoot arthritis.
- Ankle fusion followed by hindfoot-midfoot fusion.
- Progressive severe valgus deformity secondary to valgus malunion (Fig. 19.7a–c).
- Walker-dependent ambulation.
- Amputation had been offered as the only surgical option.

Reason for Failure

- Complete loss of all motion segments with pantalar fusion coupled with osteopenia and excessive valgus position of hindfoot fusion resulted in tibial stress fracture and subsequent malunion.

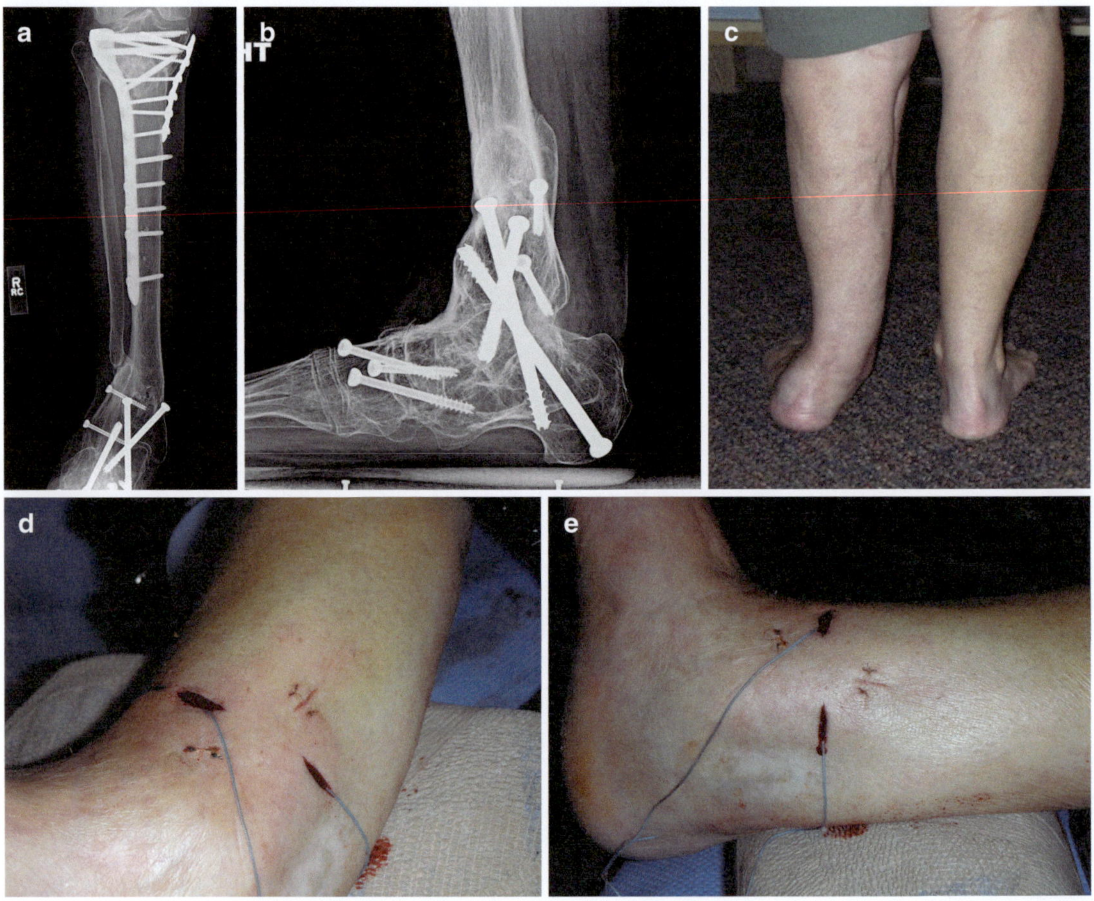

Fig. 19.7 A 67-year-old with a history of multiple lower-extremity fractures secondary to a motor vehicle accident that ultimately was treated with multiple-level ankle hindfoot and midfoot fusion. Patient then developed a progressive severe valgus malunion due to the extreme stiffness and resultant stress fracture (**a**–**c**). Because of poor soft tissues, multiple prior surgeries, and the magnitude of deformity, a staged reconstruction was chosen to minimize soft tissue stripping and allow gradual correction. In the initial stage, previously placed ankle implants were removed. Subperiosteal stripping specifically at the osteotomy site was performed with a narrow periosteal elevator, and a heavy suture was passed subperiosteal around the tibia and fibula as described by Paley and Tetsworth [29] (**d**, **e**). Gradual correction with multi-planar external fixator at 3 weeks (**f**) and 6 weeks (**g**). AP tibial alignment x-ray following removal of external fixator (**h**). One year following removal of spatial frame, ankle fusion takedown and total ankle arthroplasty are performed to restore motion and decrease tibial and midfoot stress (**i**, **j**)

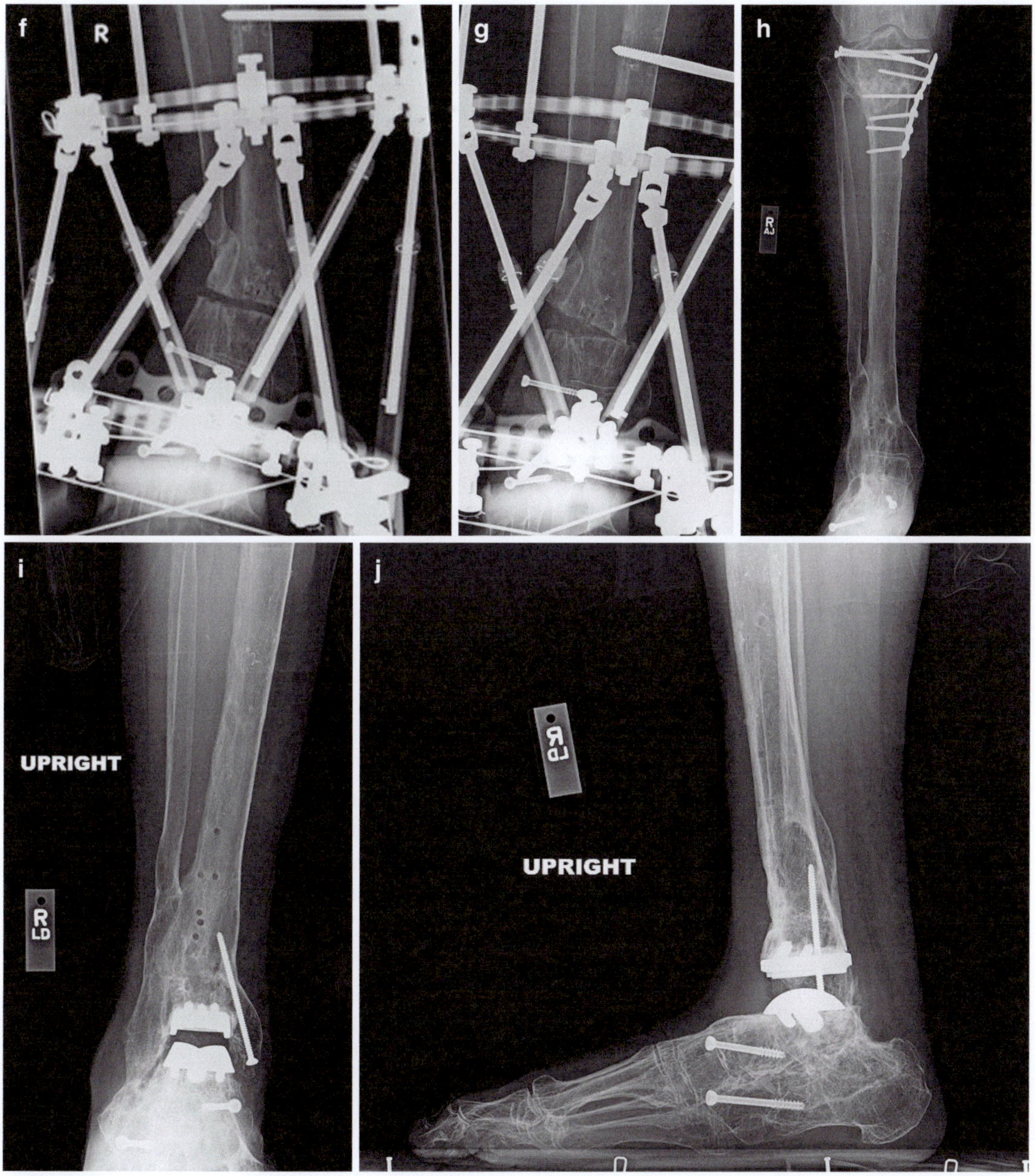

Fig. 19.7 (continued)

Surgical Plan

- Because of the severity of deformity, multiple prior surgeries resulting in extensive lateral scarring, and poor soft tissues, a limited-incision percutaneous Gigli saw osteotomy and gradual correction with external fixation were chosen [29].

Approach

- Minimal-incision percutaneous Gigli saw osteotomy at the CORA of the deformity in metaphyseal bone to maximize regenerate bone formation (Fig. 19.7d, e)

Implants

- Multi-planar external fixator (Fig. 19.7f–h)
- Fixed-bearing total ankle arthroplasty (Fig. 19.7i, j)

Pearls and Pitfalls

- It is important to be strategic in pin placement with external fixation if further surgery is planned to minimize risk of pin tract infection at site of planned open procedure (in this case ankle fusion takedown and total ankle arthroplasty).
- Restoration of motion diminished pain, improved ambulation, and avoided limb loss.
- Requires vigilant pin care and knowledge of gradual correction techniques.

Case 19.5

History

- A 63-year-old with history of infected ankle fusion nonunion.
- Previous triple arthrodesis for neuropathic foot deformity.
- An ankle fusion was performed with a locked intramedullary nail. Due to postoperative infection, the internal fixation was removed, and antibiotic-coated Steinmann pins were placed (Fig. 19.8a, b).
- Persistent drainage thru an ankle sinus track.
- Past medical history: IDDM, hypertension, and coronary artery disease.

Reasons for Failure

- Comorbidities of diabetes and neuroarthropathy
- Previous triple arthrodesis resulting in increased stress of adjacent joints
- Deep infection

Surgical Plan

- Stage 1 – debridement with aggressive removal of all nonviable tissue. Cultures of the bone and explanted device. Stabilization and infection control with antibiotic-coated ankle arthrodesis nail (Fig. 19.8c–g).
- Stage 2 – cement bead removal and application of a Taylor spatial frame (Smith-Nephew) ring external fixator. The fusion site was gradually compressed (1 mm per day) until bone contact. Rotational alignment was also gradually optimized during compression, utilizing spatial frame software. Proximal interlocking screws were placed at the time of frame removal (approximately 5 months) (Fig. 19.8h–l).

Approach

- A lateral transfibular approach to the ankle was used to expose the nonunion. The distal fibula had been previously excised, and full-thickness flaps were created anterior and posterior to the ankle. A sagittal saw was used with irrigation to create a cut in the distal tibia perpendicular to its anatomic axis. Sufficient bone was removed to create a broad, well-vascularized surface for healing. A second parallel cut was made in the residual talus with the foot held in neutral plantigrade position, also creating a broad vascularized bone surface. A 10-mm-diameter ankle fusion intramedullary nail was coated with Simplex P cement containing tobramycin and vancomycin using a silicone tube technique (Tygon SPT-3350 tubing, Saint-Gobain Corp.). This creates a smooth approximately 12-mm-diameter cement-coated stable device. A 3 cm transverse plantar incision is made just distal to the heel pad for nail insertion. Reaming is performed to 14 mm, followed by nail insertion. In this case, antibiotic-containing cement beads were placed in the bone defect. After intraoperative cultures were finalized, the spatial frame was applied as a staged procedure, with bead removal. In our current experience, this can also be performed successfully as a single-stage procedure.
- At time of frame removal, proximal interlocks were placed.
- The patient was maintained in an ankle foot orthosis (AFO) post frame removal, and a 6.5 mm screw was placed to augment fusion site stability.

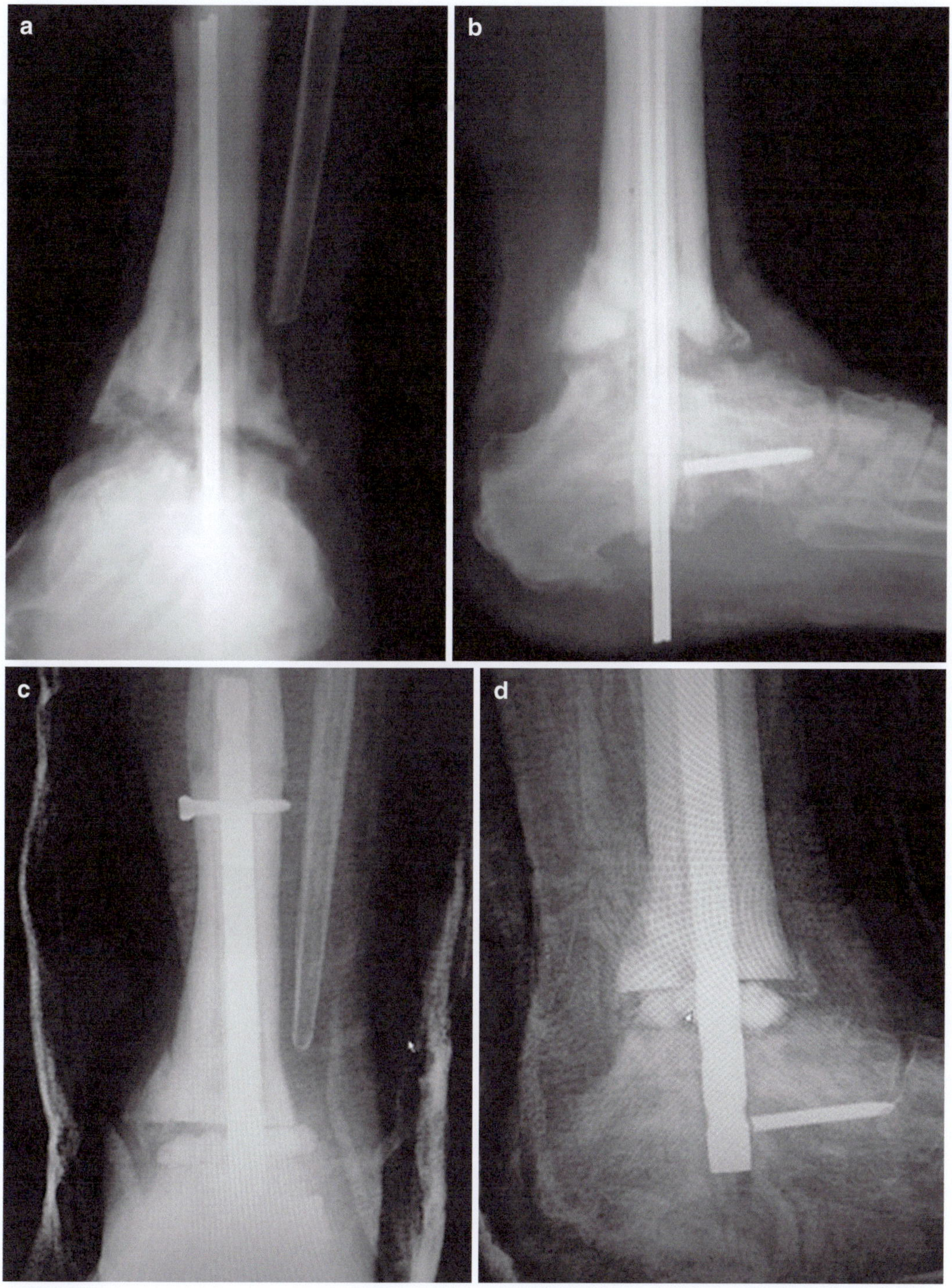

Fig. 19.8 A 63-year-old with maturity-onset diabetes and neuropathy. Multiple attempts at ankle fusion resulting in nonunion and deep infection that was treated with placement of an antibiotic-coated Steinman pin. At the time of presentation, patient had persistent draining sinus tract (**a**, **b**). Staged reconstruction with aggressive debridement of all nonviable tissue and placement of antibiotic-coated locked ankle fusion nail and antibiotic beads (**c**–**g**). Second-stage surgery to remove antibiotic beads and placement of multi-planar external fixator (**h**, **i**). Gradual compression and rotational correction until good bone apposition and provisional healing. External fixator was then removed, and interlocking screws and supplementary lag screw were placed. CT scan after external fixator removal demonstrating good bone apposition at fusion site (**j**). CT scan 7 years follow-up x-rays demonstrating solid arthrodesis (**k**, **l**)

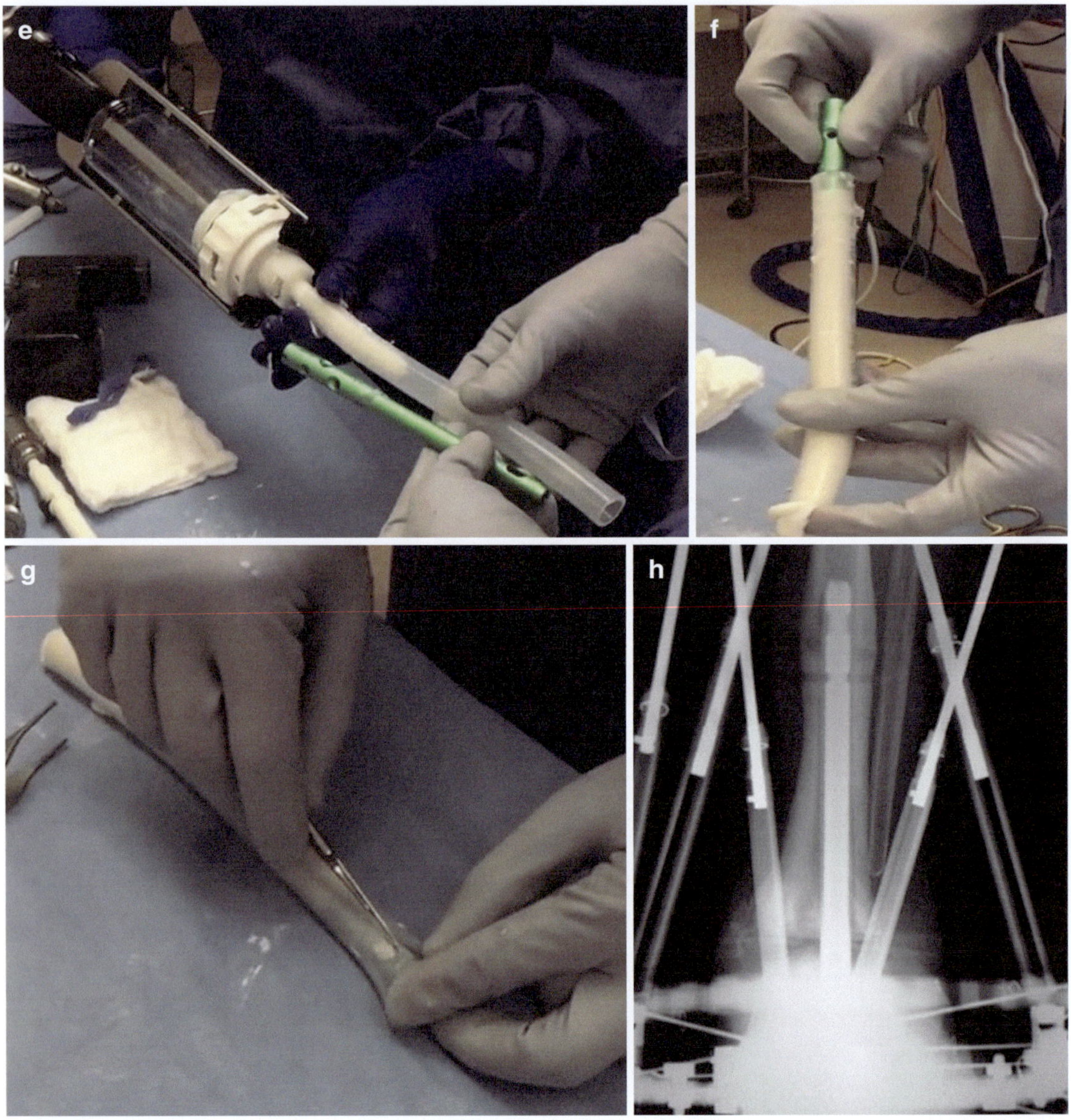

Fig. 19.8 (continued)

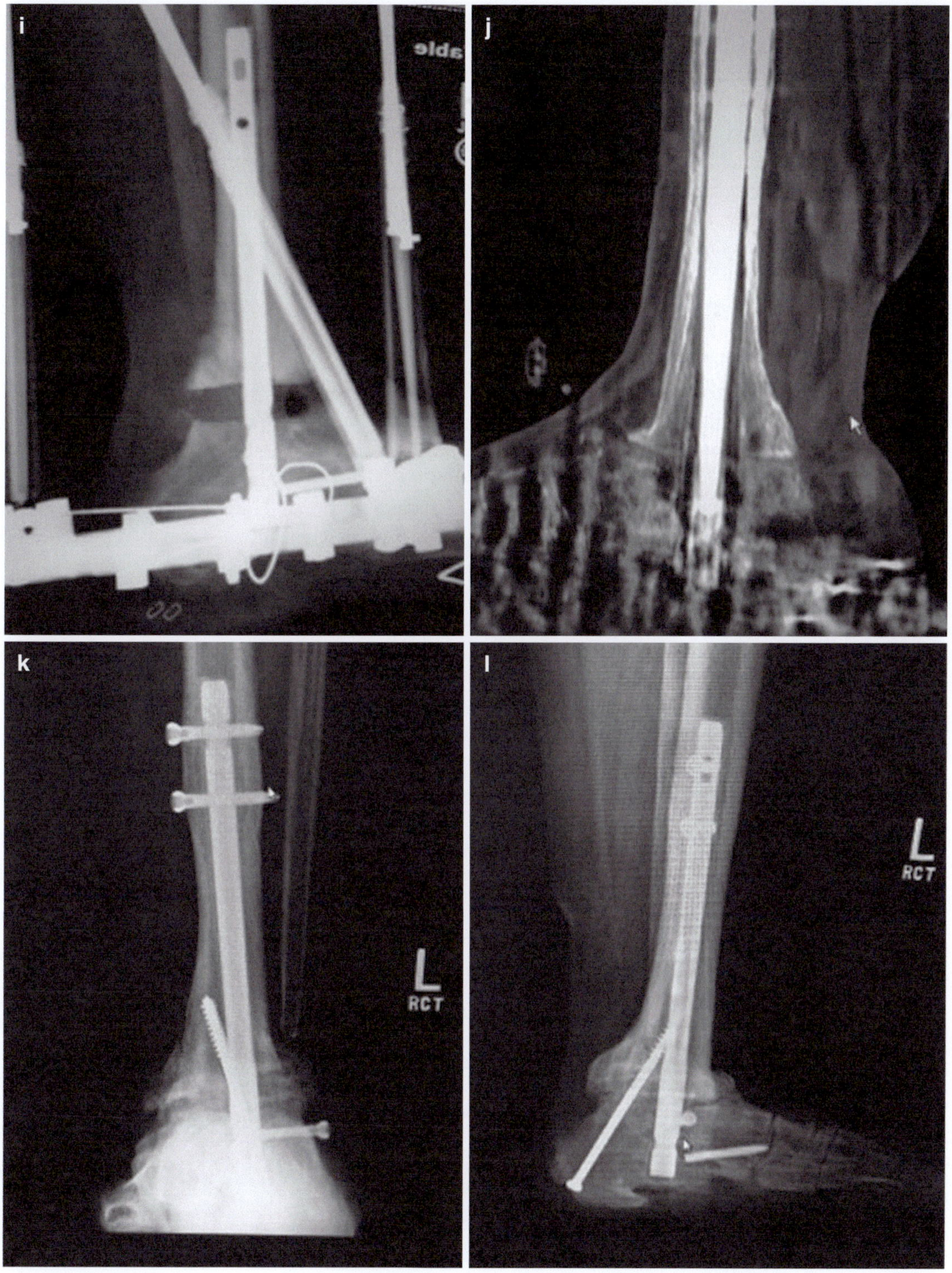

Fig. 19.8 (continued)

Implants

- Ankle arthrodesis nail
- Multi-planar external fixator

Pearls and Pitfalls

- Multi-planar external fixator used to accomplish gradual shortening and rotational deformity correction over an intramedullary nail. This is a valuable technique when bone loss is present and acute compression creates potential neurovascular or soft tissue compromise.
- The subtalar joint had been previously fused in this patient, which is important when using an ankle intramedullary nail. An unfused subtalar joint can lead to implant breakage, hindfoot bone erosion, pain, and swelling.
- An ankle fusion in a neuropathic patient can radiographically appear healed, but it is important to confirm this either on serial radiographs or with CT scan to minimize the possibility of fusion collapse. In this case, a separate screw outside the intramedullary device and an AFO were also used.
- In this patient, the spatial frame was used to accomplish gradual shortening and rotational deformity correction over an intramedullary nail. This is a valuable technique when bone loss is present and acute compression creates potential neurovascular or soft tissue compromise. Proximal interlocking can be done at time of frame removal or after alignment and compression has been achieved.
- An AFO will support the midfoot, which is placed under more stress after ankle and hindfoot fusion, and can develop neuropathic deformity. Dorsal midfoot subluxation can lead to plantar heel ulceration and subsequent below-knee amputation.

Case 19.6

History

- A 66-year-old who underwent ankle fusion 10 years ago
- Two-year history of progressive hindfoot pain due to subtalar arthritis

Reason for Failure

- Adjacent joint arthritis subsequent to ankle arthrodesis (Fig. 19.9a, b)
- Talus positioned in plantar flexion

Surgical Plan

- Conversion total ankle arthroplasty
- Simultaneous subtalar fusion
- Plantar-flexed malposition of the talus corrected thru an anterior wedge resection osteotomy that allowed talar repositioning prior to resection for talar component

Approach

- Anterior approach for total ankle arthroplasty (Fig. 19.9c, d)
- Sinus tarsi approach for subtalar joint preparation

Implants

- Cannulated headless compression screws
- Fixed-bearing total ankle arthroplasty
- Prophylactic fixation of medial column tibia

Pearls and Pitfalls

- To limit wound healing issues, use sinus tarsi approach for subtalar joint preparation to minimize soft tissue dissection.
- Equinus malunion must be addressed at time of takedown of total ankle arthroplasty to assure proper positioning of components.

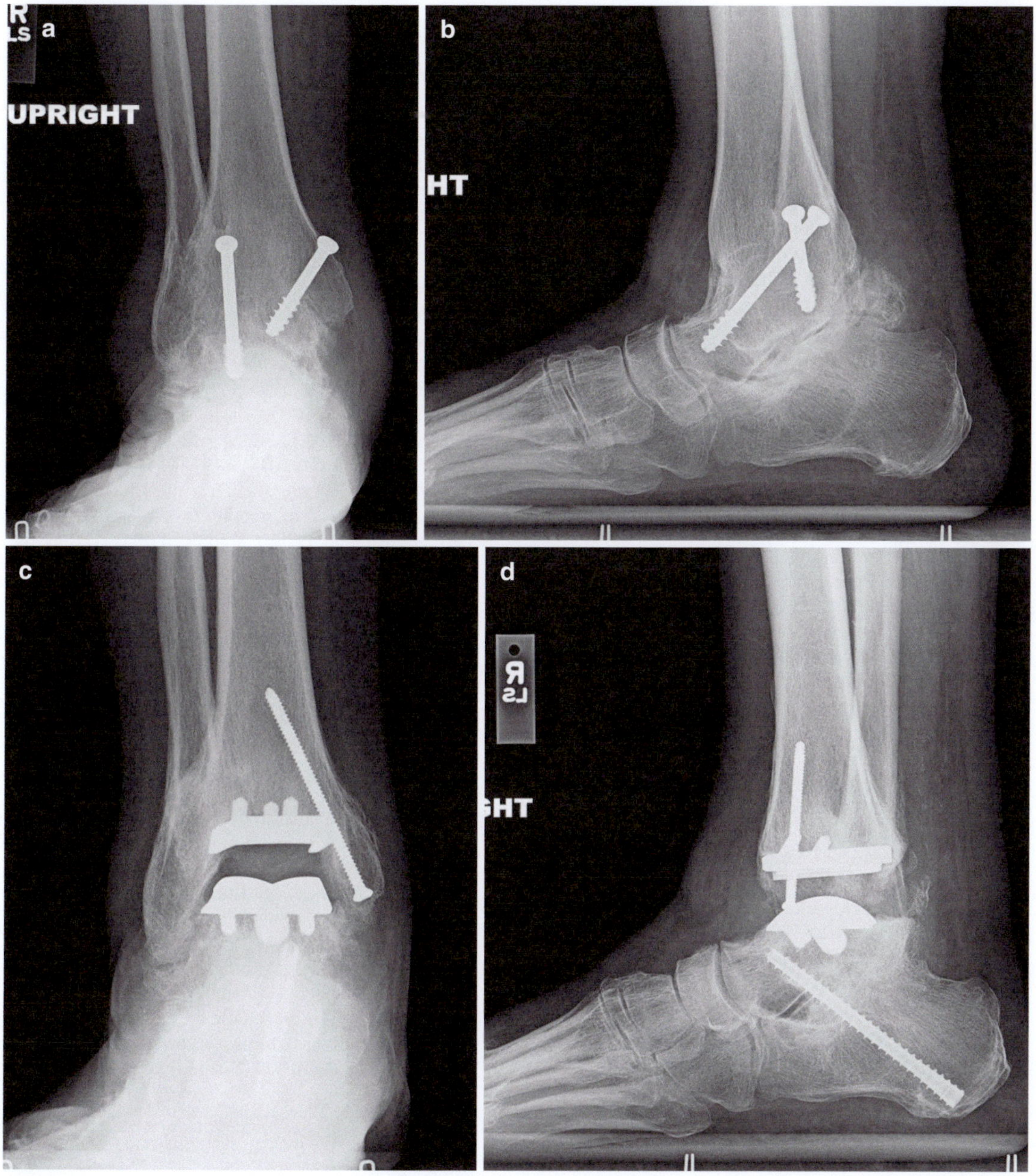

Fig. 19.9 10 years following ankle arthrodesis showing subtalar arthritis and plantar-flexed position malposition of the talus at the time of arthrodesis (**a**, **b**). Ankle fusion takedown with total ankle arthroplasty and simultaneous subtalar fusion (**c**, **d**)

References

1. Midis N, Conti SF. Revision ankle arthrodesis. Foot Ankle Int. 2002;23(3):243–7.
2. Eingartner C, Weise K. Revisionsarthrodesen des oberen Sprunggelenks revision of failed ankle arthrodeses. Oper Orthop Traumatol. 2005;17(45):481–501.
3. Easley ME, Montijo HE, Wilson JB, Fitch RD, Nunley JA 2nd. Revision tibiotalar arthrodesis. J Bone Joint Surg Am. 2008;90(6):1212–23.
4. Cheng Y-M, Chen S-K, Chen J-C, et al. Revision of ankle arthrodesis. Foot Ankle Int. 2003;24(4):321–5. http://www.pubmedcentral.nih.gov/articlerender.fcgi?artid=3235300&tool=pmcentrez&rendertype=abstract.
5. Paley D, Lamm BM, Katsenis D, Bhave A, Herzenberg JE. Treatment of malunion and nonunion at the site of an ankle fusion with the Ilizarov apparatus. J Bone Joint Surg Am. 2006;os-88(1_suppl_1):119–34.
6. Glazebrook M, Beasley W, Daniels T, et al. Establishing the relationship between clinical outcome and extent of osseous bridging between computed tomography assessment in isolated hindfoot and ankle fusions. Foot Ankle Int. 2013;34(12):1612–8.
7. Krause F, Younger ASE, Baumhauer JF, et al. Clinical outcomes of nonunions of hindfoot and ankle fusions. J Bone Joint Surg Am. 2016;98(23):2006–16.
8. Anderson JG, Coetzee JC, Hansen ST. Revision ankle fusion using internal compression arthrodesis with screw fixation. Foot Ankle Int. 1997;18(5):300–9.
9. Chalayon O, Wang B, Blankenhorn B, et al. Factors affecting the outcomes of uncomplicated primary open ankle arthrodesis. Foot Ankle Int. 2015;36(10):1170–9.
10. Cobb TK, Gabrielsen TA, Campbell DC II. Cigarette smoking and nonunion after ankle arthrodesis. Foot Ankle Int. 1994;15:64–7. https://doi.org/10.1177/107110079401500202.
11. Frey C, Halikus NM, Vu-Rose T, Ebramzadeh E. A Review of ankle arthrodesis: predisposing factors to nonunion. https://journals-ohiolink-edu.ccmain.ohionet.org/pg_99?211543556027021::NO::P99_ENTITY_ID,P99_ENTITY_TYPE:268787139,MAIN_FILE&cs=3yPhau3OiQ_ONzJK-u5G1Ml456eZhxgO4obkgVdEK8dP6MjqAHXnTs5onmGxWJmFxC9sjFwWt1knjc7yxsZkO_Q. Accessed 17 Dec 2017.
12. Thevendran G, Wang C, Pinney SJ, Penner MJ, Wing KJ, Younger ASE. Nonunion risk assessment in foot and ankle surgery. Foot Ankle Int. 2015;36(8):901–7.
13. DiGiovanni CW, Baumhauer J, Lin SS, et al. Prospective, randomized, multi-center feasibility trial of rhPDGF-BB versus autologous bone graft in a foot and ankle fusion model. Foot Ankle Int. 2011;32(4):344–54.
14. Baumhauer J, Pinzur MS, Donahue R, Beasley W, DiGiovanni C. Site selection and pain outcome after autologous bone graft harvest. Foot Ankle Int. 2014;35(2):104–7.
15. Morrey BF, Wiedeman G. Complications and long term results of ankle arthrodesis following trauma. J Bone Joint Surg Am. 1980;62(5):777–84.
16. Buck P, Morrey BF, Chao EY. The optimum position of arthrodesis of the ankle. A gait study of the knee and ankle. J Bone Joint Surg Am. 1987;69(7):1052–62. http://www.ncbi.nlm.nih.gov/pubmed/3654697.
17. Donley BG, Philbin T, Tomford JW, Sferra JJ. Foot and ankle infections after surgery. Clin Orthop Relat Res. 2001;391:162–70. http://www.ncbi.nlm.nih.gov/pubmed/11603664.
18. Myers TG, Lowery NJ, Frykberg RG, Wukich DK. Ankle and hindfoot fusions: comparison of outcomes in patients with and without diabetes level of evidence: III, retrospective comparative study. Foot Ankle Int. 2012;33(1):20–8.
19. Zanolli DH, Nunley JA, Easley ME. Subtalar fusion rate in patients with previous ipsilateral ankle arthrodesis. Foot Ankle Int. 2015;36(9):1025–8.
20. Dodwell ER, Latorre JG, Parisini E, et al. NSAID exposure and risk of nonunion: a meta-analysis of case-control and cohort studies. Calcif Tissue Int. 2010;87(3):193–202.
21. Loredo R, Rahal A, Garcia G, Metter D. Overview of imaging modalities. Imaging of the diabetic foot diagnostic dilemmas' Foot Ankle Spec. 2010;3(5):249–64.
22. Scorzolini L, Lichtner M, Iannetta M, et al. Sonication technique improves microbiological diagnosis in patients treated with antibiotics before surgery for prosthetic joint infections. New Microbiol. 2014;37(3):321–8.
23. DeVries JG, Berlet GC, Hyer CF. Predictive risk assessment for major amputation after tibiotalocalcaneal arthrodesis. Foot Ankle Int. 2013;34(6):846–50.
24. Levine SE, Myerson MS, Lucas P, Schon LC. Salvage of pseudoarthrosis after tibiotalar arthrodesis. Foot Ankle Int. 1997;18(9):580–5.
25. Shirwaiker RA, Springer BD, Spangehl MJ, et al. A clinical perspective on musculoskeletal infection treatment strategies and challenges. J Am Acad Orthop Surg. 2015;23(suppl). https://journals.lww.com/jaaos/Fulltext/2015/04001/A_Clinical_Perspective_on_Musculoskeletal.7.aspx.
26. Lareau CR, Deren ME, Fantry A, Donahue RMJ, DiGiovanni CW. Does autogenous bone graft work? A logistic regression analysis of data from 159 papers in the foot and ankle literature. Foot Ankle Surg. 2015;21(3):150–9.
27. Baumhauer JF, Pinzur MS, Daniels TR, et al. Survey on the need for bone graft in foot and ankle fusion surgery. Foot Ankle Int. 2013;34(12):1629–33.
28. DiGiovanni CW, Lin SS, Daniels TR, et al. The importance of sufficient graft material in achieving foot or ankle fusion. J Bone Joint Surg Am. 2016;98(15):1260–7.
29. Paley D, Tetsworth K. Percutaneous osteotomies. Osteotome and Gigli saw techniques. Orthop Clin North Am. 1991;22(4):613–24.

Revision Total Ankle Replacement 20

Brian Steginsky and Steven L. Haddad

Key Takeaway Points

- Within the last decade, total ankle arthroplasty has emerged as an acceptable alternative in the treatment of severe tibiotalar arthritis. However, most authors report a failure rate of 10–20% within 10 years of the index total ankle arthroplasty [1–5]. Historically, salvage of a failed total ankle arthroplasty involved either ankle arthrodesis or amputation. As implant technology and surgical techniques improve, revision arthroplasty has become an emerging surgical alternative.
- Comprehensive clinical evaluation and careful preoperative planning are critical to achieve successful outcomes after revision total ankle arthroplasty.
- The underlying reasons for component failure should be addressed. Often, this may require a two-stage procedure. We have found residual foot deformity as a major cause of early implant failure.
- Routine radiographic surveillance must be performed (at a minimum) every year following total ankle arthroplasty to monitor for the development of osteolytic cysts and impending implant failure. Severe component subsidence and delayed intervention exponentially increase the degree of difficulty of the revision arthroplasty.
- Revision total ankle arthroplasty is technically demanding and should be attempted by those with adequate experience. Referral should be considered in patients with severe component subsidence and failure.

B. Steginsky · S. L. Haddad (✉)
Orthopaedic Foot and Ankle Sugery,
Illinois Bone and Joint Institute, LLC,
Glenview, IL, USA

Introduction

First-generation total ankle arthroplasty (TAA) was associated with unacceptably high failure rates and complications. Historically, salvage of a failed total ankle arthroplasty involved either ankle arthrodesis or amputation. Within the last decade, total ankle arthroplasty has emerged as an acceptable alternative in the treatment of severe tibiotalar arthritis. However, most authors report a failure rate of 10–20% within 10 years of the index total ankle arthroplasty [1–5]. As implant technology and surgical techniques

M. J. Berkowitz et al. (eds.), *Revision Surgery of the Foot and Ankle*,
https://doi.org/10.1007/978-3-030-29969-9_20

improve, revision arthroplasty has become an emerging surgical alternative.

However, as technology and design improve with modern-generation implants, the indications for total ankle arthroplasty have expanded. As such, the number of total ankle arthroplasties being performed each year continues to increase. Greater than fifty percent of orthopedic foot and ankle surgeons have performed a TAA [6]. As acceptance of total ankle arthroplasty continues to grow, the further advancement of revision total ankle arthroplasty and surgical techniques must follow. Without co-advancement of primary and revision techniques and implants, patient reassurance that salvage of their newly placed prosthesis is feasible would generate unnecessary apprehension in those undergoing the procedure. Other surgical options following failed TAA include amputation or conversion to arthrodesis. However, salvage arthrodesis using structural bulk allograft has been associated with high rates of nonunion and inferior clinical outcomes (compared to primary arthrodesis) [7]. Finally, other options such as structural metal "fusion" implants are without scientific proof of their longevity and incorporation into surrounding bone.

Most authors report a failure rate ranging from 10% to 20% within 10 years of the index total ankle arthroplasty (with component revision as the primary endpoint) [1–5, 8]. In a large meta-analysis, survivorship of second-generation total ankle arthroplasty implants was reported to be 77% at 10-year follow-up [9]. The long-term survivorship of modern-generation implants is not yet available. Although survivorship is improving with the newer-generation implants, the failure rate of TAA still remains higher than that of other joint replacements [10]. The most frequently reported reason for revision total ankle arthroplasty is component loosening and/or subsidence [9, 10]. Other reasons for reoperation and/or revision surgery include component malposition, residual coronal plane deformity, arthrofibrosis, heterotopic ossification, ankle instability, deep infection, polyethylene failure, and persistent pain [10, 11].

Glazebrook and colleagues performed a literature review of twenty studies identifying nine main complications associated with TAA failure [12]. Complications were stratified into three groups based on their relative risk of TAA failure:

- *High grade* (deep infection, aseptic loosening, and implant failure) was associated with >50% failure rate.
- *Medium grade* (technical error, component subsidence, and postoperative fracture) was associated with <50% failure rate.
- *Low grade* (intraoperative fracture and superficial wound problems) was never associated with failure.

There is a paucity of literature on revision total ankle arthroplasty. Literature is limited by small cohorts and short-term follow-up. The Agility® prosthesis was the only FDA-approved prosthesis available in the United States until 2006; therefore, most of the US literature on revision ankle arthroplasty is limited to a single prosthesis.

DeVries et al. reviewed five patients who underwent conversion from a failed Agility® to an INBONE® with an average follow-up of 17.2 months. Two patients (40%) were converted to a tibiotalocalcaneal arthrodesis or amputation.

Williams and colleagues performed a retrospective review of 35 patients who underwent revision arthroplasty from a failed Agility® prosthesis to INBONE II® with an average follow-up of 9.1 months [13] . Revision arthroplasty was indicated in 31 patients (88.6%) for talar subsidence and/or osteolysis. Thirty-three patients required grafting procedures to fill bony deficits. Small bone deficits were packed with autograft from the tibial bone resection, cancellous allograft chips, or calcium phosphate/calcium sulfate. Large talar bony deficits were managed with femoral head allograft (4) or bone graft substitute (1). At latest follow-up, three patients had severe talar subsidence of the revision talar component (but did not require revision of the INBONE II® component). The complication rate was 31.4% in this series with the most frequent complications being intraoperative fracture (6) and wound dehiscence (2).

Ellington and colleagues performed a retrospective review of 53 patients who underwent revision total ankle replacement utilizing a custom Agility® prosthesis [14]. Forty-one patients were available for follow-up at a mean of 49.1 months. The most common indication for revision TAA was talar subsidence (63%). Five patients (12.2%) were converted to arthrodesis, and two patients (4.9%) underwent amputation. The severity of the initial talar component subsidence was determined to be a significant predictor of the revision functional outcome as measured by the American Orthopaedic Foot & Ankle Society (AOFAS) hindfoot score and Ankle Osteoarthritis Scale.

Hintermann and colleagues performed the most comprehensive review of revision total ankle arthroplasty to date. Eleven different types of prosthesis (HINTEGRA®, STAR®, Mobility®, Salto Talaris®, Agility®, ESKA®, Buechel-Pappas®, AES®, Alpha®, BOX®, Irvine®) were revised using the unconstrained, three-component HINTEGRA® system (not FDA approved for use in the United States) [10] . There were a total of 117 ankles that underwent revision TAA with a mean follow-up of 6.2 years. Seventeen patients (15%) failed revision arthroplasty; six patients were converted to arthrodesis, and eleven patients underwent a subsequent revision arthroplasty. The authors concluded that the intermediate-term results of revision TAA were similar to those after primary arthroplasty at the time of this publication.

The management of bone loss and the ability to reestablish the ankle joint center of rotation can be extremely challenging following component loosening and/or subsidence. This chapter will focus on revision total ankle arthroplasty using metal/cement augmentation to reconstitute the natural joint line level and anatomy following catastrophic failure of the index total ankle arthroplasty.

Evaluation and Surgical Planning

Thorough clinical evaluation and the appropriate diagnostic tests must be performed prior to proceeding with revision total ankle arthroplasty. Complete understanding of the reasons for failure is paramount. Often, foot balance was not appropriately achieved at the time of the index procedure, resulting in an eccentric load and early failure of the prosthesis.

All previous imaging studies, operative reports, and medical records should be obtained if possible. This information should be reviewed to determine the progression and cause of implant failure. Early intervention is preferred, as the difficulty of revision arthroplasty increases with the severity of deformity and extent of component subsidence. Index operative reports should be reviewed to determine the type of prosthesis and hardware that will be removed. Extraction of hardware should be performed efficiently and without a tourniquet, as revision arthroplasty can generate longer surgical times.

Comprehensive clinical examination is essential prior to revision surgery. Motor, sensory, and vascular deficits must be thoroughly documented. It is not uncommon for a preexisting neurovascular deficit to be present from previous surgeries. Fibrosis and scarring distort the natural anatomy, which make identification of critical neurovascular structures more challenging. Any concerns for vascular compromise should prompt further testing with ankle-brachial index, Doppler ultrasound, and/or CT angiography. Failure to do so may compromise outcomes if additional vascular violation at the time of revision results in a dysvascular extremity.

The soft tissue envelope is an important aspect of revision foot and ankle surgery that should not be overlooked. Any history of a soft tissue flap reflexively warrants preoperative consultation with a plastic surgeon, as further insult to the blood supply could potentially result in catastrophic wound problems. Obtaining the prior plastic surgical operative note allows the secondary surgeon to understand the source and location of the pedicle feeding the flap. When possible, the previous surgical incisions should be used. This is not always feasible, as revision total ankle arthroplasty requires an adequate surgical exposure. An understanding of lower extremity angiosomes and potential consequences of violating the blood supply is helpful in preventing postoperative skin necrosis. Again, consultation with a plastic surgeon is appropriate in this situation. We perform preoperative compression wraps on all patients with lower extremity edema [15, 16]. Compression wraps are started the week before surgery and changed every other day and carried into the postoperative phase at least 2 weeks to minimize tension on surgical incisions.

Limb alignment must carefully be assessed. Full-length standing radiographs or a CT scanogram should be performed if there is concern for malalignment or limb shortening. Gait should be observed for varus or valgus thrust, alignment, foot progression angle, and cadence. We routinely use a goniometer to assess hindfoot alignment and ankle range of motion. If tibiotalar joint is incongruent, we perform varus and valgus stress radiographs to determine the degree of ligament attenuation and rigidity of the deformity.

We order standard weight-bearing foot and ankle radiographs. We supplement our radiographic examination with dorsiflexion/plantarflexion radiographs of the ankle and an axial alignment view of the heel. Additionally, we obtain a weight-bearing CT scan and musculoskeletal ultrasound. We have found that a well-performed musculoskeletal ultrasound can be more helpful than MRI for preoperative surgical planning. Metal artifact limits the diagnostic value of an MRI. Furthermore, ultrasound can provide both static and dynamic information, which can be used to determine the *degree* of ligamentous attenuation and the need for a two-stage ligament reconstruction. Other tendon, ligamentous, and neurovascular structures can be visualized on ultrasound.

We use weight-bearing CT with metal subtraction protocol to examine the degree of adjacent joint arthritis, severity of component subsidence and bone loss, and residual foot and ankle deformity. The apex of the deformity must always be identified and corrected at the time of surgery. If appropriate foot balance is not achieved at the time of revision arthroplasty, then the patient is at risk for subsequent component failure through eccentric loading of the implant with gait.

As a general rule, we consider revision ankle arthroplasty in two stages for the following reasons: triple arthrodesis, revision triple arthrodesis, rotational foot deformity, deltoid ligament reconstruction with allograft, or history of deep infection. We believe that midfoot correction can be achieved at the time of revision arthroplasty.

CRP, ESR, and CBC should be obtained on any patient with a history of infection. If there is concern for an active infection involving the ankle joint, then joint aspiration and blood cultures should be performed. We order an indium-labeled tagged WBC scan if there is concern that the infection extends to the prosthesis. Infectious disease consultation is appropriate, as the infectious disease physician can develop a relationship with the patient prior to revision surgery, leading to a less apprehensive and more comprehensive approach. Antibiotics should not be administered until intraoperative cultures have been obtained, as culture-sensitive chemotherapy and thorough debridement are the foundation for eradication of the deep infection. If the infection is chronic (beyond 4 weeks), then the prosthesis is removed, and an antibiotic cement spacer is placed. Although the goal should be to convert the patient to an ankle arthrodesis or revision total ankle arthroplasty, the use of an antibiotic impregnated cement spacer has been described as a definitive treatment option for patients with low-functional demands [17]. The patient generally receives a minimum of 6 weeks of intravenous antibiotics. Inflammatory markers are followed weekly during this time period. The patient normally has an "antibiotic holiday," prior to revision surgery. If the serum inflammatory markers increase during this period, then it should be presumed that the infection has not been eradicated and repeat debridement should be considered.

Cases

Case 20.1

History

- A 55-year-old female presented with a remote history of lateral ankle instability and allograft lateral ligament reconstruction.
- Lateral ankle joint arthritis progressed after ligament reconstruction, and the patient

underwent total ankle arthroplasty with the Zimmer TM® total ankle prosthesis.

- The pain did not improve after total ankle arthroplasty. The previous surgeon performed a medial gutter debridement on two separate occasions.
- The patient complained of deep pain across the anterior ankle joint. The pain worsened with standing and ambulation. On examination, focal tenderness was elicited at the anteromedial tibial joint line.
- The patient reported significant pain relief after an intra-articular injection with 0.5% bupivacaine/1% lidocaine.
- We perform intra-articular injections under fluoroscopy to confirm appropriate placement of the anesthetic. We advocate the use of differential diagnostic injections, as they can help further localize the source of pain after routine imaging has been ordered. Occasionally, dye is used (if nonallergenic) to assess the location of the injection and potential penetration into surrounding joints.
- 8-cm scar was present over the fibula, and 3-cm scar was present over the anteromedial ankle joint (Fig. 20.1a–c). Mild pes planovalgus deformity with fixed forefoot supination was noted on clinical examination.
- Weight-bearing CT confirmed loosening of the tibial component and 3 mm of talar subsidence. We use SPECT CT to rule out implant loosening if standard CT is equivocal.

Reasons for Failure

- The Zimmer TM® instrumentation references the radius of curvature of the talus to resurface the joint through a lateral approach (Fig. 20.2a).
- The radius of curvature of the ankle joint may be variable (particularly with the severity of

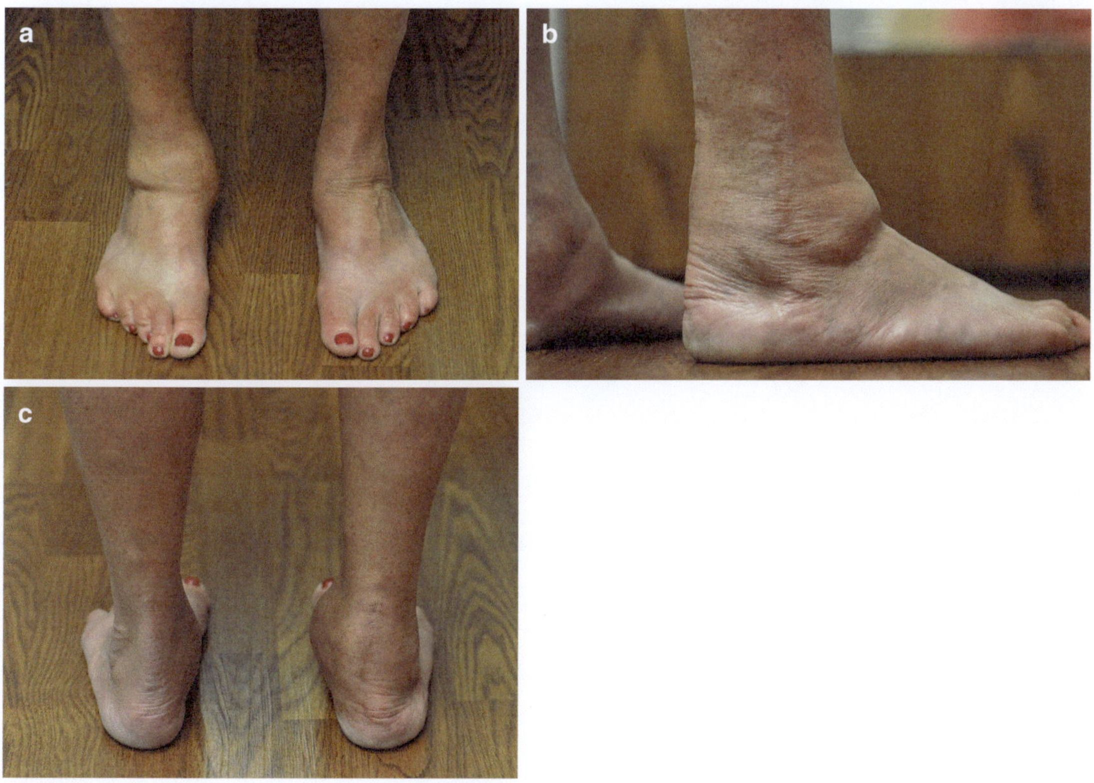

Fig. 20.1 Clinical pictures demonstrate an anteromedial ankle incision (a) used for prior medial gutter debridement and lateral (transfibular) incision used for implantation of the Zimmer TM® prosthesis (b). The hindfoot remains in slight valgus (c)

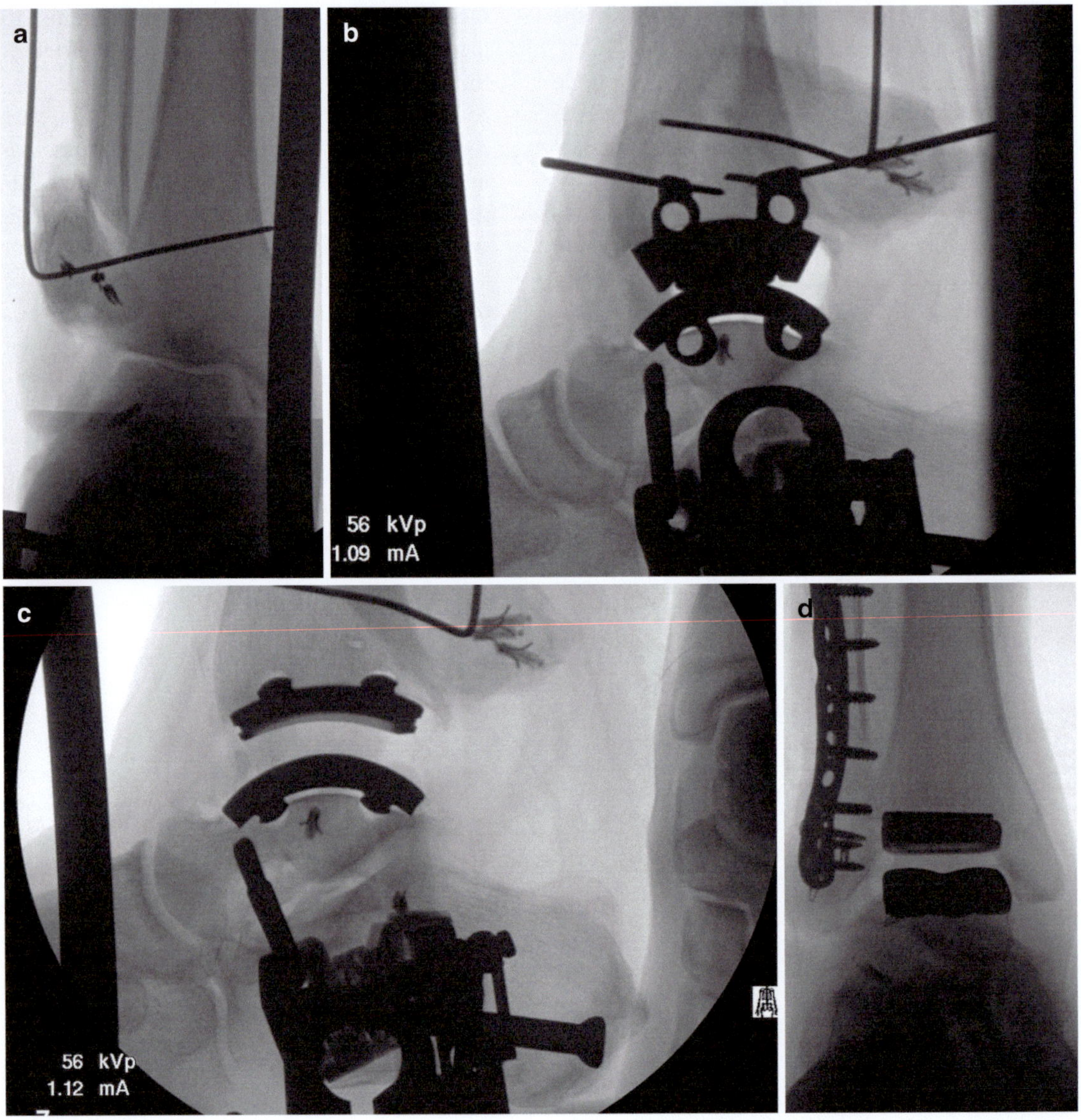

Fig. 20.2 Intraoperative images from the primary total ankle arthroplasty. The Zimmer TM® prosthesis utilizes a lateral approach (**a**). The tibial guide (**b**) and final implant (**c**) are undersized on the sagittal fluoroscopic images with posterior resection margin nearing the subtalar joint. There is insufficient anterior and posterior tibial cortical coverage. However, the tibial component appears to be maximally sized on the AP fluoroscopic image (**d**)

ankle arthritis). Therefore, components may be improperly sized in the sagittal plane (Fig. 20.2b). The lateral ankle radiograph demonstrates incomplete anterior and posterior coverage of the final tibial component (Fig. 20.2c). The tibial component appears to be maximally sized on the anterior/posterior (AP) ankle radiograph (Fig. 20.2d). Radiographic lucency at the bone and tibial component interface is present, which is indicative of component loosening and failure.

- In this case, the surgical technique and instrumentation have been associated with inadvertent violation of the dorsal cortex of the talar neck, which resulted in diminished anterior structural support for the talar prosthesis. As such, anterior talar component subsidence occurred (Fig. 20.3a).

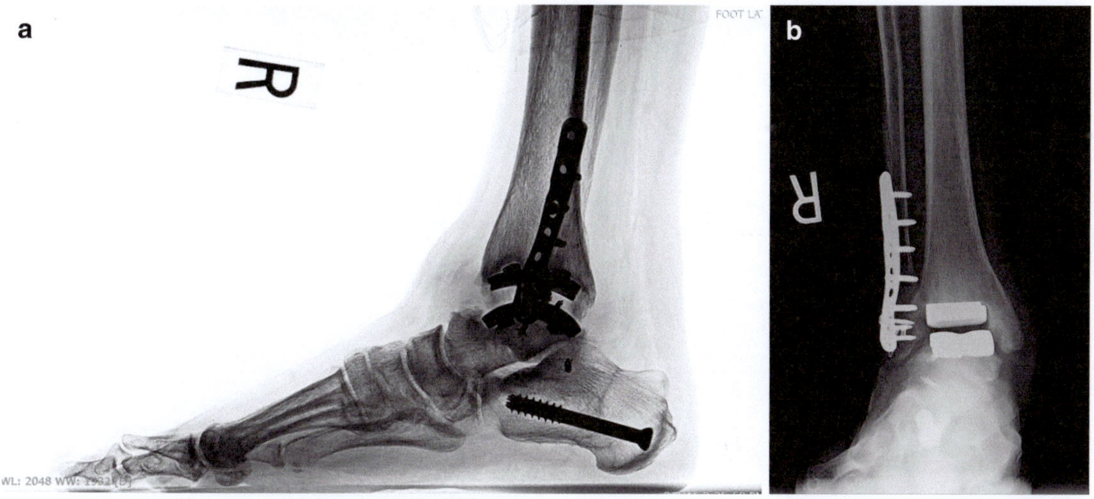

Fig. 20.3 Postoperative radiographs 2 years after primary total ankle arthroplasty. An inadvertent breech of the dorsal cortex of the talar neck at the time of joint preparation can result in diminished structural strength and subsequent talar component subsidence (**a**). AP radiograph demonstrates medial gutter impingement from what appears to be medial shift (translation) of the talar component upon the tibial component (**b**)

- The talar component was more than likely oversized due to the inability to mismatch implant sizing (tibia and talus), resulting in medial ankle gutter impingement (Fig. 20.3b). Implant overhang and gutter impingement are frequent causes of persistent pain following total ankle arthroplasty.

Preoperative Plan and Surgical Technique

- The Zimmer TM® prosthesis is the only current US total ankle system that utilizes a lateral transfibular approach. Unless the patient is being converted to an ankle arthrodesis, we prefer to avoid the transfibular approach to prevent fibular shortening and risk of fibular nonunion following revision ankle arthroplasty.
- Standard anterior approach was utilized.
- *Tibial component extraction.* Access to the anterior lip of the tibial component was achieved by carefully removing anterior tibial bone with a flexible-blade chisel. Care was taken to avoid excessive bone resection (by using the chisel from inferior to superior at the anterior tibial fixation peg) in order to preserve critical anterior tibial cortical bone for structural support. After adequate visualization of the anterior lip of the prosthesis was achieved, a bone tamp was used to mallet the tibial component free.
- *Talar component extraction.* An osteotome was used to lever the talar component free (Fig. 20.4a). If subsidence has occurred, there is often minimal bony ingrowth, and the component can easily be removed.
- *Bone resection.* The INBONE II® frame was used to perform bone cuts to provide a fresh surface for revision component ingrowth or cement interdigitation. The level of the tibial resection was just proximal to the tibial implant (Fig. 20.4b). The stemmed tibial component was implanted, and the frame was removed.
- *Gutter debridement.* Gutter debridement was performed under fluoroscopy, "unlinking" the talus from the tibia and providing an appropriate "gap" between the medial fibula/lateral talus and the lateral talus/medial malleolus (Fig. 20.4c).
- *Preparation of the talus.* The hindfoot was held in neutral with the nondominant hand, while a minimal flat talar bone surface was resected using a larger blade microsagittal saw. The INBONE II® talus component was trialed. However, we recognized that the compo-

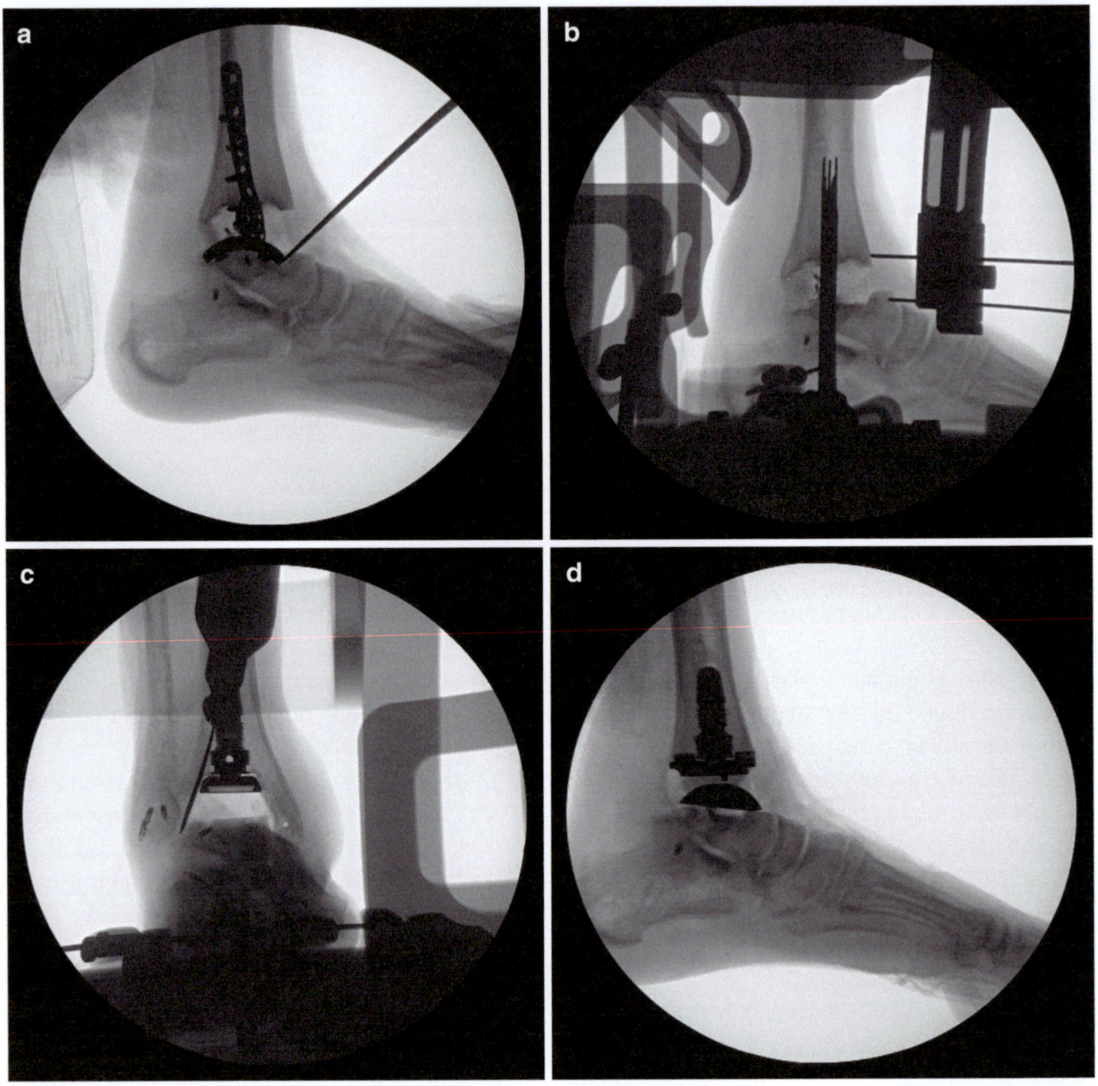

Fig. 20.4 Intraoperative fluoroscopic images from the revision total ankle arthroplasty. The talar component was extracted by using an osteotome to lever the component free from the anterior approach (**a**). The talar component is typically loose if subsidence is present. The INBONE II® frame was used to perform a tibial component cut just proximal to the level of the previous tibial component within good-quality bone (**b**). Gutter debridement is performed with a reciprocating saw to "unlink" the tibia and talus, removing all previously unresected impinging bone and acquired offending osteophytes, removing a critical source of postoperative pain (**c**). The INBONE II® talar trial component did not adequately span the residual defect from the prior talar component, and further talar bone resection would compromise the center of rotation of the ankle joint using standard implants (**d**); therefore, an INVISION® talar component was selected to provide complete talus coverage while allowing some additional talar bone resection given the capability of increasing the height of the component (**e**). Cement was used to fill the small residual contained talar defect, and the final talar component was impacted (**f**, **g**)

nent did not adequately span the anterior talar defect (Fig. 20.4d). The INVISION® component provided the additional surface contact required for support/fixation into the talus, by extending the bone-implant interface to the level of the talonavicular joint (Fig. 20.4e).

- *Cement was used to fill the talar bone void.* The defects were filled with cement to provide

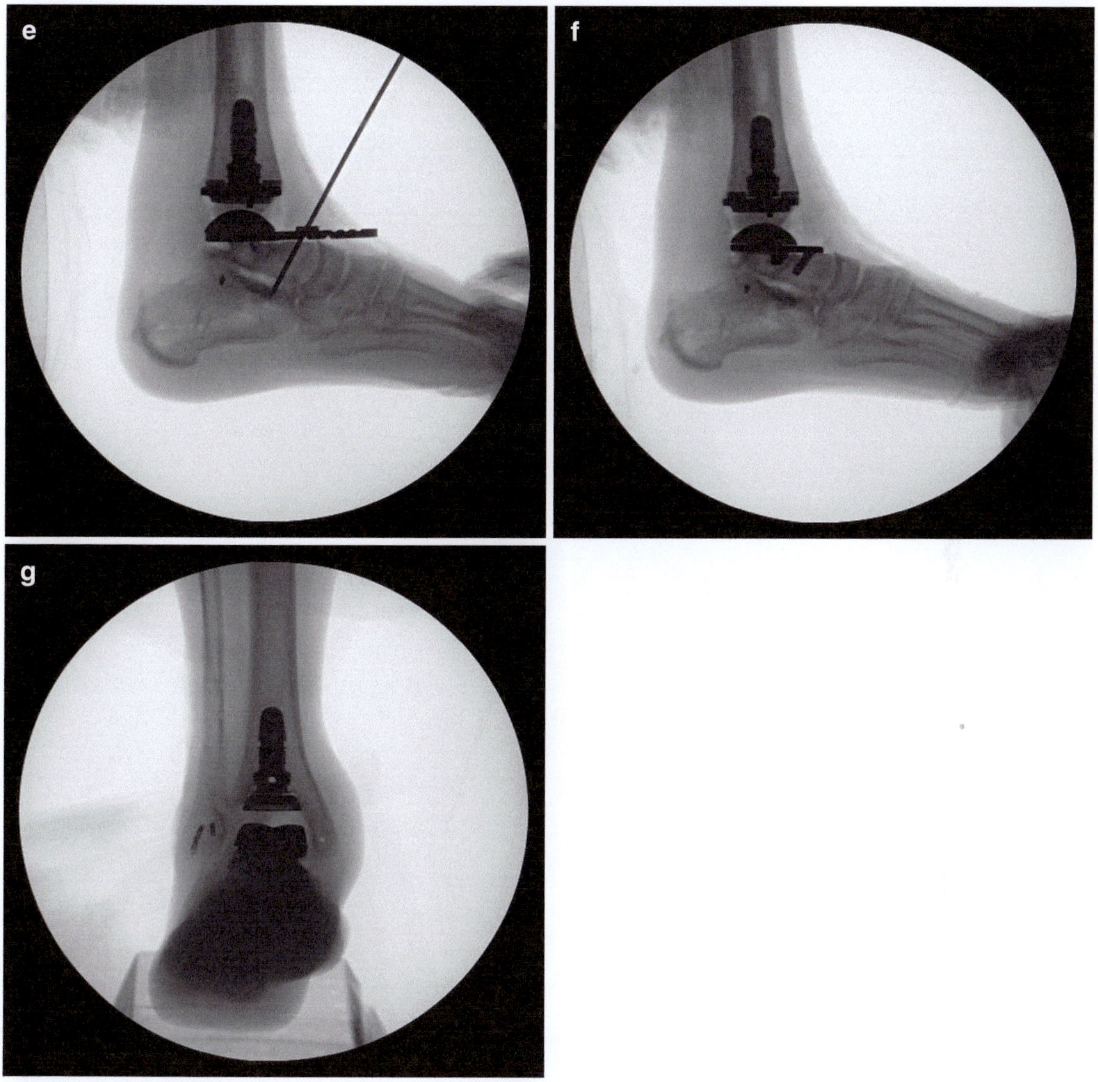

Fig. 20.4 (continued)

rotational control, and the talar component was impacted (Fig. 20.4f, g).

Case 20.2

History

A 74-year-old male underwent total ankle arthroplasty with a Salto Talaris® prosthesis for an incongruent, valgus deformity (Fig. 20.5a, b).

- Posterior talar subsidence occurred 4 months after surgery (Fig. 20.6a, b). Tibiotalar subluxation ensued, translating the weight-bearing axis through the anterior aspect of the ankle joint. Increased force transmission through the anterior ankle joint leads to significant anterior tibial component subsidence (Fig. 20.7a–c).
- Initial postoperative radiographs demonstrate that the tibial component is slightly undersized and there is lack of anterior cortical coverage. Regardless of the primary implant chosen, it is important to achieve anterior cortical coverage to minimize the risk of component subsidence.

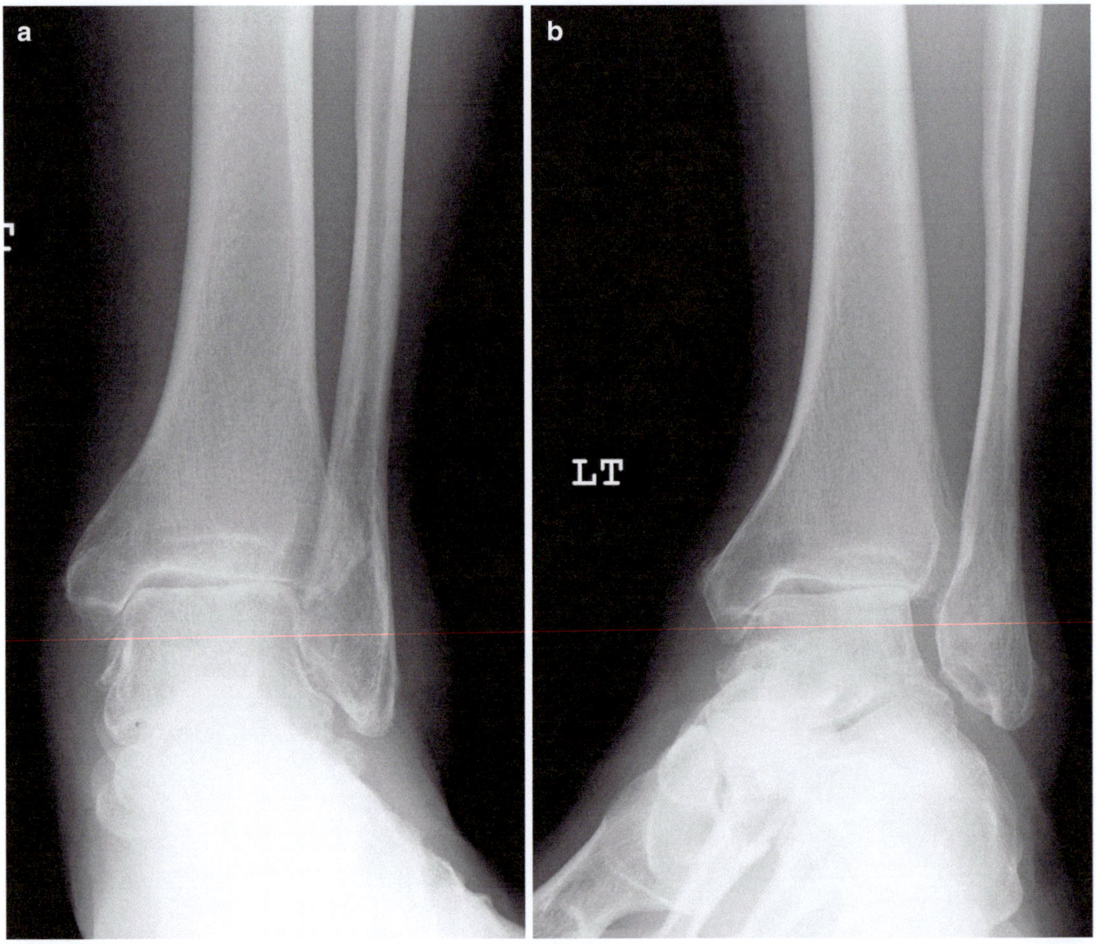

Fig. 20.5 Preoperative radiographs demonstrate a mild incongruent, valgus deformity

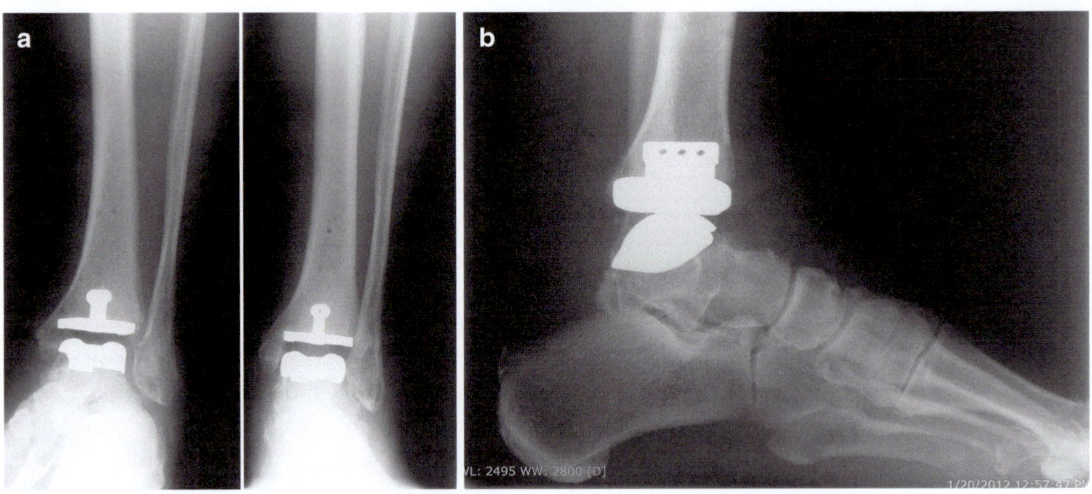

Fig. 20.6 Weight-bearing ankle radiographs 4 months following Salto Talaris® implant. The tibial tray has been placed into varus (**a**) with significant posterior talar component subsidence (**b**). Given the recent surgery, it would appear that either the talar component was cut with this alignment in the sagittal plane or early poor-quality talar bone allowed significant subsidence. The former explanation seems more likely

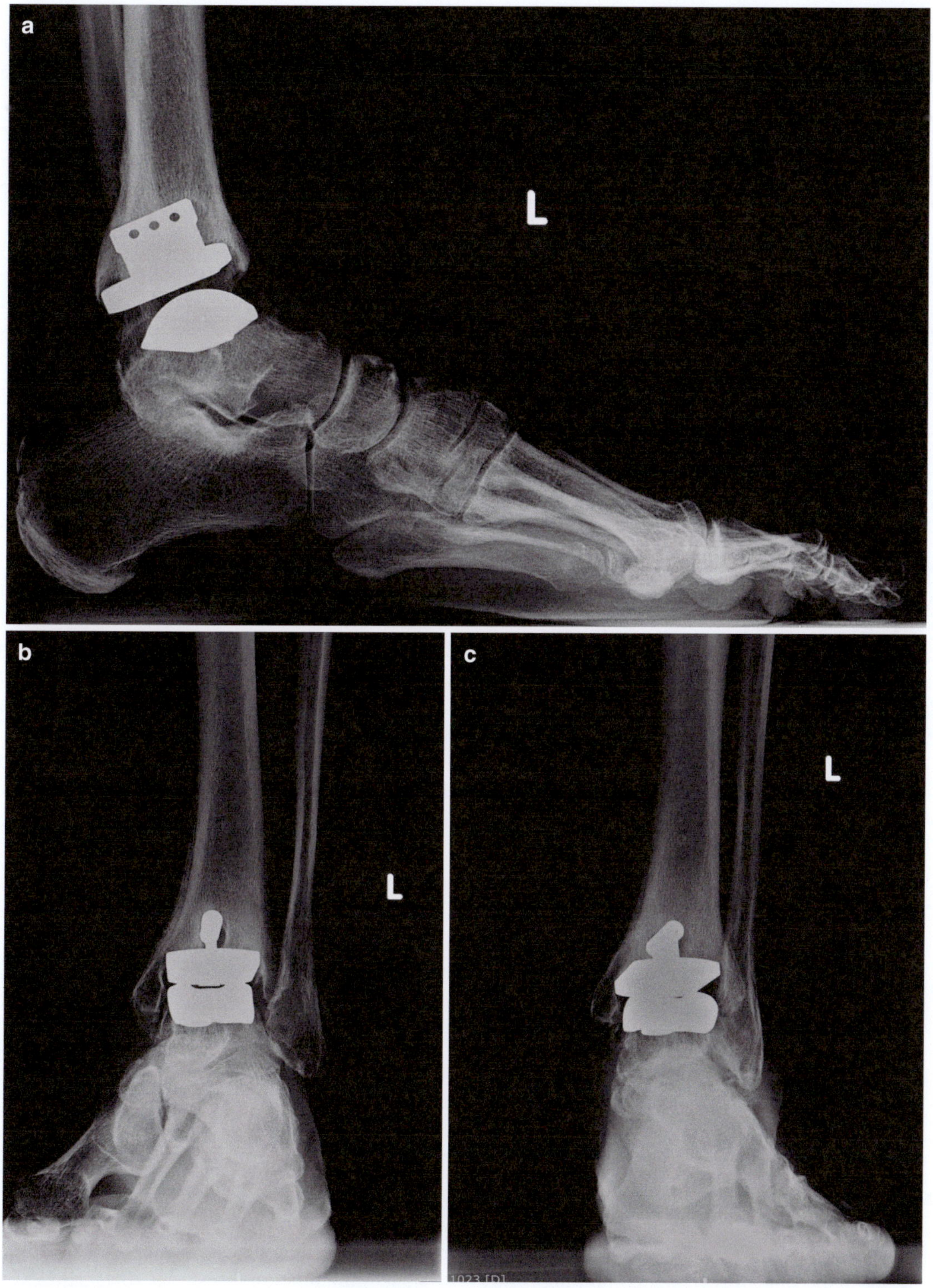

Fig. 20.7 Without early correction of the malaligned implants, eccentric anterior loading created progressive tibial component subsidence, noted on these 2-year postsurgical weight-bearing radiographs (**a**). In addition to the component subsidence, the lucency about the tibial tray is evident in the coronal plane image (**b**), particularly around the tibial tray keel. In addition, progressive subsidence has created extreme erosion of the medial malleolus, creating very little bone support medially (**b**, **c**). The lesson, of course, is to correct deformity early in the prosthesis when it is recognized

- Revision total ankle arthroplasty was performed with the INBONE II® prosthesis approximately 2 years after the index procedure (Fig. 20.8a–d).
- The INBONE II® is a fixed-bearing implant that offers metadiaphyseal tibial stem fixation. The tibial component is modular, allowing variability in the diameter and length of the tibial stem. The sulcus of the talar component imparts further coronal plane stability to the implant.
- Three years after revision arthroplasty, the patient developed osteolysis, cystic changes within the talus, and subsequent loosening of the tibial and talar components (Fig. 20.9a). These changes were not present 1 year following the index revision surgery (Fig. 20.9b).
- Despite conservative treatment, the patient reported persistent pain with activity. He underwent a second revision total ankle arthroplasty with the INVISION® prosthesis approximately 3 years after the primary revision arthroplasty with INBONE II®.

Reasons for Failure

- The primary total ankle arthroplasty (Salto Talaris®) failed because of component subsidence.
- It is important to position the tibial implant against the anterior cortex of the tibia to prevent component subsidence into the soft cancellous bone of the tibial metaphysis. Even a 1-cm resection from the subchondral bone of the tibia results in 75% less compressive resistance of the bone, highlighting the need to achieve anterior tibial cortical coverage with the index implant. It is reasonable to accept slight anterior tibial component overhang or incomplete posterior coverage in order to achieve appropriate anterior tibial cortical apposition.
- The revision total ankle arthroplasty with INBONE II® failed secondary to implant loosening, more than likely from poor-quality bone at the time of revision, complimented by the patient's age. The cystic changes and implant loosening were recognized before subsidence ensued.
- At a minimum, routine radiographic surveillance must be performed each year to monitor for osteolysis, implant loosening, and bone cyst formation. High-quality, weight-bearing, true-profile, orthogonal radiographs should be obtained to assess component alignment, position, and the bone-implant interface. If cystic changes are visible on radiographs, baseline CT should be obtained to quantify the extent of bone loss. Depending on severity and location of bone loss, CT should be performed every 3–6 months until progression has ceased, and it has been determined that the components are stable. Serial imaging is critical to document the rate of cystic progression and likelihood of impending implant failure by location of the cysts.

Preoperative Plan and Surgical Technique

- *Extraction of the tibial component.* An attempt was made to remove the tibial component of the Salto Talaris® with an osteotome. Even with the foot maximally plantarflexed, we were unable to achieve appropriate access to lever the tibial component free (Fig. 20.10a).
- The anterior cortex of the tibia was drilled proximal to the tray of the implant, and a bone tamp was used through this hole to mallet the tibial component plantarward (Fig. 20.10b, c). This technique preserved critical anterior tibial bone. We use a similar surgical technique to extract stemmed tibial components (INBONE II®) at the time of the second revision.
- Prophylactic fixation of the medial malleolus was performed with cannulated screws to prevent malleolar fracture during extraction (Fig. 20.10d, e).
- *Bone resection, gutter debridement, and talar preparation.* Similar surgical techniques were used as described in case #1. It is critical to resect poor-quality tibial and talar bone to provide appropriate structural support for component implantation (Fig. 20.10f). However, overresection will alter the joint height and potentially result in instability that cannot be corrected with a large polyethylene. The talar

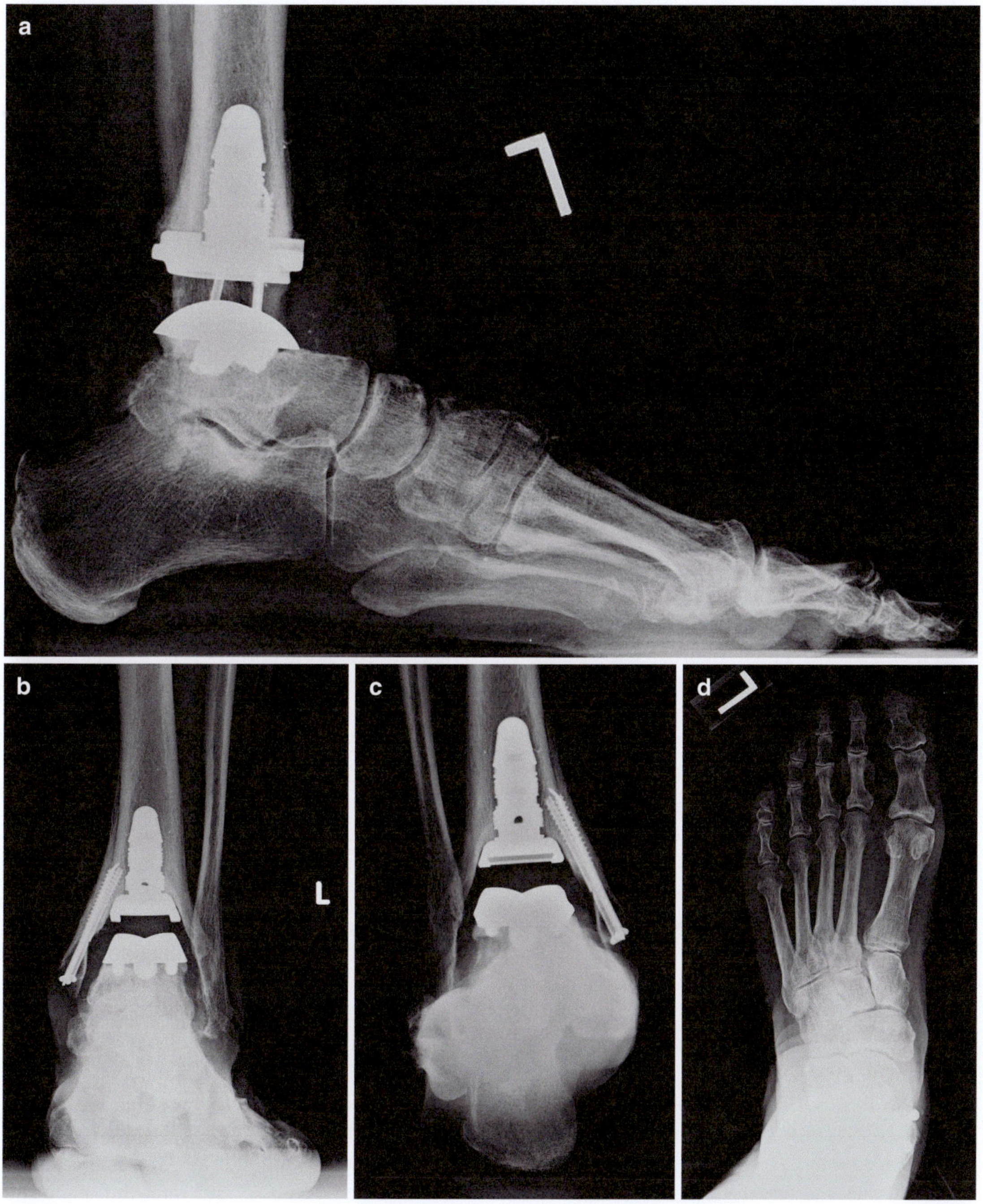

Fig. 20.8 The Salto Talaris® was revised to an INBONE II® implant (this procedure was performed before INVISION® was available). Sagittal imaging shows good anterior coverage of the distal tibia with the new implant (**a**), with preservation of residual talar bone supplementing posterior bone loss with cement. Coronal plane imaging shows reinforcement screws placed into medial malleolus prior to explanting the Salto Talaris® tibial tray (**b**). Note the increased periosteal bone growth about the medial malleolus, adding structural support. Also note the proximal placement of tibial tray due to initial poor-quality anterior tibial bone from prior subsidence. Today we would supplement with increased height tibial tray to restore center of rotation. Axial alignment view shows neutral heel alignment, beneath the prosthesis rather than in more anatomic valgus, to prevent eccentric loading of the implant (**c**). Foot radiographic series is always obtained to review for secondary deforming forces on the implant (none here) (**d**)

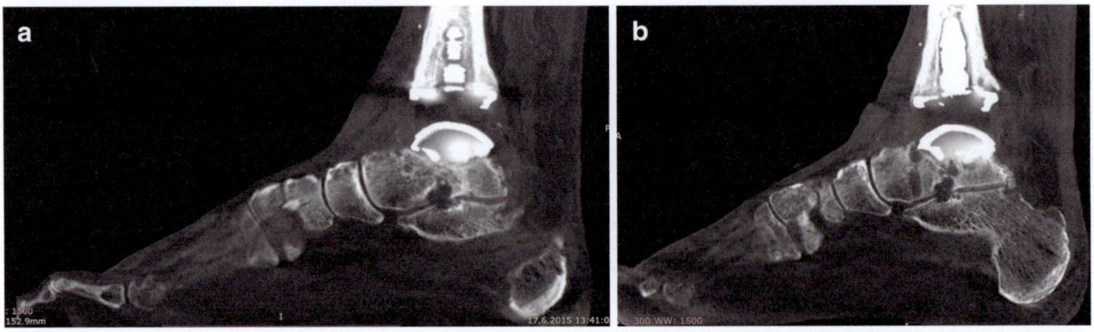

Fig. 20.9 Metal-suppressed CT scan demonstrates implant loosening and some osteolysis at 3 years after the above revision arthroplasty with INBONE II® (**a**). These cystic changes were not identifiable on the CT scan performed 1 year after revision arthroplasty (**b**)

trial component was noted to have posterior instability and dorsiflexion (Fig. 20.10g). Recognizing this, the talar trial component was repositioned and pinned at neutral with respect to the tibia to allow appropriate peg orientation (Fig. 20.10h). The talar posterior bone defect was filled with cement (Fig. 20.10i). Final fluoroscopic imaging demonstrates excellent intraoperative range of motion, balance, and implant stability (Fig. 20.10j–l).

- After components are implanted, we always obtain an intraoperative axial heel image to ensure that the calcaneus is collinear with the weight-bearing axis of the tibia. We do not strive for an anatomic 5–7 degrees of hindfoot valgus, as that may create eccentric load on the prosthesis (which is not a natural ankle). Instead, we strive to place the apex of the posterior tuberosity beneath the implant itself, especially in patients with preexisting ligament laxity. To obtain this fluoroscopic view correctly, the second toe must be aligned with the axis of the tibia in order for the image to be adequate.
- Soft tissue and structural balance of the foot and ankle must always be achieved prior to leaving the operating room. In this particular case, only a modified Brostrom lateral ligament repair was necessary to achieve balance.
- *Revision from INBONE II® to INVISION®.* The previous anterior incision was used to expose the ankle joint. The incision was carried just beyond the talonavicular joint, as adequate distal exposure is necessary when using an INVISION® talar component.
- *Extraction of the polyethylene component.* The polyethylene lock detail for the INBONE II® tibial tray is located at the superomedial and superolateral corners. The medial and lateral corners of the locking mechanism are sequentially bored using a 2.0-mm and 4.0-mm drill bit. Care must be taken to not inadvertently damage the tibial tray with the drill, particularly if the tibial component is being retained, or the lock detail may be rendered useless. An osteotome and mallet can be used to loosen the polyethylene from the tibial tray.
- *Extraction of the tibial component.* The tibial component should be levered out of the intramedullary canal with an osteotome (this is easy to perform if the stem is loose). If the stem is fixed, then a drill hole can be made at the proximal end of the stem, and a bone tamp can be used to mallet the stem free. The Morse taper of the tibial component can be disengaged, and the tibial tray is extracted. The stem is disassembled and removed using the X-Drive.
- *Modularity of the INVISION® system.* The modularity of the INVISION® prosthesis allows for restoration of the anatomic joint line by offering varying thickness of the tibial and talar components. The +4-mm tibial tray was selected after resection of the distal tibia

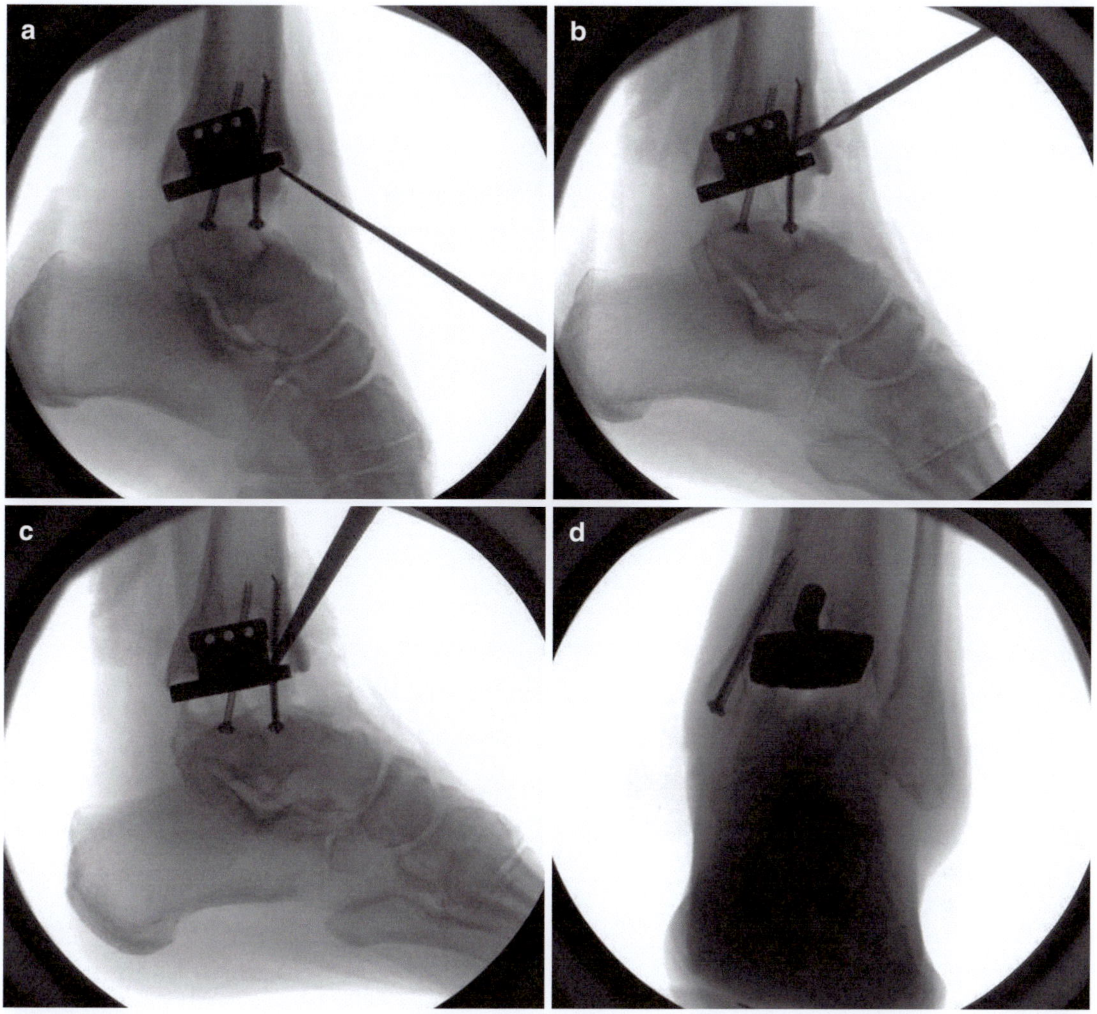

Fig. 20.10 Extraction of the Salto Talaris® prosthesis during revision surgery. It was difficult to achieve adequate exposure to lever the tibial component free, as the proximal expanded portion of the keel makes it more difficult to lever the tibial tray from proximal to distal (**a**). The anterior cortex of the tibia was thus drilled proximal to the tray of the implant, and a bone tamp was used through this hole to mallet the tibial component plantarward, allowing distal extraction (**b**, **c**). Note the provisional fixation of medial malleolus during extraction (**d**, **e**). Proposed resection margin of tibial and talar bone in sagittal plane (**f**). The tibial resection must remove all poorer-quality bone to provide good implant support. The talus has a significant posterior slope (which will be filled with cement). Talus margin resection must be limited given the more significant tibial bone resection, in order to maintain talus joint height and allow sufficient polyethylene for stability (too much talus resection, combined with more significant tibial resection, will leave too great a gap to fill with polyethylene and maintain ankle stability). In fact, posterior talar instability is present during trialing (**g**), pinned at neutral with respect to the tibia to allow appropriate talus component peg orientation (**h**) so that final implant will be neutral (**i**) with the addition of posterior cement. Excellent intraoperative range of motion of the implant despite axis alteration (**j**, **k**). Final coronal imaging demonstrates a balanced ankle implant with good stability (**l**). Medial malleolar screws left in place for stability and to maintain deltoid integrity. Note also the excellent gutter debridement to promote abovementioned flexibility

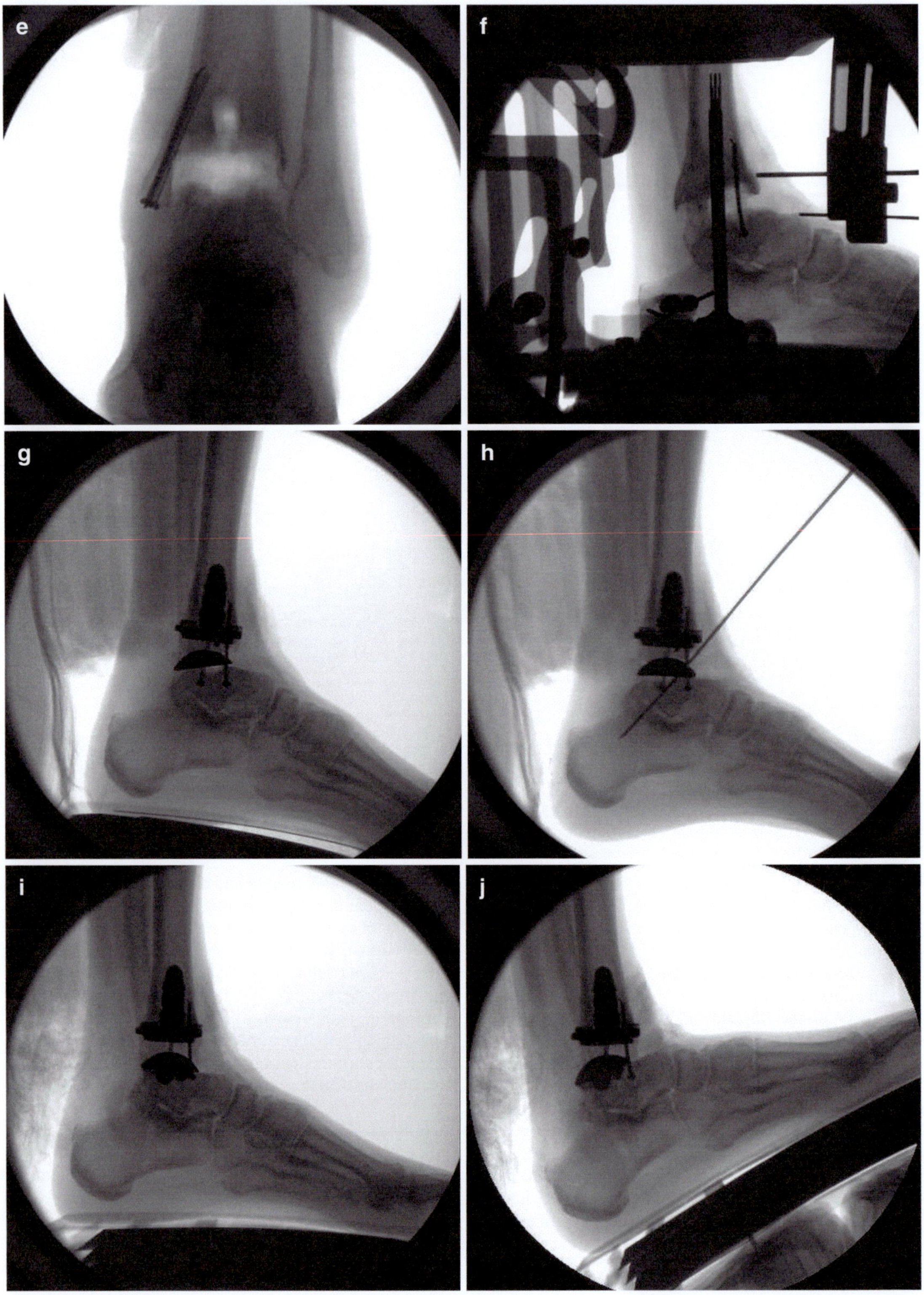

Fig. 20.10 (continued)

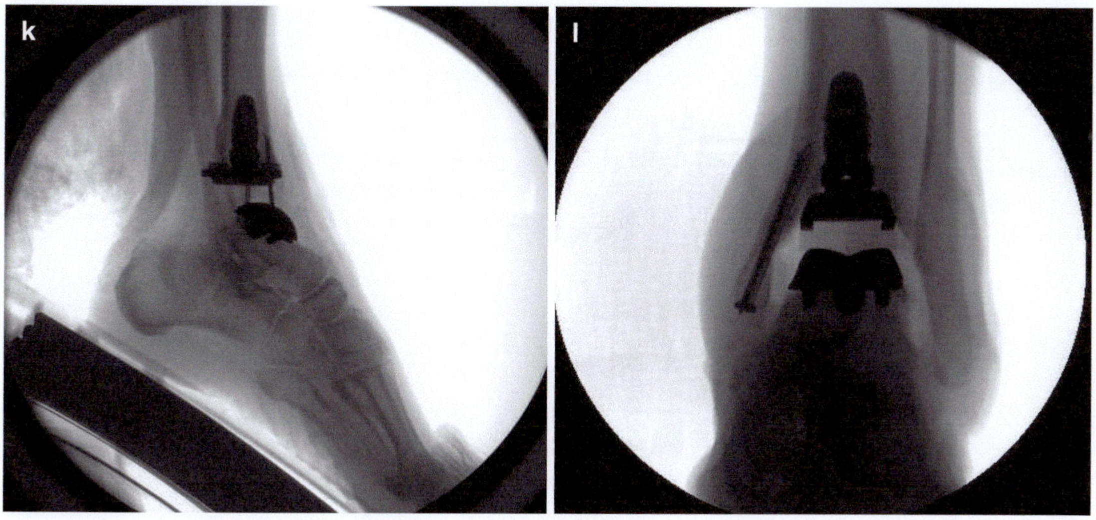

Fig. 20.10 (continued)

to achieve a good-quality bone surface for structural support (Fig. 20.11a, b). The +3-mm talar plate was used to restore talar height.

- *Talus preparation.* Minimal bone was resected using the INVISION® cutting block. The hindfoot was held in neutral, while additional talar bone was resected using a microsagittal saw. Curettes and a power burr were used to debride necrotic talar bone and define the extent of talar cysts. Talar preparation is important to achieve cement-bone interdigitation. We frequently find that small, contained, cystic talar lesions can be filled with PMMA with the implant placed overtop. Alternatively, the surgeon may utilize autograft or allograft to fill these voids. The surgical technique for large and uncontained talar defects, however, is different (see **Case 20.3**).

Case 20.3

History

- Patient is a 79-year-old female with a history of progressive medial column collapse and history of subtalar arthrodesis.
- The patient developed avascular necrosis of the talus and fragmentation of the lateral dome within 1 year of the subtalar arthrodesis.
- Lateral radiograph reveals posterior tibiotalar joint subluxation, avascular changes with secondary collapse of the talar dome, previous subtalar arthrodesis, and mild collapse of the medial longitudinal arch at the talonavicular and naviculocuneiform joints (Fig. 20.12a–h).

Preoperative Plan and Surgical Technique

- Access to the tibiotalar, transverse tarsal, and naviculocuneiform joints was performed through an extended anterior ankle incision. The skin incision was carried distal beyond the naviculocuneiform joint.
- Hardware was removed without tourniquet.
- *Joint preparation.* The transverse tarsal and naviculocuneiform joints were prepared using a power burr and rasp. The medial longitudinal arch was reduced and provisionally held in place with cannulated screw guide wires.
- The extremity was placed into the INBONE II® frame, and the tibia was prepared and implanted as previously described.
- *Preparation of the talus.* After implantation of the tibial component, the extremity was removed from the frame. The foot was held in neutral, while a freehand saw was used to resect the appropriate amount of bone and level the talar dome parallel to the tibial tray.

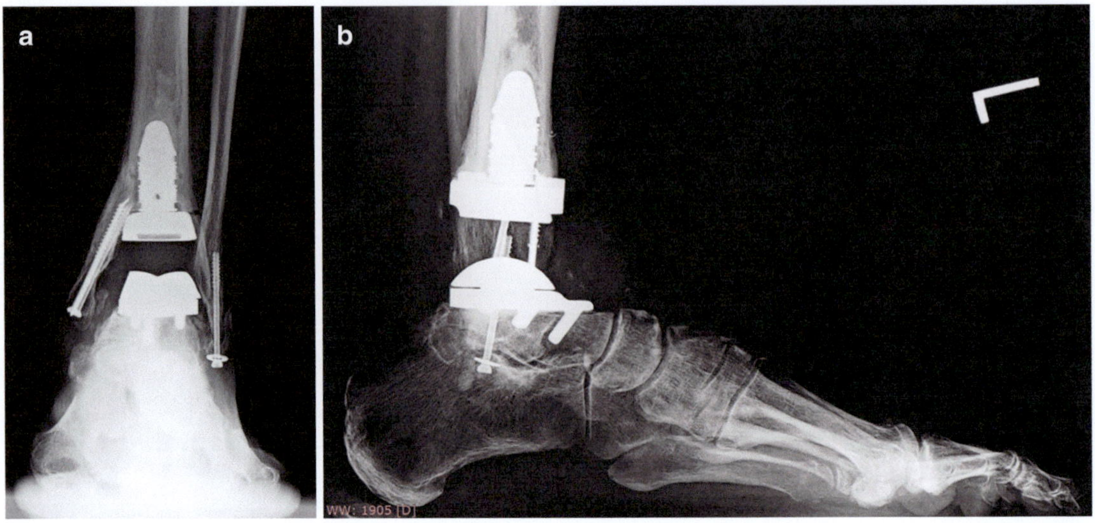

Fig. 20.11 Final weight-bearing radiographs following revision arthroplasty with the INVISION® prosthesis. Even with the thick tibial tray, it is difficult to reestablish the joint line with metal (a thicker polyethylene is required) (**a**). In addition, the thin proximal bone laterally shows asymptomatic fracturing at the lateral corner of the implant (the bone is too thin to allow fixation, and fortunately has no significant ligament attachments, and thus does not contribute to prosthesis stability). A thicker tibial stem was used to provide better proximal fixation. Sagittal plane imaging (**b**) demonstrates increased talar resection to better-quality bone, with a broader span through the talar plate. This allowed much better fixation into the talus, without compromising talar height due to the thicker implant

- Necrotic bone was removed using a burr, curettes, and pituitary.
- Coronal CT imaging revealed a chronic fracture fragment of the lateral talar body (Fig. 20.13a–c). The nonviable fragment was excised, leaving a large uncontained defect in the lateral talar dome (Fig. 20.14a, b).
- Three 4.0 cannulated screws were placed in a retrograde fashion through small plantar incisions, with the screw heads abutting the plantar calcaneus and the tips into the void left from removal of the avascular bone (Fig. 20.14c).
- It is important that these screws terminate just below the undersurface of the trial implant (Fig. 20.14d, e). Excessive screw length can prevent successful implantation of the talar component or result in tilt of the component. If the screws are too short, they will not provide enough rebar support to the cement mantle supporting a portion of the prosthesis.
- After the trial prosthesis is supported by the rebar screw fixation, the appropriately sized polyethylene and talar component can be selected by taking the ankle through range of motion and valgus/varus stress.
- We use a surgical pen to mark around the boarder of the trial talar component and peg holes. Through experience, we have found it difficult to properly position the final implant when normal talar anatomy is distorted and large bony defects are present.
- The final talar component is impacted into place. A trial polyethylene is inserted to allow range of motion of the ankle, ensuring the talar component is in appropriate axial rotation (and coronal rotation) for this patient.

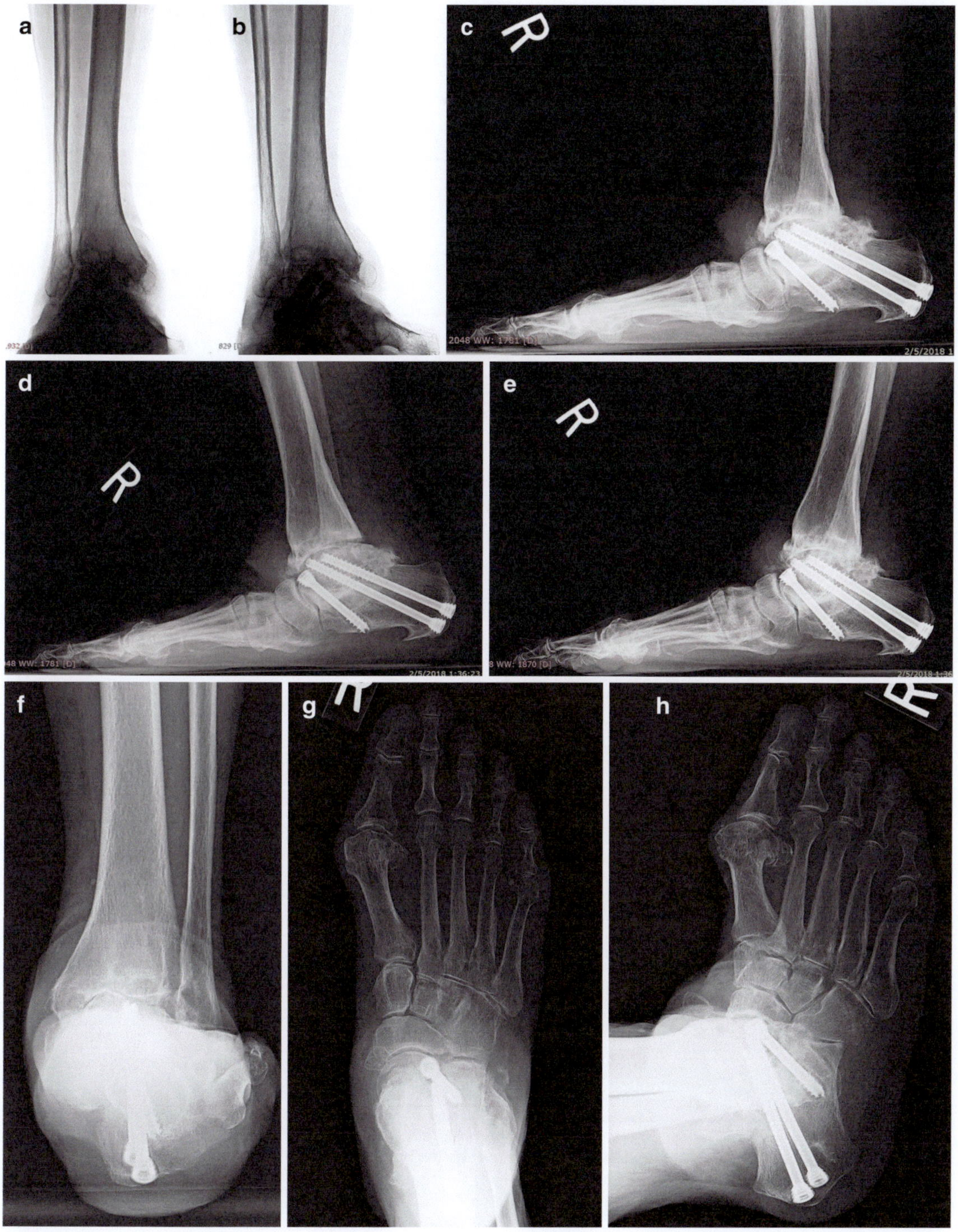

Fig. 20.12 Preoperative radiographs demonstrate avascular changes of the talus following multiple attempts at subtalar joint arthrodesis (**a**) with significant secondary ankle arthritis and residual gutter arthritis (**b**). Sagittal plane imaging demonstrates collapse of the medial longitudinal arch, with distal joint subluxation and posterior translation of the talus (**c**). Flexion/extension radiographs (**d**, **e**) demonstrate very little ankle motion. Again, weightbearing axial (hindfoot) alignment view and foot radiographs are obtained to get a thorough assessment of residual deformity (**f**–**h**)

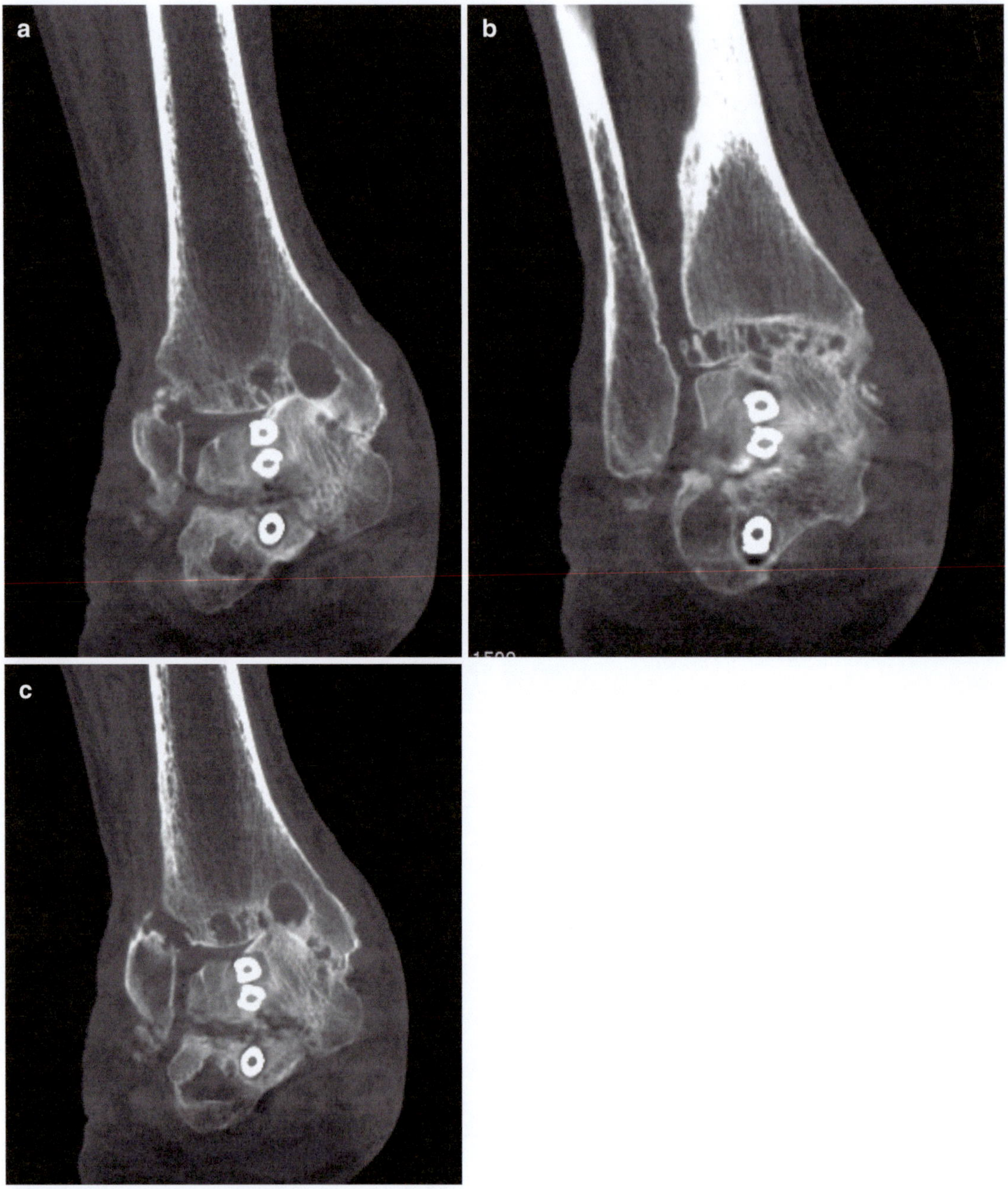

Fig. 20.13 Coronal CT imaging demonstrates dense screw placement within the talus resulting in a chronic fracture fragment of the lateral talar body. This is evident by the bony reabsorption and sclerosis present adjacent to the screws (**a**–**c**)

– An osteotome was placed into the lateral gutter, and the uncontained defect was filled with PMMA cement (Fig. 20.14f, g). It is important to pressurize the cement using a 60-mL syringe to ensure that the entire talar defect is filled. The consistency of the cement is "doughy" to prevent significant leakage during pressurization. Excess cement is removed using a freer and reciprocating saw.

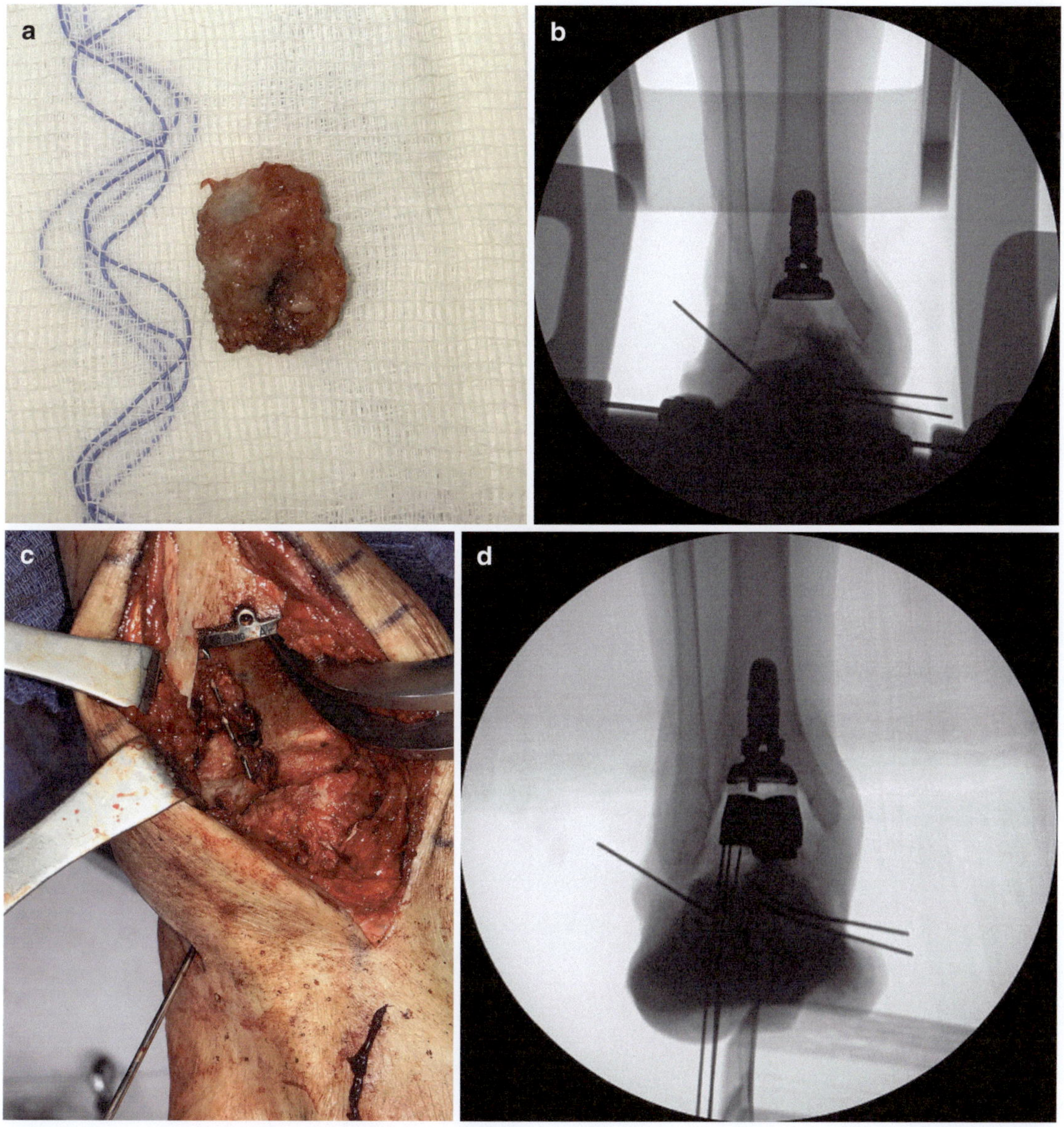

Fig. 20.14 An intraoperative photograph demonstrates the lateral talar body fragment that was excised (**a**) given its poor-quality avascular bone that would potentially collapse in the future, creating implant failure. The lateral defect is visible following tibia tray insertion and talar component preparation (to good-quality bone) (**b**). Intraoperative photo (**c**) demonstrates the guide wires placed from the plantar calcaneus into the talus defect that will guide the screws to allow the tips to create rebar within the cement. Note the cannulated screw guide wire percutaneously placed within the medial foot at the talonavicular joint to hold the joint aligned during arthrodesis (screws to be placed across this joint AFTER the talar component is inserted). Fluoroscopic images (**d**, **e**) demonstrate the placement of these guide wires (supporting the lateral prosthesis at this time), but the screws will be measured shorter than this, so they do not ultimately contact the prosthesis (they will provide rebar into the cement). The talar plate spans the uncontained lateral defect in the talus to good-quality bone (medial/anterior/posterior) (**d**, **e**). An osteotome is placed in the lateral gutter to prevent cement extravasation (**f**). The rebar screws are visible. Cement is injected using a 60-mL syringe (**g**) as a "doughy" consistency to minimize leakage. Pressure injection fills all voids. Final sagittal plane images demonstrate cement in place, with screw lengths visible (**h**, **i**). Screw fixation traverses the talonavicular, naviculocuneiform, and calcaneocuboid joints for realignment arthrodesis (prior to bone grafting). Range of motion demonstrates decent motion despite preexisting inflexibility and collapse (**j**, **k**). Final coronal plane imaging documents a neutral, stable construct, with good foot (and ankle) balance (**l**). Incisions look great at 6 days postsurgical with compression wrap protocol (**m**, **n**)

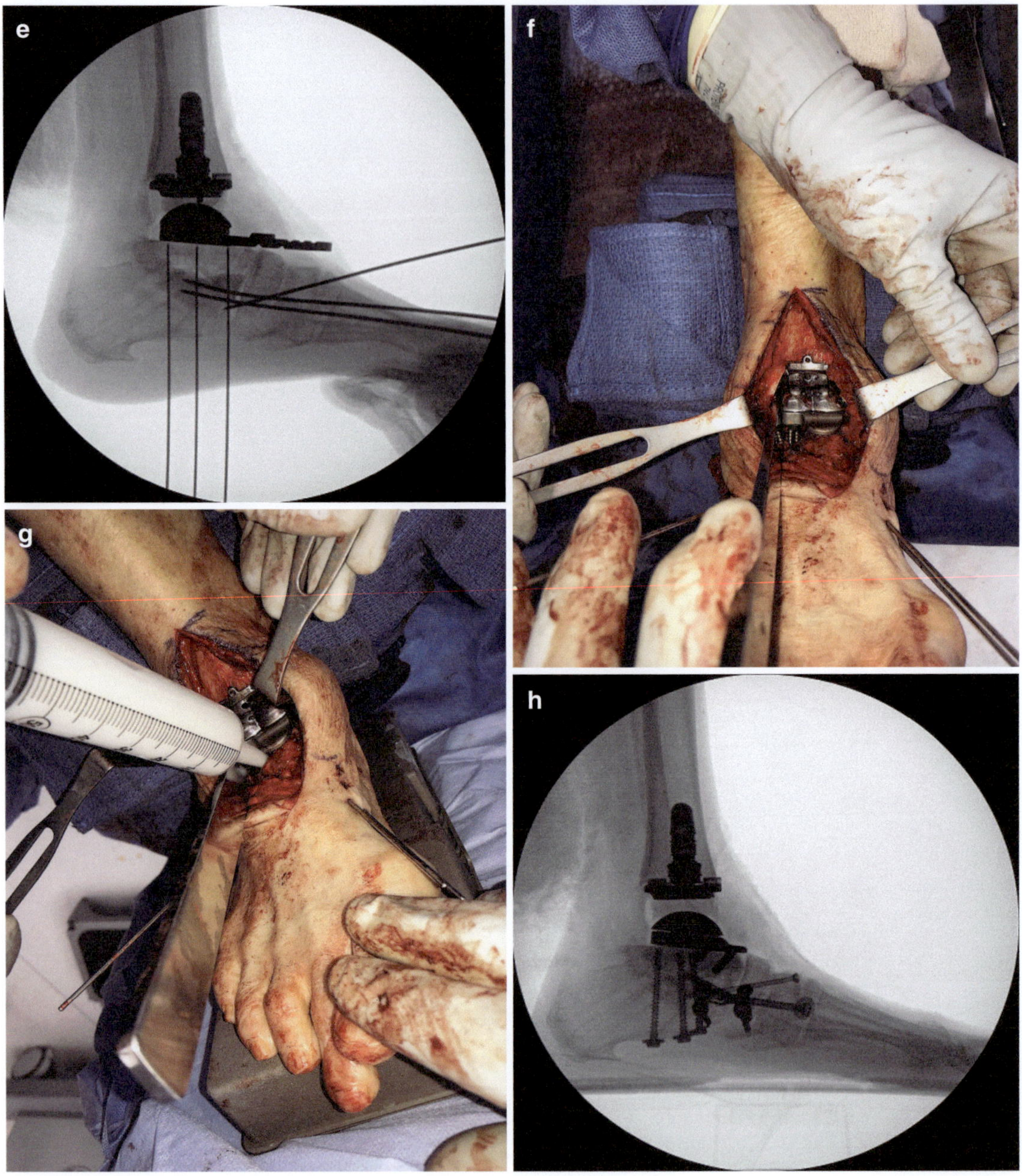

Fig. 20.14 (continued)

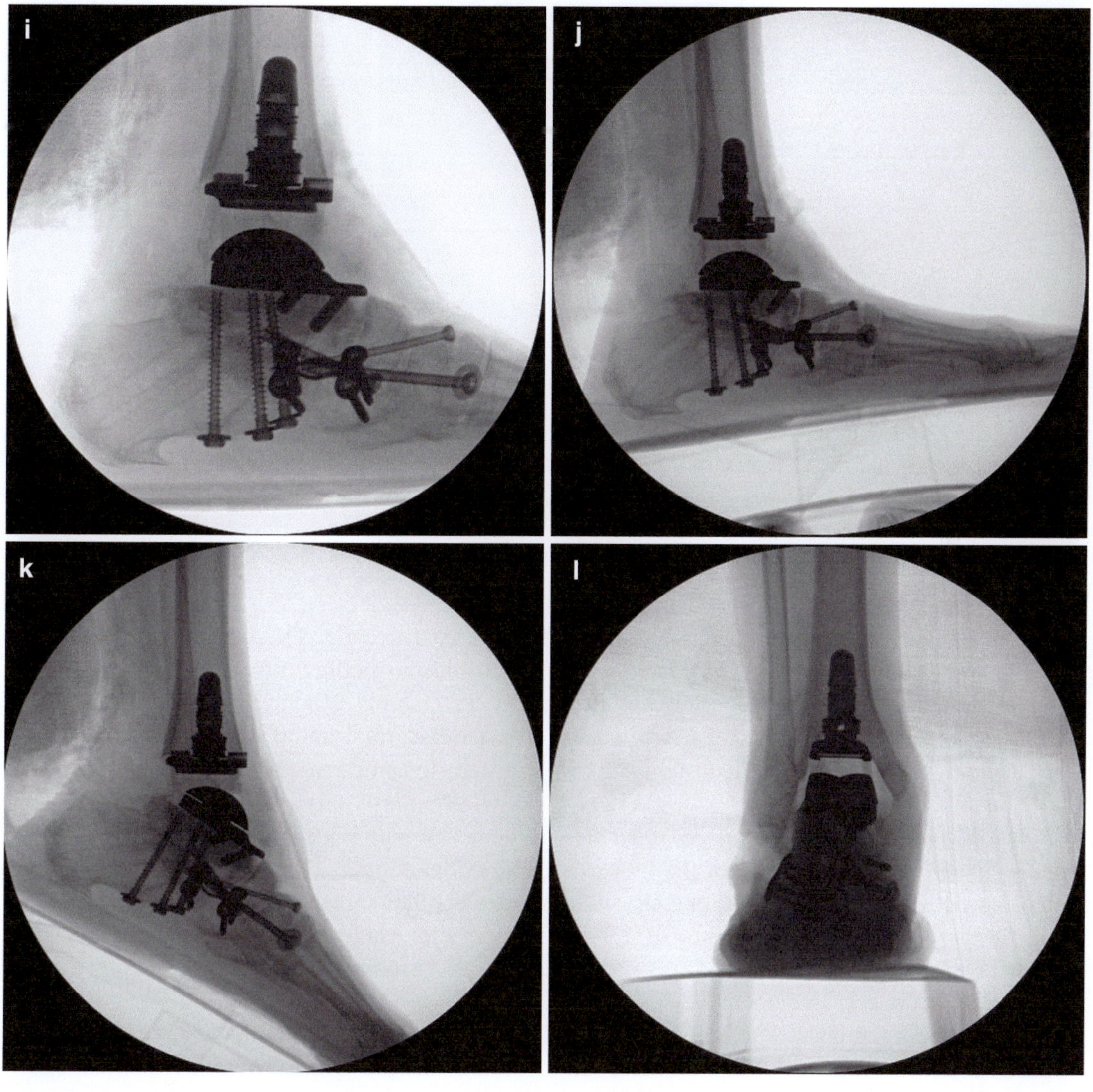

Fig. 20.14 (continued)

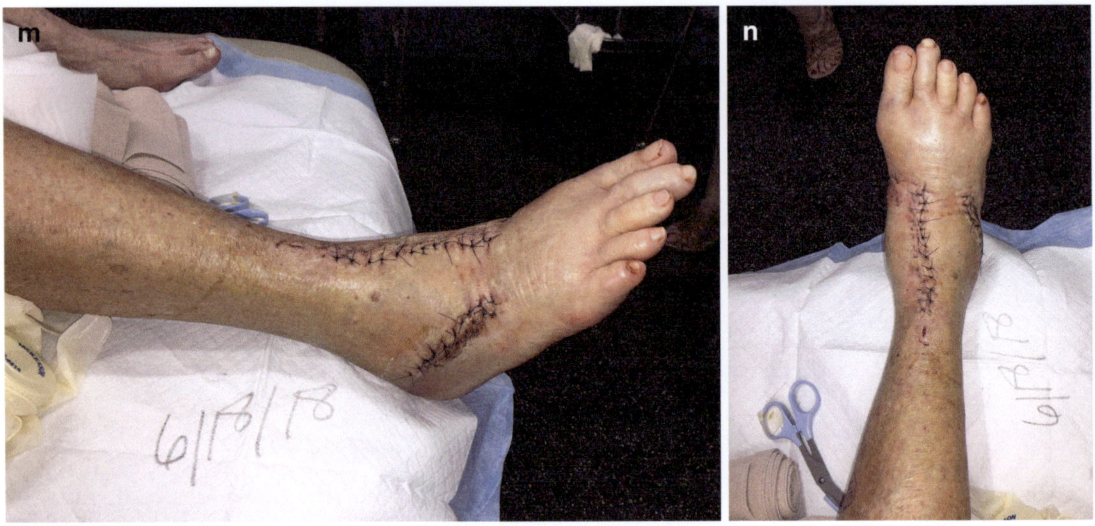

Fig. 20.14 (continued)

  - Once the cement has completely hardened, the size of the final polyethylene is selected and implanted. Final postoperative sagittal plane images demonstrate rebar screw and cement fixation of the talar component (Fig. 20.14h, i).
- *Fixation of the transverse tarsal and naviculocuneiform joints.* The balance of the foot was reassessed after implantation of the ankle prosthesis and final fixation performed with cannulated screws.
- We always assess intraoperative range of motion using a flat plate. The prosthesis demonstrates decent range of motion despite previous collapse, deformity, and ankle joint contracture (Fig. 20.14j, k). Final coronal plane imaging demonstrates a stable construct with excellent foot and ankle balance (Fig. 20.14l).
- The postoperative compression wrap protocol minimizes wound-healing complications by decreasing edema. The incisions look excellent at 6 days after an extensive reconstructive surgery (Fig. 20.14m, n).

Summary

As component technology and surgical techniques continue to advance, there has been a resurgence of interest in total ankle arthroplasty in the past decade. The number of total ankle arthroplasties being performed each year is rapidly increasing. Historically, surgical options for a failed total ankle arthroplasty have been limited to amputation or ankle arthrodesis. However, these salvage procedures have been associated with high rates of failure and/or poor clinical outcomes. Revision arthroplasty provides another salvage option in the treatment of failed total ankle arthroplasty. There is a paucity of literature on revision total ankle arthroplasty.

The surgical techniques for revision total ankle arthroplasty are continuing to evolve. We have found early success with cement/metal augmentation to restore talar height after failed arthroplasty and catastrophic component subsidence/bone loss. Only one patient required revision surgery for component subsidence at an average follow-up of 15 months. Another patient developed >2 mm of talar component subsidence, but was asymptomatic and did not require revision arthroplasty. Larger cohorts and long-term follow-up are necessary moving forward.

Disclosure Statement Brian D. Steginsky, DO: Nothing to disclose

Steven L. Haddad, MD: Consultant for Wright Medical

References

1. Karantana A, Hobson S, Dhar S. The scandinavian total ankle replacement: survivorship at 5 and 8 years comparable to other series. Clin Orthop Relat Res [Internet]. 2010 [cited 2018 Jun 8];468(4):951–7. Available from: http://link.springer.com/10.1007/s11999-009-0971-y.
2. Wood PLR, Prem H, Sutton C. Total ankle replacement: medium-term results in 200 Scandinavian total ankle replacements. J Bone Joint Surg Br [Internet]. 2008 [cited 2018 Jun 8];90(5):605–9. Available from: http://online.boneandjoint.org.uk/doi/10.1302/0301-620X.90B5.19677.
3. Henricson A, Nilsson J-Å, Carlsson Å. 10-year survival of total ankle arthroplasties. Acta Orthop [Internet]. 2011 [cited 2018 Jun 8];82(6):655–9. Available from: http://www.ncbi.nlm.nih.gov/pubmed/22066551.
4. Bonnin M, Gaudot F, Laurent J-R, Ellis S, Colombier J-A, Judet T. The Salto total ankle arthroplasty: survivorship and analysis of failures at 7 to 11 years. Clin Orthop Relat Res [Internet]. 2011 [cited 2018 Jun 8];469(1):225–36. Available from: http://www.ncbi.nlm.nih.gov/pubmed/20593253.
5. Criswell BJ, Douglas K, Naik R, Thomson AB. High revision and reoperation rates using the Agility™ total ankle system. Clin Orthop Relat Res [Internet]. 2012 [cited 2018 Jun 8];470(7):1980–6. Available from: http://link.springer.com/10.1007/s11999-012-2242-6.
6. Lau JT, Schon LC MN. Differential practice of treating ankle arthritis in a general and specialty orthopaedic society. Paper presented at: AOFAS, 20th annual summer meeting, July 29–31, 2004; Seattle.
7. Rahm S, Klammer G, Benninger E, Gerber F, Farshad M, Espinosa N. Inferior results of salvage arthrodesis after failed ankle replacement compared to primary arthrodesis. Foot ankle Int [Internet]. 2015 [cited 2018 Jun 8];36(4):349–59. Available from: http://journals.sagepub.com/doi/10.1177/1071100714559272.
8. Knecht SI, Estin M, Callaghan JJ, Zimmerman MB, Alliman KJ, Alvine FG, et al. The Agility total ankle arthroplasty. Seven to sixteen-year follow-up. J Bone Joint Surg Am [Internet]. 2004 [cited 2018 Jun 8];86-A(6):1161–71. Available from: http://www.ncbi.nlm.nih.gov/pubmed/15173288.
9. Haddad SL, Coetzee JC, Estok R, Fahrbach K, Banel D, Nalysnyk L. Intermediate and long-term outcomes of total ankle arthroplasty and ankle arthrodesis. A systematic review of the literature. J Bone Joint Surg Am [Internet]. 2007 [cited 2018 Mar 27];89(9):1899–905. Available from: http://jbjs.org/cgi/doi/10.2106/JBJS.F.01149.
10. Hintermann B, Zwicky L, Knupp M, Henninger HB, Barg A. HINTEGRA revision arthroplasty for failed total ankle prostheses. J Bone Joint Surg Am Vol [Internet]. 2013 [cited 2018 Jun 8];95(13):1166–74. Available from: http://www.ncbi.nlm.nih.gov/pubmed/23824384.
11. Jonck JH, Myerson MS. Revision total ankle replacement. Foot Ankle Clin [Internet]. 2012 [cited 2018 Jun 8];17(4):687–706. Available from: http://linkinghub.elsevier.com/retrieve/pii/S1083751512000617.
12. Glazebrook MA, Arsenault K, Dunbar M. Evidence-based classification of complications in total ankle arthroplasty. Foot Ankle Int [Internet]. 2009 [cited 2018 Jun 9];30(10):945–9. Available from: http://www.ncbi.nlm.nih.gov/pubmed/19796587.
13. Williams JR, Wegner NJ, Sangeorzan BJ, Brage ME. Intraoperative and perioperative complications during revision arthroplasty for salvage of a failed total ankle arthroplasty. Foot Ankle Int [Internet]. 2015 [cited 2018 Jun 8];36(2):135–42. Available from: http://www.ncbi.nlm.nih.gov/pubmed/25288333.
14. Ellington JK, Gupta S, Myerson MS. Management of failures of total ankle replacement with the agility total ankle arthroplasty. J Bone Joint Surg Am [Internet]. 2013 [cited 2018 Jun 9];95(23):2112–8. Available from: http://insights.ovid.com/crossref?an=00004623-201312040-00005.
15. Schipper ON, Hsu AR, Haddad SL. Reduction in wound complications after total ankle arthroplasty using a compression wrap protocol. Foot Ankle Int [Internet]. 2015 [cited 2018 Jun 17];36(12):1448–54. Available from: http://www.ncbi.nlm.nih.gov/pubmed/26231196.
16. Hsu AR, Franceschina D, Haddad SL. A novel method of postoperative wound care following total ankle arthroplasty. Foot Ankle Int [Internet]. 2014 Jul 5 [cited 2018 Jun 17];35(7):719–24. Available from: http://www.ncbi.nlm.nih.gov/pubmed/24798916.
17. Ferrao P, Myerson MS, Schuberth JM, McCourt MJ. Cement spacer as definitive management for postoperative ankle infection. Foot Ankle Int [Internet]. 2012 [cited 2018 Jun 15];33(3):173–8. Available from: http://journals.sagepub.com/doi/10.3113/FAI.2012.0173.

Index

M. J. Berkowitz et al. (eds.), *Revision Surgery of the Foot and Ankle*,
https://doi.org/10.1007/978-3-030-29969-9

L

M

MIX
Papier aus verantwortungsvollen Quellen
Paper from responsible sources
FSC® C105338
FSC
www.fsc.org

If you have any concerns about our products,
you can contact us on
ProductSafety@springernature.com

In case Publisher is established outside the EU,
the EU authorized representative is:
Springer Nature Customer Service Center GmbH
Europaplatz 3, 69115 Heidelberg, Germany

Printed by Libri Plureos GmbH
in Hamburg, Germany